Copyright © 1990 by The Telford Press, Inc.

2   3   4   5   6   7   8   9   0

THE TELFORD PRESS, INC.
Post Office Box 287, Caldwell, New Jersey 07006


Library of Congress Cataloging-in-Publication Data

Bone/[edited by] Brian K. Hall.
    p.    cm.
  Includes bibliographical references.
  Contents: v. 1. The Osteoblast and osteocyte.
  ISBN 0-936923-24-5 (v. 1)
  1. Bones.  I. Hall, Brian Keith, 1941–
  [DNLM: 1. Bone and Bones. WE 200 B7113]
QP88.2.B58    1989
599'.01852–dc20
DNLM/DLC
for Library of Congress            89-20391
                                   CIP

# BONE

## Volume 1 : The Osteoblast and Osteocyte

*Brian K. Hall*
*Department of Biology*
*Dalhousie University*
*Halifax, Nova Scotia*
*Canada*

# Contents

# Preface

This is the first of seven volumes devoted to bone. The impetus for initiating this series was not so much masochism as the desire to fill the perceived need for an up-to-date, comprehensive and authoritative treatment of all aspects of bone. Bourne's treatise, "*The Biochemistry and Physiology of Bone*", so long the benchmark encyclopoedic treatment of bone and cartilage, first appeared as a single volume in 1956, then as a four volume second edition in 1971–1976. The explosion of knowledge about bone over the past two decades has meant that "Bourne" has become a dated, albeit tremendously useful, compendium. Knese's monumental (977 pp) "*Stützgewebe and Skelettsystem*" (1979) being '*auf deutsch*' is inaccessible to the English speaker. Other annuals and series, while they deal with topics in depth, do not provide, on the one hand, the overview, and on the other, the comprehensiveness of a treatise. Bourne and Knese both treat the two major skeletal tissues, cartilage and bone. The present series concentrates on bone, primarily because cartilage has been covered in the three volumes edited by Hall (1983), and because a book, edited by Hall and Newman, and devoted to the molecular aspects of cartilage and chondrogenesis, will be published by The Telford Press in 1990.

74 chapters, written by 127 authors or coauthors are planned. That these authors are all actively engaged in basic, applied, and/or clinical research upon bone, ensures that each treatment is authoritative and up-to-date. The role of the editor has been to effect coordination, integration and synthesis of data, ideas, theories and methodologies.

The seven volumes projected for the series are organized thematically. Each volume integrates structure, function, biochemistry, metabolism, and the molecular and clinical aspects of a particular aspect of the biology of bone. Bone-forming cells are treated in volume 1; bone resorbing cells in volume 2. Volumes 3 and 4 examine the extracellular matrix of bone (what many regard as "bone" itself, although bone is, at one and the same time, a tissue, an organ and an organ system). Volume 3 concentrates on the structure of bone matrix and on bone-specific proteins; volume 4 treats mineralization (calcification) of that matrix. Volumes 5 and 6 discuss bone growth under the headings of intrinsic, extrinsic and metabolic growth control, although all three are interrelated and interconnected in their control of growth. Volume 6 also considers growth of individual skeletal units (skull, mandible, long bones and vertebrae) and the consequences of bone growth for such varied topics as body size, domestication, ageing, evolution, and paleopathology. Repair and regeneration of bone make up the final volume, whose topics include repair of fractured bones, bone grafts, bone regeneration, and the use of bone-promoting substances to augment repair and/or regeneration.

The present volume deals with **Osteoblasts and Osteocytes: the bone-forming cells**. The state of flux of knowledge about bone is amply illustrated by the fact that some experts would disagree with the seemingly innocuous phrase, bone-forming cells, for some would debate whether osteocytes are bone-forming cells (see Chapter 9). Volume 1 begins with Marijke Holtrop's superbly illustrated analysis of the ultrastructure of bone-forming cells in which she has gathered together the best of the available micrographic evidence for osteoblast and osteocyte structure. This is followed by Howie Tenenbaum's analysis of the current theories of bone cell differentiation in which he integrates theories from embryonic, adult and ectopic osteogenesis "to trace the lineage of the osteoblast." He identifies marrow, periosteum and periodontal ligament as the three principle sources of osteoblasts, and bone-derived paracrine and autocrine factors as evoking osteoblastic differentiation, a theme echoed in later chapters.

In chapter 3, Stephen Doty and Brian Schofield use the latest histochemical and microscopic techniques to provide an overview of the histochemistry and enzymology of bone-forming cells, summarising knowledge that is fundamental to understanding the metabolism of bone formation. Peter Hausckha provides, in chapter 4, a detailed and up-to-date treatment of the rapidly developing field of growth factors and growth factor effects in bone- the paracrine and autocrine factors introduced in Chapter 2. Hauschka's masterful synthesis and very extensive bibliography, organized factor by factor, provides an invaluable evaluation of this important topic. Understanding the mechanism of action of such factors requires an ability to isolate pure populations of bone-forming cells, the topic of chapter 5. As Glenda Wong states in the conclusion to her discussion of the isolation of bone-forming cells and the analysis of their behavior *in vitro:* "Studies with isolated bone cells have established bone as a fascinating model for local cellular interactions during tissue response to anabolic and catabolic stimuli."

In chapters 6 and 7 we move to syntheses of mechanisms of bone formation. This organization into separate chapters on *in vivo* and *in vitro* studies, is not because the mechanisms of bone formation are considered to differ in these two environments, but because each lends itself to the posing of different questions and to the utilization of different techniques to answer those questions. Thus David Simmons and Marc Grynpas, in analysing mechanisms of deposition of bone *in vivo* in chapter 6, emphasise the coupling of bone formation and resorption, and "the centrality of the osteoblast in all phases of bone remodeling" that has made it necessary "to redefine the osteoblasts and the coupling phenomenon."

Peter Nijweide and Elisabeth Burger in chapter 7 discuss the utility of *in vitro* methods for the study of osteoblast differentiation, matrix formation and calcification and provide a comparative analysis of several *in vitro* model systems; long bones, calvaria and periostea. Johan Heersche and Jane Aubin continue these themes in chapter 8, with their analysis of the molecules that regulate osteoblastic activity. They emphasise the role of cells from the osteoblastic lineage as mediators of bone resorption, a theme begun in chapter 6 and further developed in Volume 2.

Chapter 9 and 10 explicitly introduce the clinical perspective to bone formation. In chapter 9, Michael Parfitt evaluates bone-forming cells in optimal conditions as a basis for his analysis of bone-forming cells in non-optimal conditions, notably ageing, hormonal and vitamin deficiency. He stresses the vital need for accurate quantitation of bone formation if clinical conditions are to be adequately diagnosed, assessed and treated.

In the last chapter, David Cole and Michael Cohen discuss mutations that specifically affect bone-forming cells. Their analysis of fibrodysplasia ossificans progressiva, hypophosphatasia and osteosarcoma, highlights our understanding of the molecular and genetic basis of these mutations. Their up-to-date discussion of the role of the *c-fos* proto-oncogene in bone formation and osteosarcoma indicates how "the delineation of proto-oncogene structure and expression will undoubtedly offer important new insights into the nature of skeletal growth and development." amply illustrating the correctness of the initial decision not to separate basic and clinical studies into separate volumes.

In summary, this volume provides an up-to-date and authorititative overview of our current knowledge of bone-forming cells and of the mechanisms that control bone deposition, whether that bone is being deposited *in vivo* or *in vitro*, in the embryo or in the adult, in the skeleton or ectopically, in normality or in disease.

Halifax                                                                    Brian K. Hall
September, 1989

# 1

# Light and Electron Microscopic Structure of Bone-Forming Cells

**MARIJKE E. HOLTROP**
*Vitamin D, Skin & Bone Research Laboratory,*
*Boston University, School of Medicine,*
*Boston, Massachusetts*

## Introduction

The purpose of exploring morphology is to learn about function, since the morphological image represents the visual expression of functional activity. One tries to capture the image closest to the original by "fixing" the tissue with chemicals that bind to the molecules in the tissue and prevent chemical disintegration of the tissue molecules. The tissue needs to be cut into thin slices in order to access the inner part of the tissue and to obtain sections permeable to light or electrons; sections are about 5 μm thick for light microscopy and about 60 nm for electron microscopy. In order to be able to cut such thin sections, one needs the tissue to have a hard consistency and it is therefore, beforehand, embedded in a fluid plastic that hardens during "curing". Sections are cut on high-precision microtomes using hard steel knives for light microscopy and diamond knives for electron microscopy. In light microscopy the light travels through a condensor lens to be concentrated into a coherent bundle, then through the tissue section and subsequently through glass lenses to meet the eye of the observer or the emulsion on a photographic plate. In electron microscopy something similar happens except that electrons are used instead of light. The electrons, emitted by a tungsten filament are focused into a coherent beam by electromagnetic condensor lenses. They pass through the tissue section, the number of electrons passing through depending on the density of the structures in the tissue. In this way an "electron image" is formed that is subsequently magnified by deflection of the electrons in the beam by electromagnetic lenses. The image becomes visible when the electrons hit the surface of a fluorescent screen and make the screen light up. An image can also be obtained when the electrons hit the surface of a photographic plate and the emulsion is developed in the same way as after exposure to visible light. In both light- and electron microscopy, however, the structures in tissues and cells need treatment to enhance the visible image. For light microscopy, tissue sections are stained with stains that adhere selectively to certain compounds in the tissue, and give them a certain color. For electron microscopy, sections are "stained" with heavy metals that adhere to tissue compounds and prevent penetration, partly or completely, of the electrons, thus enhancing the contrast of the final image on the fluorescent screen or photographic plate. These artificial impacts can alter the original structure somewhat. Techniques, improved over the years, have provided images with fewer artifacts, yielding more information.

The images thus obtained are 2-dimensional representations of a 3-dimensional structure, and the visualizing ability of the mind of the observer is needed to transform the 2-dimensional image of the tissue and cells to a 3-dimensional image. For instance, circular images in tissue sections, such as mitochondria or vacuoles, represent spherical or ovoid structures; lines such as cell membranes represent surfaces; short tubules such as microtubules may represent tubules running over a long distance through the cytoplasm but appearing in the section only over a short distance; points may represent cross sections of filaments or cross sections of granules. Also, not all cell structures may be represented in the plane of section: cell images can be seen without a nucleus or other essential cell organelles. Thus, every photographic image becomes a challenge for the mind.

An electron microscopic technique for surfaces exists that yields images with the effect of shadows similar to light photography of 3-dimensional forms: scanning electron microscopy (SEM). Surfaces of tissue, for instance a bone surface, are coated with a thin metallic layer and a very fine electron beam scans the surface with high energy electrons, thereby liberating large amounts of electrons of low energy from the surface. The number of these secondary electrons varies depending on the part of the specimen surface they come from, thus forming an "electron image". They are collected and projected onto a fluorescent screen or photographic plate, thus building an image of the particular surface. The images thus obtained can supplement images from transmission electron microscopy (TEM) and thus aid in the formation of an image in the mind. In addition, structural details can be disclosed that escape the 2-dimensional image produced by TEM.

## Relationships of Bone Forming Cells in Bone Tissue

One cannot discuss the structure of a cell without looking at its environment: the way the cell relates to other cells of the same type, other cells of a different type and its relation to extracellular structures and substances. All, together, form a functional tissue of which the cell is the central unit. We will, therefore, first discuss how the bone forming cell relates and connects to its environment to form the whole of bone. Subsequently, we will look more closely at the inner machinery of the bone forming cells themselves.

We know most about osteoblasts in young fast-growing bones because function is easier to investigate when activity is high. Also, technical considerations and limitations play an important role in the choice of investigating young *vs.* old bone. Thus, most information on the structure of osteoblasts and their environment comes from fetal or newborn tissue of rats, mice, or chickens.

Bone forming activity is located in osteoblasts and osteocytes. These differ primarily in their relationship to the environment and only secondarily in structure and function. The osteoblast, the primary bone forming cell, is of course located closely opposed to the bone surface (Fig. 1). The name changes from osteoblast to osteocyte as soon as the bone forming cell is surrounded by mineralized matrix. Some authors recognize intermediate stages between these two and use the names osteocytic osteoblast (Nijweide *et al.*, 1981) or osteoid-osteocyte (Palumbo, 1986) for the bone forming cell that is completely surrounded by yet unmineralized bone matrix, and pre-osteocyte for the cell almost completely surrounded by mineralized marix (Palumbo, 1986). Such specific names seem academic but are relevant because of possible functional differences between the subcell types (Nijweide, 1981). Cells close to osteoblasts, on the side away from the bone surface, are called pre-osteoblasts. These cells distinguish themselves from osteoblasts functionally in that they are not capable of producing bone matrix yet, but they are capable of cell division, which the osteoblast is not. Morphologically, these can be distinguished from each other more by their

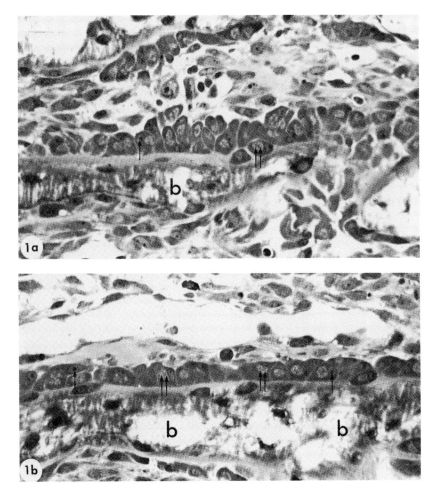

**Fig. 1** Osteoblasts, arranged in more than one layer [a] or in one layer [b], on the surface of bone trabecula in the diaphysis of a 2 week old rat tibia. The cells are plump. Most nuclei show a prominent nucleolus [arrow]. The lighter area adjacent to the nucleus represents the Golgi area [double arrow]. b: bone. Toluidine stain, x400

location than by their structure. Since these cells do not form bone, they will be given little attention in this chapter. Thus, pre-osteoblast, osteoblast, osteoid-osteocyte or osteocytic osteoblast, and osteocyte are all names for the same type of cell in different stages of development. Of all of these, only the pre-osteoblast is not capable of forming bone matrix.

Active osteoblasts cover the bone surface as a sheath of closely fitted cells, well revealed by SEM (Jones, 1974) (Fig. 2). In 2-dimensional light microscopic sections, this sheath of osteoblasts is seen as a layer of plump cells, lined up closely together along the bone surface (Fig. 1). When osteoblasts are less active, they become more elongated, with their flat surface parallel to the bone surface; their volume decreases whereas their base (the part of cell surface opposed to bone surface) increases (Fig. 3) (Zallone 1977, Marotti, 1976). At that stage, they do not necessarily cover the entire bone surface (Fig. 4). When osteoblasts are not engaged in the formation of matrix synthesis, they become very thin and elongated and leave numerous gaps and spaces between each other. These cells are commonly called bone-lining cells, inactive osteoblasts or resting osteoblasts (Fig. 5). These are commonly found on the surfaces of adult bone. In a study of bone-lining cells in adult beagles the number of cells per millimeter of trabecular bone surface in tissue sections (linear density) decreased significantly between young adult and very old dogs in the distal femur, although no decrease was seen in the distal radius (Miller *et al.*, 1980). It seems that when bone turnover decreases with age, the number of lining cells decreases as well. In adult mammals, these cells are likely the most common cells found on most types of trabecular bone (Scott, 1980). Very little, if anything, is known about these cells because of technical difficulties in preparing old bone tissue for microscopy.

Once the osteoblast has become an osteocytic osteoblast or pre-osteocyte, according to a study of osteons in dogs, the cell has already decreased in size about 30% from the mean volume of corresponding osteoblasts, no matter the size of the osteoblasts (Marotti, 1976). This process continues; the osteocyte becomes increasingly smaller, meanwhile filling the lacuna in which it is lying with bone matrix, so that the smallest osteocyte and the smallest lacunae are found far away from the bone surface (Yeager, 1975). However, if osteoblasts on the bone surface have decreased their activity and have accordingly diminished in size, young osteocytes may be smaller than older osteocytes (Fig. 6). This was shown in a study in dogs in which the accretion rate of bone matrix in osteons was correlated with the size of osteoblasts and osteocytes (Marotti, 1976).

Apart from this difference in osteocyte volume, which is reflected in the size of osteocytes in tissue sections, the size and shape of these cells in sections are also influenced by the orientation of the osteocyte in the bone

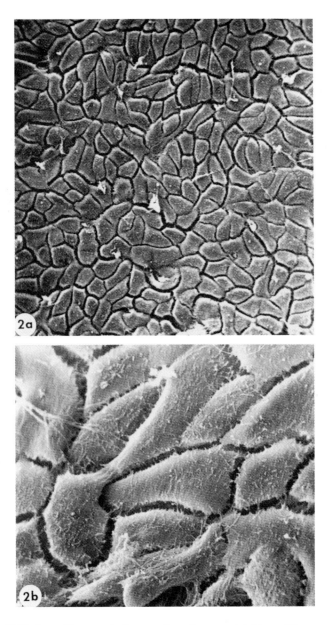

**Fig. 2**   a. Field of osteoblasts on the inner surface of a rat parietal bone. The spaces between the cells are drying artefacts. Field width 143 um. b. Cell surface detail of osteoblasts on the inner aspect of a rat parietal bone. Field height 38 um.
(from: Jones 1974).

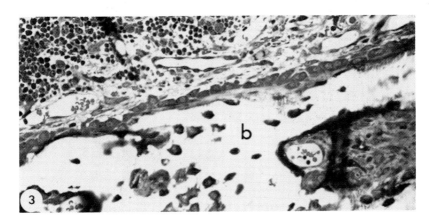

**Fig. 3**   Osteoblasts on the surface of a bone trabeculum [b] in the diaphysis of a 7 week old rat tibia. The cells are elongated. x250.

matrix. Osteocytes are elongated cells and are oriented with their long axis parallel to the collagen fibers around them. Thus, the size and shape of all osteocytes in a field of highly organized collagen fibers, for instance an osteon, will depend on whether the collagen fibers were cut longitudinally or transversely (Marotti, 1979): when cut longitudinally, the osteocyte will have an elongated shape, whereas when cut transversely, the cell will show a round or triangular shape. This is an important consideration when measurements of the osteocytes are made to investigate their function, by means of morphometry, since the stereological principles underlying this method are based on the assumption of random orientation.

Osteoblasts make contact with each other by means of small protrusions or by cell-to-cell contact, and osteoblasts and osteocytes are all connected by numerous processes running through canaliculi in the bone matrix. In this way the members of the bone cell family are all in close relation to each other, forming a functional network.

## Structure of the Osteoblast

The most striking characteristics of the active osteoblast under light microscopy is the intense staining of the cell with basic stains, indicating

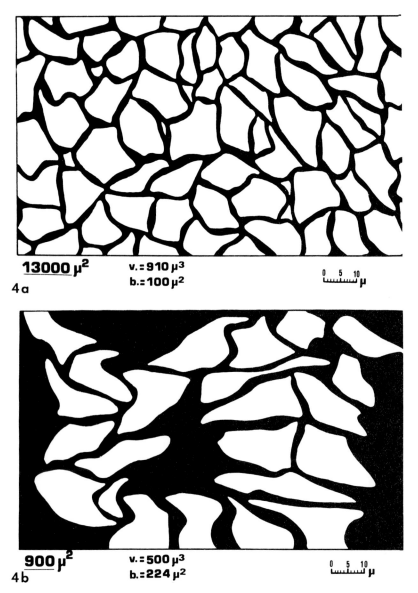

**13000 μ²**         v.: 910 μ³
4a                   b.: 100 μ²                        0  5  10
                                                       ⊔⊔⊔⊔⊔⊔⊔⊔⊔ μ

**900 μ²**           v.: 500 μ³
4b                   b.: 224 μ²                        0  5  10
                                                       ⊔⊔⊔⊔⊔⊔⊔⊔⊔ μ

**Fig. 4** Drawings of the bases of osteoblasts derived from serial sections of two growing osteons respectively at the initial (a, Haversian canal = 13,000 u²) and at the final stages of formation (b, Haversian canal = 900 u²). The intercellular spaces are black. The mean values of the cell volume (v) and of the cell base (b) are indicated below the corresponding drawing. Note the higher density and the narrower bases of osteoblasts lining the larger canal with a more active osteogenetic surface. Reduced 20%. (from: Marotti, 1976).

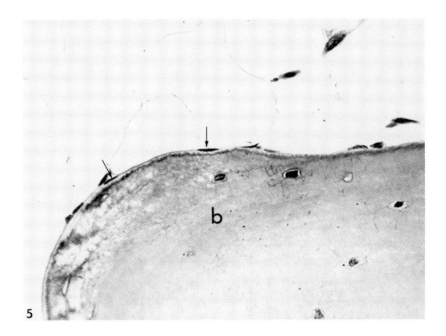

**Fig. 5** Bone lining cells on the surface of a bone spicule of a distal femur of an adult beagle. The nuclei are usually flat or ovoid. The cytoplasm usually cannot be seen in the light microscope. b: bone. x560. (from: Miller *et al*, 1980).

the presence of large amounts of RNA (Fig. 1). Inactive osteoblasts stain less intensely. In active, plump osteoblasts the nucleus is usually located eccentricly and next to it is an area that stains less intensely and corresponds to the Golgi area.

At the electron microscopic level the osteoblast was first described extensively in the 1960's (Cameron, 1961, Dudley *et al.*, 1961, Cooper *et al.*, 1966), but the improvement of techniques for fixation and embedding, and the development of more sophisticated equipment to prepare and view thin sections have greatly enhanced the images obtained in later years and disclosed finer detail of structures.

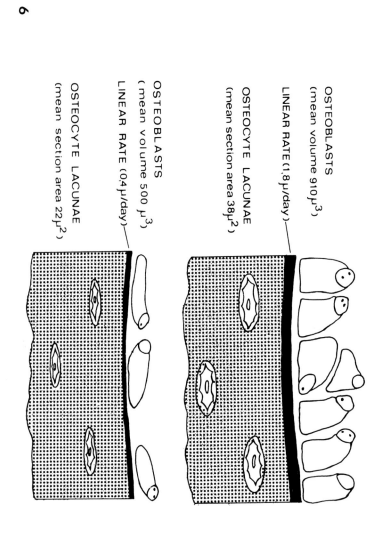

OSTEOBLASTS
(mean volume 910μ³)

LINEAR RATE (1.8 μ/day)

OSTEOCYTE LACUNAE
(mean section area 38μ²)

OSTEOBLASTS
( mean volume 500 μ³)

LINEAR RATE (0.4μ/day)

OSTEOCYTE LACUNAE
(mean section area 22μ²)

**6**

**Fig. 6**   Schematic drawing to show the possible sequence of events during bone formation: the higher the appositional growth rate, the larger the osteoblasts lining the growing surface, and consequently the larger the osteocytes encased inside the bone matrix (from: Marotti, 1976).

One osteoblast in the tibia of a chick embryo was cut in serial sections (Palumbo, 1986). Eighty seven consecutive sections were obtained from this one cell and twelve of these are shown in Figure 7. These are a beautiful demonstration of the variety of images one can obtain from one cell and aid in making the correlation between 2-dimensional pictures of sections and 3-dimensional images in the mind of the observer. A 3-dimensional reconstruction of an osteoid-osteocyte made manually and by means of a computer assisted image analyzer is represented in Figure 8. The cell processes in these figures seem to end at a short distance from the cell. It should be understood, though, that the cell processes in each individual section could be followed only for a short distance, limited by the thickness (or thinness) of the section. Cell processes that enter a section away from the cell body cannot with certainty be linked up with a cell process that is attached to the cell body in another section; these far away cross sections of cell processes are lost in the overall reconstruction. As explained earlier, and in more detail later in this chapter, these cell processes link up with other processes from other osteoblasts and osteocytes within the bone.

When viewing the overall image of osteoblasts by electron microscopy, it is striking that the cytoplasm of some cells is significantly more electrondense than that of others. It is not known what causes the greater electrondensity, nor what the significance of this difference is.

The cell seems to be occupied by three prominent, main components that reflect the main function of the cell: active synthesis of the proteins and polysaccharides of the bone matrix. These three components are: the nucleus, the Golgi area, and the rough endoplasmic reticulum (rer) (Fig. 9).

The *nucleus* is large compared to the nucleus in many other cell types and is located eccentricly in the cytoplasm. One to three well developed nucleoli can be seen in the plane of section of many osteoblasts. The exact number of nucleoli that are present in any one nucleus in total, 3-dimensionally, has not been determined.

The *rough endoplasmic reticulum* (rer) occupies another major compartment of the cell (Fig. 9). Parallel membrane sheets, represented in sections as parallel lines, are packed with ribosomes and many of these are arranged closely together in a well organized pattern. The membrane sheets separate somewhat at some places, forming cisternae. Rer and cisternae contain a moderately electrondense coarsely floccular material (Weinstock, 1975).

The *Golgi area* occupies a large space adjacent to the nucleus (Fig. 9). This area stains less intensely with basic stains in light microscopy and, since it is so large, can therefore often be vaguely recognized in light microscopic sections (Fig. 1). In electron microscopy, different structural aspects of the Golgi can be distinguished which form a functional sequence related to the synthesis of collagen. This sequence has been elucidated by

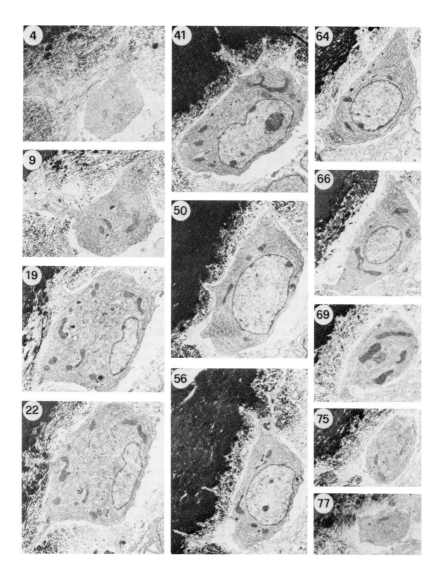

**Fig. 7** Twelve sections selected from a series of 87 consecutive sections through an osteoid-osteocyte. The number in each photograph indicates the level of the corresponding section in the whole series. The three-dimensional shape of this osteoid-osteocyte is shown in Figure 8. x2900. (from: Palumbo, 1986).

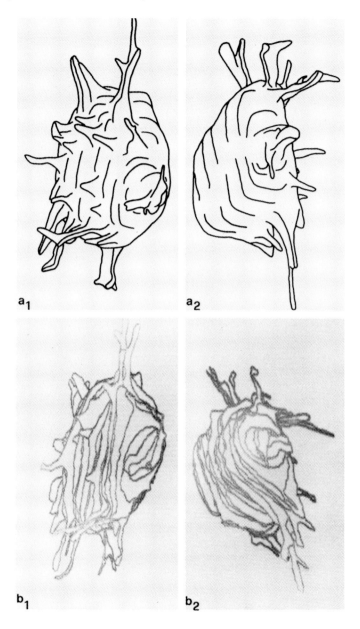

**Fig. 8** Three-dimensional reconstruction of an osteoid-osteocyte made (a) manually and (b) by means of a computer-assisted image analysis. In $a_2$ and $b_2$ the cell is rotated with respect to a, and b, by 180° on the y axis and by 90° on the z axis. The mineral facing side of the cell is the one having cytoplasmic processes. (from: Palumbo, 1986).

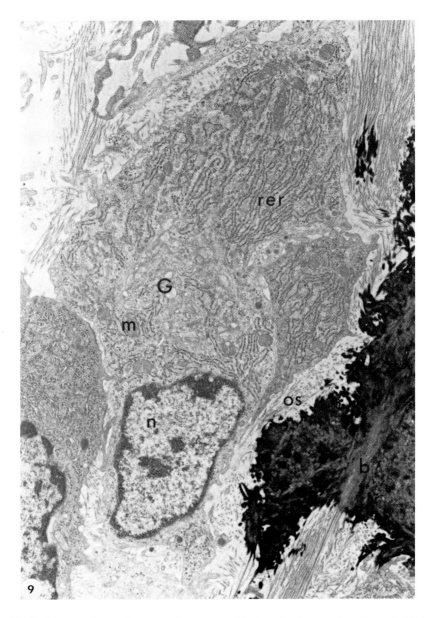

**Fig. 9** Electronmicrograph representing two osteoblasts on the bone surface. One osteoblast shows only a small part of the cell in the plane of section: the nucleus and much of the cytoplasm are not visible. The other osteoblast shows a nucleus [n], an abundance of rough endoplasmic reticulum (rer) and a large Golgi area (G) m: mitochondrion; os: osteod seam; b: mineralized bone. x9400. (from: Holtrop, 1975).

following the incorporation and transfer of $^3$H-proline, a precursor of collagen, in the cell by means of radioautography at the electron microscopic level (Weinstock 1975, Weinstock *et al.*, 1975, Leblond *et al.*, 1981) and by immunostaining with antibodies against type I procollagen coupled to electrondense horse radish peroxidase (Leblond *et al.*, 1981). The following description of the structural units of the Golgi will follow the established pathway of procollagen synthesis. Interconnected stacks of flattened saccules show dilatations which are among the most conspicious components of the Golgi. These dilatations, named "spherical portions" (Weinstock, 1975) or "spherical distentions" (Leblond *et al.*, 1981), are filled with filamentous elements, thin and irregular, with a diameter of 0.5−2 nm and without orientation (Fig. 9, 10). Flattened saccules of the Golgi also widen into cylindrical dilatations named "cylindrical portions or "cylindrical distentions" (Weinstock 1975, Leblond *et al.*, 1981). These are filled with straight slender threads, 2−3 nm thick in parallel orientation and grouped into small bundles measuring about 300 nm in length (Fig. 10) (Weinstock, 1972, 1975, Leblond *et al.*, 1981). The bundles can be so electron dense that they form rod-like structures. Elongated membrane-limited vacuoles which lie freely in the cytoplasm and have similar rod-like structures or have a fairly homogeneous content in which threads are only faintly distinguishable, are called "secretory granules" (Fig. 10). These granules may vary in length. In longer granules the bundles seem to be aligned end to end, with a total length of about 600 nm (Weinstock 1972, 1975, Scherft *et al.*, 1975, Leblond *et al.*, 1981). These granules are seen anywhere between the periphery of the Golgi area and the secretory region of the cell membrane. They seem to fuse with the cell membrane and discharge their contents by exostosis (Fig. 11) (Scherft *et al.*, 1975, Weinstock, 1975).

Electron microscopic studies of the Golgi area and the pathway of synthesis and secretion of collagen have also been described extensively by Weinstock *et al.* (1974) for the odontoblast, a cell very similar to the osteoblast. I refer the interested reader to their work.

*Mitochondria* can be found throughout the cytoplasm outside the Golgi area (Fig. 9). Occasionally, electron dense particles, about 60 nm in diameter, can be seen upon the inner membranes of the mitochondria (Fig. 12). These have been reported in osteoblasts in weanling rats (Martin *et al.*, 1970), during fracture repair of the femur of young adult rats (Gothlin, 1973), and in prenatal and postnatal humans (Kjaer, 1975). When these granules are found, they do not appear uniformly in all osteoblasts. Osteoblasts that are characterized by a greater cytoplasmic electron density in electronmicrographs seem to have the greatest number of mitochondrial granules (Martin *et al.*, 1970). Microincineration studies have proved these granules to be mineral (Martin *et al.*, 1970) and microprobe analysis has

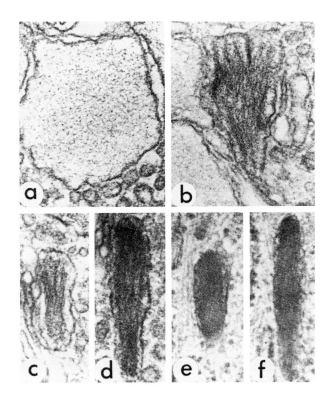

**Fig. 10** Presumed changes in the shape of distended Golgi saccules and in the organization of their content leading to the formation of secretory granules. At an early stage spherical distentions (a) contain an array of entangled threads. At a subsequent stage, the saccule becomes rectangular and the threads are aligned parallel (b) with one end closely associated with the limiting membrane (b, top). Subsequent stages involve condensation of the content into rod-like structures and the formation of Golgi secretory granules (c, d). The rod-like structures may be aligned end to end (d) Secretory granules having an electron opaque content within which filaments are no longer evident are also observed (e, f). x85,000. (from: Weinstock, 1975).

shown that these granules have a high content of calcium and phosphorus (Sutfin *et al.*, 1971).

*Microtubules* can be seen in osteoblasts in tissue that has been fixed at room temperature (Fig. 13, 14) (Holtrop *et al.*, 1971, Weinger *et al.*, 1974, Nilsen, 1980). Microtubules are labile structures and disintegrate at low temperature and under conditions known to depolymerize microtubules.

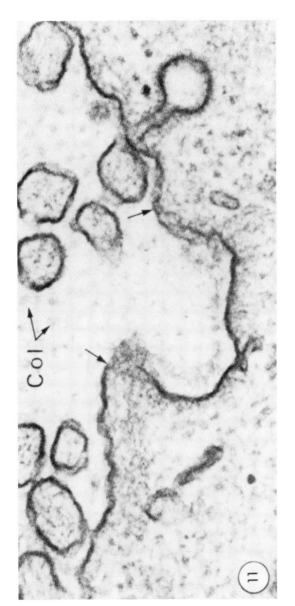

**Fig. 11**  Late stage of secretory granule discharge into the pre-bone. The membrane of the granule is continuous with the apical plasmalemma in the region between the arrows. Electron dense accumulations adjacent to the external surface of the membrane resemble filament bundles in cross-section. Collagen fibrils [col] are visible beyond. x145,000. (from: Weinstock, 1975).

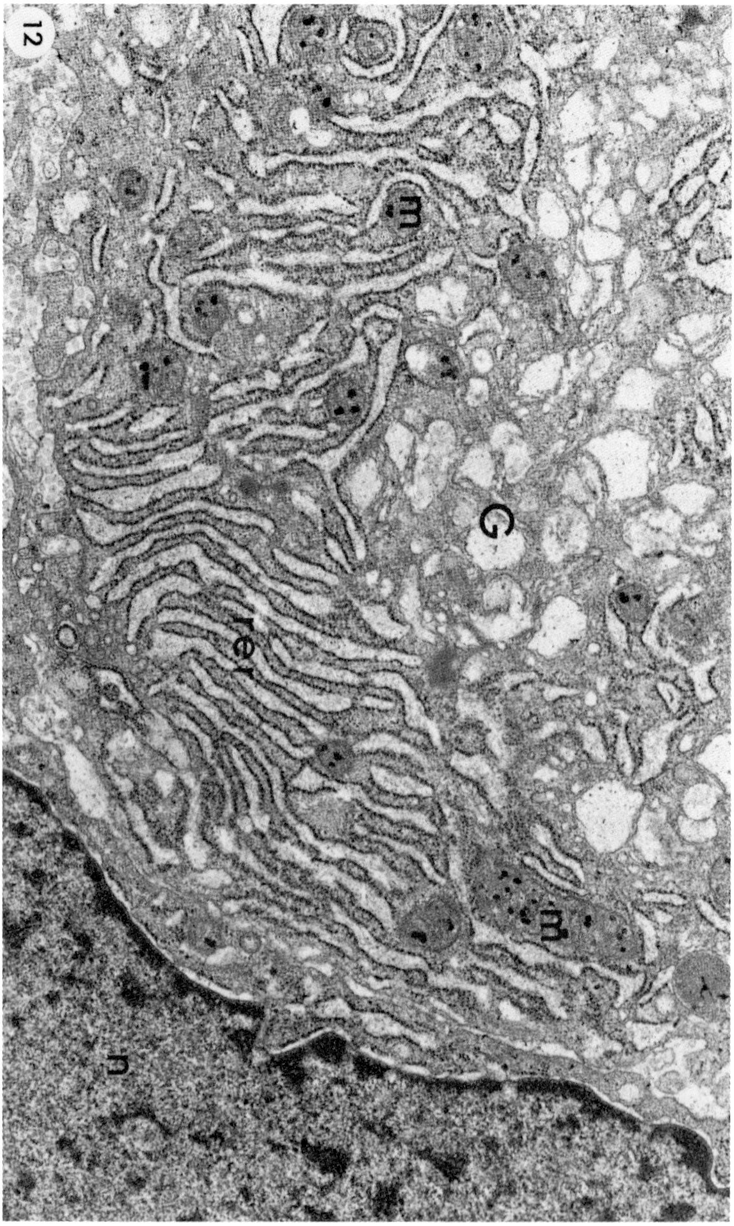

Marijke E. Holtrop

**Fig. 12** Part of an osteoblast showing dense granules in the mitochondria. m: mitochondrion; rer: rough endoplasmic reticulum; G: Golgi area; n: nucleus.

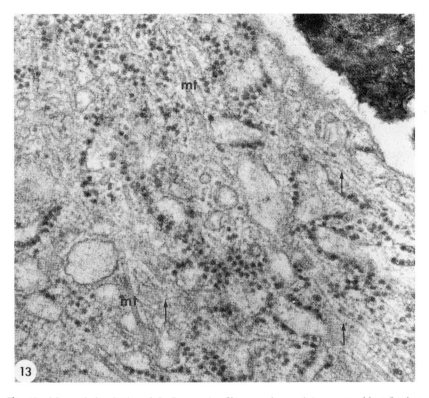

**Fig. 13** Microtubules (mt) and 5–7 nm microfilaments (arrows) in an osteoblast fixed at room temperature. x66,000.
[from Holtrop, 1971].

The loss of microtubules has been correlated with an increase of 9 to 11 nm filaments. Bundles of 10 nm filaments were indeed demonstrated in osteoblasts in tissue fixed at 0°C (Fig. 15) (Gothlin *et al.*, 1970, Weinger *et al.*, 1974, Stanka, 1975). Microtubules have a diameter of about 24 nm and usually appear to run singly, although sometimes small clusters of microtubules are seen running parallel to each other. It is not clear whether there is any orientation of the microtubules relative to cell organelles or cell

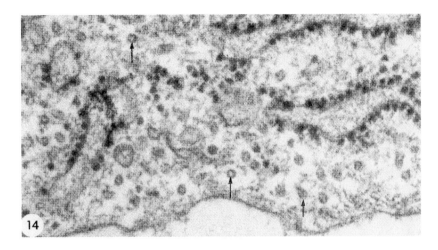

**Fig. 14**   Cross sections of microtubules in an osteoblast fixed at room temperature. x86,000.

polarity. Microtubules are seen in a sufficient number of osteoblast sections to assume that they are present in every cell, but it is difficult to assess their number, partly because they can be seen only when cut longitudinally or in cross section, and those cut tangentially are missed.

*Microfilaments* with a diameter of 5 to 7 nm occur in small numbers and are randomly distributed through the cytoplasm (Fig. 13), or form bundles that run parallel along the cell membrane and extend into protrusions (Fig. 16) (Holtrop *et al.*, 1971, Weinger *et al.*, 1974, Stanka, 1975). Bundles of parallel microfilaments are numerous in osteoblast processes (see below). These filaments are actin-like, as has been demonstrated by their binding to heavy meromyosin (King *et al.*, 1975) and by indirect immunofluorescence (Nilsen, 1980).

*Lysosome* like bodies do occur in osteoblasts, although not frequently (Scott *et al.* 1971, Thyberg *et al.*, 1975). They are dense spherical bodies bounded by a membrane and they contain a homogeneous material. Sometimes, variable amounts of inclusion material can be found within these dense bodies (Thyberg *et al.*, 1975). They have been identified as lysosomes

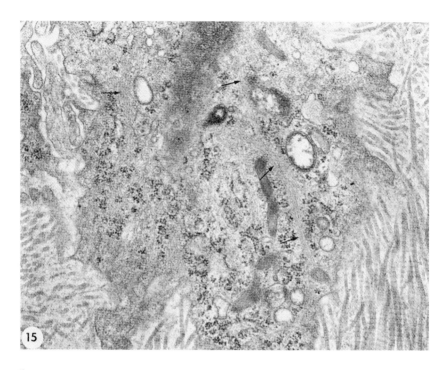

**Fig. 15**   10 nm filaments in an osteoblast fixed at 0°C. x17,600 (from: Weinger *et al.*, 1974).

by histochemistry (Gothlin *et al.* 1973, Hanker *et al.* 1973, Jande *et al.* 1975, Thyberg 1975, Thyberg *et al.*, 1975).

*Glycogen* has been reported as a prominant cytoplasmic constituent in osteoblasts from fetal rats and is located in compacted form at one or both poles of the cell (Scott *et al.*, 1971). However, osteoblasts from post-natal tissue do not show an appreciable amount of glycogen (Thyberg *et al.*, 1975).

*Lipid droplets* have been described in fetal rat osteoblasts, concommittant with the process of disappearance of glycogen (Scott *et al.*, 1971). Lipid droplets have also been reported in young adult rats (Gothlin *et al.*, 1970) but are not a usual constituent of the cell.

*Centrioles* (Tonna *et al.*, 1972) and *solitary cilia* (Tonna *et al.*, 1972, Stanka,

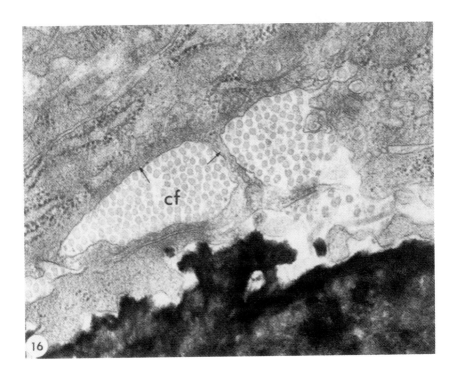

**Fig. 16** Microfilaments, 5—7 nm in diameter, along the cell membrane and in protrusions of an osteoblast. cf: cross section of collagen fibres.

1975; Nilsen, 1977) have been encountered in osteoblasts, but are extremely rare. Nothing is known about their function.

Inactive osteoblasts, resting osteoblasts or lining cells have very little cytoplasm compared with their active counterpart, and have an elongated shape parallel to the bone surface (Fig. 17). They usually contain small amounts of rer, free ribosomes, and a few mitochondria (Luk *et al.*, 1974 a, Miller *et al*, 1980)

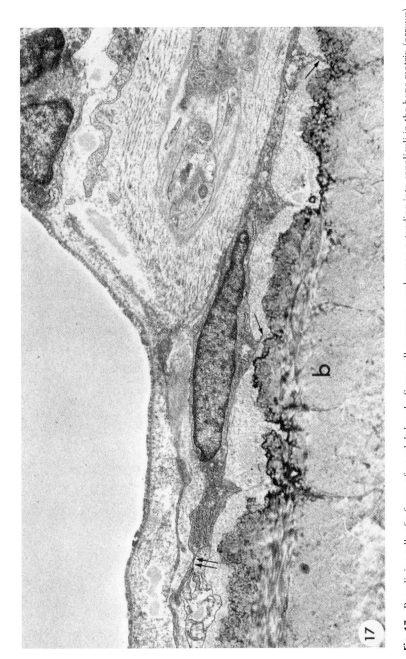

**Fig. 17** Bone lining cells of a femur of an adult beagle. Some cell processes can be seen extending into canaliculi in the bone matrix (arrows). A junction between bone lining cell processes can also be observed (double arrow). b: bone. x8,900. (from: Miller *et al.*, 1980).

## Structure of the Osteocyte

Young osteocytes that have just been encased in mineralized matrix resemble osteoblasts in every respect: the nucleus has prominent nucleoli, the cytoplasm is taken up by large areas of rer and Golgi area, mitochondria are present throughout the cytoplasm and microtubules, microfilaments, and occasional lysosomes are demonstrable (Fig. 18). As more mineralized matrix is laid down and the cell becomes located deeper within the bone, changes in morphology gradually occur: the cell becomes smaller, at the expense of the cytoplasm, so that the nucleus becomes the outstanding feature of the cell (Fig. 19). Yet, all the cell organelles previously mentioned are still clearly present, giving the cell the machinery for synthesizing matrix (Baylink *et al.*, 1971). The lacuna of the osteocyte has meanwhile also diminished in size and the space between osteocyte and mineralized bone matrix varies. At times the osteocyte is closely surrounded by mineralized matrix (Fig. 20); at other times variable space is left between cell and mineralized matrix that is filled with collagen fibers and can be regarded as osteoid (Fig. 21). In young tissue, these are the characteristic features of the osteocyte. In bone tissue where osteocytes have a longer life span, as in the osteons of compact bone in adult animals, other types of osteocytes have been recognized as well. The osteocyte described above has been regarded as corresponding to the formative stage of the cell. A subsequent phase would be a resorptive stage (Fig. 22), followed by a degenerative stage (Fig. 23) (Jande *et al.*, 1971, 1973, Jande, 1971, Luk *et al.*, 1974 b). In the resorptive stage (Fig. 22) little rer is left, but the Golgi, although greatly diminished, is still clearly present and lysosomes have become more frequent (Baud, 1968, Scott, 1971, Jande *et al.*, 1971, Jande, 1971). More osteoid is seen outside the osteocyte and this has been interpreted as a sign of resorption (Jande *et al.*, 1971). However, this could also be explained by the cell decreasing in size and not keeping pace with the formation of mineralized matrix. One could also argue that the pictures of "resorbing and degenerating" osteocytes develop when the fixative can not penetrate into the bone quickly enough to preserve the deep lying osteocytes adequately. Nevertheless, these images of osteocytes have been associated with the concept of "osteocytic osteolysis", an active resorptive function of osteocytes under certain metabolic requirements (Belanger *et al.*, 1967, Belanger, 1969, Jande *et al.*, 1973). This concept finds support in the finding that young chicks treated with parathyroid hormone have a decreased number of formative osteocytes and an increased number of resorptive osteocytes (Jande, 1972) and also by the finding that under different circumstances of immobilization of rat tibiae and subsequent osteoporosis the number of enlarged osteocytes increased significantly, which was prevented by para-

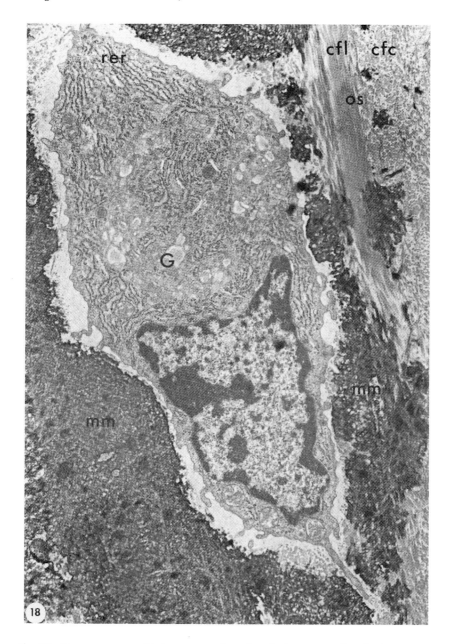

**Fig. 18** Young osteocyte with large areas of rough endoplasmic reticulum (rer) and Golgi area (G), mm: mineralized matrix; os: osteoid; cfl: collagen fibres cut longitudinally. cfc: collagen fibres in cross section.

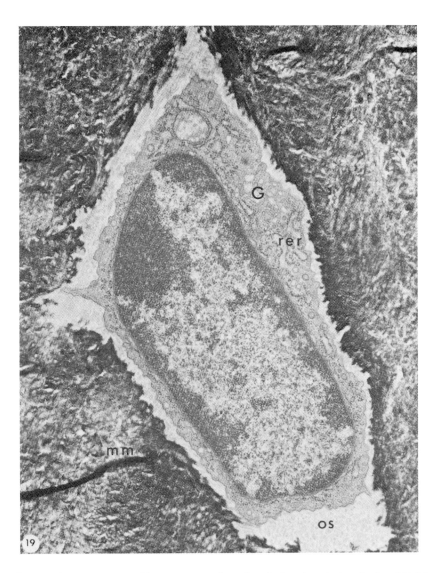

**Fig. 19** Mature osteocyte with sparse areas of rough endoplasmic reticulum (rer) and Golgi area (G). mm: mineralized matrix; os: osteoid. x14,400. (from: Holtrop, 1975).

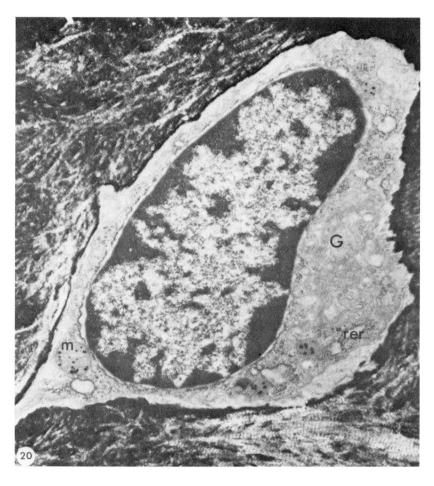

**Fig. 20** Osteocyte closely surrounded by mineralized matrix. Mitochondria [m] show dense granules. rer: rough endoplasmic reticulum: G: Golgi area. x13,800. (from Holtrop, 1971).

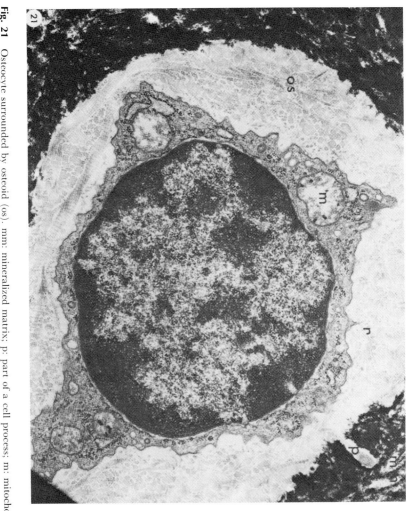

**Fig. 21** Osteocyte surrounded by osteoid (os). mm: mineralized matrix; p: part of a cell process; m: mitochondrion.

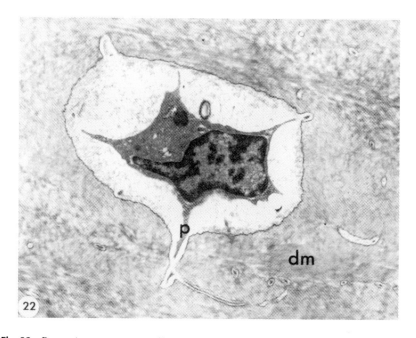

**Fig. 22**   Resorptive osteocyte. p: cell process; dm: demineralized matrix. x7,100. [Courtesy of Dr. G.T. Simon, McMaster University, Hamilton, Canada].

thyroidectomy (Krempien, 1976). These experiments indeed point to a resorptive function for osteocytes in addition to the well established formative function of these cells.

Lipid droplets and glycogen have been seen in osteocytes (Baud, 1968), and centrioles and cilia have been found rarely (Tonna, 1972, Luk *et al.*, 1974 b; Nilsen, 1977).

## Structure of the Connecting Cell Processess

Osteocytes are connected with each other and also with osteoblasts on the bone surface by means of cell processes that meet with each other or

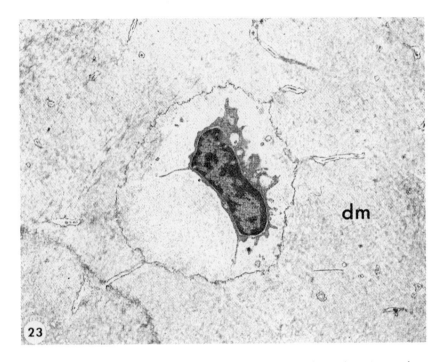

**Fig. 23** An osteocyte in an early stage of degeneration with several vacuoles in its cytoplasm. dm: demineralized matrix. x6,000. (from Luk *et al.*, 1974b).

with a cell body (Fig. 24). The cell processes travel through canaliculi in the bone matrix, sometimes over great distances. With good fixation they can be shown to fill up the canalicular space completely, leaving no space between process and bone matrix. Osteoblasts are also connected with each other, either cell to cell or by means of short protrusions.

Bone cell processes consist mainly of microfilaments, 5–7 nm in diameter, that run in a tight bundle parallel to the long axis of the cell process (Figs 25, 26). At the interface of the cell process and cell body the filaments spread out and continue along the cell membrane for a short distance (Fig. 25). The filaments occupy most of the space in the cell process, but sometimes some smooth vesicles or clusters of ribosomes can be seen

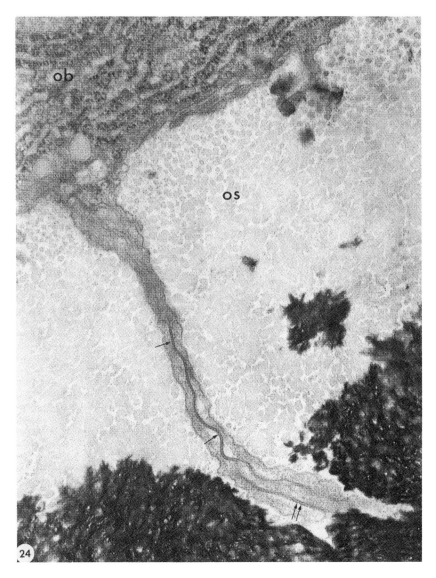

**Fig. 24** Cell process of an osteoblast (ob) meeting side-to-side with a cell process of an osteocyte. All along the area of contact the membranes form a specialized junction. The plane of section intersects the undulating junctional plane twice. (Single and double arrows). os: osteoid seam. x31,000. (From: Holtrop *et al.*, 1971).

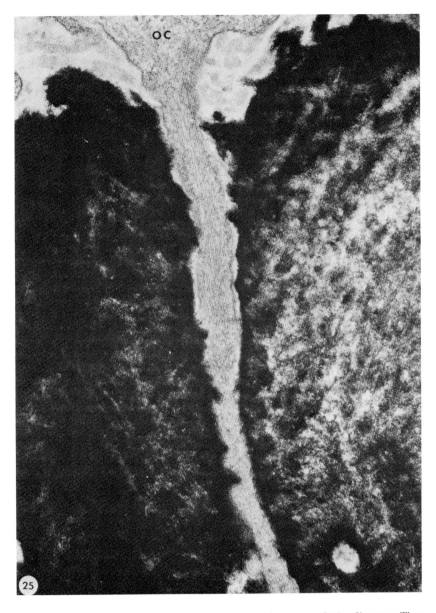

**Fig. 25**  Cell process of an osteocyte (oc) containing an abundance of microfilaments. These filaments are clearly visable in the first part of the process where they run roughly in the plane of section. More periferally they become fuzzy when the direction of the filaments and the plane of section do not coincide anymore. x52,600. (from: Weinger, *et al.*, 1974).

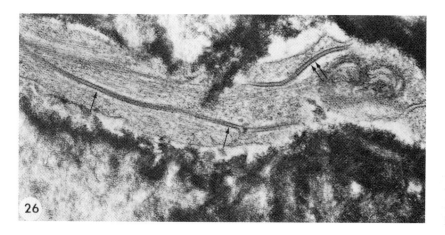

**Fig. 26** Two cell processes meet and form a side-to-side junction. The plane of section intersects the junctional plane twice, thus showing two cross sections (single and double arrows). The process is filled with microfilaments that run roughly parallel to the junction. x6,400. (from: Weinger *et al.*, 1974).

(Weinger *et al.*, 1974). Where the processes or bodies of two bone cells meet, the opposing membranes form a special junction that has been described as a tight junction by several investigators (Holtrop *et al.* 1971, Whitson 1972, Furseth 1973, Weinger *et al.*, 1974; Stanka, 1975). The junction is characterized by an enhanced electron density of the inner leaflets of the opposing membranes with dense cytoplasmic material along the membrane, and an apparent fusion of the outer leaflets that shows up with routine fixation as a row of regularly spaced globules (Fig. 26, 27). When improved fixation was obtained by removal of the superficial layers of the periostium and post-fixation in uranyl acetate, the outer leaflets appeared as a solid dense line (Figs 28) (Holtrop *et al.*, 1971, Weinger *et al.*, 1974). Later, Doty (1981) showed that the outer leaflets of the opposing membranes are not completely fused but show a gap of 2 nm. Using lanthanum as an extracellular marker, he demonstrated that bridging components exist in the gap region between the two outer leaflets of the membranes, classifying this junction as a gap junction. The importance of this finding lies in the fact that gap junctions are involved in intercellular

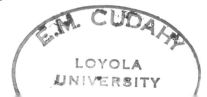

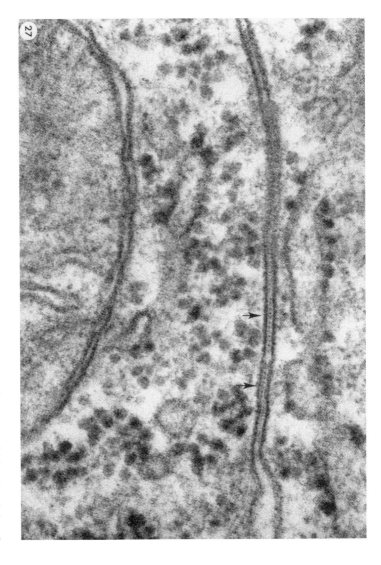

**Fig. 27** Detail of a junction between two osteoblasts. The inner leaflets of the membranes are thickened and show fuzzy material alongside in the cytoplasm. The outer membranes of the junction appear as a row of globules. x153,400. (from: Weinger *et al.*, 1974).

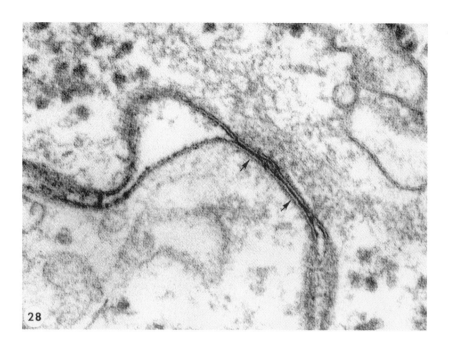

**Fig. 28**  Junction between two osteoblasts, fixed after removal of the superficial layers of the periosteum and after post fixation with uranyl acetate, thus allowing for improved preservation of the junction. The outer membranes now appear as a solid line, x156,000. (from: Holtrop *et al.*, 1971).

communication. Indeed, dyes injected into a single osteoblast on rat calvaria were transmitted to numerous surrounding cells (Jeansomme *et al.*, 1979).

Cell processes of two bone cells meet sometimes end-to-end, but more usually side-to-side, thus forming an extended area of membrane contact (Figs 24, 26). Moreover, the junctional plane is often undulating, both in longitudinal and transverse direction, thus greatly extending the area of cell contact (Figs 24, 26). Sometimes, one cell process is invaginated into another and the entire circumference of membrane contact shows the structure of the junction (Fig. 29).

Thus, the structural characteristics of the cell processes and their junctions reveal a functional interrelationship between all bone cells.

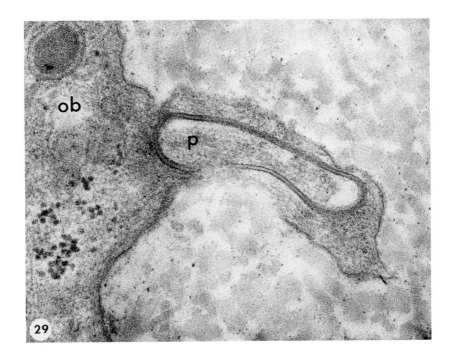

**Fig. 29** Invagination of a cell process (p) into a protrusion of an osteoblast (ob). Along the complete circumference of membrane contact a junction can be seen. x58,000. (from: Holtrop *et al*, 1971).

## Conclusion

The morphology of bone cells at the light and electron microscopic level teaches us that all bone forming cells are connected to form a functional unit. The osteoblasts on the cell surface with their abundant rer and extensive Golgi area are well equipped for the synthesis of extracellular proteins and polysaccharides, the building blocks of bone matrix. The cell processes connecting the osteoblasts on the bone surface to the osteocytes deep in the mineralized bone matrix show the morphological characteristics of structures that enable active transport: microfilaments in the processes presumably facilitate cytoplasmic flow, and extended gap junctions enable cell-to-cell communication and interaction. In this way osteocytes can be alive and functional cells. It has been suggested that osteocytes play a role in calcium homeostasis. Such questions remain to be answered definitively.

## References

Baud, C. A. (1968). Submicroscopic structure and functional aspects of the osteocyte. *Clin. Orthop.*, **56**: 227–236.

Baylink, D. J., and Wergedal, J. E. (1971). Bone formation by osteocytes. *Am. J. Physiol.*, **221**: 669–678.

Belanger, C., and Semba, T. (1967). Technical approaches leading to the concept of osteocytic osteolysis. *Clin. Orthop.*, **54**: 187–196.

Belanger, L. F. (1969). Osteocytic osteolysis. *Calcif. Tissue Res.*, **4**: 1–12.

Boyde, A., Jones, S. J., Binderman, I, and Harrell, A. (1976). Scanning electron microscopy of bone cells in culture. *Cell. Tissue Res.*, **166**: 65–70.

Cameron, D. A. (1961). The fine structure of osteoblasts in the metaphysis of the tibia of the young rat. *J. Biophys. Biochem. Cytol.* **9**: 583–595.

Cooper, R. R., Milgram, J. W., and Robinson, R. A. (1966). Morphology of the osteon. An electron microscopic study. *J. Bone Joint Surg.*, [AM] **48**: 1239–1271.

Doty, S. B. (1981). Morphological evidence of gap junctions between bone cells. *Calcif. Tissue Int.*, **33**: 509–512.

Dudley, H. R., and Spiro, D. (1961). The fine structure of bone cells. *J. Biophys. Biochem. Cytol.*, **11**: 627–649.

Furseth, R. (1973). Tight junctions between osteocyte processes. *Scand. J. Dent. Res.*, **81**: 339–341.

Gothlin, G. (1973). Electron microscopic observations on fracture repair in the rat. *Acta Pathol. Microbiol. Scand.*, [A] **81**: 507–522.

Gothlin, G., and Ericsson, J. L. (1970). Electron microscopic studies of cytoplasmic filaments and fibers in different cell types of fracture callus in the rat. *Virchows Arch.*, [Cell Pathol] **6**: 24–37.

Gothlin, G., and Ericsson, J. L. (1973). Fine structural localization of acid phosphomono-esterase in the osteoblasts and osteocytes of fracture callus. *Histochemie*, **35**: 81–91.

Hanker, J. S., Dixon, A. D., and Smiley, G. R. (1973). Acid phosphatase in the Golgi apparatus of cells forming extracellular matrix of hard tissues. *Histochemie*, **35**: 39–50.

Holtrop, M. E. (1975). The ultrastructure of bone. *Annals of Clinical and Laboratory Science*, **5**: 264–271.

Holtrop, M. E., and Weinger, J. M. (1971). Ultrastructural evidence for a transport system in bone. In: R. V. Talmage, P. L. Munson (eds): *Calcium, Parathyroid Hormone and the Calcitonins.* Excerpta Medica, Amsterdam 365–374.

Jande, S. S. (1971). Fine structural study of osteocytes and their surrounding bone matrix with respect to their age in young chicks. *J. Ultrastruct. Res.*, **37**: 279–300.

Jande, S. S. (1972). Effects of parathormone on osteocytes and their surrounding bone matrix. *Z. Zellforsch.*, **130**: 463–470.

Jande, S. S., and Belanger, L. F., (1971). Electron microscopy of osteocytes and the pericellular matrix in rat trabecular bone. *Calcif. Tissue Res.*, **6**: 280–289.

Jande, S. S., and Belanger, L. F. (1973). The life of cycle of the osteocyte. *Clin. Orthop. Rel. Res.*, **94**: 281–305.

Jande, S. S., and Grosso, W. T. (1975). Acid phosphatase in Golgi vesicles of osteoblasts. *Experientia*, **31**: 223–225.

Jeansonne, B. G., Feagin, F. F., McMinn, R. W., Shoemaker, R. L, and Rehm, W. S. (1979). Cell to cell communication of osteoblasts. *J. Dent. Res.*, **58**: 1415–1423.

Jones, S. J. (1974). Secretory territories and rate of matrix production of osteoblasts. *Calcif. Tiss. Res.*, **14**: 309–315.

King, G. J., and Holtrop, M. E. (1975). Actin-like filaments in bone cells of cultured mouse calvaria as demonstrated by binding to heavy meromyosin. *J. Cell Biol.*, **66**: 445–451.

Kjaer, I., and Matthiessen, M. E. (1975). Mitochondrial granules in human osteoblasts with a reference to one case of osteogenesis imperfecta. *Calcif. Tiss. Res.*, **17**: 173–176.

Krempien, B., Manegold, Ch., Ritz, E., and Bommer, J. (1976). The influence of immobilization on osteocyte morphology. *Virchows Arch. A. Path. Anat. and Histol.*, **370**: 55–68.

Leblond, C. P., and Wright, G. M. (1981). Steps in the elaboration of collagen by odontoblasts and osteoblasts. *Methods Cell Biol.*, **23**: 167–189.

Luk, S. C., Nopajaroonsri, C., and Simon, G. T. (1974a). The ultrastructure of endosteum: a topographic study in young adult rabbits. *J. Ultrastruct. Res.*, **46**: 165–183.

Luk, S. C., Nopajaroonsri and Simon, G. T. (1974b). The ultrastructure of cortical bone in young adult rabbits. *J. Ultrastruct. Res.*, **46**: 184–205.

Marotti, G. (1976). Decrement in volume of osteoblasts during osteon formation and its effect on the size of the corresponding osteocytes. In: *Bone Histomorphometry*, P. J. Meunier (ed), 385–397.

Marotti, G. (1979). Osteocyte orientation in human lamellar bone and its relevance to the morphometry of periosteocytic lacunae. *Metab. Bone Dis. and Rel. Res.*, **1**: 325–333.

Marotti, G., Zallone, A. Z., and Ledda, M. (1976). Number, size, and arrangement of osteoblasts in osteons at different stages of formation. *Calcif. Tiss. Res.*, Suppl to vol 21 96–101.

Matthews, J. L., and Martin, J. H. (1971). Intracellular transport of calcium and its relationship to homeostasis and mineralization. An electron microscope study. *Am. J. Med.*, **50**: 589–597.

Martin, J. H., and Matthews, J. L. (1970). Mitochondrial granules in chondrocytes, osteoblasts and osteocytes. An ultrastructural and microincineration study. *Clin. Orthop.*, **68**: 273–278.

Miller, S. C., Bowman, B. M., Smith, J. M., and Jee, W. S. S. (1980). Characterization of endosteal bone-lining cells from fatty marrow bone sites in adult beagles. *Anat. Rec.*, **198**: 163–173.

Nijweide, P. J., Plas, A. van der, and Scherft, J. P., (1981). Biochemical and histological studies on various bone cell preparations. *Calif. Tiss. Int.*, **33**: 529–540.

Nilsen, R. (1977). Electron microscopic studies on heterotopic bone formation in guinea pigs. *Arch. Oral Biol.*, **22**: 485–493.

Nilsen, R. (1980). Microfilaments in cells associated with induced heterotopic bone formation in guinea pigs. An immunofluorescence and ultrastructural study. *Acta Pathol. Microbiol. Scand.*, [A] **88**: 129–134.

Palumbo, C. (1986). A three-dimensional ultrastructural study of osteoid-osteocytes in the tibia of chick embryos. *Cell Tiss. Res.*, **246**: 125–131.

Pawlicki, R. (1975). Bone caniculus endings in the area of the osteocyte lacuna. Electron-microscopic studies. *Acta. Anat.*, (Basel) **91**: 292–304.

Scherft, J. P., and Heersche, J. N. M. (1975). Accumulation of collagen-containing vacuoles in osteoblasts after administration of colchicine. *Cell Tiss. Res.*, **157**: 355–365.

Scott, B. L, and Glimcher, M. J. (1971). Distribution of glycogen in osteoblasts of the fetal rat. *J. Ultrastr. Res.*, **36**: 565–586.

Stanka, P. (1975). Occurrence of cell junctions and microfilaments in osteoblasts. *Cell Tiss. Res.*, **159**: 413–422.

Sutfin, L. V., Holtrop, M. E., and Ogilvie, R. E. (1971). Microanalysis of individual granules with diameters less than 1000 Angstroms. *Science*, **174**: 947–949.

Thyberg, J. (1975). Electron microscopic studies on the uptake of exogenous marker particles by different cell types in the guinea pig metaphysis. *Cell Tiss. Res.*, **156**: 301–315.

Thyberg, S., Nilsson S., and Friberg, U. (1975) Electron microscopic and enzyme cytochemical studies on the guinea pig metaphysis with special reference to the lysosomal system of different cell types. *Cell Tiss. Res.*, **156**: 273–299.

Tonna, E. A., and Lampen, N. M. (1972). Electron microscopy of aging skeletal cells. I. Centrioles and solitary cilia. *J. Gerontol.*, **27**: 316–324.

Weinger, J. M., and Holtrop, M. E. (1974). An ultrastructural study of bone cells: the occurrence of microtubules, microfilaments and tight junctions. *Calcif. Tis. Res.*, **14**: 15–29.

Weinstock, M. (1972). Collagen formation — observation on its intracellular packaging and transport. *Z. Zellforsch. Mikrosk Anat.*, **129**: 455–470.

Weinstock, M. (1975). Elaboration of precursor collagen by osteoblasts as visualized by radioautography after [3H]proline administration. In: *Extracellular matrix influences on gene expression*. H. C. Slavkin, R. C. Greulich (eds). Academic Press; New York, San Francisco, London 119–128.

Weinstock, A., Bibb, C., Burgeson, R. E., Fessler, L. I., and Fessler, J. H. (1975). Intracellular transport and secretion of pro-collagen in chick bone as shown by E. M. radioautography and biochemical analysis. In: *Extracellular matrix influences on gene expression*. H. C. Slavkin, R. C. Greulich (eds). Academic Press 321–330.

Weinstock, M., and Leblond, C. P. (1974). Synthesis, migration, and release of precursor collagen by odontoblasts as visualized by radioautography after [3H]proline administration. *J. Cell Biol.*, **60**: 92–127.

Yeager, V. L., Chiemchanya, S., and Chaiseri, P. (1975). Changes in size of lacunae during the life of osteocytes in osteons of compact bone. *J. Gerontology*, **30**: 9–14.

Zallone, A. Z. (1977). Relationships between shape and size of the osteoblasts and the accretion rate of trabecular bone surfaces. *Anat. Embryol.*, **152**: 65–72.

# 2

# Cellular Origins and Theories of Differentiation of Bone-forming Cells

## H. C. TENENBAUM
*Mount Sinai Hospital Research Institute
and Faculty of Dentistry,
University of Toronto
Toronto, Canada*

## Introduction

The goal of this chapter will be to highlight information regarding the putative origins of bone-forming cells; osteoblasts. In this regard, the tissue sources of osteoblasts will be discussed. This discussion shall also include information regarding the cellular sources of the osteoblastic cell. In discussing the cellular sources of osteoblasts, it will also become necessary to search for methods of identifying osteoblastic precursor cells, as well as osteoblasts themselves. Following the discussion regarding the identity, as well as tissue and cellular origins of the osteoblast cell, some of the mechanisms whereby osteoblastic precursors are induced to differentiate into osteoblasts will be addressed.

## Marrow

There now seems to be little doubt that bone marrow serves as a major source of osteogenic cells. There are two major cellular elements within marrow and they belong to a haemopoietic group and to a stromal group. (Owen, 1982, 1985).

The haemopoietic group of cells is primarily responsible for giving rise to blood cells such as lymphocytes, erythrocytes, granulocytes, megakaryocytes and monocytes (Owen, 1978; 1980). Interestingly, the circulating monocytes are identical to tissue macrophages which are therefore thought to be derived from the aforementioned blood borne cells. Moreover, the osteoclast (a bone resorbing cell) is probably derived from these cells and can be said to be derived from the haemopoietic group of marrow cells (Stutzman and Petrovic, 1982) Alternatively, the osteoblast is derived from the stromal group of cells within the marrow (Owen, 1978, 1980, 1982, 1985; Stutzman and Petrovic, 1982).

It is believed that, within the marrow, there is a developmental pathway along which a cell must travel before it becomes an osteoblast. A population of cells called stromal stem cells has been postulated to exist in the marrow, which, by definition, is self-renewing (Owen, 1982). It is from these stromal stem cells that subsequent osteogenic precursor cells may develop. While stem cells would have the capacity to self-renew and, therefore, have an unlimited number of divisions, the more developed precursor cells would not. (See Fig. 1)

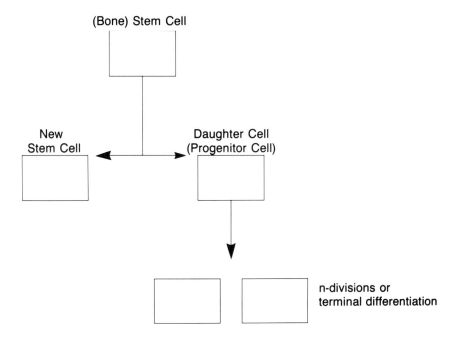

**Fig. 1** This diagram describes the developmental pathway along which cells must traverse during differentiation. The stem cell, by definition, is self renewing. The progenitor cell derived from the stem cell ultimately gives rise to a terminally differentiated cell.

At least two levels of differentiation have been implicated in the precursor bone cells. Cells demonstrating this phenomenon have been called Determined Osteoprogenitor Cells (DOPC) and Inducible Osteoprogenitor Cells (IOPC) (Owen, 1985). It is believed that the IOPC is a more immature form of the DOPC. IOPCs may be induced to differentiate further or mature into DOPCs. The DOPC would ultimately develop into an osteogenic cell.

Some interesting features of these cells are that, while both are probably found in marrow, IOPCs may be found in other areas such as muscle or soft connective tissues (Gray and Speak, 1979; Urist et al., 1983). IOPCs and DOPCs probably have a limited number of divisions and are therefore not self-renewing (Stutzman and Petrovic, 1982). Thus, if for some reason marrow is depleted of stem cells, it would ultimately lose its osteogenic capacity as the DOPC population diminished.

Methods of Establishing that Osteogenic Cells are Derived from Marrow

Two basic forms of investigation have been undertaken in order to demonstrate the osteogenic potential of marrow. Specifically, either an *in vitro* approach or an *in vivo* approach has been used. The *in vivo* investigations can be subdivided further into marrow depletion/regeneration studies or marrow transplantation studies (Amsel and Dell, 1972; Ashton *et al.*, 1984, 1985; Bab *et al.*, 1984, 1986; Budenz and Bernard, 1980; Friedenstein *et al.*, 1974, 1976; Howlett *et al.*, 1986, Luria *et al.*, 1987; Mardon *et al.*, 1987; Owen *et al.*, 1987; Tibone and Bernard, 1982).

Marrow Depletion/Regeneration

Investigations utilizing the marrow depletion/regeneration technique have demonstrated not only the osteogenic potential of marrow but also a sequence of events ultimately leading to new bone and marrow formation (Friedenstein *et al.*, 1974, 1976; Owen, 1980).

After removal of the marrow in a long-bone, a blood clot will fill the depleted cavity. This is apparently followed by a proliferation of connective tissue from or near bone surfaces. Following the proliferation step, differentiation of new osteoblasts, presumably derived from the previously proliferating cells, occurs and these osteoblasts subsequently synthesize new bone trabeculae. After the trabeculae have formed, reconstruction and reorganization ultimately result in the complete regeneration of marrow. This sequence of events takes about thirty days and has been subdivided into four stages by Owen (1980; See Table 1). A potential conclusion from the aforementioned studies is that the regenerating marrow must contain bone progenitor cells as new bone trabeculae are formed during the regeneration process. However, as stated above, the proliferating cells giving rise to osteoblasts are apparently located on or near bone at its endosteal surface and may not, therefore, be, strictly speaking, "marrow cells". In order to circumvent this problem, marrow transplantation studies were developed (Owen, 1980).

Marrow Transplantation Studies

Experimental evidence from marrow transplantation studies has confirmed further that cells with osteogenic capacity reside therein. A sequence of events, not dissimilar to that occurring in the marrow depletion studies, has been described (Owen, 1980; see Table 1). Marrow explants have been implanted either subcutaneously or within permeable, membrane-bound diffusion chambers (Amsel and Dell, 1972; Ashton *et al.*, 1984; Bab *et al.*, 1984, 1986; Budenz and Bernard, 1980; Friedenstein *et al.*, 1974; Mardon *et al.*, 1987). Following transplantation of marrow into an ectopic site, necrosis

Table 1

Approximate time sequence of events during tissue regeneration

| Stage | Time (days) | After removal of marrow from cavity | After transplantation of marrow to ectopic site |
|-------|-------------|-------------------------------------|------------------------------------------------|
| 0 | 0 | Removal of marrow from cavity | Transplantation of marrow to ectopic site |
| 1 | 0–2 | Blood clot fills depleted region of cavity | Necrosis of hemopoietic cells; stromal cells survive |
| 2 | 2–7 | Proliferation of connective tissue from bone surfaces | Proliferation of surviving stromal tissue |
| 3 | 7–10 | Differentiation of cells into osteoblasts<br>Formation of bone trabeculae<br>Reconstruction of sinusoidal microcirculation<br>Arrival of hemopoietic stem cells | Differentiation of cells into osteoblasts<br>Formation of bone trabeculae<br>Reconstruction of sinusoidal microcirculation<br>Arrival of hemopoietic stem cells |
| 4 | 10–30 | Resorption of trabecular bone<br>Hemopoietic marrow reestablished | Bone trabeculae remodeled to form ossicle with hemopoietic marrow enclosed |

From M.E. Owen (1982)

of the haemopoietic cells takes place while the stromal cells, from which osteoblasts are derived, survive. After proliferation of the stromal cells takes place, differentiation of osteoblasts follows.

The osteoblasts ultimately form bone trabeculae. In some studies, both bone and cartilage are formed (Budenz and Bernard, 1980). If marrow is placed in a diffusion chamber, the development of bone (or cartilage) is not followed by marrow regeneration as a new marrow microcirculation network cannot be established (Budenz and Bernard, 1980) and because the haemopoietic stem cells have died (Friedenstein et al., 1974, 1982; Owen, 1980). However, when implanted subcutaneously, new marrow can form, thus resulting in complete regeneration of an ossicle. These data also suggest that, while the haemopoietic stem cell is migratory and probably blood borne, the stromal stem cell and preosteoblast cell is non-migratory. This assumption is based on the observation that, whether marrow is implanted subcutaneously or not, the hematopoietic stem cell (HSC) will necrose. Thus, there must be an exogenous source of HSC which is responsible for repopulating the transplanted marrow. Moreover, the stromal cells within the implant must provide the appropriate microenvironment which will support new marrow growth from newly arrived HSC of the host. Other evidence for this hypothesis has been obtained by the use of "radio-chimeras" as described by Friedenstein and Kurolesova (1971).

Clearly, the marrow depletion/regeneration studies, along with marrow transplantation studies, demonstrate that osteogenic precursor cells are contained in the marrow. Further studies have been carried out to determine the location of the osteogenic precursor cells within the marrow. Data reported by Ashton et al. (1984) indicates that, when marrow explants are separated into core, intermediate and endosteal zones (See Fig. 2), different osteogenic potential is demonstrated on diffusion chamber implantation. Specifically, marrow explants obtained from the endosteal and intermediate regions are more highly osteogenic and must therefore contain more osteo-progenitor cells, than the core region.

In trying to establish the location of the osteoprogenitor cell within marrow, it becomes apparent that the above described in vivo studies have some significant limitations. For example, the precise identity of the osteo-progenitor cells as determined from strictly in vivo investigation may be difficult to ascertain. Moreover, the conditions required to induce full differentiation of the osteoprogenitor cell cannot be studied in vivo. Therefore, in vitro methods have been developed for the study of marrow's osteogenic potential and the osteogenic potential of cells derived therefrom.

## In Vitro Studies of Osteogenic Potential of Marrow

Early attempts at inducing marrow-derived cells to differentiate into osteoblasts met with limited success. There was no doubt that cells with osteoblastic characteristics could be grown from marrow or composites of trabecular bone and marrow. One interesting study reported by Ashton et al. (1985) showed that cultured cells derived from human marrow demon-strated some distinct osteoblastic features, such as high alkaline phosphatase activity, which was stimulated by 1,24 Dihydroxyvitamin $D_3$ and inhibited by parathyroid hormone. These cells could also be induced to produce increased levels of osteocalcin when treated with 1,25 dihydroxyvitamin $D_3$. In spite of the osteoblastic characteristics demonstrated in vitro, these cells were incapable of forming bone, even if implanted within diffusion chambers in vivo. Thus, while the above noted cells fulfilled some criteria as osteoblasts or osteoblastic precursor cells, they could not be shown to be osteogenic. One reason for this might be that the appropriate bone formation conditions were not established in vitro. However, this would not explain the diffusion chamber results. It is likely then, that in this in vitro experiment, the cells selected for their ability to survive in culture had lost the ability to completely express their potential phenotype.

Investigators came closer to the elusive goal of inducing marrow or

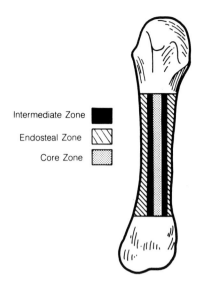

Intermediate Zone
Endosteal Zone
Core Zone

**Fig. 2** This is a schematic representation of a marrow space showing the regions referred to by Ashton *et al.* (1984). As noted in the text, osteogenic potential is greatest in the endosteal zone.

marrow-derived cells to form bone *in vitro*, as demonstrated in a paper reported by Howlett *et al.* (1986). In this study, fibroblastic cells were isolated from cell suspensions of marrow and then put into tissue culture. After one to two weeks in culture, the formation of nodules was observed in confluent cultures. Using various analytical techniques such as alkaline phosphatase, and von Kossa histochemistry, as well as x-ray dispersive microanalysis and electron microscopy, it was suggested that these nodules contained bone-like tissue as well as osteoblast-like cells. Specifically, some cells were positive for alkaline phosphatase within the nodules (as well as some others remote from nodules) which were shown to contain hydroxy-apatite and cross-banded collagen. Some of the mineralization appeared to be associated with cellular debris and other products of cellular degeneration. In fact, these appeared, to the authors, to be the initial sites for mineraliz-ation with calcification of collagen occurring secondarily. In addition, some regions of these cultures contained no matrix. In view of the above, it might be tempting to conclude that marrow cells were capable of forming bone *in vitro*. However, the tissue formed may only distantly resemble bone, thus leaving the question of marrow osteogenic potential without the participation of a live host still open.

Recent and convincing evidence regarding the above, was reported by Luria *et al.* (1987). These investigators placed whole marrow explants in an organ culture milieu whereupon osteodifferentiation and osteoid formation occurred. In the presence of Na-β-glycerophosphate, mineralized bone was produced as already shown in other systems (Tenenbaum *et al.*, 1982, 1987). The tissue formed demonstrated histochemical, histological and ultrastructural features completely consistent with those of bone formed *in vivo*. Thus, this study provides unequivocal evidence that cells from marrow, without interaction of exogenous factors supplied by a living host, are fully capable of osteogenic differentiation, and phenotypic expression.

## Periosteum and Mesenchyme

### Periosteum

It has long been established that, aside from bone marrow, another very important source of osteoprogenitor cells is the periosteum (Fell, 1932, 1969; Fitton Jackson and Smith, 1957; Gaillard, 1934; Goldhaber, 1966; Nijweide *et al.*, 1975, 1982; Tenenbaum and Heersche, 1986). Mesenchymal tissue from which periosteum is derived has also been shown to contain osteogenic cells (Marvaso and Bernard, 1977). While periosteum is an important source of osteogenic cells in fetal and post-fetal bone development, mesenchymal tissue is principally involved in bone formation in the fetal organism.

Some of the earliest studies on the osteogenic capacity of periosteum were reported by Dame Honour Fell in the 1930's (Fell, 1932). She showed unequivocally that explants of periosteum grown on natural undefined culture media were capable of forming osteoblast-like cells which, in turn, produced osteoid. The osteoid formed did not mineralize readily and thus form bone. This does not mean that osteoblastic differentiation did not take place but rather that the conditions allowing subsequent reproducible mineralization of osteoid produced *in vitro* to occur *in vitro* had not been established. Work reported by others also confirmed indirectly or directly Fell's findings (Fitton-Jackson and Smith, 1957; Gaillard, 1934; Goldhaber, 1966; Nijweide *et al.*, 1975, 1982; Tenenbaum, and Heersche, 1986).

Further and very elegant extensions of the earlier studies were done by Nijweide and Van der Plas (1975). In these studies, it was shown quite clearly that osteogenic precursor cells reside in the periosteum. This was done by culturing periosteal tissues, initially devoid of differentiated osteo-blasts, in which osteoblast and osteoid formation was demonstrated after 4 days. Thus, since osteoid formation occurred in these cultures, *de novo* differentiation of osteoblasts must have occurred *in vitro* (Fig. 3). The osteoprogenitor cells in the cultured periosteum are fibroblastic in appearance

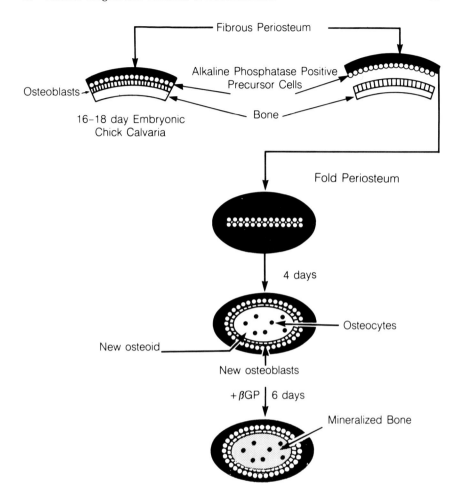

**Fig. 3** This figure depicts the Chick Periosteal Osteogenesis model. Periosteum is stripped off the 16–18 day old embryonic chick calvaria and folded with the osteogenic cells on the inside. Within 4 days new osteoblasts have developed and have produced osteoid. If β-glycero-phosphate is contained in the medium, mineralized bone is formed two days later.

and are virtually indistinguishable from other fibroblastic cells in the fibrous portion of the periosteum (Tenenbaum and Heersche, 1986). However, if periosteal tissues are histochemically-stained for alkaline phosphatase activity, a thin layer of cells originally subjacent to the fully differentiated osteoblasts will be identified that produce significant levels of alkaline phosphatase activity and yet are fibroblastic in morphology (Tenenbaum and Heersche, 1986). These cells could be identified as osteoprogenitor cells and will ultimately give rise to osteoblasts *in vivo* or *in vitro* under the appropriate conditions. The mechanisms behind the induction of osteoblastic differentiation of these osteoprogenitor cells will be discussed in a following section.

An interesting feature of periosteum is that not all periosteal tissues possess the same osteogenic potential. For example, the ectocranial periosteum derived from embryonic chick calvariae is highly osteogenic *in vitro*, under permissive conditions, whereas the endocranial periosteum is not. Teleologically speaking, this is because there is more growth of bone on the ectrocranial side. It is not known how this is accomplished but apparently fewer osteoprogenitor cells reside in the endocranial tissue. Alternatively, periosteum derived from embryonic chick long bones seems to be just as osteogenic as ectocranial periosteum (i.e., similar growth characteristics, Pal, 1984). Clearly, periosteum contains determined osteoprogenitor cells located near the bone surface but there may also be inducible osteoprogenitor cells farther away from the bone surface which would not, for example, demonstrate marked alkaline phosphatase staining. Whether osteogenic stem cells are contained in periosteum is not known for certain. One final interesting feature of periosteum is that it also contains chondroprogenitor cells. Cartilage formation can be induced in periosteum under conditions of low oxygen tension (Thorogood, 1979) and following exposure to glucocorticoids in serum-free culture conditions (Heersche *et al.*, 1984). Tissues taken from younger fetal sources are more likely to develop cartilage. This would indicate that, as the fetus matures, the majority of periosteal chondroprogenitor cells may be lost while the osteoprogenitor cells are retained.

Mesenchyme

Mesenchyme is an embryonic connective tissue responsible for the initial formation of embryonic flat or intramembranous bones (Thorogood, 1979) and ultimately, periosteum. The osteogenic potential of mesenchyme is obvious *in vivo* and for this reason, mesenchymal tissues have been used to study factors affecting osteodifferentiation *in vitro*. Based on studies reported by Tyler and Hall (1977) and others (Hall, 1981; Hall *et al.*, 1983; Johnson, 1980; Tyler and McCobb, 1980; Van Exan and Hall, 1984) it would appear that mesenchymal tissue certainly contains a complement of determined osteoprogenitor cells.

When mesenchymal tissues are cultured appropriately, osteodifferentiation will occur and osteoid formation will take place. One of the most fascinating aspects of mesenchymal osteogenesis has been described for mandibular mesenchyme and it is the requirement for prior interaction between mesenchyme and epithelium if subsequent osteogenesis is to occur *in vitro* (and likely *in vivo*) (Hall, 1980; Hall *et al.*, 1983; Tyler and McCobb, 1980; Van Exan and Hall, 1984). This inductive interaction implies the presence in mesenchyme of inducible osteoprogenitor cells. If these cells are not exposed to epithelium or its products, osteogenesis will not occur, demonstrating that the determined osteoprogenitor cells of mesenchyme are derived from the inducible osteoprogenitor cells previously exposed to some "epithelial factor(s)". Recent evidence suggests that inducible osteoprogenitor cells can be switched on by, for example, fluoride without the benefit of previous inductive tissue interaction with epithelium (Hall, 1987).

## Soft Connective Tissue and Muscle

In the foregoing discussion, it is apparent that tissues intimately associated with bone in fetal and post-fetal life contain cells with osteogenic potential. In general, as discussed, it is speculated that at least two distinct populations of osteoprogenitor cells exist. Those cells which, under permissive circumstances, mature directly into bone cells were called determined osteoprogenitor cells (DOPC). The other population needs some form of induction whereupon DOPC arise and fully differentiate and were called inducible osteoprogenitor cells (IOPC).

It is not surprising that tissues closely associated with bone contain DOPC and IOPC; however, of great interest is that tissues remote from the skeleton also contain IOPC. This phenomenon has been demonstrated repeatedly by various investigators. In general, when demineralized bone or dentine powder is implanted subcutaneously or intramuscularly into a host animal, a sequence of endochondral ossification will occur in that animal adjacent to the implant (Nogami and Urist, 1975; Reddi, 1972a, b; Reddi and Huggins, 1972; Urist *et al.*, 1971, 1981). This is called matrix-induced endochondral ossification. This phenomenon will not occur if mineralized bone is implanted. The unmineralized bone powder can be implanted directly or within a diffusion chamber, and when a diffusion chamber is used, the sequence of endochondral ossification will take place outside of the chamber (Fig. 4). A similar sequence of events (stopping at cartilage formation) can be shown *in vitro* (Sampath *et al.*, 1984; Seyedin *et al.*, 1986). These experiments show quite clearly that inducible osteoprogenitor cells reside in many soft connective tissues and in muscle. These cells would not normally become osteogenic and, if not exposed to an inducing agent (released from demineralized bone?), would continue throughout post-fetal life to produce fibrous tissues. This will be discussed further in the last section of this chapter.

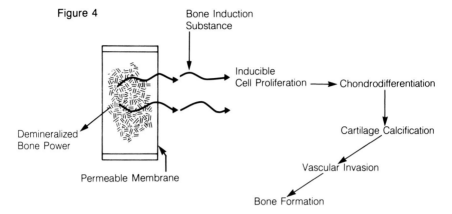

**Fig. 4**  This schematic diagram describes how subcutaneously implanted demineralized bone powder induces bone formation. An inducing substance diffuses out of the demineralized bone and crosses the permeable membrane of the implanted chamber containing the powder.

This inductive substance then triggers the cascade of events depicted on the right. Note that while bone formation does occur ultimately, it is cartilage formation that occurs first.

## Periodontal Ligament

Periodontal ligament (PDL) is the connective tissue interface between tooth and bone. The embryonic origin of the PDL is the dental follicle (Gaunt *et al.*, 1971). It is believed that, while the tooth and ligament is fundamentally contained by either the maxillary or mandibular bones, the source of bone and bone cells initially lining the tooth socket is, in fact, separate and distinct from the surrounding bone. Indeed, upon extraction of a tooth, the bone in the area resorbs (Boucher *et al.*, 1975). The reasons for this are largely unknown but could be related to the fact that the periodontal ligament is a source pf osteoblasts. During orthodontic tooth movement, new bone formation can be stimulated in various regions within the PDL. Generally, tension in the area will ultimately lead to recruitment of new osteoblasts. According to Roberts *et al.* (1982) the osteoprogenitor cells that respond to orthodontic loading reside throughout the periodontal ligament. Roberts *et al.* (1982) have also tentatively identified a small fibroblastic (IOPC) precursor cell which ultimately gives rise to the osteoprogenitor cell (DOPC). A series of at least two divisions is required for this to occur.

Other studies have shown that, if the PDL is wounded gently, new osteoblast precursor cells are detected primarily in perivascular locales

(Gould *et al.*, 1977, 1980). These cells probably also pass through an IOPC and DOPC maturation scheme as they develop into bone-producing cells (McCulloch and Melcher, 1982, 1983).

Interesting recent evidence has shown that some osteoprogenitor cells residing in the PDL may have migrated originally from adjacent endosteal spaces (McCulloch *et al.*, 1988).

The osteogenic potential of PDL has been demonstrated by the above noted studies *in vivo*; however, cells from the PDL have not yet been shown to possess osteogenic potential *in vitro*.

## Identification of osteogenic cells

The unambiguous identification of osteogenic cells is hampered by the failure to identify specific cellular markers for those cells. Methods have been developed that permit investigators to trace and potentially identify putative osteogenic precursor cells within various tissues. Autoradiographic techniques have been used to localize cells *in vivo* or *in vitro* that have taken up $^3$H-Thymidine ($^3$H-Tdr) and are preparing to divide. Once cells have taken up $^3$H-Tdr, they can be followed over an appropriate period of time. For example, if an animal is given a single dose of $^3$H-Tdr, all cells in the S-phase of the cell cycle will take up this marker. These cells can be identified using radioautography. In order to localize bone progenitor cells, it is possible to determine, after a single $^3$H-Tdr dose, the initial location of labelled cells that over a period of time become labelled osteoblasts. This has been shown in the periodontal ligament (PDL) of mice (McCulloch and Melcher, 1982, 1983). After wounding the PDL, it was shown that, after a single dose of $^3$H-Tdr, labelled cells were found perivascularly (Gould *et al.*, 1977, 1980). After a period of days (no further $^3$H-Tdr given), these labelled cells had disappeared; however, labelled osteoblasts were observed. This indicates that bone progenitor cells are capable of migrating and do go through at least one division prior to differentiating.

In view of the fact that it is possible to label the progeny of osteoblasts with $^3$H-Tdr, others have tried to use this as a tool to aid in identifying other features of osteoprogenitor cells. This would permit identification of osteoprogenitor cells with or without radioactive label. To this end, Roberts *et al.* (1982) have suggested that nuclear size can be used as a cell kinetic marker for osteoblast differentiation in the periodontal ligament. They have suggested that preosteoblasts have large nuclei ($> 170$ $\mu m^3$) whereas the fibroblastic precursors of preosteoblasts have smaller nuclei ($< 80$ $\mu m^3$). By observing changes in nuclear volume, it is possible to follow the kinetics of cellular differentiation without the use of radioactive labels.

Other methods of tentatively identifying osteoprogenitor cells have relied on the isolation of bone tissue and cell specific macromolecules. Termine *et al.* (1981) first identified osteonectin as a bone-specific protein. However, newer studies indicate that osteonectin is found in a wide variety of cells, including periodontal ligament and other dental tissues (Tung *et al.*, 1985). The foregoing notwithstanding, osteonectin may still be a useful bone cell marker if only skeletal tissues are examined. Jundt *et al.* (1987) demonstrated that osteonectin can be immunolocalized in active bone cells but also apparently in osteoprogenitor cells. The osteoprogenitor cells were always close to bone but still demonstrated fibroblastic morphology and were otherwise indistinguishable from fibroblasts. The enzyme alkaline phosphatase demonstrates very similar features, thus making it a potentially useful histochemical bone cell and osteoprogenitor cell marker (Tenenbaum and Heersche, 1986). Another potentially useful marker for osteogenic cells may be the so-called bone sialoprotein (Fisher *et al.*, 1983).

## Theories of Bone Cell Differentiation

As can be seen from the foregoing sections of this chapter, numerous studies have been undertaken to study and understand the cellular origins of bone cells. Differentiation schemes have been presented that identify osteoprogenitor cells and follow them through their development into osteoblasts (Fig. 5). Other investigations have been carried out in order to identify and quantify some of the biochemical/physiological properties of osteoblasts and their progenitors.

However, such studies do not address a central question in bone biology. That is, what is the mechanism behind the induction of osteodifferentiation. How is an IOPC or DOPC signalled to differentiate and become, ultimately, an osteoblast?

Several theories have been put forth that attempt to answer the above questions. For example, it has been postulated that the oxygen concentration of a local tissue plays a vital role in signalling bone cell differentiation. Some studies suggest that osteodifferentiation is favored in cases where a low oxygen concentration is present (Brighton *et al.*, 1976; Gray and Hamblen, 1976; Hall, 1969; Heppenstall *et al.*, 1976). Other studies may suggest the opposite (Thorogood, 1979) or no relationship (Tenenbaum and Heersche, 1986).

Other investigators have suggested that osteodifferentiation can be induced by various electromagnetic phenomena.

Electrical osteogenesis is a term used to describe bone formation induced by the presence of electric currents or electromagnetic fields (Baranowski

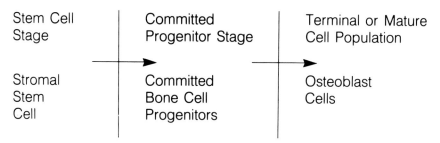

**Fig. 5**  This diagram, as proposed by Owen (1978), can be related to the information in Figure 2. A stromal stem cell is proposed which divides and thus regenerates itself and produces a committed bone cell progenitor. The progenitor cells can divide further and result in the production of osteoblast cells. The progenitor population is not self renewing and the osteoblast population is terminally differentiated and incapable of dividing.

*et al.*, 1983; Brighton *et al.*, 1985, 1986; Lavine and Grodzinsky, 1987). Non-union fractures have been induced to heal by the use of electromagnetism (Bassett *et al.*, 1976). It is hypothesized that bone formation brought about by movement is the result of piezo-electric forces created by the bending of bone surfaces (Shamos and Lavine, 1964). *In vitro* studies of electromagnetic field effects on bone-forming cells have been difficult to interpret (Lavine and Grodzinsky, 1987), and thus the mechanisms behind electrically induced osteogenisis are not understood.

## Factors that Regulate Bone Cell Differentiation

In discussing factors that regulate bone cell and differentiation, it is essential to address homeostatic mechanisms governing bone growth and metabolism.

The homeostasis of bone is regulated to a large degree by systemic influences expressed through the endocrine system (Canalis, 1983). The processes of bone resorption (calcium mobilization) and bone formation (calcium accretion) are closely tied to the systemic requirement for calcium balance by the endocrine system. Parathyroid hormone, which is primarily responsible for the maintenance of systemic calcium balance, is capable of inducing both bone formation and resorption (Parfitt, 1980; Tam *et al.*, 1982). For example, an excess of parathyroid hormone can have serious effects on skeletal mass by producing both osteoporosis and osteosclerosis (Gennant et al., 1975).

Clearly, bone metabolism and, particularly, bone resorption are influenced to a great degree by systemic factors (for a review, see Raisz and Kream, 1983a, b). It has been suggested, however, that local homeostasis of bone cannot be entirely regulated systemically but must also be under the control of local factors (Drivdahl et al., 1982; Puzas et al., 1981).

Baron et al. (1977) have described a local bone remodelling sequence involving a bone resorption phase, a reversal phase, and a bone formation phase. It is hypothesized that during the reversal phase, new osteoblasts are being recruited and that this recruitment is signalled by a factor (or factors) released locally during the resorption phase. Locally available factors must be involved in remodelling phenomena secondary to mechanical stress, disuse osteoporosis and the connective tissue diseases, rheumatoid arthritis and periodontitis (Canalis, 1983).

## Bone Cell and Tissue Derived Growth Factors

### Bone Cell Released Factors

It has been shown that paracrine factors can regulate the proliferation of fibroblast cells (Gospodarowicz et al., 1987). Further, it has been suggested that bone cells also can produce growth factors. Canalis et al. (1980) demonstrated that conditioned-medium derived from cultured rat calvariae or from bone-cell cultures was capable of stimulating $^3$H-Thymidine incorporation into DNA and $^3$H-Proline incorporation into collagen in cultures of fetal rat calvariae. A similar phenomenon was described by Drivdahl et al. (1982). Other investigators have data showing that rat or human osteosarcoma cells may produce a growth factor (Heldin et al., 1980; and Chapter 4).

### Bone Tissue Released Factors

In other studies, it has been shown that factors, derived directly from bone tissue using both denaturing and non-denaturing extraction procedures, can induce cell proliferation. In particular, Wergedal et al. (1985) have isolated a factor from human bone which stimulates proliferation in bone-derived cells. Canalis and Centrella (1985), Puzas and Brand, (1985) and Hauschka et al. (1985) have isolated bone matrix factors which are mitogenic for bone-derived cells as well as for other mesenchymal cell types such as 3T3 fibroblasts or NRK cells.

## Bone Derived Factors and Osteodifferentiation

The studies previously referred to focus primarily on cell proliferation and protein synthesis but do not address the question of bone cell differentiation. This question was approached by Urist *et al.* (1973) and Reddi and Huggins (1972) who showed that subcutaneously-implanted bone matrix will ultimately induce metaplastic changes in mesenchymal cells (IOPC's), leading to endochondral ossification in host rats or rabbits (See figure 4). Recent work by Sampath *et al.* (1984) and Muthukumaran *et al.* (1985) has demonstrated that these factors can induce muscle cells to become chondrogenic, but not osteogenic. Canalis *et al.* (1985) have shown that a partially purified protein with similar activity to that described by Sampath *et al.* (1984) and called Bone Morphogenetic Protein (BMP) (obtained from M. Urist) can stimulate DNA synthesis in calvarial or fibroblast cultures.

## Deficiencies of the Model Systems Used to Evaluate Growth/ Differentiation Factors

Clearly, there is ample evidence to suggest that there are growth/proliferation factors produced by bone cells or contained in bone tissues. It is also likely that inhibitory factors are present (Puzas *et al.*, 1981; Canalis and Centrella, 1985). However, the regulation of osteogenesis involves more than modulation of cell proliferation. Osteogenesis encompasses osteodifferentiation, matrix synthesis and mineralization. If factors which promote or inhibit osteogenesis are to be isolated, model systems which demonstrate osteogenesis must be employed. Moreover, while proliferation is an important parameter to study and since it usually precedes differentiation, it cannot be concluded that proliferation leads *a priori* to differentiation or is synonymous with differentiation. In order to determine whether a factor does stimulate bone growth and cellular differentiation, other parameters related to bone cell differentiation, such as alkaline phosphatase activity, bone matrix synthesis and mineralization should be studied. The bone and tissue culture systems discussed above are obviously not unequivocally osteogenic and their use would thus seem inappropriate for the study of differentiation of bone cells.

Another shortcoming of the model systems reviewed above is that they have not been well-defined, either morphologically or in terms of cell and tissue kinetics. Only gross biochemical studies, such as $^3$H-Thymidine incorporation or $^3$H-Proline incorporation have been done. These data provide little insight into the heterogeneity of the cell populations that proliferate, differentiate and synthesize bone. A similar problem is associated with cell cultures using more defined cell populations. The exact lineage and identity of the cells responding to manipulation is not known.

Many of the problems alluded to above can be circumvented by the use of *in vitro* osteogenesis, osteodifferentiation models. These systems will be discussed in chapters 5 and 7 of this book. However, for the purpose of highlighting further concepts regarding mechanisms of osteodifferentiation, a description here of some experiments done with the chick periosteal osteogenesis model will be discussed.

## Microenvironment

Utilizing a chick periosteal culture technique, Nijweide and Van der Plas (1975) first showed that by placing osteogenic precursors within a microenvironment created by folding the periosteum, osteodifferentiation ensued (See Figs 3 & 6). Thus, it might be assumed that osteogenic precursor cells require a microenvironment in order to differentiate. However, it was also possible to explain the phenomenon by suggesting that the oxygen concentration within the folded periosteum was decreased, thus permitting or promoting differentiation (Brighton *et al.*, 1976; Gray and Hamblen, 1976; Hall, 1969; Heppenstall *et al.*, 1976). Another explanation would state that the increased cell-to-cell contact created by folding the periosteum was responsible for inducing osteodifferentiation.

In order to explore this question, further experiments were designed in an attempt to create a microenvironment without folding the periosteal tissue (Tenenbaum and Heersche, 1986). Some periosteal explants were cultured folded with the osteogenic cells within the fold, (as described by Nijweide) as positive controls. However, other periostea were cultured unfolded, one group with the osteogenic layer away from the medium and another group with the osteogenic layer facing the medium (Fig. 6). (All explants were maintained at the gas/liquid interface). The purpose behind these manipulations can be explained in the following way.

When tissues are cultured in an organ culture system, a thin film of liquid will form via capillary action over the top of the tissue. It seems likely that, within this film of fluid, even a limited number of cells might condition their surroundings. Therefore, explants cultured with the osteogenic layer of cells facing the air phase might be able to create a microenvironment, whereas, if this layer of cells is cultured facing the culture medium, they would be under "diffusing" conditions and thus not able to create a microenvironment (Fig. 6).

Moreover, the cells in the osteogenic layer facing the air or gas phase would not be exposed to the low oxygen concentration that might be

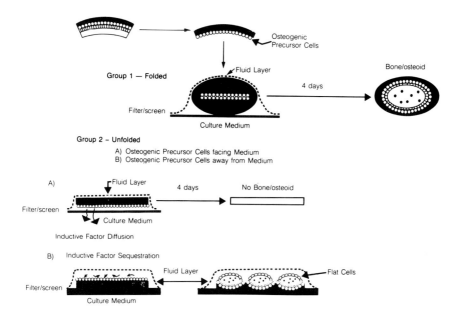

**Fig. 6** This flow diagram demonstrates the concepts of microenvironment formation and suggests how a microenvironment might help to trap factors capable of inducing osteodifferentiation.

present within a folded periosteum, thus indirectly addressing the question of oxygen concentration.

In these experiments, differentiation of osteoblasts was observed when explants were cultured with the osteogenic side facing the air phase while no osteodifferentiation occurred when similar periostea were cultured with the osteogenic layer facing the medium. As expected, osteogenesis took place in the folded explants.

Taken together, these findings would confirm that a microenvironment was required for osteodifferentiation and that bone cell differentiation was not related in this case to oxygen concentration or increases in cell-to-cell contact.

To state that a microenvironment is required for osteodifferentiation is obviously an oversimplification. Further studies have been done to explore the nature of a microenvironment and these were based on the hypothesis that cellularly-produced osteoinductive factors must be trapped and concentrated within a putative microenvironment. Until an as yet unknown critical concentration of these also unknown factors near osteoprogenitor cells is reached, differentiation of those cells will not occur.

In an attempt at preliminary characterization of these putative osteo-inductive factors, further experiments with unfolded periosteal explants were performed. In these studies, unfolded periostea were cultured with their osteogenic layer of cells facing the culture medium. As discussed above, these cells would thus be placed under diffusing conditions and therefore concentration of inductive factors could not take place. In order to trap osteoinductive factors without changing the oxygen concentration or increasing cell-to-cell contact, Diaflo® membranes were interposed between the osteogenic cells and the culture medium. Molecular weight, cut-off pore-sizes, ranging from 1000 daltons to 300,000 daltons were used. The results obtained showed that, when very large pore-sizes ($> 300,000$ D) were used, diffusion of osteoinductive factors away from osteoprogenitors still took place, thus not allowing differentiation. However, as the pore-size approached 100,000 daltons, osteodifferentiation occurred, thus suggesting that osteoinductive factors were being trapped in the artificially-created microenvironment (Fig. 7). These findings not only supported the micro-environment hypothesis but also indicated that the osteoinductive factors operating in the chick periosteum probably range in size somewhere between 100,000 and 300,000 daltons.

Based on the above findings, it might be possible to speculate about the possible identity of osteoinductive factors based on molecular weight esti-mates. It must be stressed that even low molecular weight growth/differen-tiation factors could aggregate and thus give the mistaken impression of a larger molecular weight factor.

Some factors that could be involved in osteoinduction here are the following larger molecular weight molecules; fibronectin (400,000 daltons), collagen (285,000 daltons), procollagen peptides (100,000 daltons) and possibly proteoglycans greater than 100,000 daltons.

Fibronectin, for example, has been localized immunohistochemically in the matrix of haversian bone and this molecule is known to induce pheno-typic changes in malignant cell lines (Yamada and Olden, 1978) as well as being involved in the early stages of endochondral ossification (Weiss and Reddi, 1980). Other evidence indicates that fibronectin (as well as collagen) is associated with terminal differentiation of odontoblasts (Lesot et al., 1981). Exogenously-added fibronectin may also have an organizing effect on myoblasts in vitro (Chiquet et al., 1981).

Collagens, proteoglycans and/or hyaluronic acid have also been implicated as important factors regulating differentiation. Kosher and Church (1975) demonstrated that in vitro somite chondrogenesis could be stimulated by type II collagen. In addition, they demonstrated that procollagen, as well as proteoglycans, were also capable of stimulating chondrogenesis in vitro.

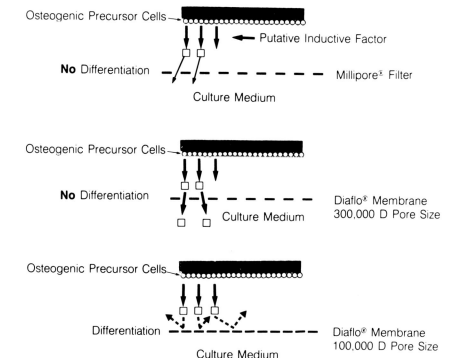

**Fig. 7** In this figure it is shown how, by interposing Diaflo® membranes between osteogenic cells and the culture medium, a molecular weight estimate can be made for the putative osteoinductive factors. The molecular weight estimate of these factors is less important in this experiment than the demonstration that they actually must exist.

Weiss and Reddi (1980) demonstrated mesenchymal cell proliferation in response to implantation of "collagenous bone matrix". Collagen, however, was not the only component of the collagenous bone matrix. There is some tantalizing but indirect evidence that hyaluronic acid may have osteostimulative properties *in vitro* as well (Fitton-Jackson, 1970). When bone explants were treated with hyaluronidase, osteogenesis was inhibited. As well, changes in hyaluronate levels may influence cellular condensation in mesenchyme (Shur *et al.*, 1982).

Some well known growth factors unlikely to be involved in differentiation in the chick model would include, insulin-like growth factors (4,000 D), skeletal growth factor (12,000 D, Drivdahl *et al.*, 1982) and bone morphogenetic protein (23,000 D, Urist *et al.*, 1981).

## Bone Induction by Bone Morphogenetic Protein or Cartilage Induction Factor

In the foregoing section, it was shown that it is highly probable that biochemical factors may play an important role in the induction of osteo-differentiation. However, the actual role played by the identified and un-identified factors is largely unknown, and discussion in this realm could be considered to be highly theoretical.

The biological role for bone morphogenetic protein (BMP) is not known but its ultimate biological effect is well-characterized (Nogami and Urist, 1970; Urist and Strates, 1971; Urist et al., 1981, 1983). Historically, it has been shown that following subcutaneous implantation of demineralized bone powder (DBP) in host animals, a sequence of endochondral ossification is induced (Nogami and Urist, 1975; Reddi, 1972, 1981; Reddi and Huggins, 1972; Urist and Strates, 1971; Urist et al., 1981, 1983). This phenomenon will occur when DBP is implanted directly subcutaneously or is contained within Millipore chambers and implanted intramuscularly. As host cells could be induced to form bone on the outside of Millipore chambers containing DBP, Urist and Strates (1971) concluded that an osteoinductive agent was diffusing across the Millipore filters. It was hypothesized that this agent was stimulating soft connective tissue IOPC's to differentiate into mature osteoblasts. This putative agent accordingly was named Bone Morphogenetic Protein (Fig. 4). This protein has been purified from Human and Bovine bone (Urist et al., 1983, 1984) and is being studied further for its potential clinical use in the area of bone regeneration.

A protein with similar activity has been isolated and characterized by Seyedin et al (1986). It has been named Cartilage Induction Factor (C.I.F.) and is homologous with Transforming Growth Factor β. This factor will induce a sequence of endochondral ossification if implanted in host animals (Seyedin et al., 1986). Other studies performed in vitro have demonstrated that C.I.F. (and other probably related bone-derived factors) can induce the formation of cartilage but not bone in, for example, muscle explants (Sampath et al., 1984).

Perhaps the name C.I.F. may be more appropriate than BMP for these factors do not appear to stimulate bone formation directly. It would appear that C.I.F. or BMP probably stimulate soft connective tissue inducible chondroprogenitor cells to differentiate first. This is then followed by the well-documented sequence of cartilage formation, cartilage calcification, vascular invasion, resorption of calcified cartilage and then finally the induction of new bone formation.

In view of the above, consideration should be given to the possibility that direct bone inductive agents may be found not necessarily or not only in bone itself but, perhaps, also in calcified (or non-calcified?) cartilage. There is already some evidence that subcutaneously-implanted, calcified cartilage will induce new bone formation and thus it would seem logical to extend the search for bone differentiation induction factors from bone to cartilage as well (Moskalewski *et al.*, 1975; Thyberg and Moskalewski, 1979).

## Conclusion

In this chapter, we have attempted to trace the lineage of the osteoblast. In so doing, various *in vivo* and *in vitro* studies have been discussed. These have shown that multiple tissues are capable of giving rise to osteoblasts but that the three principle ones are marrow, periosteum and periodontal ligament. Other soft connective tissues have "osteo-competent" cells but these seem to require exogenously-added inductive agents.

The methods used to identify and trace the lineage of osteoblasts have also been discussed but, as yet, unequivocal osteoblastic or osteoprogenitor markers have not been identified.

Finally in this chapter, we have attempted to highlight some of the theories regarding the mechanisms behind osteodifferentiation. Special emphasis was placed on the potential importance of bone derived paracrine or autocrine factors in this regard. Investigations whose purpose is to identify and purify osteoinductive factors is likely to be very fruitful in the future.

## References

Amsel, S., and Dell, E. S. (1972). Bone formation by hemopoietic tissue: separation of preosteoblast from hemopoietic stem cell function in the rat. *Blood*, **39**: 267−273.

Ashton, B. A., Abdullah, F., Cave, J., Williamson, M., Sykes, B. C., Couch, M., and Poser, J. W. (1985). Characterization of cells with high alkaline phosphatase activity derived from human blood and marrow: preliminary assessment of their osteogenecity. *Bone* **6**: 313−319.

Ashton, B. A., Allen, T. D., Howlett, C. R., Eagelsom, C. C., Hattori, A., and Owen, M. E. (1980). Formation of bone and cartilage by marrow stromal cells in diffusion chambers *in vivo*. *Clin. Orthop. Rel. Res.* **151**: 294−307.

Ashton, B. A., Eagelsom, C. C., Bab, I., and Owen, M. E. (1984). Distribution of fibroblastic colony-forming cells in rabbit bone marrow and assay of their osteogenic potential by an *in vivo* diffusion chamber method. *Calc. Tissue Intern.*, **36**: 83−86.

Bab, I., Ashton, B. A., Gazit, D., Marx, G., Williamson, M. C., and Owen, M. E. (1986). Kinetics and differentiation of marrow stromal cells in diffusion chambers *in vivo*. *J. Cell Sci.*, **84**: 139–151.

Bab, I., Ashton, B. A., Syftestad, G. T., and Owen, M. E. (1984). Assessment of an *in vivo* diffusion chamber method as a quantitative assay for osteogenesis. *Calc. Tissue Intern.*, **36**: 77–82.

Baranowski, T. J. Jr., Black, J., Brighton, C. T., and Friedenberg, Z. B. (1983). Electrical osteogenesis by low direct current. *J. Orthopaedic Res.*, **1**: 120–128.

Baron, R., Saffan, J. L., and Duflot-Vignery, A. (1977). Alveolar bone remodelling in the rat: normal status and effects of PTX and PTH on the remodelling sequence and the osteoclastic pool. *Calc. Tissue Res.*, **22** (suppl.) 502–504.

Bassett, C. A. L., Pawluk, R. J., and Pilla, A. A. (1974). Augmentation of bone repair by inductively-coupled electromagnetic fields. *Science*, **184**: 575–577.

Boucher, C. O., Hickey, J. C., and Zarb, G. A. (1975). *"Prosthodontic Treatment for Edentulous Patients"* C. V. Mosby, St. Louis.

Brighton, C. T., Fox, J. L., and Seltzer, D. (1976). *In vitro* growth of bone and cartilage from rat periosteum under various oxygen tensions. 22nd Annual ORS, Branoff Place Hotel, New Orleans, Louisiana, January 28–30.

Brighton, C. T., Hozak, W. J., Brager, M. D., Windsor, R. E., Pollack, S. R., Vreslovic, E. J., and Kotwickm, J. E. Fracture healing in the rabbit fibula when subjected to various capacitively coupled electrical fields. *J. Orthopaedic Res.*, **3**: 331–340 (1985)

Brighton, C. T., and Hunt, R. M. (1986). Ultrastructure of electrically induced osteogenesis in the rabbit medullary canal. *J. Orthopaedic Res.*, **4**: 27–36.

Budenz, R. W., and Bernard, G. W. (1980). Osteogenesis and leukopoiesis within diffusion chamber implants of isolated bone marrow subpopulations. *Amer. J. Anat.*, **159**: 455–474.

Canalis, E. (1983). The hormonal and local regulation of bone formation. *Endocrine Rev.*, **4**: 62–77.

Canalis, E., and Centrella, M. (1985). Purification of bone-derived growth factor (BDGF) from cultured fetal rat calvariae. *Proc. Amer. Soc. Bone Mineral Res.*, abstract 8.

Canalis, E., Centrella, M., and Urist, M. R. (1985). Effect of partially purified bone morphogenetic protein on DNA synthesis and cell replication in calvarial and fibroblast cultures. *Clin. Orthop. Rel. Res.*, **198**: 289–296.

Canalis, E., Peck. W. A. and Raisz, L. G. (1980). Stimulation of DNA and collagen synthesis by autologous growth factor in cultured fetal rat calvaria. *Science*, **210**: 1021–1023.

Chiquet, M., Eppenberger, H. M., and Turner, D. C. (1981). Muscle morphogenesis: evidence for an organizing function of exogenous fibronectin. *Devel. Biol.*, **88**: 220–234.

Davidson, D., and McCulloch, C. A. G. (1986). Proliferative behaviour of periodontal ligament cell populations. *J. Periodontal Res.* **21**: 414–428.

Drivdahl, R. H., Howard, G. A., and Baylink, D. J. (1982). Extracts of bone contain a potent regulator of bone formation. *Biochem. Biophys. Acta*, **714**: 26–33.

Fell, H. B. (1932). The osteogenic capacity *in vitro* of periosteum and endosteum isolated from the limb skeleton of fowl embryos and young chicks. *J. Anat. Lond.*, **66**: 157–180.

Fell, H. B. (1969). The effect of environment on skeletal tissue in culture. *Embryologia*, **10**: 181–205.

Fisher, L. W., Whitson, S. W., Avioli, L. V., and Termine, J. D. (1983). Matrix sialoprotein of developing bone. *J. Biol. Chem.*, **258**: 12723–12727.

Fitton-Jackson, S. (1970). Environmental control of macromolecular synthesis in cartilage and bone: morphogenetic response to hyaluronidase. *Proc. R. Soc. Lond. B*, **175**: 405–453.

Fitton-Jackson, S., and Smith, R. H. (1957). Studies on the biosynthesis of colagen. I. The growth of fowl osteoblasts and the formation of collagen in tissue culture. *J. Biophys. Biochem. Cytol.*, **3**: 897–912.

Friedenstein, A. J., Chailakhyan, R. K., Latsinik, N. Y., Panasyuk, A. F., and Keiliss-Borok, I. V. (1974). Stromal cells responsible for transferring the microenvironment of the hemopoietic tissues. *Transplantation*, **17**: 331–340.

Friedenstein, A. J., Gorskaya, U. F., and Kulagina, N. N. Fibroblast precursors in normal and irradiated mouse hematopoietic organs. *Exp. Hematol.*, **4**: 267–274 (1976)

Friedenstein, A. J., and Kuralesova, A. I. (1971). Osteogenic precursor cells of bone marrow in radiation chimeras. *Transplantation*, **12**: 99–108.

Friedenstein, A. J., Latsinik, N. V., Grosheva, A. G., and Gorskaya, U. F. (1982). Marrow microenvironment transfer by heterotopic transplantation of freshly isolated and cultured cells in porous sponges. *Exp. Hematol.*, **10**: 217–227.

Gaillard, R. J. (1935). Developmental changes in composition of body fluids in relation to growth and differentiation of tissue cultures. *Proroplasma*, **23**: 145–174.

Gaunt, W. A., Osborn, J. W., and Ten Cate, A. R. (1971). *"Advances in Dental Histology"* 2nd ed, pp. 110–113. John Wright & Sons, Bristol.

Gennant, H. K., Baron, J. M., Straus, F. H. (1975). Osteosclerosis in primary hyperparathyroidism. *Amer. J. Med.*, **59**: 104–113.

Goldhaber, P. (1966). Remodelling of bone in tissue culture. *J. Dental Res.* (Suppl. to No. 3). **45**: 490–499.

Gospodarowicz, D., Weseman, J., Moran, J. S., and Lindstrom, J. (1976). Effect of fibroblast growth factor on the division and fusion of bovine myoblasts. *J. Cell Biol.*, **70**: 395–405.

Gould, T. R. L., Melcher, A. H., and Brunette, D. M. (1977). Location of progenitor cells in periodontal ligament of mouse molar stimulated by wounding. *Anat. Rec.*, **188**: 133–142.

Gould, T. R. L., Melcher, A. H., and Brunette, D. M. (1980). Migration and division of progenitor cell populations in periodontal ligament after wounding. *J. Periodont. Res.* **15**: 20–42.

Gray, D. H., and Hamblen, D. L. (1976). The effects of hyperoxia upon bone in organ culture. *Clin. Orthop. Rel. Res.*, **119**: 225–230.

Gray, D. H., and Speak, K. S. (1979). The control of bone induction is soft tissues. *Clin. Orthop. Rel. Res.*, **143**: 245–250.

Hall, B. K. (1969). Hypoxia and differentiation of cartilage and bone from common germinal cells *in vitro*. *Life Sciences*, **8**: 553–558.

Hall, B. K. (1981). The induction of neural crest-derived cartilage and bone by embryonic epithelia: an analysis of the mode of action of an epithelial-mesenchymal interaction. *J. Embryol. Exp. Morph.*, **64**: 305–320.

Hall, B. K. (1987). Sodium fluoride as an initiator of osteogenesis from embryonic mesenchyme *in vitro*. *Bone*, **8**: 111–116.

Hall, B. K., Van Exan, R. J., and Brunt, S. L. (1983). Retention of epithelial basal lamina allows isolated mandibular mesenchyme to form bone. *J. Craniofac. Gen. Devel. Biol.*, **3**: 253–267.

Hauschka, P. V., Lafrati, M. D., Doleman, S. E., Sullivan, R. C., and Klagsbrun, M. (1985). Bone matrix-derived growth factors (BDGF) resolved by heparin affinity chromatography. *Proc. Amer. Soc. Bone Mineral Res.*, Abstract 7.

Heersche, J. N. M., Pitaru, S., Aubin, J. E., and Tenenbaum, H. C. (1984). Corticosteroid-induced expression of cartilage phenotype in cultured membrane bone periosteum. In *Endocrine Control of Bone and Calcium* (D. V. Cohn, T. Fujita, J. T. Potts, and R. V. Talmage, eds), pp 147–150. Intern. Congress Series, Exerpta Medica, Amsterdam.

Heldin, C. H., Westermark, B., and Wasteson, J. (1980). Chemical and biological properties of a growth factor from human-cultured osteosarcoma cells: resemblance with platelet-derived growth factor. *J. Cell Physiol.*, **105**: 235−246.

Heppenstall, R. B., Goodwin, C. W., and Brighton, C. T. (1976). Fracture healing in the presence of chronic hypoxia. *J. Bone Jt. Surg.*, **58A**: 1153−1156.

Howlett, C. R., Cavé, J., Williamson, M., Farmer, J., Ali, S. Y., Bab, I., and Owen, M. E. (1986). Mineralization in *in vitro* cultures or rabbit marrow stromal cells. *Clin. Orthop. Rel. Res.* **213**: 251−263.

Johnson, D. R. (1980). Formation of marrow cavity and ossification in mouse limb buds grown *in vitro. J. Embryol. Exp. Morph.*, **56**: 302−327.

Jundt, G., Berghäuser, K-H., Termine, J. D., and Schulz, A. (1987). Osteonectin- a differentiation marker of bone cells. *Cell Tissue Res.*, **248**: 409−415.

Kosher, R. A., and Church, R. L. (1975). Stimulation of *in vitro* somite chondrogenesis by procollagen and collagen. *Nature*, **258**: 327−329.

Lavine, L. S., and Grodzinsky, A. J. (1987). Current concepts review: electrical stimulation of repair of bone. *J. Bone Jt. Surg.*, **69A**: 626−63.

Lesot, H., Osman, M., and Ruch, J-V. (1981). Immunofluorescent localization of collagens, fibronectin and laminin during terminal differentiation of odontoblasts. *Devel. Biol.*, **82**: 371−381.

Luria, E. A., Owen, M. E., Friedenstein, A. J., Morris, J. F., and Kuznetsow, S. A. (1987). Bone formation in organ cultures of bone marrow. *Cell Tissue Res.*, **248**: 449−454.

Mardon, H. J., Bee, J., von der Mark, K., and Owen, M. E. (1987). Development of osteogenic tissue in diffusion chambers from early precursor cells in bone marrow of adult rats. *Cell Tissue Res.*, **250**: 157−165.

Marvaso, V., and Bernard, G. W. (197 ). Initial intramembranous osteogenesis *in vitro. Amer. J. Anat.*, **149**: 453−468.

McCulloch, C. A. G., and Melcher, A. H. (1982). Continuous labelling of the periodontal ligament of mice. *J. Periodont. Res.*, **18**: 231−241.

McCulloch, C. A. G., and Melcher, A. H. (1983a). Cell density and cell generation in the periodontal ligament of mice. *Amer. J. Anat.*, **167**: 43−58.

McCulloch, C. A. G., and Melcher, A. H. (1983b). Cell migration in the periodontal ligament of mice. *J. Periodont. Res.*, **18**: 339−352.

McCulloch, C. A. G., Nemeth, E., Lowenberg, B. and Melcher, A. H. (1988). Paravascular cells in endosteal spaces of alveolar bone contribute to periodontal ligament cell populations. *Anat. Rec.*, (in press).

McCulloch, C. A. G., Tenembaum, H. C., Fair, C. A., and Birek, C. (1988). Site-specific regulation of osteogenesis: maintenance of discrete levels of phenotypic expression *in vitro. Anat. Rec.*, (in press).

Moskalewski, S., Malejczyk, J., and Osiecka, A. (1986). Structural differences between bone formed intramuscularly following the transplantation of isolated calvarial bone cells or chondrocytes. *Anat. & Embryol.*, **175**: 271−277.

Muthukumaran, N., Sampath, T. K., and Reddi, A. H. (1985). Comparison of bone induction proteins or rat and porcine bone matrix. *Biochem. Biophys. Res. Commun.*, **131**: 37−41.

Nijweide, P. J., Burger, E. H., Hekkelman, J. W., Herrmann-Erlee, M. P. M., and Gailard, P. J. (1982). Regulatory mechanisms in the development of bone and cartilage: the use of tissue culture techniques in the study of the development of embryonic bone and cartilage: a perspective. In: *Factors and Mechanisms Influencing Bone Growth* (A. D. Dixon and B. G. Sarnat, eds), pp. 457−480. Alan R. Liss Inc., New York.

Nijweide, P. J., and van der Plas, A. (1975). Embryonic chicken periosteum in tissue culture: osteoid formation and calcium uptake. *Proc. K. Ned. Akad. Wet.*, **C78**: 410−417.

Nogami, H., and Urist, M. R. (1975). Transmembrane bone matrix gelatin-induced differentiation of bone. *Calc. Tissue Res.*, **19**: 153−164.

Owen, M. E. (1978). Histogenesis of bone cells. *Calc. Tissue Res.*, **25**: 205−207.

Owen, M. E. (1980). The origin of bone cells in the postnatal organisms. *Arthritis & Rheumatism*, **23**: 1073−1080.

Owen, M. E. (1982). Bone growth at the cellular level: a perspective. In: *Factors and Mechanisms Influencing Bone Growth* (A. D. Dixon and B. G. Sarnat, eds), pp. 19−28. Alan R. Liss Inc., New York.

Owen, M. E. (1985). Lineage of osteogenic cells and their relationship to the stromal system. In: *Bone and Mineral Research* (W. A. Peck, ed), pp. 1−25. Elsevier Science Publisher, Amsterdam.

Owen, M. E., Cavé, J., and Joyner, C. J. (1987). Clonal analysis *in vitro* of osteogenic differentiation of marrow CFU-F. *J. Cell Sci.*, **87**: 731−738.

Pal, T. (1986). *The effects of dexamethasone on the in vitro differentiation of bone and cartilage.* M. Sc. Thesis, University of Toronto, Toronto, Canada.

Parfitt, A. M. (1976). The actions of parathyroid hormone on bone: relation to bone remodelling and turnover, calcium homeostasis, and metabolic bone disease. Part III of IV parts: PTH & osteoblasts, the relationship between bone turnover and bone loss, and the state of the bones in primary hyperparathyroidism. *Metabolism*, **25**: 1033−1069.

Puzas, J. E., and Brand, J. S. (1985). Heterotopic bone in metabolically active and contains a potent stimulator and inhibitor of cell proliferation. *Proc. Amer. Soc. Bone Mineral Res.*, abstract 13.

Puzas, J. E., Drivdahl, R. H., Howard, G. A., and Baylink, D. J. (1981). Endogenous inhibitor of bone cell proliferation. *Proc. Soc. Exp. Biol. Med.*, **166**: 113−122.

Raisz, L. G., and Kream, B. E. (1983a). Regulation of bone formation (first of two parts). *New Engl. J. Med.*, **309**: 29−34.

Raisz, L. G., and Kream, B. E. (1983b). Regulation of bone formation (second of two parts). *New Engl. J. Med.*, **309**: 83−89.

Reddi, A. H. (1981). Cell biology and biochemistry of endochondral bone development. *Collagen & Rel. Res.* **1**: 209−226.

Reddi, A. H., and Huggins, C. (1972a). Biochemical sequences in the transformation of normal fibroblasts in adolescent rats. *Proc. Natl. Acad. Sci. USA.*, **69**: 1601−1605.

Reddi, A. H., and Huggins, C. (1972b). Citrate and alkaline phosphatase during transformation of fibroblasts by the matrix and minerals of bone. *Proc. Soc. Exp. Biol. Med.*, **140**: 807−810.

Roberts, W. E., Mozsary, P. G., and Klingler, E. (1982). Nuclear size as a cell-kinetic marker of osteoblast differentiation. *Amer. J. Anat.*, **165**: 373−384.

Sampath, T. K., Nathanson, M. A., and Reddi, A. H. (1984). *In vitro* transformation of mesenchymal cells derived from embryonic muscle into cartilage in response to extracellular matrix components of bone. *Proc. Natl. Acad. Sci. USA*, **81**: 3419−3423.

Seyedin, S. M., Thompson, A. Y., Bentz, H., Rosen, D. M., McPherson, J. M., Conti, A., Siegel, N. R., Gallupi, G. R., and Piez, K. A. (1986). Cartilage-inducing factor-A. Apparent identity to transforming growth factor- β *J. Biol. Chem.*, **261**: 5693−5695.

Shamos, M. H., and Lavine, L. S. (1964). Physical bases for bioelectric effects in mineralized tissues. *Clin. Orthop. Res. Res.*, **35**: 177−188.

Shur, B. D., Vogler, M., and Kosher, R. A. (1982). Changes in endogenous cell surface galactosyltransferase activity during *in vitro* limb bud chondrogenesis. *Exp. Cell Res.*, **137**: 229−237.

Stutzman, J. J., and Petrovic, A. G. (1982). Bone cell histogenesis: the skeletoblast as a stem cell for preosteoblasts and for secondary-type prechondroblasts. In: *Factors and Mechanisms*

*Influencing Bone Growth* (A. D. Dixon and B. G. Sarnat, eds), pp. 29—45. Alan R. Liss Inc., New York.

Tam, C. S., Heersche, J. N. M., Murray, T. M., and Parsons, J. A. (1982). Parathyroid hormone stimulates the bone apposition rate independently of its resorptive action: differential effects of intermittent and continuous administration. *Endocrinology*, **110**: 506—512.

Tenenbaum, H. C., and Heersche, J. N. M. (1982). Differentiation of osteoblasts and formation of mineralized bone *in vitro*. *Calc. Tissue Res.*, **34**: 76—79.

Tenenbaum, H. C., and Heersche, J. N. M. (1986). Differentiation of osteoid-producing cells *in vitro*: possible evidence for the requirement of microenvironment. *Calc. Tissue Intern.*, **38**: 262—267.

Tenenbaum. H. C., and Palangio, K. (1987). Phosphoethanolamine- and fructose 1,6-diphosphate-induced calcium uptake in bone formed *in vitro*. *Bone and Mineral*, **2**: 201—210.

Termine, J. D., Kleinman, H. K., Whitson, S. W., Conn, K. M., McGarvey, M. L., and Martin, G. R. (1981). Osteonectin: a bone-specific protein linking mineral to collagen. *Cell*, **26**: 99—106.

Thorogood, P. V. (1979). *In vitro* studies on skeletogenic potential of membrane bone periosteal cells. *J. Embryol. Exp. Morph.*, **54**: 185—207.

Thyberg, J., and Moskalewski, S. (1979). Bone formation in cartilage produced by transplanted epiphyseal chondrocytes. *Cell Tissue Res.*, **204**: 77—94.

Tibone, K. W., and Bernard, G. W. (1982). A new *in vitro* model of intramembranous osteogenesis from adult bone marrow stem cells. In: *Factors and Mechanisms Influencing Bone Growth* (A. D. Dixon and B. G. Sarnat, eds), pp. 107—123. Alan R. Liss Inc., New York.

Tung, P. S., Domenicucci, C., Wasi, S., and Sodek, J. (1985). Specific immunohistochemical localization of ostenonectin and collagen types I and III in fetal and adult porcine dental tissues. *J. Histochem. Cytochem.*, **33**: 531—540.

Tyler, M. S., and Hall, B. K. (1977). Epithelial influences on skeletogenesis in the mandible of the embryonic chick. *Anat. Rec.*, **188**: 229—240.

Tyler, M. S., and McCobb, D. P. (1980). The genesis of membrane bone in the embryonic chick maxilla: epithelial-mesenchymal tissue recombination studies. *J. Embryol. Exp. Morph.*, **56**: 269—281.

Urist, M. R., Conover, M. A., Lietze, A., Triffit, J. T., and DeLange, R. J. (1981). In: Hormonal Control of Calcium Metabolism. (D. V. Cohn, R. V. Talmage and J. L. Mathews, eds), pp. 307—314. International Congress Series, Exerpta medica, Amsterdam.

Urist, M. R., Delange, R. J., and Finerman, G. A. M. (1983). Bone cell differentiation and growth factors. *Science*, **220**: 680—686.

Urist, M. R., Huo, Y. K., Brownell, A. G., Hohl. W. M., Buyske, J., Lietze, A., Tempst, P., Hunkapiller, M., and DeLange, R. J. (1984). Purification of bovine bone morphogenetic protein by hydroxyapatite chromatography. *Proc. Natl. Acad. Sci. USA*, **81**: 371—375.

Urist, M. R., Iwata, H., Ceccoiit, P. L., Dorfman, R. L., Boyd, S. D., McDowell, R. M., and Chien, C. (1973). Bone morphogenesis in implants of insoluble bone gelatin. *Proc. Natl. Acad. Sci. USA*, **70**: 3511—3515.

Urist, M. R., and Strates, B. S. (1971). Bone morphogenetic protein. *J. Dental Res.*, **50**: 1392—1406.

Van Exan, R. J., and Hall, B. K. (1984). Epithelial induction of osteogenesis in embryonic chick mandibular mesenchyme studied by transfilter tissue recombination. *J. Embryol. Exp. Morph.*, **79**: 225—242.

Weiss, R. E., and Reddi, A. H. (1980). Influence of experimental diabetes and insulin on matrix-induced cartilage and bone differentiation. *Amer. J. Physiol.*, **238**: E200—E207.

Wergedal, J. E., Mohan, S., and Baylink, D. J. (1985). Human skeletal growth factor (SGF) is produced by human osteoblast-like cells. *Proc. Soc. Amer. Bone Mineral Res.* abstract 81.

Yamada, K. M., and Olden, K. (1978). Fibronectins-adhesive glycoproteins of cell surface and blood. *Nature*, **275**: 179–184.

# 3

# Histochemistry and enzymology of bone-forming cells.

**STEPHEN B. DOTY**
*Department of Anatomy and Cell Biology,*
*College of Physicians & Surgeons of Columbia University,*
*New York, New York*


*AND*


**BRIAN H. SCHOFIELD**
*Orthopaedic Research Laboratory,*
*The Johns Hopkins University School of Medicine,*
*Baltimore, Maryland*

**Introduction**

Understanding the biology of the bone-forming cells, the osteoblast and osteocyte, has developed slowly because of the difficulty in biochemical analysis of cells derived from *in vivo* sources. This is due to the presence of the associated calcified matrix and the potential source of non-bone cells from marrow or surrounding connective tissues. Therefore, for many years, the histochemical study of bone cells was necessary to monitor and define the results of biochemical analyses. More recently, enzyme cytochemistry and electron microscopy has widened our knowledge of bone cell activity. Immunocytochemistry is becoming a powerful adjunct to the molecular biological approach investigating osteoblasts both *in vivo* and *in vitro*. In the future, techniques such as *in situ* hybridization will provide more understanding of bone cell function, especially the osteocyte population which is difficult to study except by *in vitro* methods. The present study has utilized the latest histochemical and microscopic techniques to produce a deeper understanding of the biology of the bone-forming cells.


**General Procedures**

The microscopic localization of enzyme activity to cellular structures requires: a) Stabilization of the structure to be examined without destroying all of the associated enzyme activity. Aldehyde fixatives and freeze-fixation are the two most commonly used methods; b) The deposition of an insoluble reaction product at the cellular sites of enzyme activity. For phosphatase histochemistry, for example, a heavy metal complex is formed between lead or cerium and free phosphate which is liberated from a hydrolyzed substrate. By utilizing different substrates, the reaction product can be an organic compound instead of a heavy metal; c) The product must be visible by microscopy. Light microscopy usually depends on color constrasts whereas electron microscopy depends on density contrast. In order for an organic deposit to be seen by electron microscopy, additional treatment to increase its electron density is required; d) The enzyme reaction is most easily carried out on demineralized bone samples. Not only are calcified samples difficult to work with, but mineral can cause artifactual deposition of heavy metal reaction products. We find that EDTA buffered to neutral pH, when used at 4°C, preserves many enzyme activities while decalcifying mineralized samples.

The various enzymatic methods used in this study are described in detail elsewhere (Doty and Schofield, 1984).

## Cell Surface Associated Enzyme Histochemistry

### Histochemical Results

At neutral and alkaline pH, the osteoblast demonstrates phosphatase activity along the cell membrane on the exterior surface (Fig. 1). Several substrates can be used to show this membrane reaction: betaglycero-phosphate, p-nitrophenylphosphate, phosphoserine, and adenosine tri-phosphate, (ATP). The ATPase activity may be due to alkaline phospha-tase removing monophosphate groups from ATP since true ATPase is inactivated by glutaraldehyde. However, if very brief fixation with low levels of glutaraldehyde or fixation with paraformaldehyde only is employed, a membrane-bound enzyme which hydrolyzes ATP in the presence of an alkaline phosphatase inhibitor (levamisole) is demonstrable. This ATPase activity is inhibited by the presence of pCMB (p-chloro-mercuri-benzoic acid) and is apparently not due to an alkaline phosphatase but to an ecto-ATPase.

Osteoblasts and very young osteocytes (those at the outer surface of trabecular bone) possess alkaline and neutral phosphatase activity on their cell membranes (Fig. 2). Old osteocytes (those deeply buried within trabeculae or in compact bone) do not exhibit cell membrane alkaline phosphatase. If, however, a mild fixation schedule is employed (4% para-formaldehyde perfused for 30 minutes), there is strong 5'-nucleotidase activity in the osteocyte lacunae and membranes (Fig. 3a and 9) as well as on the osteoblast cell membranes (Fig. 3c). This nucleotidase reaction occurs at neutral pH, is not eliminated by levamisole (an alkaline phos-phatase inhibitor) but is inhibited by pretreatment of the tissue with con-canavalin A (Fig. 3b). Alkaline phosphastase continues to be active following glutaraldehyde fixation and is stimulated by the addition of zinc ion to the incubation media. 5'-nucleotidase is inhibited by both these treatments. These results indicate that the osteocyte population demonstrates only 5'nucleotidase activity whereas osteoblast cell membranes contain alkaline phosphatase and 5'nucleotidase activities.

The distribution of enzyme activity on exterior cell membranes is relatively uniform except that the membrane, when closely apposed to bone matrix, tends to show slightly less activity. The reaction products appear initially as discrete "dots" or vesicle-shaped deposits along the surfaces of the mem-brane (Fig. 4). As the reaction progresses, the dots coalesce into a uniform layer of reaction product on the cell surface. Should the cells be in close contact, the reaction appears dense and uniformly fills the space between the cells. At points where cells in contact form a junctional complex or an

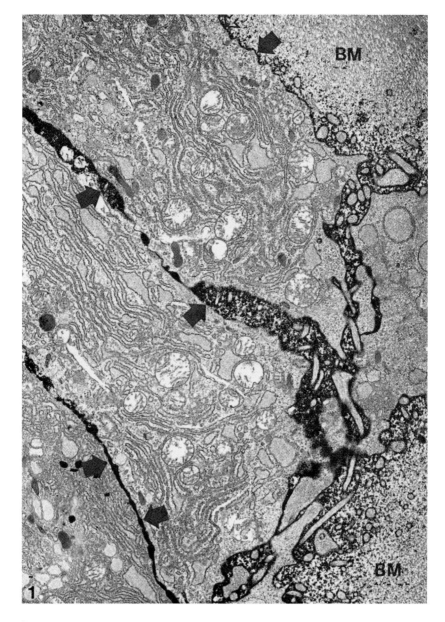

**Fig. 1**  A typical demonstration of alkaline phosphatase activity (arrows) displayed on the external cell surface of osteoblasts. This reactivity was produced at pH 9.5 using b-glycerophosphate as substrate and zinc ion as an enzyme activator.

BM = bone matrix, decalcified                                  Magnification: 9,600x

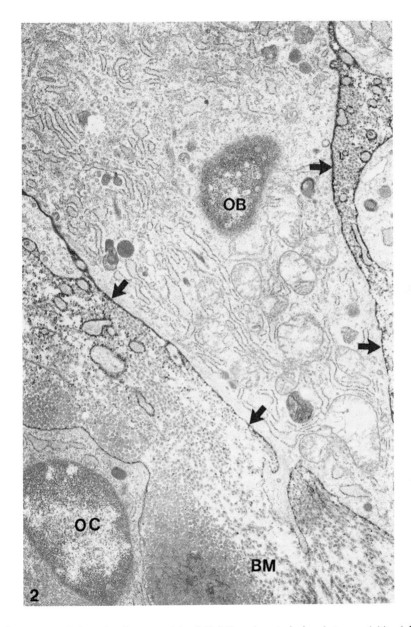

**Fig. 2** The alkaline phosphatase activity (pH 9.5) and neutral phosphatase activities (pH 7.2) tend to show loss of reaction product (arrows) very quickly as an osteoblast (OB) on the surface of bone converts to an osteocyte (OC) buried within the bone matrix (BM).

Magnification: 12,000x

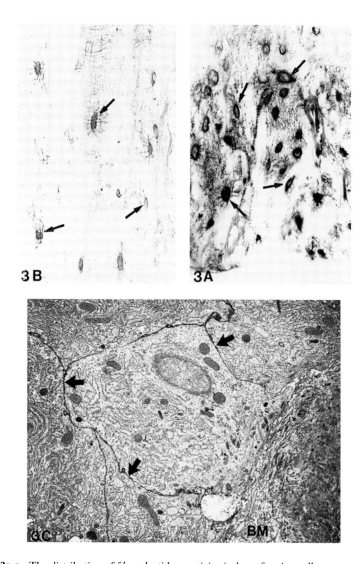

**Fig. 3a-c** The distribution of 5'-nucleotidase activity in bone-forming cells.
**Fig. 3a** Dense reaction product is visualized within osteocytes (arrows) and the canalicular system which permeates the bone matrix. Magnification: 812x
**Fig. 3b** Pretreatment of bone tissue with Cancanavalin A (0.1 mg/ml) inhibits the 5'-nucleotidase activity in most osteocytes (arrows). Magnification: 812x
**Fig. 3c** If cerium is used as a capture agent in place of lead ion, a 5'-nucleotidase activity can be seen along the osteoblast membrance (arrows). The presence of lead ions inhibits this activity. Magnification: 5,265x
BM = bone matrix

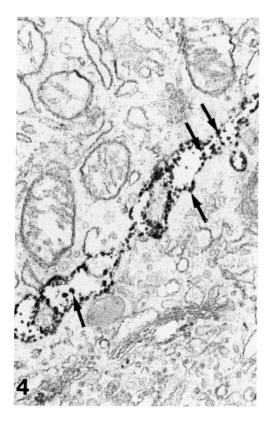

**Fig. 4** Alkaline phosphatase activity on osteoblast cell membranes during the initial stages of the reaction show punctate deposits along the membranes (arrows). With further incubation times, the reaction "fills in" and appears as a solid line of reaction product as seen in Figure 1.
Magnification: 31,600x

apparent gap junction, the reaction product is absent (Fig. 5). On the free surfaces of cells where no cell-cell contact exists, the reaction product is more diffuse (Fig. 6). Apparent reactivity also exists within the osteoid layer (new bone not yet mineralized) (Fig. 8). Alkaline phosphatase reactivity is frequently associated with matrix vesicles, but at many other locations within the osteoid, matrix vesicles are not apparent. Reaction product is

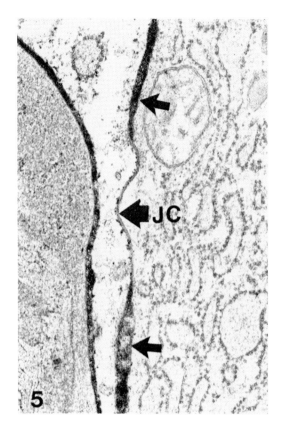

**Fig. 5** Osteoblasts form specialized gap junctional complexes (JC) between adjacent cells. Alkaline phosphatase reaction is absent from the junction (large arrow) but present along either side (small arrows).

Magnification: 42,000x

also present on the surface of cytoplasmic extensions of the osteoblasts. Those cytoplasmic projections which are not encased in matrix (Fig. 8) have the strongest alkaline phosphatase reactivity and those that extend towards the osteocytes, the least. In the case of 5′-nucleotidase, which is found on osteocytes as well as osteoblasts, enzyme activity is present on the

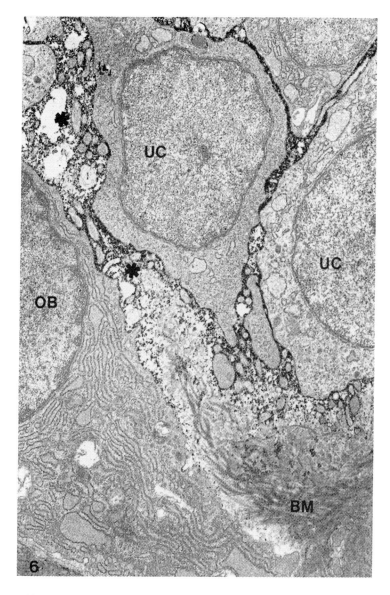

**Fig. 6** Alkaline phosphatase enzyme activity (asterisks) is found diffusely spread between bone cells when they are not in close contact. Cells adjacent to osteoblasts (OB) but which may not be fully differentiated (UC) nor situated on bone matrix (BM) may also demonstrate alkaline phosphatase activity. This diffuse reaction can sometimes also be seen at the light microscopic level (see Figure 10).

Magnification: 12,525x

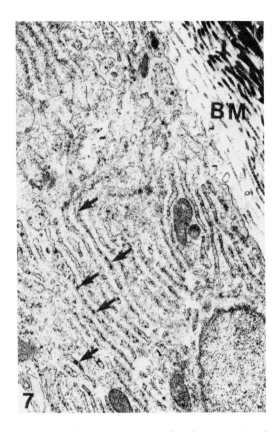

**Fig. 7** An electron micrograph showing glucose-6-phosphatase reaction (arrows) within the rough endoplasmic reticulum.
BM = bone matrix                                                        Magnification: 15,700x

osteocyte canaliculi (canaliculi contain cytoplasmic extensions from the body of the osteocyte) (Fig. 9).

It is assumed that alkaline phosphatase, like other cell products and all other cell-membrane-associated enzymes, is synthesized in the cell, perhaps

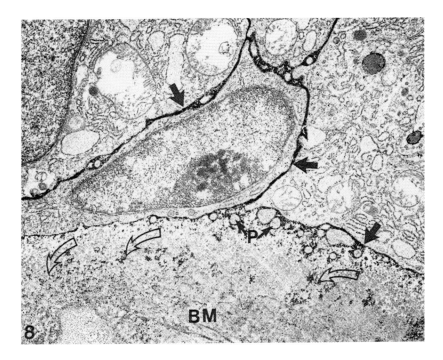

**Fig. 8** Alkaline phosphatase activity (black arrows) on osteoblast membranes may be diffusely spread through the bone matrix underlying these cells. This diffuse reaction is not scattered through the entire volume of osteoid but appears organized along a "front" (open curved arrows). The reaction is also associated with recognizable cell structures such as cytoplasmic projections (P).

BM = bone matrix                                                  Magnification: 11,680x

packaged in the Golgi, and carried to the cell surface by vesicles. The "vesicular" distribution of early-forming reaction product would suggest that this does occur. However, we seldom find any such enzyme activity in the endoplasmic reticulum or the Golgi complex using standard histochemical techniques. It may be that the enzyme is not active while within the cytoplasmic compartments. Intracellular distribution of alkaline phosphatase activity has been demonstrated in other cell types (Tokumitsu and Fishman, 1983) and may eventually be intracellularly localized in osteoblasts. It is interesting that the NADP reactivity which we will describe later, which also appears along the external cell membrane of the osteoblasts, is strongest within the Golgi complex. This suggests that intracellular enzymes which are secreted onto the cell surface or released during secretory activity may continue to show activity along the exterior of the cell membrane.

For light microscopy, alkaline phosphatase is often visualized using an azo dye method (Fig. 10). This method shows very dramatically that there is a layer of cells immediately adjacent to the endosteal osteoblasts which contain strong alkaline phosphatase activity yet by electron microscopy these cells are not always osteoblast-like in their structure (Fig. 6). These cells may be part of the marrow cell population or a stem cell population which differentiates into functioning osteoblasts. If so, it is interesting to note that they already have alkaline phosphatase activity before they reach the bone surface.

When very brief fixation is used to preserve osteoblast structure, it is possible to demonstrate a cell-membrane-associated 5'-nucleotidase activity. This reaction is inhibited by the presence of glutaraldehyde in the fixative, by fixation in 4% para-formaldehyde for longer than 60 minutes, and by the presence of lead ions in the incubation mixture. If cerium is used to capture the phosphate liberated by the enzyme activity and brief paraformaldehyde perfusion fixation is used, the 5'-nucleotidase activity can be localized on the external surface of the cell membranes (Fig. 3c). This reactivity is not inhibited by levamisole but is inhibited by concanavalin A and, therefore, is not due to alkaline phosphatase.

Brief fixation also preserves glucose-6-phosphatase reactivity within the endoplasmic reticulum of the osteoblast population (Fig. 7). Similar treatment does not produce a reaction in the endoplasmic reticulum of osteocytes, suggesting that there is truly a lower metabolic activity in osteocytes compared to osteoblasts.

There are also bone-forming cells associated with the vascular supply of compact diaphyseal bone (Figs 11a & b). These cells possess the same cell-membrane-associated enzyme activities as endosteal and periosteal osteoblasts. The adjacent vessels consist of endothelial cells which contain an ATPase (Fig. 11c) which is only preserved by brief 4% p-formaldehyde fixation and is inhibited by glutaraldehyde. The vascular endothelium of blood vessels in the marrow cavity also shows 5'-nucleotidase activity when mild fixation is used.

Cell surfaces can be stained by the lanthanides such as lanthanum

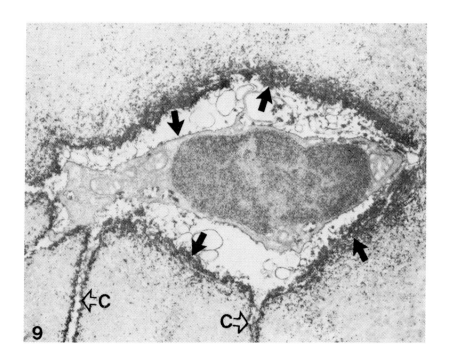

**Fig. 9** 5'-nucleotidase localized along the canaliculi (C) which extend between cells. This electron micrograph illustrates cell membrane reaction not evident in the light micrograph (Figure 3a).

Magnification: 14,800x

chloride or terbium. These positively charged, electron-dense markers are located in patterns very similar to alkaline phosphatase reactions. Cationic ferritin also binds to these same cell surfaces as well as collagen fibrils (Fig. 12). Thus, the phosphatase activities are apparently located in the same areas where binding sites exist for positively charged ions.

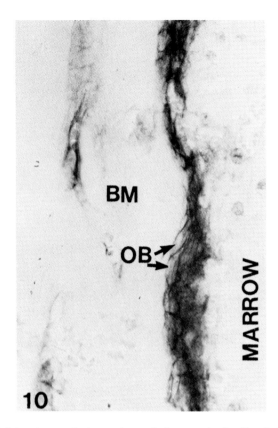

**Fig. 10** In this light micrograph, the azo dye method was used to localize alkaline phosphatase activity (pH 8.5) in osteoblasts. The reaction is strong along the osteoblast (OB) membranes, but additional reactivity can be seen in a cell layer immediately adjacent to these osteoblasts. BM = bone matrix                                    Magnification: 1,200x

## Cellular Functions Associated with the Histochemical Results

Alkaline phosphatase activity has historically been associated with new bone formation (Bourne, 1943; McLean and Urist, 1961) and has been shown by many workers to exist within the osteoblast population (Burstone, 1960; Bernard, 1978). This enzyme activity has also been associated with matrix vesicles as a mechanism to initiate mineralization in calcifying

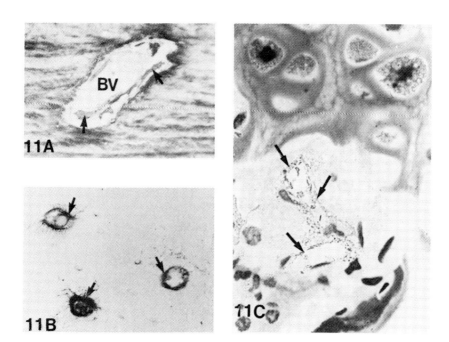

**Fig. 11a–c**
**Fig. 11a**   This light micrograph demonstrates the presence of bone cells (arrows) arranged around a blood vessel (BV) deep within the bone matrix. Magnification: 1,840x
**Fig. 11b**   Bone cells associated with the blood vessels will continue to demonstrate alkaline phosphatase activity (arrows) as long as the vessels continue to function. Magnification: 960x
**Fig. 11c**   This light micrograph demonstrates the ATPase activity of the endothelial cells of blood vessels within bone. The ATPase activity (arrows) is stimulated by calcium ion and appears to be specific for vascular endothelium. Magnification: 2,400x

cartilage and rapidly growing bone (Anderson, 1969). As we demonstrated in the previous section, the alkaline phosphatase of bone can hydrolyze many substrates and release monophosphate. Even phosphotyrosine phosphate which may be involved in the cellular differentiation process can be dephosphorylated by alkaline phosphatase (Swarup, *et al.*, 1981; Burch, *et al.*, 1985). Therefore, the fine structural localization of these enzyme activities has not been very helpful in defining their precise biochemical

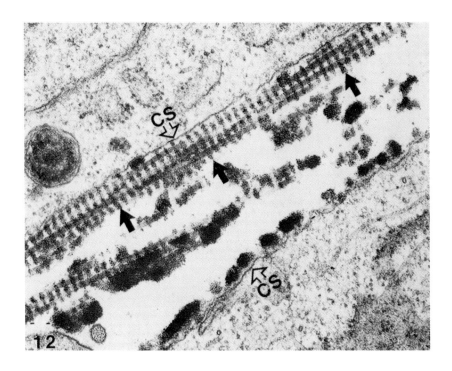

**Fig. 12** Cationic ferritin binds to the cell surfaces of collagen secreting cells and to collagen fibrils along regular binding sites (arrows). The binding occurs across several fibrils in a regular pattern and extends to the cell surface (CS).

Magnification: 48,000x

function. Documentation of alkaline phosphatase distribution intracellularly under differing conditions of bone matrix synthesis and/or matrix mineralization would help in determining the importance of this enzyme activity. For example, new enzyme may be synthesized within the osteoblasts prior to new matrix synthesis if the alkaline phosphatase is truly important in some phase of matrix formation. The same argument could be used if the enzyme has a functional role in the process of mineralization of matrix.

Because alkaline phosphatase and neutral phosphatases are localized to cell surfaces which also show binding affinities for positively charged molecules, the relationship between alkaline phosphatase and calcium transport may be an important one (Ramp, 1975; Haiech and Demaille, 1983). If calcium transport in bone requires the presence of alkaline phosphatase, then calcium movement at the osteocyte level is either nonexistent or below our limits of detection. On the other hand, the ATPase which is localized to the endothelial cells of the blood vessels in bone is strongly stimulated in the presence of calcium ion (Doty, 1985). Thus, calcium movement into or out of the blood may be regulated by an ATPase at the level of the endothelial cell whereas calcium used for mineralization may be regulated by alkaline phosphatase associated with the osteoblasts.

The bone-lining cell is found on older bone surfaces where no apparent bone-forming activity is taking place. The function of these cells is not presently understood (Miller and Jee, 1987); but at this time, we have found no cell-membrane-associated phosphatase activity.

The role of 5'-nucleotidase in the osteocyte population is presently not understood. In a discussion of this enzyme function in cartilage cells, it was postulated that as 5'-nucleotidase activity increased the adenylate cyclase activity decreased (Rodan, et al., 1977). These authors suggested that this enzyme is part of a complex involved in the "flow of intercellular information". Dornand, et al. (1980), have shown that 5'-nucleotidase activity may effect intracellular cyclic AMP levels. However, other studies such as that of Carraway, et al. (1979), have shown that nucleotidase activity and its inhibition with concanavalin A was related to cytoskeletal function in these cells. Osteocytes contain numerous cytoskeletal elements as seen by electron microscopy and perhaps their nucleotidase activity is involved in some type of "information flow", whether chemical (e.g., cyclic nucleotides) or mechanical (e.g., cytoskeletal integrity), mediated through the osteocyte network in bone.

Adenylate cyclase has been localized to osteoblast membranes in calvaria but has not been detected in osteocytes deep in bone (Walzer, 1980). Davidovitch, et al. (1977), have indicated that cyclic AMP levels correlate inversely with collagen production by osteoblasts. Our histochemical results indicate that osteocytes have reduced metabolic activity compared to the osteoblast population. Therefore, the adenyl cyclase and/or cyclic AMP levels in osteocytes may be quite low. This activity is difficult to demonstrate with present histochemical methods and may require the development of immunocytochemical methods.

## Enzyme Histochemistry Associated with the Golgi Complex

### Histochemical Results

Saccules of the Golgi complex contain enzymes which will hydrolyze pyridoxal-5-phosphate, thiamine pyrophosphate (Fig. 13a) b-nicotinamide adenine dinucleotide phosphate (NADP), b-glycerophosphate (Fig. 14), trimetaphosphate, cytidine monophosphate, and uridine diphosphate at pH 5.0. We have found no Golgi saccule activity at neutral pH (including uridine diphosphatase activity which is strongly reactive in the Golgi of cartilage cells). Connections between saccules and the terminal buds of forming granules show a continuation of reaction product (Figs 14 and 15) so that we may assume that isolated granules with reaction product have originated from the saccules. The collagen-containing, large vesicles or granules (Fig. 13b) seldom contain these enzyme activities although they will occasionally exhibit acid phosphatase or other lysosomal enzyme activity (Fig. 16). These large granules also stain with silver staining techniques (Fig. 17) which also stain extracellular collagen. The same granules contain carbohydrates which can be stained with lectin conjugates (Fig. 18). It is not possible at this time to relate a specific function to these histochemical results.

As a result of silver staining, and the lectin binding of the collagen-containing secretory granules, we have noted that these granules tend to be localized in specific regions of the osteoblast. The osteoblast is somewhat polarized in relation to the underlying collagen along the bone matrix/cell interface. We often find a large number of granules concentrated at the point where the cytoplasmic projections bud off from the main body of the osteoblast (Fig. 19a). However, we have not observed these granules within the cytoplasmic projections which are buried within the matrix. This would suggest that very few, if any, secretory granules travel into the deep matrix by means of the cytoplasmic projections which are buried in bone. The cytoplasmic projections which are not buried in bone but extend along the surface of the matrix do, however, contain many collagen-containing granules (Fig. 19b).

In an occasional osteoblast, the Golgi complex is not found as a single complex of saccules. Rather, some saccules are distributed in various areas of the cytoplasm in small groupings of 3−5 saccules (Fig. 20). These portions of Golgi also show enzyme activities but at what appears to be a reduction in reaction product.

In osteocytes (Fig. 21), only the Golgi of recently formed osteocytes show the same strong staining patterns as the functioning osteoblasts. However, the numbers of secretory granules are reduced almost to zero. Secretory

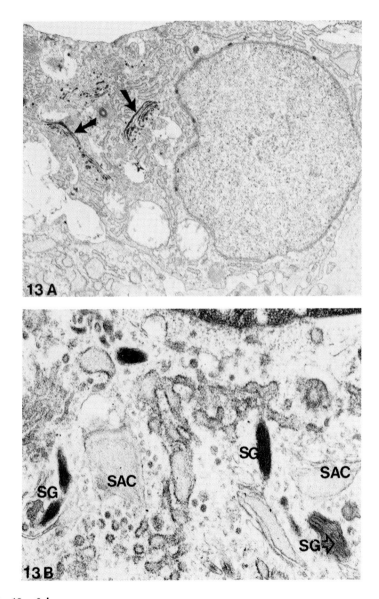

**Fig. 13 a & b:**

**Fig. 13a**   The thiamine pyrophosphatase activity (arrows) in osteoblasts is localized to the saccules of the "trans" face of the Golgi complex. This region of the Golgi is where the procollagen molecules are collected. Magnification: 13,160x

**Fig. 13b**   The procollagen containing saccules (SAC) are condensed into densely stained secretory granules (SG) which will be transported to the cell surface. Magnification: 27,510x

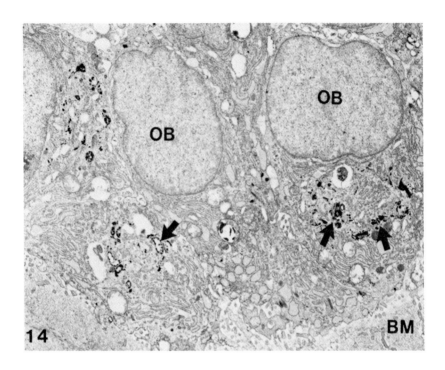

**Fig. 14** Acid glycerophosphatase activity (arrows) is shown in a group of osteoblasts. The Golgi saccules and lysosomes contain dense reaction product when b-glycerophosphate is used as substrate at pH 5.0.
OB = nuclei of osteoblasts          BM = bone matrix          Magnification: 5,120x

granules have not been found in the cytoplasmic extensions originating from osteocyte bodies.

## Cell Functions Related to Histochemical Results

The Golgi system functions to glycosylate procollagen prior to secretion and to package this material into granules for secretion at the cell surface.

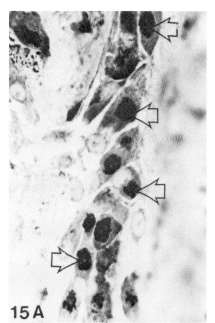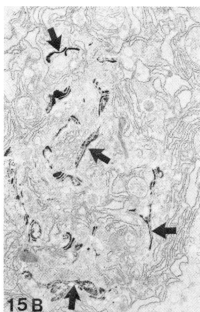

**Fig. 15 a & b**
**Fig. 15a** Nicotinamide dinucleotide (NADP) is hydrolyzed at pH 5.0 in the Golgi saccules (arrows) of osteoblasts. Magnification: 2,400x
**Fig. 15b** This electron micrograph demonstrates that NADPase activity (arrows) is found in the Golgi lamellae and the enlarged saccules derived from the lamellae. Magnification: 10,000x

These collagen-containing granules may be targeted for either the cell membrane or the lysosomes (Farquhar, 1985). Intracellular degradation of collagen prior to the normal secretary process can be an important regulatory function of lysosomal activity. In fibroblasts, the intracellular degradation of collagen may reach very significant percentages of normal collagen

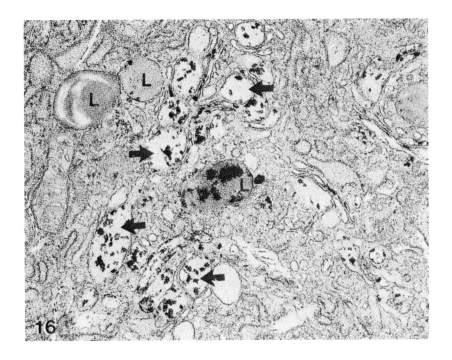

**Fig. 16** Acid glycerophosphatase activity is found within most components of the Golgi apparatus. This electron micrograph demonstrates reaction product within the saccules, the mature lysosomes (L), and the procollagen-containing terminal saccules (arrows).

Magnification: 46,400x

synthesis (Rennard, *et al.,* 1982; Beinkowski, 1983). It seems reasonable that in the bone-forming cells, if the secretory granule is not targeted to reach the cell membrane, lysosomal activity may degrade this material and, thus, regulate the amount of collagen synthesis and secretion by these cells. We have noted that some osteoblast secretory granules containing collagen precursors also may contain enzyme activity normally confined to lyso-

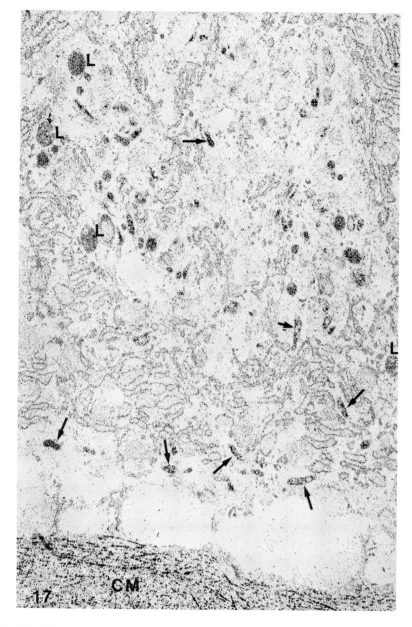

**Fig. 17**   When silver methanimine is used to stain osteoblasts, the secretory granules (arrows) and the lysosomes (L) as well as the collagen matrix (CM) are all densely stained.

Magnification: 13,800x

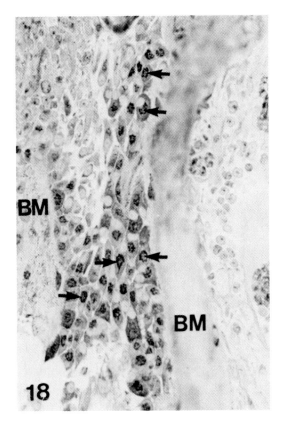

**Fig. 18** The lectin from *Tetragonolobus purpureas*, conjugated to horseradish peroxidase, will complex with carbohydrates in the Golgi apparatus (arrows). This staining pattern looks very similar to the NADP reaction seen with enzyme histochemistry (see Figure 15). Nuclei of the osteoblasts are unstained in this preparation.
BM = bone matrix                                                    Magnification: 800x

somes. This could be an indication of an intracellular degradation process. However, degradation of terminal telopeptides is also a normal step in the formation of procollagen (Prockop, *et al.*, 1979); and these peptides may be packaged with the procollagen during the Golgi packing process.

The Golgi saccules exhibit some specificity to different enzyme substrates.

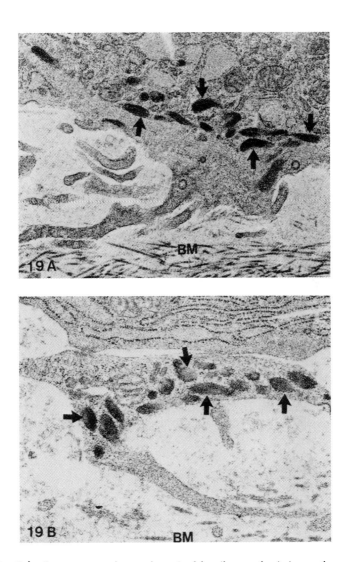

**Fig. 19 a & b** Secretory granules can be stained by silver methanimine or the conjugated lectins.

**Fig. 19a** This figure shows these granules (arrows) accumulated at the base of cytoplasmic projections which extend into the adjacent bone matrix (BM). However, we do not find that these granules are released via these projections. Magnification: 20,025x

**Fig. 19b** The cytoplasmic extensions which are parallel and adjacent to the existing bone matrix (BM) often contain large numbers of secretory granules (arrows). Magnification: 37,500x

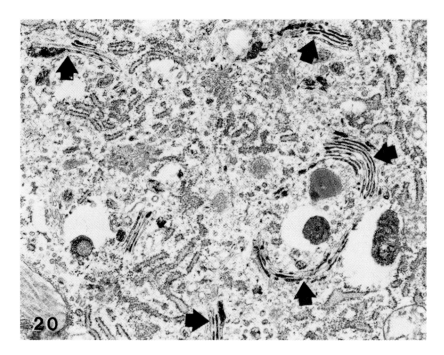

**Fig. 20**  The Golgi apparatus within this osteoblast is fragmented into several series of lamellae (arrows); however, the enzyme activity for NADPase is still present. Magnification: 19,760x

Whereas acid glycerophosphate and cytidine monophosphate are hydrolyzed in all saccules, thiamine pyrophosphatase activity appears only in the "trans" face of the saccule complex. The NADP reaction products are found in the medial saccules of the Golgi complex and in the vesicles forming at the ends of the medial saccules. Pyridoxal-5′-phosphatase produced a similar reaction. We noted previously (Doty and Mathews, 1971) that in osteogenesis imperfecta tarda deficient collagen synthesis by osteoblasts was accompanied by altered Golgi histochemistry.

As the Golgi secretory granules condense into dense secretory granules, their staining characteristics change; and it becomes possible to use their silver-staining and lectin-binding characteristics to follow these granules as they move through the cytoplasm. The micrographs shown in the previous

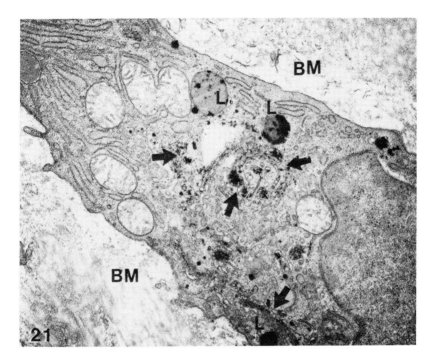

**Fig. 21** This osteocyte, embedded in bone matrix (BM), continues to show acid glycerophosphatase activity (arrows) within the Golgi apparatus and lysosomes (L). Magnification: 18,800x

sections indicate that the preference is for these granules to move towards the bone matrix/cell interface. Thus, these granules are "targeted" and do not randomly drift through the cytoplasm. The mechanism of this targeting process is unknown. Others (Ehrlich, *et al.*, 1974; Scherft and Heersche, 1975; Fernandez-Madrid, *et al.*, 1980) have shown that disruption of the cytoskeletal system eventually inhibits collagen secretion so we might infer that cytoskeletal integrity is important for this movement and targeting of collagen-containing granules.

Binding of the lectin from *Tetragonolobus purpureas* (Fig. 18) and the findings of Weinstock (1979) suggests that alpha-L-fucose is a unique sugar attached either to the procollagen molecule or part of a noncollagenous protein. Deeply buried osteocytes do not show this binding ability and

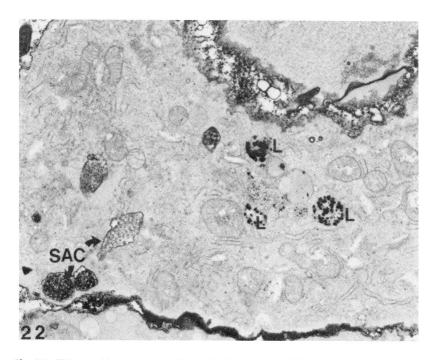

**Fig. 22**   This osteoblast was stained for acid phosphatase activity to demonstrate lysosomes (L) and stained for precollagen material within Golgi saccules (SAC) using tannic acid and osmium tetroxide.

Magnification: 13,600x

seldom show any of the more specific histochemical reactions for Golgi. Occasionally, acid, glycero-phosphatase activity can be found in some of the saccules; but, in general, osteocytes exhibit significantly reduced enzyme histochemical activities as compared to osteoblasts.

## Enzyme Histochemistry Associated with Lysosomes

### The Lysosomal Population

Dense, single-membrane-bound bodies which contain acid phosphatase activity are fairly abundant in the osteoblast and osteocyte population.

These are typical lysosomal bodies as described in many other cell types. Other membrane-bound (nonlysosomal), dense bodies which are obviously derived from the Golgi complex also contain some of the same lysosomal enzymes. This can be seen in Figure 16 in which an obvious Golgi-derived granule, which contains collagenous-like material, also contains acid phosphatase activity. However, the typical lysosome does have a uniform and dense central matrix so that morphological distinctions can be made. Even when the secretory granule condenses down to form a very dense body, it no longer retains a large spherical shape as does the typical lysosome. Thus, size and overall shape must be used to define lysosomes in osteoblasts and osteocytes.

Using the aryl sulfatase reaction, many small primary vesicles are localized around the Golgi complex, which also contains this enzyme activity. Mature lysosomes also contain this enzyme activity so it is not known whether the small primary vesicles carry the enzyme to mature lysosomal bodies or whether the small vesicles are contributing to some Golgi function.

Lysosomal bodies are always found within the osteocyte population. In mature rat bone, every osteocyte will contain some reactive lysosomes. Lysosomal enzyme activity is not found along the lacunae surface surrounding the osteocyte, suggesting that these enzymes are not secreted into the surrounding matrix or, alternatively, that the enzyme is secreted in such low concentrations that it is not detectable by these methods. The low level of metabolic activity in the osteocyte may help explain the long-lived nature of these cells.

## Histochemical Studies

Two isoenzymes of acid phosphatase have been found in odontoblasts using inhibitors or enzyme stimulators which permit such discrimination (Hamerstrom, et al., 1971; Anderson and Toverud, 1979). Using pyridoxal-5'-phosphate as substrate, it has been possible in osteoblasts to distinguish lysosomal acid phosphatase activity from Golgi acid phosphatase (Coleman, et al., 1980). With NADP as substrate, at pH 5.0, the enzyme activity is associated with the lamellae and saccules of the Golgi (Fig. 15); and the lysosomes are not reactive. In cases where a particular substrate produces a weak lysosomal reaction, pretreatment with an ammonia solution will eliminate the lysosomal staining while preserving the Golgi reaction (Coleman, et al., 1980). Therefore, these techniques may be used either as indicators of cellular synthetic processes associated with Golgi function or of cellular degradative processes associated with lysosomal function. It is also possible to combine techniques whereby lysosomes and procollagen containing saccules are stained in the same cells (Fig. 22). This combination of techniques may help to deliniate specific functions of these organelles. These types of studies, combined with biochemical studies of collagen synthesis in bone-forming cells, would greatly help our understanding of the cell biology of bone formation.

Other enzyme activities found in osteoblasts and osteocytes include a phosphamidase activity with a maximum activity at pH 6.0. This activity is not due to a phosphomonoesterase function, as seen with acid glycerophosphatase activity, but due to a phosphoprotein phosphatase activity. We reported that osteoclasts showed strong reactivity at pH 7.2 (Doty and Schofield, 1972) but the lysosomes of osteoblasts and osteocytes were also active. The importance of this function is unknown but does indicate the variable hydrolytic potential in lysosomes of the bone-forming cells. Osteoblast and osteocyte lysosomes contain sulfatase activity, phosphodiesterase activity, nonspecific esterase activity, cathepsin B, and dipeptidyl peptidase II activity. It is interesting that this dipeptidyl peptidase activity is strongly present in lysosomes of osteoblasts and osteocytes but largely absent in osteoclasts (Sannes, et al., 1982). Electron microscopic localization of this enzyme activity in osteoblasts indicates it is definitely confined to the lysosomal population (Doty and Schofield, 1984).

In some tissues, discrimination can be made between the Golgi apparatus and a GERL system as described by Novikoff and Novikoff (1977). Because of the complex series of enzyme activities in the osteoblast at neutral and acidic pH, we have not been able to identify a GERL system in bone-forming cells.

# References

Anderson, H. C. (1969). Vesicles Associated with Calcification in the Matrix of Epiphyseal Cartilage. *J. Cell Biol.*, **41**: 59–72.

Anderson, T. R., and Toverud, S. U. (1979). Purification and Partial Characterization of Two Acid Phosphatases from Rat Bone. *Calcif. Tissue Int.*, **27**: 219–226.

Bernard, G. W. (1978). Ultrastructural Localization of Alkaline Phosphatase in Initial Intramembraneous Osteogenesis. *Clin. Orthop. Rel. Res.*, **135**: 218–225.

Bienkowski, R. S. (1983). Intracellular Degradation of Newly Synthesized Secretory Proteins. *Biochem. J.*, **214**: 1–10.

Bourne, G. (1943). The Distribution of Alkaline Phosphatase in Various Tissues. *Quart. J. Exptl. Physiol.*, **32**: 1–20.

Burch, W. M., Hamner, G., and Wuthier, R. E. (1985). Phosphotyrosine and Phosphoprotein Phosphatase Activity of Alkaline Phosphatase in Mineralizing Cartilage. *Metabolism*, **34**: 169–175.

Burstone, M. S. (1960). Hydrolytic Enzymes in Dentinogenesis and Osteogenesis. In: Calcification in Biological Systems (R. F. Sognnaes, editor), AAAS, Washington D.C., 217–243.

K. L. Carraway, R. C. (1979). Doss, J. W. Huggins, R. W. Chesnut, and Carraway, C. A. C. Effects of Cytoskeletal Perturbant Drugs on Ecto 5'-nucleotidase, A Concanavalin-A Receptor. *J. Cell Biol.*, **83**: 529−543.

Coleman, R. A., Schofield, B, H, and McDonald, D. F. (1980). Selective Localization of a Golgi Apparatus Acid Phosphotase Isoenzyme in Bone Using Pryidoxal-5'- Phosphate. *J. Histochem Cytochem.*, **28**: 115−123.

Davidovitch, Z., Montgomery, P. C., and Shanfield, J. L. (1977). Cellular Localization and Concentration of Bone Cyclic Nucleotides in Response to Acute PTE Administration. *Calcif. Tiss. Res.*, **24**: 81−91.

Dornand, J., Bonnafous, J. C., and Mani, J. C. (1980). 5'-Nucleotidase-Adenylate Cyclase Relationships in Mouse Thymocytes. *FEBS Letters*, **110**: 30−34.

Doty, S. B. (1985). Localization of Calcium Stimulated Adenosine Triphosphatase Activity in Blood Vessels of the Skeleton. *Physiologist*, **28**: 5125−5126.

Doty, S. B., and Mathews, R. S. (1971). Electron Microscopic and Histochemical Investigation of Osteogenesis Imperfecta Tarda. *Clin. Orthop. Rel. Res.*, **80**: 191−201.

Doty, S. B., and Schofield, B. H. (1984). Ultrahistochemistry of Calcified Tissues. In: Methods of Calcified Tissue Preparation (G. R. Dickson, Editor), Elsevier Science Publisher, 149−198.

Ehrlich, H. P., Ross, R., and Bornstein, P. (1974). Effects on Antimicrotubular Agents on the Secretion of Collagen. *J. Cell Biol.*, **62**: 390−405.

Farquhar, M. G. (1985). Progress in Unraveling Pathways of Golgi Traffic. *Ann. Rev. Cell Biol.*, **1**: 447−488.

Fernandez-Madrid, F., Noonan, S., Riddle, J., Karvnoen, R., and Sasaki, D. (1980). Intracellular Processing of Procollagen Induced by the Action of Colchicine. *J. Anat.*, **130**: 229−241.

Haiech, J., and Demaille, J. G. (1983). Phosphorylation and the Control of Calcium Fluxes. *Phil. Trans. Royal Soc. Lond.*, B, **302**: 91−98.

Hammerstrom, L. E., Hanker, J. S., and Toverud, S. V. (1971). Cellular Differences in Acid Phosphatase Isoenzymes in Bone and Teeth. *Clin. Orthop. Rel. Res.*, **78**: 151−162.

McLean, F. C., and Urist, M. R. (1961). Bone, An Introduction to the Physiology of Skeletal Tissues. University of Chicago Press, Chicago, Illinois, 226.

Miller, S. C., and Jee, W. S. S. (1987). The Bone Lining Cell: A Distinct Phenotype? *Calcif Tissue Int.*, **41**: 1−5.

Novikoff, A. B., and Novikoff, P. M. (1977). Cytochemical Contributions to Differentiating GERL from the Golgi Apparatus. *Histochem. J.*, **9**: 525−551.

Prokop, D. J., Kivirikko, K. I., Tuderman, L., and Guzman, N. A. (1979). The Biosynthesis of Collagen and its Disorders. *J. Biochem.*, **301**: 13−23 and 77−85.

Ramp, W. K. (1975). Cellular Control of Calcium Movements in Bone. Interrelationships of the Bone Membrane, Parathyroid Hormone, and Alkaline Phosphatase. *Clin. Orthop. Rel. Res.*, **106**: 311−322.

Rennard, S. I., Stier, L. E., and Crystal, R. G. (1982). Intracellular Degradation of Newly Synthesized Collagen. *J. Invest. Dermatol.*, **79**: 77s−82s.

Rodan, G. A., Bourret, L. A., and Cutler, L. S. (1977). Membrane Changes During Cartilage Maturation. Increase in 5'-Nucleotidase and Decrease in Adenosine Inhibition of Adenylate Cyclase. *J. Cell Biol.*, 493−501.

Sannes, P. L., Schofield, B. H., and McDonald, D. F. (1986). Histochemical Localization of Cathepsin B, Dipeptidyl Peptidase I and Dipeptidyl Peptidase II in Rat Bone. *J. Histochem. Cytochem.*, **34**: 983−988.

Scherft, J. P., and Heersche, J. N. M. (1975). Accumulation of Collagen-Containing Vacuoles in Osteoblasts after Administration of Colchicine. *Cell Tiss. Res.*, **157**: 353−365.

Swarup, G., Cohen, S., and Garbes, D. L., (1981). Selective Dephosphorylation of Proteins Containing Phosphotyrosine by Alkaline Phosphatase. *J. Biol. Chem.*, **256**: 8197—8201.

Tokumitsu, S. I., and Fishman, W. N. (1983). Alkaline Phosphatase Biosynthesis in the Endoplasmic Reticulum and Its Transport Through the Golgi Apparatus to the Plasma Membrane. *J. Histochem. Cytochem.*, 647—655.

Walzer, C. (1980). An Attempt at Localizing Adenylate Cyclase in Rat Calvaria. Influence of Sodium Fluoride and Parathyroid Hormone. *J. Histochem.*, **68**: 281—296.

Weinstock, M. (1979). Radioautographic Visualization of $H^3$-Fucose Incorporation into Glycoprotein by Osteoblasts and Its Deposition into Bone Matrix. *Calcif. Tiss. Intl.*, **27**: 177—185.

# 4

# Growth Factor Effects in Bone

**PETER V. HAUSCHKA**
*Department of Oral Biology and Pathophysiology*
*Harvard School of Dental Medicine, and*
*Department of Orthopaedic Surgery*
*Children's Hospital Medical Center*
*Boston, Massachusetts*

*Author's Note:* For the reader's convenience, references have been cited alphabetically under the appropriate topic headings of the table of contents, and by individual growth factor within Section III (Properties of Growth Factors). Consecutive numbering provides unequivocal reference access.

*Abbreviations*

IGF        Insulin-like growth factor
EGF        Epidermal growth factor
TGF-α      Transforming growth factor-alpha
TGF-β      Transforming growth factor-beta
PDGF       Platelet-derived growth factor
aFGF       Acidic fibroblast growth factor
bFGF       Basic fibroblast growth factor
SGF        Skeletal growth factor (IGF-II)
IL-1       Interleukin-1
TNF        Tumor necrosis factor
GH         Growth hormone
PTH        Parathyroid hormone
DBP        Demineralized bone powder
kDa        Kilodalton


## Introduction

The current information explosion in the related fields of polypeptide growth factors and oncogenes has provided new insight into the mechanisms controlling cell proliferation and differentiation. This new knowledge applies to all tissues, and it is particularly relevant to bone. It has been widely recognized that skeletal form and function are regulated by a complex interplay between *systemic* hormonal signals and *local* factors [Canalis(1,2), Nijweide *et al.* (364), Raisz (369)]. Bone is a complex connective tissue comprised of many cell types: mesenchymal cells, chondrocytes, osteoblasts, osteocytes, osteoclasts, macrophages, monocytes, other leukocytes, endothelial cells, hematopoietic marrow cells, and neurons--to mention a few. All of these may respond to circulating endocrine substances as well as secreting their own growth-regulating factors. The abundance of each cell type and its secretory activity varies significantly with developmental age, bone type (endochondral *vs.* intramembranous) and anatomical location. The osteoblast, which plays a central role in bone biology [Rodan and Martin (407)], operates at the interface between the mineralized extracellular matrix [Jones *et al.* (359)] and the complex environment created by these other cells and their products. In keeping with the focus of this book, this chapter is primarily concerned with polypeptide growth factor effects on osteoblasts, but will address other factors and cell types where appropriate.

## I. Growth Factors and Their Relevance to Bone Growth

Skeletal enlargement or enhanced anabolic metabolism *per se* are not necessarily the outcome when bone growth factors are studied in osseous systems, particularly where multiple possible target cell types are present. Clearly, skeletal growth can be stimulated by direct infusion of insulin-like growth factor I (IGF-I) or growth hormone (GH) which elevates IGF-I [Isaksson *et al.* (46), Schlechter *et al.* (65), Schoenle *et al.* (68)]. However, depending on the developmental stage, a substance such as epidermal growth factor (EGF) may have stimulatory or inhibitory effects on the formation of mineralized bone nodules in vitro [Antosz *et al.* (128)], while EGF stimulates bone resorption in other models [Cohen (87), Tashjian and Levine (118), Tashjian *et al.* (192)]. With rapidly expanding data on growth factor effects, it is important to draw distinctions between several stages of bone development which are active subjects for bone growth factor research:

(a) *normal embryonic bone development*: including all the pathways leading from migration and differentiation of mesenchymal cells to the formation of bone by intramembranous or endochondral processes (Fig. 1);

(b) *bone cells in vitro*: wherein osseous cell types are maintained or propagated in isolated culture conditions to define phenotypic properties and hormonal responsiveness. Rapidly proliferating, transformed clonal osteosarcoma cell lines may provide an incomplete picture of normal osteoblasts operating in a complex mineralized extracellular matrix. Primary and secondary cultures of osteoprogenitor cells and "normal" osteoblasts, while not necessarily homogeneous, enable modeling of the synthesis and mineralization of bone matrix and the consequential feedback on phenotypic expression;

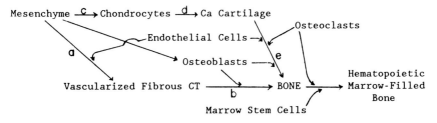

**Fig. 1** Alternate developmental routes leading to bone by intramembranous (a, b) or endochondral (c, d, e) ossification. *In vivo* models for studying osteoinduction [Howes *et al.* (412); Kapur and Reddi (413); Reddi (415); Sampath *et al.* (417); Urist *et al.* (421, 422)] typically take the endochondral pathway following exposure of mesenchymal cells to osteoinductive protein preparations. Clearly, growth factors could affect bone development, growth, and remodelling by operating on any of the target cell populations at critical times.

(c) *osteoinduction*: a process which normally occurs in embryonic bone development, but which may also be elicited in ectopic sites by implantation of suitable nonvital materials containing bone morphogenetic protein (BMP) [Urist *et al.* (421,422), Yoshikawa *et al.* (425,426), Rosen *et al.* (416)] or osteogenic protein [Sampath *et al.* (417)].Osteoinduction is distinguished by *de novo* bone formation, whereas osteoconduction, creeping substitution and osteointegration involve migration of bone-forming cells from a pre-existing bone site to implanted matrices, powders, and prosthetic devices;

(d) *fracture healing*: a repair process wherein most of the normal bone development pathway (Fig. 1) is recapitulated. Abnormal healing leading to reduced mechanical strength or ossification failure (nonunion) may result from imbalanced cellular proliferation, inadequate blood circulation, or improper physical loading of the healing fracture;

(e) *skeletal growth and resorptive remodeling*: the amplification of existing bone involving the interplay of osteoclastic resorption with intramembranous and endochondral bone formation. This is subject to regulation by genetic, nutritional, and hormonal conditions, as well as to local physical stresses which stimulate remodeling according to Wolff's Law [Glimcher (3)];

(f) *skeletal pathology*: the abnormalities of skeletal hard tissues which are are attributable to altered bone cell function including: elevated osteoclastic activity or imbalanced or reduced osteoblastic activity in osteoporosis, enhanced metabolic states in Paget's disease, and complex cellular responses in bone to a wide variety of endocrine (eg. Cushing's disease) and neoplastic disorders (eg. malignant hypercalcemia [Mundy *et al.* (106)] and enhancement of bone growth by prostatic carcinoma [Koutsilleris *et al.* (307−309)].

The above areas are bound together by the common thread of osteoblastic and osteoclastic biology. As we attempt to extrapolate and adapt findings involving growth factors from each of these areas to practical medical technology, we must recognize the limitations of our experimental models.

## II. General Features of Receptor-Mediated Growth Factor Action

The wide variety of growth factors which may be of relevance to bone are depicted along with their identified plasma membrane receptors in Fig. 2., For each growth factor type there is a characteristic receptor with distinct properties of ligand specificity and post-binding signalling events [see Section III and reviews [Bradshaw and Prentis (7); Carpenter (8); Deuel (11)]]. A complex chain of events couples the initial binding of a factor by its specific receptor to the cellular response of proliferation or modulation of phenotypic expression. For the most thoroughly studied receptors such as insulin and EGF, these events include: 1) ligand binding; 2)activation of receptor

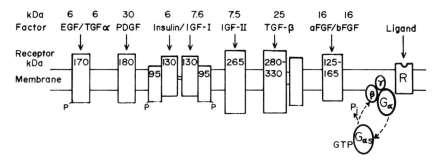

**Fig. 2** Growth factors and their membrane receptors. The known polypeptide growth factors, with molecular weights indicated, are shown interacting with specific high molecular weight membrane receptors. The appropriate monomeric or oligomeric structure is indicated for each receptor. Growth factor binding to the extracellular domain is translated into an intracellular signal via a transmembrane conformational change. For some receptors this stimulates auto-phosphorylation of tyrosine residues. The G protein complex shown at the right is a common pathway for intracellular signalling by a variety of hormonal ligand-receptor (R) complexes. There may be interactions between the G protein system and growth factor signalling pathways in certain situations (see text).

protein kinase; 3) receptor tyrosine autophosphorylation; 4) changes in gene transcription [eg. c-myc and c-fos [Barber *et al.* (5); Bradshaw and Prentis (7); Rollins and Stiles (15)]]; 5) elevated sugar and ion transport; 6) endocytosis of receptor-ligand complexes; 7) activation/inhibition of intra-cellular enzymes [Ballard *et al.* (4)]; 8) phosphorylation of receptor serine and threonine sites; 9) altered synthesis of RNA, DNA, protein, and lipid; 10) maximal down-regulation of the receptor; 11) cell proliferation. The time course for these events ranges from seconds (steps 1–3) to minutes (steps 4–8) to hours (steps 9–11), as reviewed by Rosen (16). Receptor numbers per cell are typically in the $10^3-10^5$ range, with ligand dissociation constants between 2 pM and 10 nM.

Autophosphorylation by an intrinsic tyrosine kinase is not yet a proven property of all growth factor receptors [Bradshaw and Prentis (7); Carpenter (8)]. The G protein complex (Fig. 2) is another common pathway for intracellular signalling [Gilman (12); Limbird (13)]. Ligands such as PTH or alpha$_2$-adrenergic agonists bind to their specific receptors (R). Through altered interaction with the $[G_{alpha}]\cdot[G_{beta}\cdot G_{gamma}]$ complex in the membrane, $G_{alpha}$ dissociates, binds GTP, and acts transiently to either stimulate or inhibit adenylate cyclase (causing fluctuations in intracellular cAMP, protein kinase, etc.). Also, stimulation of phosphoinositidase results in hydrolysis of phosphatidylinositol 4, 5-bisphosphate to yield diacylglycerol and phosphatidylinositol 1,4,5-triphosphate, a bifurcating pathway allowing complex second messenger signalling through $Ca^{2+}$ and protein kinase C [Berridge (6); Gilman (12)]. There are also other possible intracellular targets for $G_{alpha}$-GTP [Limbird (13)]. Interestingly, some growth factor effects in osteoblasts appear to involve the G protein pathway [Gutierrez et al. (92); Centrella et al. (140); Noda et al. (165), Rodan et al. (278)].

### Growth Factor Effects on the Cell Cycle

The cell cycle (Fig. 3) describes all typical diploid eukaryotic cells, where daughter cells from a mitotic event, M, traverse the $G_1$ phase prior to entering another round of DNA replication, S. Cells may pause transiently in a prolonged $G_1$ state, or may actually stop cycling and enter $G_0$. The availability of specific growth factors is a critical determinant in the cycling behavior of cells. Elegant studies of the serum and growth factor requirements of proliferating cells in culture [Clemmons et al. (10); Stiles et al. (19), Rollins et al. (238)] identified *competence* factors (eg. PDGF) which would induce $G_0$-arrested cells to enter $G_1$, and *progression* factors (eg. IGF-I) which would facilitate the traverse of the cell cycle. Exposure of quiescent 3T3 cells to PDGF for as little as 30 min induces the state of competence [Singh et al. (18)]. TGF-β has also been implicated in a prolonged prereplicative ($G_0$-$G_1$) stage prior to entry into S [Shipley et al. (17)]. Autocrine stimulation of proliferation can also be caused by TGF-beta-mediated induction of c-sis mRNA, where the endogenously produced PDGF-like activity is the actual mitogenic stimulus [Leof et al. (14)].

Terminal differentiation is the possible fate of certain cell types which are deprived of essential growth factors. The MM14 mouse muscle myoblast is such a cell. Deprivation of aFGF for as little as $2-3$ hr causes commitment to myotube differentiation and precludes reentry to the cell cycle [Clegg et al. (9)]. Differentiated expression of most cell types is associated with $G_0$ or a prolonged $G_1$ phase, and is typically suppressed if mitogenic and nutritional factors are adequate to maintain proliferative cycling. For example, TGF-β can suppress adipogenic transformation of fibroblasts by preventing entry into $G_0$ [Ignotz and Massague (152)]. In normal embryonic development, differentiation is typically correlated with cessation of proliferation. Application of these principles to osteoblasts is discussed in Section V below.

A key issue in growth factor biology is the similarity between certain oncogene products and growth factors or their receptors. The initial discovery involving the SSV v-sis gene product and its 90% homology to the B chain of PDGF provided a rational mechanism for viral transformation and

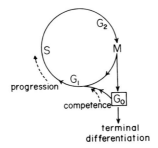

**Fig. 3** The cell cycle.

neoplasia involving autocrine growth factor stimulation [Bradshaw and Prentis (7); Doolittle *et al.* (215); Heldin and Westermark (223); Waterfield *et al.* (245)]. Subsequently, many other oncogenes have been identified, and the cellular analogs of some, such as c-fos and c-myc, are sensitive to growth factor stimulation [Barber *et al.* (5); Rollins and Stiles (15)].

## Complexity of Growth Factor Action

Receptor-mediated cellular responses are sensibly dependent on all "reactants" in the total process. The regulatory aspects of membrane receptors are as critical to the overall cellular response to a growth factor as the presence of the factor itself. For growth factors the complexity echoes all the variables known to pharmacologists and endocrinologists. First are variations in *growth factor concentration* involving production rate [Leof *et al.* (14); McCarthy *et al.* (56); Mohan *et al.* (59); Wahl *et al.* (198)], self-stimulation of growth factor production [Van Obberghen-Schilling *et al.* (197)], sequestration by extracellular matrix [Folkman *et al.* (265); Gospodarowicz and Tauber (340); Hauschka *et al.* (341−2); Baird and Ling (392)], activation of latent forms [O'Connor-McCourt and Wakefield (167); Wakefield *et al.* (200)], carrier and binding proteins [Daughaday *et al.* (33); Wilkins and D'Ercole (77); Pfeilschifter *et al.* (174); Huang *et al.* (226)], proteinase modification [Klagsbrun *et al.* (269)], and catabolism and clearance [O'Connor-McCourt and Wakefield (167)]. The second important component is the *growth factor receptor* which may vary in abundance and affinity [Carpenter (8); Chinkers and Garbers (87); Petkovich *et al.* (174); Wakefield *et al.* (199)], ligand specificity [Gill *et al.* (91); Cheifetz *et al.* (143); Heldin *et al.* (224)], internalization/catabolism/recycling kinetics [Carpenter (8); Rosen (16); Keating and Williams (227)], and ligand-dependent downregulation [Carpenter (8); Deuel (11); Wakefield *et al.* (19)]. The third variable is *synergism/antagonism* involving common receptors and intracellular signalling mechanisms [Inman and Colowick (154); Roberts *et al.* (178); Keating and Williams(227); Baird and Durkin (377); Centrella *et al.* (379; Globus *et al.* (381); Massague *et al.* (382)], growth factor regulation of receptors for a second factor [Assoian (130); Massague (159)], and G protein effects [Noda *et al.* (166)]. Finally, the *state and environment of the target cell* is important: growth conditions [Robey *et al.* (181); Centrella *et al.* (379)], modulation by other cell types [Pfeilschifter *et al.* (173); Manishen *et al.* (399); Van der Plas and Nijweide (409)], and presence of extracellular matrix [Gospodarowicz and Tauber (340); Hauschka *et al.* (341−2); Linkhart *et al.* (343); Pacifici *et al.* (321); Baird and Ling (392); Barnes and Colowick (393)] can affect the response.

## III. Properties of Growth Factors

A comprehensive review of each growth factor is beyond the scope of this chapter. The reference list should be consulted for information beyond the brief outlines of properties which follow. The current wealth of protein and nucleic acid sequence data has disclosed many important relationships within growth factor families, as well as more obscure homologies with other proteins. Table 1 summarizes the rapidly expanding information regarding growth factor heterogeneity.

### Insulin and Insulin-like Growth Factors [IGF-I and IGF-II (SGF)]

#### Molecular Properties

Insulin (6 kDa) is a disulfide-bonded molecule consisting of a 21 amino acid residue (res) A chain and a 30 res B chain. Proteolytic excision of a 30−35 res C peptide from proinsulin leads to the active form of insulin [King and Kahn (49)]. Circulating forms of nonsuppressible, insulin-like activity [Rinderknecht and Humbel (62); Zapf *et al.* (78, 79)] were isolated and sequenced. IGF-I (7.6 kDa) consists of 70 res in a single chain with 3 internal disulfide bonds [Rinderknecht and Humbel (62)]. There exists strong homology with the A and B chains of insulin, but a 12 res C peptide is very different from the proinsulin C peptide, and IGF-I has an 8 res COOH-terminal extension compared to proinsulin [Rinderknecht and Humbel (62)]. IGF-II (7.5 kDa) is a 67 res polypeptide with 45 res identical to IGF-I [Rinderknecht and Humbel (63)]. The multiplication

**Table 1.**
Heterogeneity within the Major Growth Factor Families

| Family | # | Common Forms | # | Other Related Sequences |
|--------|---|--------------|---|--------------------------|
| IGF | 3 | Insulin, IGF-I, IGF-II | >6 | somatomedin A, $NH_2$ truncated IGF-I relaxin, NGF, other SGFs, MSAs |
| EGF | 2 | EGF, TGF-a | >13 | HMW forms of TGF-a (89, 97 res) vaccinia VGF, tPA, proteinase domains, LDLr, proEGF, lin-12, notch |
| TGF-β | 4 | TGF-β11, -β12, -β22, -β3 | 3 | latent TGF-β, inhibins A and B, MIS, decapentaplegic locus, BMPs? |
| PDGF | 5 | AB, BB, AA, A*A*, v-sis | ? | HMW PDGFs from macrophages |
| FGF | 2 | aFGF, bFGF | >3 | HMW and truncated FGFs, IL-1, MMTV (int-2), hst |

stimulating activity (MSA) from rat liver cell cultures is virtually identical (93% homology) to human IGF-II [Marquardt *et al.* (54)]. Of particular relevance to bone is the recent finding that skeletal growth factor [Farley and Baylink (38); Mohan *et al.* (57, 58)] is homologous, if not identical, to IGF-II [Mohan *et al.* (59)]. The gene structures for the IGFs have been determined [Soares *et al.* (72)]. A trailing E peptide which is proteolytically cleaved from the pro-IGF-II molecule may be involved in potentiating IGF-II activity [Hylka *et al.* (45)]. There are several known binding proteins for IGFs which may regulate biological activity [Daughaday *et al.* (33); Hossenlopp *et al.* (44); Povoa *et al.* (61); Wilkins and D'Ercole (77)] and may be growth hormone-dependent [Ernst *et al.* (37); Povoa *et al.* (61)].

## Receptors

Insulin and IGF-I have distinct but homologous membrane receptors [Carpenter (8); Hollenberg (43)] consisting of two alpha chains (130 kDa) which specifically bind the ligand, and two beta chains (95 kDa) with activatable tyrosine kinase activity. Two alpha-beta heterodimers are disulfide crosslinked to form the ~450 kDa native receptor [Carpenter (8); King and Kahn (49); O'Hare and Pilch (60)]. The IGF-II receptor is single chain of 220−265 kDa [Carpenter (8); King and Kahn (49)] which has recently been implicated in a distinct and puzzling second function; the binding of mannosyl moieties in proteins [Roth (64)]. IGF-II is not known to be mannosylated. Expression of receptors for IGF-I and -II has been traced in the developing mouse limb [Baumick and Bala (22)].

*Biological Activity*

Longitudinal bone growth is apparently controlled by growth hormone (GH) through its stimulation of IGF-I (somatomedin C) production by the liver [Ashton *et al.* (20); Daughaday *et al.* (32); D'Ercole (34); Schoenle *et al*; (68)]. Recent studies in the GH-deficient *lit/lit* mouse [Mathews *et al.* (55)] showed a 10-fold increase in liver IGF-I mRNA, but most non-hepatic tissues did not show GH-dependent IGF-I expression. Bone may be an exception [Ernst and Froesch (36); Stracke *et al.* (73)]. Infusion studies with GH and IGF-I in rats attribute endochondral bone growth to local somatomedin production [Schlechter *et al.* (65)]. While production of IGF-I has been demonstrated for fibroblasts [Adams *et al.* (21)] and bone cells [Blatt *et al.* (25); Canalis *et al.* (27, 29); Ernst and Froesch (36); McCarthy *et al.* (56)], the issue is less clear for chondrocytes [Kato *et al.* (48); Shen *et al.* (69)]. SGF (IGF-II) is produced by isolated osteoblasts [Mohan *et al.* (59); Strong *et al.* (74); Wergedal *et al.* (75)] at about 40 times the rate of IGF-I production. In bone matrix, IGF-II is abundant and about 10-fold more concentrated than IGF-I [Frolik *et al.* (40); Mohan *et al.* (57)]. There are clear mitogenic effects of insulin [Barnes and Sato (23); Hayashi *et al.* (41)] and IGFs [King and Kahn (49), Marquardt *et al.* (54)] on a variety of cell types in tissue culture. For insulin, the protein structural requirements for mitogenesis are somewhat less stringent than those for stimulation of glucose oxidation [King and Kahn (49)].

*Effects in Bone*

There have been extensive studies of insulin [Canalis *et al.* (2); Ernst and Froesch (35); King and Kahn (49); Kream *et al.* (50); Levy *et al.* (52); Whitson *et al.* (76)]; IGF-I [Bennett *et al.* (24); Canalis (26,28); Canalis *et al.* (27); Ernst and Froesch (35); Hock *et al.* (42); Schmidt *et al.* (66,67); Stracke *et al.* (73)]; and IGF-II (SGF) [Farley *et al.* (39); LaTour *et al.* (51); Linkhart *et al.* (53); Mohan *et al.* (58)] in bone organ culture and isolated osteoblasts, as well as utilizing bone markers *in vivo* [Catherwood *et al.* (30), Schlechter *et al.* (65), Sibonga *et al.* (71)]. Generally, there is a dose-dependent stimulation of osteoblastic proliferation and enhanced collagen biosynthesis. IGF-I is about 10 times more potent as a mitogen than insulin [Ernst and Froesch (35)]. IGF-I (and perhaps IGF-II) are unusual in that bone cell replication and differentiation are simultaneously stimulated [Canalis (1); Farley *et al.* (39); Mohan *et al.* (58)]. Insulin alone does not alter osteocalcin production in cultured fetal rat calvaria, but insulin enhances $1,25(OH)_2$ vitamin $D_3$ stimulation of osteocalcin [Lian *et al.* (102)]. IGF-I receptors are modulated by glucocorticoids [Bennett *et al.*

(24)] and PTH [Ituarte *et al.* (47)]; PTH [McCarthy *et al.* (56)] and $\beta_2$-microglobulin [Centrella *et al.* (31)] also stimulate IGF-I production, with synergistic effects on bone formation [Si *et al.* (70)]. The anabolic effect of PTH on bone has been a longstanding puzzle in bone biology. Given the target specificity of PTH for osteoblasts, the PTH-dependent upregulation of IGF-I production and receptor levels [McCarthy *et al.* (56)] may explain the phenomenon through autocrine effects of IGF-I on osteoblasts.

## Epidermal Growth Factor (EGF) and Transforming Growth Factor-$\alpha$ (TGF-$\alpha$)

### Molecular Properties

EGF and TGF-$\alpha$ are discussed together because of their homologous structures, common membrane receptor, and related biological activities. EGF (53 amino acid res) and TGF-$\alpha$ (50 res) are related, 6.0 kDa polypeptides with three intramolecular disulfide crosslinks. Murine EGF and human EGF (urogastrone) share 70% sequence homology, while rat TGF-$\alpha$ is 33% homologous to mEGF and 44% homologous to hEGF [Cohen and Carpenter (90); Marquardt *et al.* (104); Twardzik *et al.* (122)]. Protein sequences related to EGF have been described in a host of evolutionarily divergent molecules including: vaccinia virus growth factor VVGF [Twardzik *et al.* (123)], blood coagulation factors VII, IX, X, and protein S, tissue plasminogen activator, LDL receptor, *C. elegans* lin-12, and *D. melanogaster* notch locus. The latter contains 36 separate EGF-like domains. The enormous 130 kDa (1207 res) human proEGF precursor from which EGF (53 res) is proteolytically excised contains up to 8 EGF-related sequences with unknown fate or function [Bradshaw and Prentis (7); Carpenter (8); Bell *et al.* (81)]. Glandular kallikreins may play a role in proEGF processing [Isacksson *et al.* (99)]. TGF-$\alpha$ is derived from a much smaller precursor (160 res) which is glycosylated and palmitoylated, providing anchorage as a transmembrane protein. Extracellular proteolytic cleavage apparently generates TGF-$\alpha$ and related peptides [Bringman *et al.* (84)].

### Receptor

EGF and TGF-$\alpha$ both bind to the EGF receptor [Todaro *et al.* (120)], a large (1186 res) polypeptide with prototypic membrane receptor structure including an NH$_2$-terminal extracellular growth factor ligand domain, a hydrophobic transmembrane segment, and an intracellular protein-tyrosine kinase domain [Carpenter (8); Twardzik (124)]. Homology between the

COOH-terminal half of the EGF receptor and the protein product of the avian erythroblastosis v-erbB oncogene was a keystone in the experimental data bridging growth factors and neoplastic cellular transformation [Carpenter (8)]. Transfection of normal cells with the v-erbB oncogene can produce a transformed, tumorigenic phenotype, whereas transfection with the full-length EGF receptor gene permits EGF to stimulate normal mitosis [Pierce et al. (111)] or transformation [Velu et al. (125)] depending on the target cell.

Regulation of the EGF receptor population on the cell surface depends on ligand concentration, with EGF-receptor complexes being internalized for subsequent EGF degradation and receptor recycling [Gill et al. (91)]. The internalization process has been visualized in A-431 cells [Carpentier et al. (85)]. Glycosylation [Moseley and Suva (105)] and phorbol esters or vitamin $K_3$ [Cohen (87)] can alter EGF receptor function. The receptor appears to recognize the conserved COOH-terminal region of EGF and TGF-$\alpha$ [Lazar et al. (101)]. Osteoblast-like cells appear to express the EGF receptor, thereby being candidates for modulation by EGF and TGF-$\alpha$ [Ng et al. (108); Shupnik and Tashjian (116)]; there are examples of non-responsive cells with deficiencies in receptor activity [Ibbotson et al. (98)] or EGF-induced $Ca^{2+}$ uptake [Shupnik and Tashjian (116)].

*Biological Activity*

The effects of EGF on neonatal mouse development were originally described for eyelid opening and tooth eruption [Cohen (89)]. EGF has mitogenic effects on a variety of adult tissues [Carpenter (8); Cohen and Carpenter (90)]. Maternal sources of EGF (transplacental, milk) are probably important for early development, since EGF mRNA is apparently not produced by fetal mouse tissues; the earliest appearance is $11-14$ days postpartum [Popliker et al. (112)]. Functional EGF receptors appear by the 9th day of gestation, but it may be TGF-$\alpha$, the "fetal" form of EGF, which activates these early receptors [Popliker et al. (112); Twardzik (122, 124)]. TGF-$\alpha$ was originally isolated as the smaller of two polypeptides produced by cultured tumor cells and virally transformed cells [Todaro et al. (120); Twardzik et al. (122)]. Both factors reversibly promoted anchorage independent growth of normal cells. TGF-$\alpha$ was found to act through EGF receptors, while TGF-$\beta$ has a distinct mode of action discussed below. Consistent with the mitogenic effects of EGF and TGF-$\alpha$, cellular differentiation may be attenuated by these factors [Adashi et al. (80); Yoneda et al. (127)].

The relative biological activities of TGF-$\alpha$ and EGF are not identical, despite the sharing of the EGF receptor. TGF-$\alpha$ is a more potent angiogenic mediator [Schreiber et al. (114)], stimulator of bone resorption [Ibbotson et *al.* (98); Mundy *et al.* (106); Tashjian and Levine (118)], and antagonist of osteoblastic phenotypic expression [Ibbotson *et al.* (98)] than EGF. Until recently, the only known sources of TGF-α production in adult humans were tumor cells, with TGF-α being a potential cause of the hypercalcemia of malignancy [Ibbotson *et al.* (97, 98); Mundy *et al.* (106); Stern *et al.* (117); Tashjian *et al.* (119)].

*Effects in Bone*

   EGF and TGF-α are examples of factors which can affect bone in organ culture and osteoblasts *in vitro*, but due to the lack of known sources in normal bone tissue and their apparent absence in bone matrix (Table 2), these factors have been principally of endocrinological interest. However, the recent discovery of TGF-α production by activated diploid human macrophages [Madtes *et al.*, 1988 (103)] should stimulate further work on EGF/TGF-α effects in bone. The effects of EGF and/or TGF-α in bone organ cultures include: mitogenic stimulation of periosteal fibroblasts and osteoblasts, decreased synthesis of type I collagen and alkaline phosphatase [Canalis 1985 (1); Hurley *et al.*, 1988 (96)], failure of EGF to stimulate osteocalcin and EGF opposition of the $1,25(OH)_2$ vitamin $D_3$ upregulation of osteocalcin [Lian *et al.* (102)], and increased bone resorption [Canalis (1); Tashjian and Levine (118); Tashjian *et al.* (192)]. Effects on cultured osteoblastic cells include increased DNA synthesis [Ng *et al.* (107; Tsunoi (121)], decreased collagen synthesis [Hata *et al.* (93); Hiramatsu *et al.* (94); Kumegawa *et al.* (100); Osaki *et al.* (109)], increased prostaglandin $E_2$ synthesis [Hirata *et al.* (95); Yokota *et al.* (126)], altered intracellular $Ca^{2+}$ [Boland *et al.* (83)], and increased collagenase and collagenase inhibitor synthesis [Chikuma *et al.* (86); Chua *et al.* (88); Partridge *et al.* (110)]. EGF and TGF-α also lower the responsiveness of osteoblastic adenylate cyclase to PTH [Bernier *et al.* (82); Gutierrez *et al.* (92)], similar to the findings for other growth factors [see below, and Hauschka *et al.* (342)]. This creates a particularly complex situation with regard to bone resorption. PTH-like peptides produced by cancer cells are another recognized cause (along with TGF-α) of the hypercalcemia of malignancy [Mundy *et al.* (106)] and must act on the osteoblast to stimulate osteoclastic resorption [Rodan and Martin (407)]. EGF stimulates synthesis of a PTH-like factor in the human SAOS-2 osteosarcoma [Rodan *et al.* (113)], yet both EGF and tumor-derived TGF-α should attenuate the response of osteoblasts to PTH-like factors. *In vivo* infusion of EGF in mice at doses adequate to cause significant gastric and pancreatic hyperplasia failed to cause hypercalcemia [Shevrin *et al.* (115)]. Thus, in addition to ligands for the EGF receptor, there are probably other factors which enhance bone resorption in the hypercalcemia of malignancy.

## Transforming Growth Factor-β (TGF-β)

### Molecular Properties

As originally characterized, TGF-β from human platelets [Assoian et al. (129)], human placenta [Frolik et al. (149)], and bovine kidney [Roberts et al. (179)] was a 25 kDa protein comprised of two identical subunits cross-linked by disulfide bonds. The 112 amino acid subunit originates by proteolytic excision from the COOH-terminus of a putative 391 amino acid precursor [Derynck et al. (145)]. Two cartilage induction factors (CIF-A and CIF-B) isolated from bovine bone [Seyedin et al. (187)] were found to have related NH₂-terminal sequences. CIF-A was shown to be identical to TGF-β, and this form is now called TGF-β 1 [Seyedin et al. (188)]. CIF-B, now designated TGF-β 2, represented a new form with 71% sequence identity to TGF-β 1 [Cheifetz et al. (143); Segarini et al. (186); Seyedin et al. (189)]. A heterodimer isolated as a minor TGF-β component from porcine platelets contains both TGF-β 1 and 2 chains and is known as TGF-β 1.2 [Cheifetz et al. (143)]. A third TGF-beta polypeptide sequence (TGF-β 3) has recently been deduced from a human rhabdomyosarcoma cDNA sequence [Ten Dijke et al. (193)]. The 112 amino acid sequence of this molecule is probably derived from a 412 amino acid precursor and shares about 80% sequence identity with type TGF-β 1 and -β 2. The form of TGF-β 1 originally secreted from platelets is biologically latent [Wakefield et al. (200)]. It consists of mature TGF-β 1 (25 kDa), the remainder of the precursor (74 kDa), and an unidentified 135 kDa protein species.

Other factors whose amino acid sequences place them in the TGF-β family [see Cheifetz et al. (143) and Sporn et al. (190)] include inhibin/activin [Ling et al. (158)], Mullerian inhibitory substance (MIS) [Cate et al. (135)], BSC-1 inhibitor [Tucker et al. (195)], the transcript of the decapentaplegic gene complex in *Drosophila* [Padgett et al. (171)], and perhaps several osteoinductive proteins [Wozney et al. (416); Sampath et al. (417)].

### Receptors

The high affinity receptor for TGF-β is a 280−330 kDa glycosylated membrane protein which occurs as a 565−615 kDa disulfide-linked oligomer containing at least one ligand binding site [Massague (160)]. Distinct 85 kDa and 65 kDa receptor species have also been observed for TGF-β [Cheifetz et al. (143)]. The 280 kDa receptor displays high affinity for both TGF-β1 and 2, and occupancy of this receptor correlates with the degree of bioactivity in several different cellular assays; maximum biological response may occur at 10−50% receptor occupancy [Tucker et al. (196); Wakefield et al. (199)]. The 85 and 65 kDa receptors have about 10-fold greater affinity for TGF-β 1 than for TGF-β 2 [Cheifetz et al. (143)]. Other studies have described three classes of TGF-β receptors, one of which is highly selective for TGF-β 1 [Segarini et al. (186)].

Receptors for TGF-β are universally present on some 35 different cell lines [Wakefield et al. (199)]. The dissociation constant $K_d$ typically ranges from 1−60 pM, with 600−81,000 receptors/cell. The osteoblastic TGF-β receptor is distinguished by its extremely high affinity (2.2 pM) [Robey et al. (181)]. Interestingly, there is a very strong inverse correlation between receptor number and affinity (fewer receptors-higher affinity) such that virtually the same number of TGF-β molecules are bound per cell at any given ambient TGF-β concentration [Wakefield et al. (199)]. TGF-β receptors are susceptible to down-regulation by TGF-β itself, perhaps as a result of internalization of the receptor-ligand complex [Frolik et al. (148); Wakefield et al. (199)], but the ~2-fold extent of downregulation is minor compared to the effects of EGF, PDGF, IGF-1 and insulin on their own receptor levels. $^{125}$I-TGF-β is degraded by lysosomal proteinases after binding to NRK cells [Frolik et al. (148)].

Viral transformation has modest effects on TGF-β receptor properties, but the total variation in TGF-β binding is only 2−3−fold [Wakefield et al. (199)]. The quantitative TGF-β binding is also essentially unaltered by a variety of agents which are known to modulate the responses of cells to TGF-β (EGF, PDGF, retinoic acid, phorbol ester TPA, and epinephrine) [Wakefield et al. (199)]. In contrast, while TGF-β binds exclusively to its own receptor types, it can affect EGF receptor levels, in turn altering its biological activity, since many cells require EGF or TGF-α to respond to TGF-β [Assoian (130); Massague (159); Petkovich et al. (172)].

## Biological Activity

As early as 1981, Roberts et al. (178) recognized that two distinct classes of cellular transforming growth factors (TGFs) existed in both normal and neoplastic tissues. One type (TGF-alpha) was competitive with EGF for EGF receptors and was not potentiated by EGF in soft agar assays for anchorage-independent colony formation. The other type (TGF-β) was not competitive with EGF but was potentiated by EGF to induce colony formation. The range of biological activities attributed to TGF-β has expanded dramatically in the past few years and is the subject of several excellent reviews [Cheifetz et al. (143); Sporn et al. (190); Sporn and Roberts (191)]. TGF-β is known for its antiproliferative effects on cells, particularly epithelial cells [Tucker et al. (195)], but inhibition is also common for mesenchymal cells such as fibroblasts, endothelial cells, and T- and B-lymphocytes [Roberts et al. (180); Sporn et al. (190)]. In many cases the antiproliferative effects correlate with enhanced cellular differentiation

[Ignotz and Massague (153)], but even a transient exposure to TGF-β can block the commitment to adipogenic differentiation of 3T3 fibroblasts [Ignotz and Massague (152)]. In one example where TGF-β blocks the mitogenic stimulation of mink lung epithelial cells by EGF or insulin, an early mitogen-dependent event involving activation of a protein kinase for ribosomal protein S6 is unaffected by TGF-β. Thus the antiproliferative effect of TGF-β appears to operate distal to the receptors for other growth factors [Like and Massague (157)].

Osteoblasts and Schwann cells are unusual in that they exhibit a proliferative response to TGF-β [Centrella *et al.* (137, 138); Sporn *et al.* (190)]. In part this response may be a consequence of the ability of TGF-β to stimulate extracellular matrix synthesis and inhibit matrix degradation [Ignotz and Massague (153); Overall *et al.* (170); Pfeilschifter *et al.* (177); Sporn *et al.* (190)]. It is also known that TGF-β can enhance both its own expression [VanObberghen-Schilling *et al.* (197)] and that of other growth factors including PDGF-like factors [Leof *et al.* (14); Moses *et al.* (161)] and macrophage and monocyte factors including interleukin 1 [Assoian *et al.* (131); Wahl *et al.* (198)]. Thus, to establish TGF-β as a mitogen, the secondary effects of other growth factors must first be ruled out [Roberts *et al.* (180)]. In the standard quantitative assay for TGF-β activity, NRK cell colony formation in soft agar requires both TGF-β and EGF. Events associated with cellular proliferation such as enhanced glucose uptake are triggered by EGF [Inman and Colowick (154)]. The bifunctional regulatory effects of TGF-β which span the entire range of overt mitogenesis to chalone-like inhibition are believed to be a manifestation of "...the total set of growth factors and their receptors...operant in the cell at a given time" rather than from intrinsic pleitropic effects of the TGF-β peptide itself [Roberts *et al.* (180)].

Immunohistochemical studies of the distribution of TGF-β 1 in the developing mouse embryo have demonstrated the abundance of this factor in mesenchyme and mesenchymally derived tissues [Ellingsworth *et al.* (147); Heine *et al.* (150)]. TGF-β 1 is most evident in focal areas of epithelial-mesenchymal interaction and during periods of morphogenesis and remodelling. Pronounced angiogenic activity is also coupled with intense staining for TGF-β 1 [Heine *et al.* (150)]. Both TGF-β 1 and 2 appear to act interchangeably in most systems, but a specific role has been discovered for TGF-β 2 in muscle induction in the amphibian embryo [Rosa *et al.* (182)]. TGF-β 1 is about 100-fold more potent than TGF-β 2 in its inhibition of the proliferation of hematopoietic progenitor cells; the type I TGF-β receptors on the sensitive cells bind TGF-β 1 some 20-fold more avidly than TGF-β 2 [Ohta *et al.* (168)].

The potent effects of TGF-β on incisional wound healing [Mustoe *et al.* (162)] involve a variety of cellular responses to this factor. Enhanced collagen biosynthesis and fibrogenesis [Ignotz and Massague (153); Rossi *et al.* (185); Seyedin *et al.* (188); Sporn *et al.* (190)] is amplified both by the TGF-β dependent chemotaxis of fibroblasts and mononuclear cells, and by the autocrine and paracrine effects of growth factor production by these cells [Leof *et al.* (14); Mustoe *et al.* (162); Wahl *et al.* (198)]. TGF-β 1 and 2 also can suppress the respiratory burst of activated macrophages, and thus may perform an important negative feedback function in wound healing and inflammatory events [Tsunawaki *et al.* (194)]. TGF-β has also been shown to operate as a potent immunosuppressive agent [Sporn *et al.* (190)].

Perhaps the most intriguing aspect of TGF-beta biology is the recent discovery of a latent form of the factor in platelets [Wakefield *et al.* (200)], macrophages [Assoian *et al.* (131)], and bone [Pfeilschifter *et al.* (173−177)]. This 220−235 kDa latent TGF-beta, as characterized from platelets, appears to be a delivery complex which releases active TGF-β 1 upon transient acidification [Wakefield *et al.* (200)]. Osteoclastic bone resorption involves local acidification, and may correlate with local activation of latent TGF-β [Pfeilschifter *et al.* (174)]. It is not known whether the high levels of TGF-β extractable from bone matrix occur as a true latent form, analogous to the platelet complex, or in association with other binding proteins. Importantly, free TGF-β also binds to alpha$_2$-macroglobulin which may act as a clearance mechanism to mop up excess factor escaping into the blood plasma [O'Connor-McCourt and Wakefield (167); Wakefield *et al.* (200)]. Endogenous production of TGF-β and $\alpha_2$-macroglobulin by many cell types, along with the presence of $\alpha_2$-macroglobulin in serum, severely complicates the interpretation of experiments with exogenous TGF-β.

*Effects in Bone*

The abundance of TGF-β in bone matrix [Seyedin *et al.* (187−189)] and its production by cultured bone tissue [Centrella and Canalis (136, 139)] and osteoblasts [Robey *et al.* (181)] heralded the intense investigation of TGF-β effects on isolated bone cells. The effects observed on osteoblastic cells depend on TGF-β dose, culture density, serum concentration, and cell origin, as might be expected from the above discussion of latent TGF-β and TGF-β-$\alpha_2$-macroglobulin complexes. For normal osteoblast-like cells from rodent calvaria, TGF-β enhances proliferation [Centrella *et al.* (137, 138, 141)] and tends to reduce the phenotypic expression [Antosz *et al.* (128); Elford *et al.* (146), Hauschka *et al.* (342); Noda and Rodan (163); Rosen *et al.* (183)]. However, proliferation of normal osteoblasts [Robey *et al.* (181)] and osteosarcoma-derived clonal osteoblastic cell lines [Ibbotson *et al.* (151); Noda and Rodan (163); Pfeilschifter *et al.* (176)] can be inhibited by TGF-β, in concert with enhanced expression of some characteristic proteins including Type I collagen [Centrella *et al.* (138, 141); Noda and Rodan

(163); Wrana *et al.* (201, 202)], alkaline phosphatase [Noda and Rodan (163); Pfeilschifter *et al.* (176)], osteonectin [Noda and Rodan (164)], osteopontin [Noda *et al.* (166)], phosphoproteins [Kubota *et al.* (156), Wrana *et al.* (202)] and proteinases and their inhibitors [Overall *et al.* (170); Pfeilschifter *et al.* (177); Wrana *et al.* (201)]; osteocalcin expression is generally decreased [Hauschka *et al.* (342); Noda *et al.* (166a)], although long-term studies with TGF-β and FGF showed an increase in osteocalcin [Globus *et al.* (381)]. It is significant that TGF-β does not uniformly suppress all of the phenotypic characteristics of osteoblasts when it enhances proliferation, and *vice versa* [see Table 3]. The osteoblastic estrogen receptor is also modulated by TGF-β [Komm *et al.* (155)], and PTH is observed to exert some of its effects on osteoblasts by modulating TGF-β activity [Centrella and Canalis (139); Centrella *et al.* (142)]. Bone organ culture studies suggest that TGF-β mediates the stimulatory effects of mechanical stress on bone cell proliferation [Burger *et al.* (133)]. TGF-β effects on chondrocytes [Rosen *et al.* (183); Rosier *et al.* (184)] and synovial fibroblasts [Brinckerhoff (132)] are analogous to those on osteoblasts. The complex kinetics of TGF-β concentration changes in osteoinductive implants have been recently reported [Carrington *et al.* (134)].

Bone resorption is stimulated by TGF-β in a prostaglandin-dependent fashion [Tashjian *et al.* (192)]. At the same time, bone matrix is a rich depository of TGF-β (see above), and TGF-beta is apparently released from resorbing bone [Pfeilschifter *et al.* (173)], release which is enhanced by bone resorbing agents including PTH, $1,25(OH)_2$ vitamin $D_3$, and interleukin 1 [Pfeilschifter and Mundy (175)]. Both TGF-β 1 and 2 inhibit osteoclastic activity [Oreffo *et al.* (169)] and macrophage activity [Tsunawaki *et al.* (194)], while monocytes are chemotactically attracted to TGF-β [Wahl *et al.* (198)]. Long-term effects of TGF-β on marrow cultures include the inhibition of osteoclast formation [Chenu *et al.* (144)]. Clearly in need of further study, the mechanisms by which various bone cell types cope with the multiple forms of TGF-β [free, matrix-bound, latent, and complexed with $\alpha_2$-macroglobulin] are critical to the understanding of bone physiology.

## Platelet-Derived Growth Factor (PDGF)

### Molecular Properties

PDGF was originally characterized from human platelets and behaved as a 28−35 kDa heterodimer comprised of a disulfidebonded A chain (~14 kDa) and B chain (~17 kDa) [Antoniades and Williams (203); Deuel and Huang (212); Raines and Ross (235)]. Extensive sequence identity (~90%) between the protein product of the simian sarcoma virus transforming gene (p28$^{v\text{-}sis}$) and the PDGF B chain was a major breakthrough in unravelling the complex mechanisms of oncogenic transformation and autocrine growth regulation [Antoniades (204); Betsholtz *et al.* (207); Deuel *et al.* (214); Doolittle *et al.* (215); Heldin and Westermark (223); Waterfield *et al.* (245)]. The A chain [Betsholtz *et al.* (208); Bonthron *et al.* (209)] and B chain [Rao *et al.* (236)] are the products of two different genes located on human chromosomes 7 and 22, respectively. The 211 amino acid residue A chain precursor contains a 20 residue signal peptide and a 66 residue propeptide; the mature A chain is 125 residues [Betsholtz *et al.* (208)]. The B chain gene (*c-sis*, the cellular analog of the v-sis oncogene) codes for a protein of 240 residues, with 20 residues in the signal peptide, 60 residues in the propeptide, and 160 residues in the mature B chain [Betsholtz *et al.* (208)]. There is about 40% sequence homology between the A and B chains [Betsholtz *et al.* (208)], and a distant relationship has been demonstrated between the long 3' untranslated regions of the mRNAs for the A and B chains [Hoppe *et al.* (225)]. Heterogeneity in the PDGF chains on SDS-polyacrylamide gels may be due to variable glycosylation of the A chain, anomalous proteolytic cleavage, and alternative mRNA splicing [Betsholtz *et al.* (208); Bonthron *et al.* (209)]. The A chain from a transformed glioma cell line is longer and more basic than the A chain from endothelial cells [Bonthron *et al.* (209); Collins *et al.* (211); Tong *et al.* (244)]. Antisera to PDGF or synthetic peptides mimicking portions of the A and B chains reveal a variety of high molecular weight PDGF-like proteins which occur in complex intracellular processing and secretion by various cell types [Graves *et al.* (219); Niman *et al.* (232)]. The human macrophage is noted for its production of several forms of PDGF, 37−39 kDa and 12−17 kDa, which are different from the platelet ∼31 kDa AB heterodimer [Shimokado *et al.* (240)]; the rat macrophage also produces a PDGF homologue [Kumar *et al.* (228)]. In addition to the AB heterodimer form of PDGF in human platelets, there are BB homodimers in porcine platelets [Stroobant and Waterfield (242)], AA homodimers in human osteosarcoma cells [Betsholtz *et al.* (208), Heldin *et al.* (222)], and the 28 kDa v-sis homodimer in transformed cells [Robbins *et al.* (237)].

## Receptors

The PDGF receptor is a 160−180 kDa glycosylated transmembrane protein comprised of a single 1067 residue polypeptide chain [Pike *et al.* (234); Yarden *et al.* (247)]. There are many similarities to the EGF receptor in terms of domain organization, but the PDGF receptor lacks cysteine-rich sequences in the extracellular domain, and its tyrosine kinase domain is interrupted by unrelated sequences [Carpenter (8); Yarden *et al.* (247)]. The v-kit oncogene exhibits some homology to the PDGF receptor [Besmer *et al.* (206); Yarden *et al.* (247)]. Recent studies suggest that at least two different PDGF receptors exist [Heldin *et al.* (224); Hart *et al.* (221)]. The A type receptor (125 kDa with a minor 160 kDa component) binds AA, AB, and BB forms of PDGF. The B type receptor (160 and 175 kDa) binds BB strongly, AB weakly, and AA not at all [Heldin *et al.* (224)]. It is likely that the B type receptor is more important in eliciting the mitogenic response to PDGF [Heldin *et al.* (224)]. Transformation by the v-sis gene product appears to require the PDGF receptor [Leal *et al.* (229)]. *Intracellular* PDGF receptors in v-sis transformed NRK cells provide a novel pathway for autocrine stimulation which is resistant to intervention by PDGF antisera [Keating and Williams (227)].

The PDGF receptor in Swiss 3T3 cells is half-saturated at about 60 pM PDGF (2 ng/ml), while the activation of glycogen synthase is half-maximal at 6 pM PDGF [Chan *et al.* (210)], and half-maximal receptor autophosphorylation occurs at 3 nM PDGF [Pike *et al.* (234)]. Receptors for PDGF have also been characterized in human osteosarcoma cells, and are coexpressed with PDGF activity [Betsholtz *et al.* (207), Graves *et al.* (218)].

*Biological Activity*

PDGF is perhaps the most abundant growth factor in serum at ~15−50 ng/ml, originating from platelet alpha granules during blood coagulation [Antoniades *et al.* (204)]. Platelet-poor plasma is essentially devoid of PDGF and was used to demonstrate the unique role of PDGF as a progression factor in promoting the proliferation of quiescent cells [Graves *et al.* (216); Scher *et al.* (239); Stiles *et al.* (19)]. The early events in PDGF-dependent mitogenesis include receptor autophosphorylation, expression of c-myc and c-fos [Rollins and Stiles (15)] and selective stimulation of protein synthesis [Scher *et al.* (239)]. Antibody to the $PIP_2$ phosphatidylinositol metabolite can block mitogenesis if injected intracellularly [Matuoka *et al.* (231)]. Not all PDGF-inducible genes are coordinately expressed; growth conditions are an important variable, with c-myc responding best to PDGF in cycling cultures [Rollins *et al.* (238)]. In the MG63 human osteosarcoma cell line with apparently normal PDGF receptors, PDGF induces c-myc mRNA expression but this fails to couple to mitogenesis [Womer *et al.* (246)]. Fibroblasts from individuals with Werner's syndrome (premature senescence) also have a defective response to PDGF [Bauer *et al.* (205)].

Beyond its role in autocrine stimulation of transformed cells [Antoniades (204); Betsholtz *et al.* (207); Heldin and Westermark (223)], PDGF has many potential functions in the growth regulation of normal cells, especially those of mesenchymal origin [Deuel and Huang (212); Raines and Ross (235)]. As with other growth factors, the processes of 1) localized release and 2) inactivation of excess factor are critical to the mechanism of action. Many normal diploid cell types are known to produce some form of PDGF activity, including activated monocytes [Martinet et al. (230)], macrophages [Kumar et al. (228); Shimokado et al. (240)], and other cells mentioned above. Endothelial cells, which are typically nonresponsive to PDGF [eg. Raines and Ross (235)], secrete PDGF-like activity preferentially through their basal surface [Zerwes and Risau (248)]. PDGF release is countered by an inactivation pathway wherein PDGF is covalently complexed with $\alpha_2$-macroglobulin [Huang et al. (226)].

In mitogenesis assays, PDGF AB and BB species are equally potent, while the AA homodimer is relatively ineffective [Heldin et al. (224); Nister et al. (233)]. PDGF also exhibits chemotactic activity for monocytes, neutrophils [Deuel et al. (213)], smooth muscle cells, and fibroblasts [Zerwes and Risau (248)], where again the AB and BB forms are more active than AA [Nister et al. (233)]. The AA form can actually inhibit AB-dependent chemotaxis; one activity of the AA homodimer involves modulation of the EGF receptor [Nister et al. (233)].

*Effects in Bone*

Early studies of PDGF effects on bone organ culture showed stimulation of cell replication, collagen, and non-collagen protein synthesis [Canalis (1)]. Bone resorption is also stimulated by PDGF in a prostaglandin-dependent fashion [Tashjian et al. (243)]. PDGF was also recently found to stimulate the osteoinductive response to demineralized bone powder implants in older rats [Howes et al. (412)]. Addition of PDGF to normal calvarial osteoblasts *in vitro* causes dose-dependent mitogenic stimulation [Hanks et al. (220); Hauschka et al. (341, 342)]. Some osteoblastic proteins are upregulated by PDGF [Hanks et al. (220)] in a manner analogous to the fibroblastic response [Scher et al. (239)], while phenotypically characteristic proteins, including alkaline phosphatase and osteocalcin, are downregulated [Hauschka et al. (341, 342)]. The osteoblast mitogen(s) synthesized by macrophages may involve some form of PDGF [Peck et al. (322); Rifas et al. (325)].

Historically, osteosarcoma cells were an early focal point of PDGF research because of their production of, and response to, PDGF-like activity [Graves et al. (216–219); Heldin et al. (222)]. Parallels drawn for PDGF effects between normal osteoblasts and osteosarcoma cells may be inappropriate because of the variable endogenous production of PDGF A chain, v-sis gene product, and other immunoreactive PDGF forms by different osteosarcoma lines. To date there has been no demonstration of PDGF production by normal osteoblasts, although these cells apparently have PDGF receptors judging from their responsiveness to PDGF [Hauschka et al. (341, 342)].

Properties which deserve further study in osteoblasts are prostaglandin production and the EGF receptor, both of which are altered by PDGF in osteosarcoma cells [Shupnik *et al.* (241)].

## Acidic Fibroblast Growth Factor (aFGF) and Basic Fibroblast Growth Factor (bFGF)

### Molecular Properties

The FGFs represent a family of related growth factors which apparently arose by gene duplication and evolutionary divergence from a common ancestral protein. The two major types are differentiated by their isoelectric points: aFGF (pI = 5−7) and bFGF (pI = 9.6) [Bradshaw and Prentis (7); Thomas and Gimenez-Gallego (258); Thomas (259)]. aFGF occurs in bovine brain as a 140 amino acid residue, major form (15.9 kDa) and a 134 residue species (15.2 kDa) missing 6 $NH_2$-terminal residues [Esch *et al.* (249); Gimenez-Gallego *et al.* (251); Huang *et al.* (266); Thomas (259)]. The human aFGF is also 140 residues, but differs at 11 positions from bovine aFGF [Gautschi-Sova *et al.* (250)]. bFGF occurs in bovine brain as a 146 residue species [Esch *et al.* (264)], and the human bFGF gene codes for a molecule of identical size [Abraham *et al.* (261)]. Observed molecular weights for bFGF are typically in the 18−20 kDa range [Lobb and Fett (254), Klagsbrun *et al.* (269), Sullivan and Klagsbrun (284)]. Several truncated variants of bFGF result from acid proteinase cleavage during isolation [Esch *et al.* (264), Klagsbrun *et al.* (269)]. An oversize bFGF with 8 additional residues at the $NH_2$-terminus has been isolated from human benign prostatic hyperplastic tissue [Story *et al.* (283)], and a 157 residue placental bFGF with an 11 residue $NH_2$-terminal extension has been identified [Sommer *et al.* (282)]. The observation of at least 5 different bFGF mRNA species by Northern blot analysis of fibroblasts suggests the possibility that alternative mRNA splicing is a source of bFGF heterogeneity and diversity [Kurokawa *et al.* (270)]. Sequence comparison shows 55% identity between bovine aFGF and bFGF. There is also significant homology between the FGFs and interleukin 1-beta, and to a lesser extent IL-1−alpha [Bradshaw and Prentis (7); Gimenez-Gallego *et al.* (251)]. Several oncogenes (hst, Kaposi's, int-2) are also homologous to the FGF sequences [Marx (272)]. A plethora of FGF-like mitogens from different sources (brain, eye, endothelial cells, cartilage, bone, and tumors) have been classified as aFGF-like and bFGF-like by heparin affinity and antibody cross-reactivity [Lobb *et al.* (254); Schreiber *et al.* (257); Shing *et al.* (280); Sullivan and Klagsbrun (284); Hauschka *et al.* (341); Klagsbrun *et al.* (268)].

*Receptors*

The receptor for aFGF has been characterized in 3T3 fibroblasts and mouse muscle MM14 myoblasts [Olwin and Hauschka (255)]. A single receptor class exhibits a $K_d$ of 45 pM (3T3) or 10 pM (MM14), with 60,000 (3T3) or 2000 (MM14) receptors per cell. The receptor size is 165 kDa by SDS-PAGE. Importantly, both bFGF and aFGF compete with equal affinity for this receptor [Olwin and Hauschka (255)]. Preliminary studies with several osteoblastic cell types have corroborated the equivalent affinity for aFGF and bFGF ($K_d$ = 20−60 pM; receptor number 10,000−32,000/cell) [Hauschka *et al.* (342)]. Slightly different properties have been described for the hamster BHK-21 bFGF receptor [Neufeld and Gospodarowicz (276)]. A 90 kDa phosphotyrosine-containing protein is found after FGF treatment of Swiss 3T3 cells [Coughlin *et al.* (263)], and other work has ruled out the involvement of polyphosphoinositide hydrolysis and protein kinase C activation in FGF-stimulated mitogenesis [Magnaldo *et al.* (271)]. Synthetic peptides mimicking regions of bFGF have allowed identification of the receptor-binding and heparin-binding domains of this protein [Baird *et al.* (262)].

*Biological Activity*

FGFs are strong mitogens for a variety of mesenchymal cell types: fibroblasts, chondrocytes, osteoblasts, myoblasts, smooth muscle cells, glial cells, and endothelial cells [reviewed by Gospodarowicz *et al.* (252), Thomas (259)]. Half-maximal activity is typically in the range 0.05−5 ng/ml. Sources of FGFs include neural tissue [see above], endothelial cells [Guenther *et al.* (253); Schreiber *et al.* (257)], and normal cells and tumor cells [Klagsbrun *et al.* (268); Moscatelli *et al.* (275)]. There are also major stores of bFGF in cartilage [Sullivan and Klagsbrun (284)], and of both FGFs in bone matrix, where osteoblasts may be responsible for their biosynthesis [Hauschka *et al.* (341, 342)].

Heparin affinity is a key property of the FGFs. Heparin affinity chromatography has streamlined FGF purification and permitted classification of growth factors [Lobb *et al.* (254); Shing *et al.* (280); Sullivan and Klagsbrun (284)]. aFGF, which is generally less active as a mitogen than bFGF *in vitro*, attains equivalent potency in the presence of soluble heparin [Thomas (259)]. The heparin requirement for aFGF potentiation has been reduced to a simple heparin pentasaccharide [Uhlrich *et al.* (260)]. *In vivo* storage of FGFs apparently involves basement membrane structures which are rich in heparan sulfate and other glycosaminoglycans [Folkman *et al.* (265); Baird and Ling (392)]. Mechanisms for release involving heparinase or other agents are clearly important in the overall scheme of FGF action [Baird and Ling (392)].

A focal point of FGF action is angiogenesis [Folkman *et al.* (265); Montesano *et al.* (274)], and this pathway offers hope for intervention in all forms of human disease which involve deficient or excessive neovascularization. TGF-β opposes some of the enhancing effects of bFGF on plasminogen activator release by capillary endothelial cells [Saksela *et al.* (279)]. Mitogenic stimulation of chondrocyte proliferation by FGF is enhanced by TGF-β [Kato *et al.* (267)]. In chondrocytes, IL-1-mediated proteinase release is greatly enhanced by bFGF [Phadke (277)]. A final interesting activity of bFGF is its ability to substitute with high specificity for the morphogenic action of the ventrovegetal (VV) factor in *Xenopus* development [Slack *et al.* (281)].

## Effects in Bone

Mitogenesis is the principal effect of aFGF and bFGF added to bone organ cultures [Canalis (1)] and calvaria-derived osteoblast-like cells [Hauschka *et al.* (341, 342); Rodan *et al.* (256)]. aFGF stimulation of osteoblastic DNA replication is half-maximal at 0.75 ng/ml (47 pM), is enhanced by heparin and IGF-I, and is dependent on the serum concentration. Globus *et al.* (381) found bFGF to be a much more potent mitogen for bovine osteoblastic cells than aFGF [$ED_{50}$ 60 pg/ml and 2 ng/ml, respectively]. Two phenotypic hallmarks of osteoblasts, alkaline phosphatase and PTH-responsive adenylate cyclase, are both decreased strongly by aFGF and mixed BDGF preparations containing FGFs [Hauschka *et al.* (341, 342); Rodan *et al.* (256)]. In the ROS 17/2.8 rat osteosarcoma line, bFGF stimulates proliferation only in the absence of serum, and mRNA levels are reduced for alkaline phosphatase, type I collagen, and osteocalcin, while osteopontin is increased [Rodan *et al.* (278); see Miller and Puzas (273) for other results with UMR and ROS cells]. Interestingly, pertussis toxin (PT) has opposite effects on these parameters, and since bFGF negates the PT effect if both are added together, the bFGF apparently acts distally to the known GTP-binding proteins [Rodan *et al.* (278)]. The recent finding of enhanced osteocalcin formation in bovine osteoblast-like cells treated simultaneously with bFGF and TGF-beta [Globus *et al.* (381)] stands in contrast to the above data, but may reflect the longer assay period (6 days) where an expanded cell population begins to reexpress its differentiated phenotype.

Other Factors

*Interleukin-1 (IL-1)*

Among the regulatory products (monokines) secreted by cells of the monocyte-macrophage lineage, IL-1 is known to exert powerful effects on bone [Dinarello (295); Gowen *et al.* (299); Krane *et al.* (310)]. Sources of IL-1 in bone include monocytes/macrophages [Beresford *et al.* (285); Dinarello (295); Pacifici *et al.* (321)] and osteoblasts [Hanazawa *et al.* (301); Hughes *et al.* (303)]. Monocytic contact with bone matrix surfaces enhances IL-1 production [Pacifici *et al.* (321)]. IL-1 is the most potent known stimulator of bone resorption *in vitro*. Recent work has shown that human osteoclast activating factor (OAF) is identical to IL-1-β [Dewhirst *et al.* (294)]. IL-1-α increases the number of active osteoclasts on bone surfaces [Boyce *et al.* (289)] and enhances multinucleated cell formation in human marrow cultures synergistically with $1,25(OH)_2$ vitamin $D_3$ [Hughes *et al.* (303)]. IL-1-α was several-fold more potent than IL-1-β in stimulating mouse calvaria resorption [Bosma *et al.* (288)], while IL-1-β was more potent as a resorption stimulus in another study [Stashenko *et al.* (330)]. Both factors elevate $PGE_2$ levels, which mediates the resorptive effect, but IL-1-α is unique in that a portion of its resorption-stimulating activity is resistant to indomethacin treatment [Bosma *et al.* (288)]. The short-term ($\leq 7$ days) bone resorbing effects of IL-1-α *in vivo* are also relatively unaffected by indomethacin [Boyce *et al.* (289)]. IL-1, TNF, and lymphotoxin act synergistically in bone resorption [Stashenko *et al.* (330)]. Feedback effects have been noted between glucocorticoids and IL-1 [Besedovsky *et al.* (287)], and this may also have an impact on bone resorption.

With regard to osteoblasts, the net effect of IL-1 is to suppress the phenotypic parameters of bone formation [Beresford *et al.* (285); Canalis (291), Stashenko *et al.* (331, 332)]. IL-1 suppression of collagen synthesis by cultured fetal rat calvaria is synergistically enhanced by TGF-α [Hurley *et al.* (304)]. *In vitro* effects on osteoblasts are serum-dependent, and recombinant IL-1-β can stimulate DNA synthesis in serum-free conditions [Rifas *et al.* (326)]. The critical role of the osteoblast in facilitating bone resorption [Rodan and Martin (407)] probably involves low molecular weight osteoblastic signals which activate osteoclasts [McSheehy and Chambers (317)]. Osteocalcin (bone Gla protein, BGP) and its peptide fragments have been investigated as a possible signal for monocyte recruitment and osteoclast activation [Malone *et al.* (316); Mundy and Poser (320); Lian *et al.* (312); Hauschka (302); Webber *et al.* (336)]. However, the strong suppression of osteocalcin production by IL-1-α and IL-1-β [Stashenko *et al.* (332)]

argues against a role for intact osteocalcin in IL-1—stimulated bone resorption. IL-1-$\beta$ is also observed to elevate TGF-$\beta$ production 4-fold, which could account for some of the IL-1 effects on bone resorption and formation [Rifas *et al.* (326)].

## Tumor Necrosis Factor (TNF)

TNF-alpha from monocytes is homologous to TNF-$\beta$ (lymphotoxin) secreted by lymphocytes [Pennica *et al.* (323)]. By analogy to IL-1, the major effects of TNF on bone are to stimulate resorption and suppress formation [Bertolini *et al.* (286), Stashenko *et al.* (330—332)]. TNF-stimulated resorption involves osteoblasts [Thompson *et al.* (334)]. TNF generally inhibits osteoblastic bone formation and mineralization *in vitro* [Bertolini *et al.* (286), Stashenko *et al.* (332)] and suppresses the response to osteoinductive implants *in vivo* [Yoshikawa and Takaoka (337)]. In contrast, a human osteosarcoma line is mitogenically stimulated by TNF [Kirstein and Baglioni (306)]. TNF has other effects with relevance to bone, including its ability to stimulate angiogenesis [Liebovich *et al.* (313)] and to enhance production of granulocyte/macrophage colony-stimulating factor (GM-CSF) by endothelial cells [Broudy *et al.* (290)].

## $\beta_2$-Microglobulin

One of the bone-active factors (BDGFs) produced by fetal bone cultures was found to be $\beta_2$-microglobulin [Canalis *et al.* (292)]. This protein, which is also a minor serum component, was shown to upregulate the IGF-1 receptor and IGF-1 mRNA, as well as to potentiate the effects of IGF-1 on osteoblastic DNA synthesis [Centrella *et al.* (31)]. $\beta_2$-microglobulin is probably not a bone cell mitogen with the capacity for solitary action [Jennings *et al.* (305)].

## Prostatic Mitogens

The remarkable skeletal consequence of prostatic carcinoma has stimulated interest in potential bone growth factors of prostatic origin. Several mitogens have been isolated and shown to be active on osteoblasts and fibroblasts [Koutsilleris *et al.* (307—309)]. These factors may be similar to those produced by osteoblasts [Linkhart *et al.* (314)]. Benign prostatic hyperplastic tissue produces an NH$_2$-terminal extended form of bFGF [Story *et al.* (283)] which probably accounts for some of the bone-active substances from prostatic cancer.

*Miscellaneous Factors*

Macrophages are known to produce factors which stimulate osteoblasts [Peck *et al.* (322); Rifas *et al.* (325)]. These factors are distinct from IL-1 [Estes *et al.* (297)], but they may be related to PDGF [Kumar *et al.* (228); Shimokado *et al.* (240)]. GTP-binding proteins appear to play a role in regulation of osteoblastic function, apparently by coupling to a variety of membrane receptors [Strewler *et al.* (333)]. Heparin has important effects on bone resorption [Glowacki (300)], and there is a vast clinical bibliography on heparin-induced osteoporosis. Some heparin effects must also be considered to operate through potentiation of aFGF activity [Rodan *et al.* (256); Thomas and Gimenez-Gallego (258)].

*Hematopoietic Factors*

The essential role of bone in providing a home for hematopoietic marrow is an anatomical fact, yet little is known about the biological basis for this interdependence. Establishment of functional bone marrow involves stem cell colonization and proliferation. A variety of specific colony-stimulating factors (CSFs) are required [Metcalf (319); Sachs (327)]. The local production of CSFs by nonhematopoietic cells has been addressed [Chan and Metcalf (293)], and several groups have identified the osteoblast as a likely source. Murine osteoblasts produce CSFs which can affect hematopoiesis [Washington *et al.* (335)], macrophage CSF (M-CSF) was demonstrated in osteoblastic conditioned medium [Elford *et al.* (296)], and both a CSF and a differentiation factor are produced by MC3T3-E1 cells [Shiina-Ishimi *et al.* (328)]. Osteoblastic products other than the common mitogens mentioned above may interact with bone marrow cells in important ways. The abundant matrix protein osteocalcin exhibits CSF activity in marrow cultures [Povolny *et al.* (324)]. In the other direction, osteogenic marrow stromal cells [Owen and Friedenstein (365)] in the endosteal cavity may benefit from growth factors produced by marrow. Healing marrow has been shown to produce osteogenic growth factors [Gazit *et al.* (298)].

## IV Growth Factors in Bone Matrix and Osseous Sources of Growth Factors

Bone is unique because of its abundant mineralized extracellular matrix which may sequester growth factors and modulate their biological action through complex modes of release and presentation to responding cells. Extracellular matrix accounts for about 90% of the total weight of compact bone and is composed of microcrystalline calcium phosphate resembling hydroxyapatite (60%) and fibrillar type I collagen (27%). The remaining 3% consists of minor collagen types and other proteins including osteocalcin, osteonectin, matrix Gla protein, phosphoproteins, sialoproteins and glyco-proteins, as well as proteoglycans, glycosaminoglycans, and lipids. Osteo-blasts are principally responsible for biosynthesis of this complex matrix. Additional levels of compositional and biological complexity are imposed by: 1) matrix adsorption of numerous plasma proteins; 2) osteoclastic remodelling of calcified cartilage during endochondral bone development; 3) the capillary network with its associated endothelial cells and basement membranes; and 4) hematopoietic marrow and blood borne cells including monocytes, the apparent precursors of multinucleated osteoclasts which resorb bone, and other leukocytes which may regulate resorption via mono-kines and lymphokines.

Extraction of growth factors from bone matrix typically requires deminer-alization with HCl or EDTA [Hauschka *et al.* (341)], but this is not adequate evidence to establish the mineralized extracellular matrix as the precise locus of these growth factors. In fact, some or all of these activities could be associated with the cells (osteoblasts, osteocytes, osteoclasts, mesenchymal cells, capillary endothelial cells, monocytes/macrophages, and less abundant types) normally present in compact bone of membranous or endochondral origin. Marrow elements, cartilage, and periosteum are typi-cally excluded by bone powder preparation procedures, and pre-extraction hypotonic washing removes trapped blood and many cytosolic components without releasing appreciable growth factor activity [Hauschka *et al.* (341)]. Ultimate access of aqueous solvents to the growth factors, whether associated with cells, extracellular organic matrix, or hydroxyapatite, requires dissol-ution of the bulk matrix by demineralization. Comparison of various extrac-tion protocols showed that bovine bone powder yielded the greatest total mitogenic activity when extracted with 0.5M EDTA at neutral pH [Hauschka *et al.* (341)]. This result should not be misconstrued as proof for direct binding of growth factors to mineral crystals. In a preliminary study of $^{125}$I-aFGF binding to bone powder fractions, HCl-demineralized bone demonstrated a binding capacity equal to that for whole bone powder [K. Choi and P. V. Hauschka (unpublished)].

How will it be possible, ultimately, to identify and quantitate all the growth factors present in bone matrix? Any growth factor is necessarily defined by a bioassay (eg. quiescent fibroblast mitogenesis), but the activity may show target cell specificity and may not apply to another cell of interest such as the osteoblast. Prerequisites for the study of any single growth factor include: 1) solubilization by a non-destructive extraction technique which simultaneously avoids losses from adsorption and proteo-lysis; 2) a specific screening bioassay with immunity to interference or synergism by other growth factors present in complex samples; and 3)

**Table 2.**

Growth Factor Levels and Sources in Bone

| Factor | Matrix Conc. ng/g dry bone | $ED_{50}$ ng/ml | Osseous Source | | Obl Receptor |
|--------|----------|--------|-----|-------|---------|
| | | | Obl | Other | |
| IGF-I (Sm-C) | 85−170 | 6−100 | + | + | + |
| IGF-II (SGF) | 1260−1750 | 2−3 | + | + | + |
| EGF | 0 | 0.4−200 | ? | ? | + |
| TGF-alpha | 0 | 0.5−30 | ? | ? | + |
| TGF-beta | 400−460 | 0.04−3 | + | + | + |
| PDGF | 50−70 | 3−100 | + | + | + |
| aFGF | 0.5−12 | 0.1−5 | + | + | + |
| bFGF | 40−80 | 0.06−5 | + | + | + |
| IL-1 | | | + | + | + |
| CSF's | + | | + | + | |
| Beta$_2$-mic | | >50,000 | ? | + | |
| Osteogenin | + | | ? | + | |
| BMP | + | | ? | + | |

Osseous sources include proven biosynthesis in cultured osteoblastic cells (Obl), and either biosynthesis by bone organ cultures or extractability from bone matrix (Other). See text for individual references.

precautions for removal of binding proteins and activation of latent factor (eg. with low pH). Because item #2 is virtually unattainable, fractionation and partial purification (eg. heparin-Sepharose) is worthwhile prior to bioassay.

The informative technique of chromatography on heparin-Sepharose, permitting classification of growth factors based on their empirically defined affinity [Lobb et al. (254); Klagsbrun et al. (268); Shing et al. (280)], has been applied to the isolation and partial purification of several bone derived growth factors. The variety of growth factors in bone matrix has been displayed in the heparin-Sepharose chromatogram of an EDTA extract of fetal calf mandible, where at least six separate peaks of mitogenic activity are evident [Hauschka et al. (341)]. The most interesting variation in the BDGF elution pattern was the dramatic shift in relative abundance of two forms of bFGF-like activity eluting at 1.5 and 1.7M NaCl. In adult bovine femur the 1.7M bFGF is abundant, while the 1.5M bFGF species predominates in fetal calf mandible [Hauschka et al. (341)]. Differences stemming from bone maturity and membranous (mandible) vs. endochondral (femur) developmental origin probably account for this observation. Although the exposure of a single factor to proteolytic degradation, or aggregation of a factor with different "carrier" proteins, could theoretically account for multiple peaks in bone, this is unlikely for several reasons. It is now clear that the variety of BDGF's truly represent different types of polypeptide growth factors according to the criteria set forth previously (Hauschka *et al.* 1986). Application of heparin affinity techniques to characterize pathological alteration of growth factor profiles in any tissue resulting from nutritional, metabolic, or hereditary disorders now appears very promising.

The presence of multiple types of polypeptide growth factors in the mineralized extracellular matrix of bone is now well established by work from numerous laboratories (see Table 2) [Canalis *et al.* (338); Hauschka *et al.* (341, 342); Linkhart *et al.* (343); Mohan *et al.* (345); Onizawa (346); Seyedin *et al.* (187−189); Triffitt (388)]. These factors were originally referred to as bone-derived growth factors (BDGFs) [Canalis (1)], but this historical term now encompasses virtually all of the familiar polypeptide growth factors. Dentin matrix also contains at least 3 different growth factors, including IGF-1, PDGF-like, and FGF-like activities [Finkelman *et al.* (339); C. Glass and Hauschka (unpublished)]. In addition to the growth factors shown in Table 2, bone contains chemotactic factors [Landesman and Reddi (311); Lucas *et al.* (315); Malone *et al.* (316); Minkin *et al.* (318); Somerman *et al.* (329)].

Table 2 indicates growth factor concentrations in bone matrix, possible osseous sources of the factors, and the potential for receptor-mediated osteoblastic response. Detailed information regarding the biosynthetic origins of the various growth factors is provided in Section III above. It is fairly certain that osteoblastic cells propagated *in vitro* can produce IGF-I, IGF-II, aFGF, bFGF, TGF-beta 1, TGF-beta 2, IL-1, and CSFs. There is some question regarding PDGF. Most studies of PDGF-like activity have involved osteosarcoma cell lines which are known to express the v-sis oncogene [Betsholtz *et al.* (207, 208), Graves *et al.* (216−219); Heldin *et al.* (222, 223)]. The MG63 human osteosarcoma line does not express v-sis and does not secrete PDGF-like activity [Hauschka *et al.* (341, 342)]. However, a recent study of conditioned medium from normal rat osteoblast-like cells demonstrated PDGF activity by heparin-Sepharose chromatography and immuno-precipitation [Mallory *et al.* (344)]. Wong *et al.* (391) have shown that the late-released cells from collagenase-digested mouse calvaria are the major source of endogenous growth factors, and that both early (fibroblastic) and late (osteoblastic) populations are responsive to these growth factors. Thus, the osteoblast remains a likely candidate for biosynthesis of many of the polypeptide growth factors found in bone matrix (Table 2). The growth factor contributions from other indigenous cell types, and the sequestration from blood circulating through bone, add to the total complexity of these substances in bone matrix. Pathologically derived factors, such as those from tumors, could also lodge in the bone matrix. In a sense, the *origin* of the BDGFs is a moot point, since it has no bearing on their presence in the matrix or their potential regulatory actions on bone cells. Bone exhibits the most complex spectrum of growth factor activities of any tissue yet described.

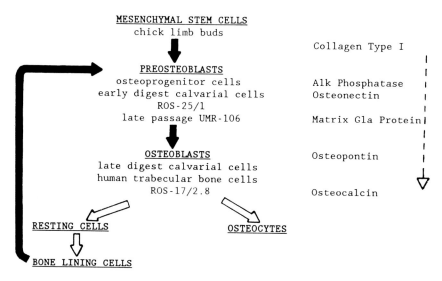

**Fig. 4**  The osteoblastic lineage. Stages of differentiation defined by histological criteria are underlined. The solid arrows indicate the likely progressions which involve cell division. The open arrows indicate progressions which probably do not involve mitosis. Under each stage are indicated the cell types with the most closely related phenotypic properties *in vitro*. At the right is the probable sequence of expression of "osteoblast specific" markers during differentiation and maturation. The various phenotypic properties may be differentially sensitive to proliferation rate, extracellular matrix, hormonal signals, and growth factor activities. Thus it is unclear from the disparate properties of many osteoblastic cell types whether the phenotypic characteristics are normally expressed in a *linear progression* (eg. − −→) or a *branched pathway* as differentiation proceeds.

In bovine bone powder free of blood and cartilage contamination the volume concentration of mitogens is hundreds of times greater than in serum.

## V. Target Cells for Growth Factors within the Osteoblastic Lineage

The osteoblastic lineage (Fig. 4) is of mesenchymal origin [Nijweide *et al.* (364); Owen and Friedenstein (365); Tenenbaum (374) and see chapter 2]. Histological definitions of cells within the lineage focus on morphology and topological orientation to the mineralized extracellular matrix [Jones *et al.* (359); Miller and Jee (363); Nijweide *et al.* (364)]. Biochemical and physiological definitions of bone cell phenotypes are in their infancy [Aubin *et al.* (347); Aufmkolk *et al.* (348); Bellows *et al.* (349); Beresford *et al.* (350); Catherwood *et al.* (351); Chen *et al.* (352–354); Ecarot-Charrier *et al.* (355); Feyen *et al.* (356); Gerstenfeld *et al.* (357); Hamilton *et al.* (358); Kodama *et al.* (360); Majeska *et al.* (361); Manolagas *et al.* (362); Partridge *et al.*

(366, 367); Peck and Rifas (368); Robey and Termine (370); Rodan *et al.* (371); Rosen and Luben (372); Sakamoto and Sakamoto (373); Wong (375); Yoon *et al.* (376)]. In general, only the mesenchymal stem cell (osteoprogenitor cell) and preosteoblast are considered to have high mitotic activity. The remaining cells normally do not divide, yet under appropriate stimulus, all cells including the osteoblast, osteocyte, resting osteoblast, and bone lining cell are capable of proliferation [Miller and Jee (363)]. Osteoblast-like cells can be propagated in primary culture, and osteocytes apparently revert to osteoblastic behavior if released from trabecular bone [Peck and Rifas (368); Robey and Termine (370)]. Referring to the cell cycle (Fig. 3), osteoblasts and osteocytes are likely to be in a prolonged $G_1$ or $G_0$ state *in vivo*, but probably do not undergo terminal differentiation.

## Osteoblast differentiation and phenotypic expression

Many phenotypic characteristics have been identified for osteoblast-like cells in culture, including: a) biosynthesis of type I collagen, b) high alkaline phosphatase specific activity, c) PTH-dependent adenylate cyclase activation, d) prostaglandin $E_2$ production, e) biosynthesis of osteonectin, osteopontin, other bone phosphoproteins, proteoglycans, and collagenase, and f) $1,25(OH)_2$ vitamin $D_3$-dependent production of osteocalcin and matrix Gla protein (see Chapters 5 & 7). Some of these properties, particularly the former, are expressed by virtually all primary osteoblasts, clonal osteoblast lines, and osteosarcoma cells in culture. However certain properties such as osteocalcin, osteopontin, and matrix Gla protein synthesis may be more volatile aspects of the phenotype, requiring suitable culture conditions for expression [Gerstenfeld *et al.* (357); Rodan *et al.* (371)] (see Fig. 4). In normal bone development the temporal sequence of expression of "bone specific" markers parallels the stages of osteoblastic differentiation (Fig. 4). Osteocalcin appears to be a "late" marker [Rodan *et al.* (371)], characteristic of mature osteoblasts and the ROS 17/2.8 osteosarcoma line. Importantly, osteocalcin mRNA is the last of several osteoblastic markers to be expressed in developing rat calvaria [Yoon *et al.* (376)], coinciding with the approximate onset of mineralization.

## VI. Phenotypic Modulation of Osteoblasts by Growth Factors

Experimental results concerning polypeptide growth factor effects in bone must be clearly differentiated with regard to the model system in which they have been studied: 1) *in vivo*; 2) *in vitro* bone organ culture; or 3) *in vitro* bone cell (osteoblast) culture. The dilemma faced by researchers in this field should be apparent to the reader cognizant of the information in Sections III and IV: mechanistic interpretation of *in vivo* and organ culture

**Table 3.**
Phenotypic Responses of Osteoblastic Cells *in Vitro*

| | Calvarial Osteoblasts | | | | | ROS 17/2.8 Osteosarcoma | | |
| --- | --- | --- | --- | --- | --- | --- | --- | --- |
| | *TGF-β* | *bFGF* | *aFGF* | *PDGF* | *BDGFs** | *TGF-β* | *bFGF* | *PTH* |
| Proliferation | +/− | + | + | + | + | − | +/0 | |
| Alk phosphatase | − | − | − | − | − | + | − | |
| PTH stim cAMP | | − | − | | − | | | |
| Collagen Type I | + | | | | | + | | |
| Osteocalcin | +/− | − | − | − | − | − | − | + |
| Osteopontin | + | | | | | + | + | − |
| Mineralization | − | | | | | | | |

* Mixed total growth factors (BDGFs) extracted from bovine bone matrix by EDTA [Hauschka *et al.* (341)]. Composition reflected in Table 2. See text for references to individual studies.

experiments is severely complicated by the plethora of cell types and growth factors, whereas extrapolation of *in vitro* osteoblastic responses to the complex *in vivo* milieu is hazardous. Complete description of the biological functions of growth factors which are relevant to bone will ultimately depend on many specific bioassays involving individual and mixed specific cell types *in vitro*, as well as *in vivo* animal models for skeletal development, osteoinduction, fracture healing, and remodeling. Fundamental work with fetal rat calvaria showed that EGF, FGF, PDGF,and IGF-I generally stimulated cellular proliferation, EGF and FGF depressed formation of the collagenous extracellular matrix, while PDGF and IGF-I stimulated collagen synthesis [Canalis (1), Canalis *et al.* (2)]. PDGF, EGF/TGF-α, and TGF-β also play a role in bone resorption in organ culture, as they stimulate calcium release by a prostaglandin-mediated mechanism [Tashjian and Levine (118); Tashjian *et al.* (119, 192, 243)].

Phenotypic properties of osteoblastic cells are useful in monitoring the responses to growth factors. However, it is essential to recognize the very different basal states of differentiation and expression for various model cell types (Fig. 4). A summary table of the growth factor responses of normal osteoblastic cells freshly isolated from bone, and the ROS 17/2.8 osteosarcoma cell line reveals some major differences (Table 3). In particular, TGF-β has opposite effects on proliferation, alkaline phosphatase, and osteocalcin, but parallel effects on collagen and osteopontin [Centrella *et al.* (138); Noda *et al.* (164−166), Robey *et al.* (181); Wrana *et al.* (201, 202)]. Even for normal rat calvarial osteoblasts comparing term fetal material to newborn, there is a 3- to 5-fold decrease in the mitogenic sensitivity to TGF-β during a one day period [Centrella *et al.* (138)]. The hazards inherent in extending these findings to osseous tissue *in vivo* are obvious. Studies with primary rat osteoblast-like cells exposed either to the mixed growth factors present in bone extracts, or to pure TGF-β, or heparin-purified PDGF, aFGF, or bFGF from bovine bone have shown a general dose-dependent mitogenic effect. Phenotypic changes which accompany the BDGF-induced wave of proliferation include decreased osteocalcin secretion and a reduction in $1,25(OH)_2$-vitamin $D_3$-stimulated osteocalcin synthesis, reduced alkaline phosphatase specific activity, and decreased cAMP responsiveness to PTH [Hauschka et al. (341, 342)].

Target cell specificity is an issue of great importance in bone where so many factors and cellular responses are possible. Most of the growth factors found in bone matrix are generally active on mesodermally derived cells, but several factors have apparent target cell selectivity for stimulation of fibroblasts (F), chondrocytes (C), osteoblasts (O), and capillary endothelial cells (E). A typical example is PDGF which is mitogenic for F and O but not E [Hauschka et al. (341)]. Other suggestions of target cell specificity include: endothelial cell-derived growth factor (ECDGF) [O, but not F or C [Guenther et al. (253)]]; macrophage-derived growth factor (MDGF) [O and C, but not F [Rifas et al. (325)]]; prostatic tumor factor [O, but not F [Koutsilleris et al. (307)]; and IGF-II(SGF) [O and C, but not F [Farley and Baylink (38); Mohan et al. (57)]]. The failure of IGF-II to act on fibroblasts in the latter study is puzzling in view of the potency of IGF-I and IGF-II on fibroblasts observed by others [King and Kahn (49)]. Similar criticism could apply to the other specificity studies. ECDGF and prostatic tumor factor contain forms of FGF which should act on fibroblasts, while MDGF contains PDGFs and IL-1, which should also affect fibroblasts in addition to osteoblasts. Further substantiation of these findings with well defined assay systems is important. A growth factor with osteoblastic specificity would be an extremely significant scientific development.

While mitogenesis is often the focus of interest in growth factors, of equal importance is the potential hormonal action by which specific differentiated functions of *non-proliferating* cell populations may be regulated. Typical of many cell types, for the osteoblast the states of proliferation vs. differentiation are often at odds. Growth factor enhancement of some osteoblastic functions are shown in Table 3. Growth factors may also regulate osteoblastic collagenase [Sakamoto and Sakamoto (373)] similar to their elevation of this enzyme in fibroblasts. Of particular relevance to bone may be the enhanced protein kinase activity and the intracellular $Ca^{2+}$ mobilization accompanying growth factor stimulation of cells. Such stimulation could provide for the special needs of mineralizing tissues involving calcium phosphate mineral deposition and the prolific biosynthesis and secretion of phosphorylated proteins into the extracellular matrix.

## VII. Multiple Growth Factor Effects: Synergism / Antagonism

The possible responses to mixtures of growth factors expand geometrically with the ever lengthening lists of growth factor species (Table 1), carrier proteins, target cells, and membrane receptors. At present there are a number of clear binary and ternary effects of growth factor combinations. Perhaps the first example of synergism was the distinction drawn by Stiles and colleagues between *competence* and *progression* factors in serum [see Section II; Rollins *et al.* (238); Stiles *et al.* (19)]. Certain growth factors such as PDGF provide the competence for quiescent cells to escape $G_0$ or a prolonged $G_1$ phase, while other growth factors such as IGF-I speed the progression through the cell cycle. Concurrent availability of both types of factors would insure proliferation, provided that the nutritional environment is complete. With the knowledge now available regarding autocrine production of growth factors by osteoblasts and other cell types, it is difficult to pinpoint the exact growth factor requirements for maintenance of proliferating vs. differentiated populations. A recent study of the MG63 human osteosarcoma showed that IGF-I was mitogenic, and that the competence factor PDGF failed to enhance this mitogenesis despite its induction of c-myc [Womer *et al.* (246)]. PDGF thus appears to be uncoupled for mitogenesis in MG63 cells. It is not known whether constitutive production of FGF-like activity by MG63 cells [Hauschka *et al.* (341, 342)] might provide the necessary competence factor in this system.

Synergism between TGF-β and EGF (or TGF-α) is well known, and the standard assay for TGF-β involving anchorage-independent growth of NRK cells in soft agar invokes this phenomenon [Roberts *et al.* (179); Inman and Colowick (154); Massague (159)]. Other studies have shown a requirement for IGFs and PDGF in the TGF-β transformation of normal fibroblasts [Massague *et al.* (382)]. It has been postulated that full mitogenic stimulation by the complete set of growth factors (EGF, IGFs, and PDGF) is a prerequisite for the transforming action of TGF-β [Massague *et al.* (382)]. For osteoblastic cells, TGF-β can enhance the mitogenic effects of aFGF and bFGF [Globus *et al.* (381)], while for capillary endothelial cells TGF-β antagonizes mitogenesis by FGF [Baird and Durkin (377).]

The growth factor cocktail (see Table 2) derived from bone matrix extracts [Hauschka *et al.* (341, 342); Linkhart *et al.* (343)] or from cultured bones and bone cells [Canalis *et al.* (1, 2); Mallory *et al.* (344); Wong *et al.* (391)] is generally mitogenic for osteoblastic cells. In fact, the combined application of a bovine bone extract with other known growth factors stimulated osteoblastic DNA synthesis to a greater extent than the known growth factors alone [Linkhart *et al.* (343)]. Much of this complex synergy depends on TGF-β. The mitogenic effects of EGF, bFGF, and TNF-α on rat osteoblastic cells are inverted by shifting the TGF-β concentration from 0.04nM to 0.4nM [Centrella *et al.* (379)]. Robey *et al.* (181) have documented the importance of serum concentration on TGF-β effects. With bovine osteoblastic cells, TGF-β potentiates the mitogenic effects of aFGF and bFGF [Globus *et al.* (381)].

In other model systems TGF-β has been observed to interfere with the actions of FGF-class growth factors. Capillary endothelial cell mitogenesis by aFGF and bFGF is inhibited by TGF-β [Baird and Durkin (377)]. Production of plasminogen activator, induced by bFGF treatment of capillary endothelial cells, is also suppressed by TGF-β [Saksela *et al.* (279)]. Lymphocyte mitogenesis triggered by IL-1 is blocked by TGF-β [Wahl *et al.* (390)].

Finally, hormones and other agents have a critical impact on growth-factor-dependent events. Retinoic acid, an inducer of terminal differentiation, suppresses c-myc expression and upregulates EGF receptors [Sporn *et al.* (387)]. Glucocorticoids such as hydrocortisone enhance the mitogenic response of osteoblastic cells to mixed autocrine growth factors [Wong *et al.* (391)]. PTH modulates TGF-β effects in rat calvarial osteoblast cultures [Centrella *et al.* (140−142)] and has profound effects on autocrine IGF-I production and IGF-I receptor levels [McCarthy *et al.* (56)].

## VIII. Possible Mechanisms for Activation, Release, and Presentation of Growth Factors in Bone

Faced with the challenge of numerous growth factors provided by its bone matrix environment, as well as by autocrine, paracrine, and endocrine sources, the osteoblast may display a variety of responses. Limiting our consideration to the *local* environment, we must make clear distinctions between 1) *matrix growth factor activation/release*, and 2) *local growth factor biosynthesis*.

Clearly, a strong case can be made for the existence of high levels of many growth factors in bone matrix (see Table 2 and Section IV). The volume concentration of total bone growth factor activity shown in Table 2 is at least 1000 growth factor units (GFU) per $cm^3$, assuming an average density of 1.9 $g/cm^3$ for bone powder. A concentration of 5 GFU/ml *in vitro* causes half-maximal mitogenic stimulation [Hauschka *et al.* (341)]. Thus bone matrix harbors about 100 times more mitogenic activity than would be required to cause maximal mitogenic stimulation of BALB/c 3T3 fibroblasts, capillary endothelial cells, and osteoblasts [Hauschka *et al.* (341, 342)]. If TGF-β is considered, its level of ~400 ng/g bone powder [Seyedin *et al.* (187−189)] is also about 1000-fold greater than the 0.6−1.5 ng/ml necessary for osteoblastic stimulation [Centrella *et al.* (138); Robey *et al.* (181)]. A similar excess is observed for IGFs in bone matrix [Frolik *et al.* (40); Mohan *et al.* (59)]. While the growth factor activity in bone appears high, especially in contrast with the 50−100 GFU/ml (principally PDGF) for calf serum, it is modest in comparison with the 20,000 GFU of aFGF/g wet weight of bovine brain [Giminez-Gallego *et al.* (251); Lobb *et al.* (254)], and the 30,000 GFU of hepatoma GF activity/g packed human hepatoma cells [Klagsbrun *et al.* (268)]. Obviously, the bone matrix must play an important role in sequestering and masking its growth factors, since the cells of bone are not continuously proliferating. Another factor is the dose-dependence of the osteoblastic response. While TGF-$\beta$ is mitogenic, this response vanishes at non-optimal cell densities and growth factor concentrations [Centrella *et al.* (138); Robey *et al.* (181)]. Hence the tremendous level of TGF-$\beta$ in bone (Table 2) may be incapable of osteoblastic stimulation, except under "wound healing" situations where osteoblastic cell density on matrix surfaces is reduced.

By what mechanisms might the abundant growth factor content of bone matrix be exposed, activated, and/or released to act locally on responsive cells? *Mechanical* and *cell mediated* processes are both important, and in turn are subject to hierarchical control by genetics, age, functional loading, and endocrine status.

## Mechanical Phenomena

Fracture is a simple event whereby bone matrix surfaces are instantaneously exposed to a new population of cells. Immediate dissolution of surface components could allow leaching of growth factors and establishment of chemoattractant gradients prior to the colonization of these surfaces by cells. Eventually the cell-mediated processes would take over as newly recruited osteoclasts initiate their resorption [Glowacki (300)]. The involvement of growth factors in a rat femur fracture repair model is under intensive study [Bolander (410)].

In the normal mechanical loading cycles to which bones are exposed during routine muscular contraction, exercise, and weight-bearing, microstrain (microfracture) displacements are known to occur. As with gross fractures, these small imperfections could release growth factors and initiate a local biological response involving osteoclasts and/or osteoblasts [Burr *et al.* (397)]. The long-term effect of microfracture repair has been developed into a "mechanostat" theory [Frost (401)] which could be the underlying basis for Wolff's Law. Piezoelectric and electromechanical consequences of stressing the skeleton also have direct effects on the migration of bone cells [Ferrier *et al.* (400)], but the relationship to growth factors is unknown (see Volume 7 of this series).

## Osteoclastic Cell-Mediated Phenomena

The interplay between osteoblasts and osteoclasts in bone resorption is well recognized [Rodan and Martin (407), and see Chapter 8]. The osteoblast plays an essential, permissive role in initiating resorption [McSheehy and Chambers (317)]. The osteoclast has garnered much attention because of 1) its direct role in bulk dissolution of bone matrix (with a high growth factor content) and 2) the *coupling phenomenon* which links local osteoblastic proliferation and bone formation with the osteoclastic resorption lacuna [Howard *et al.* (403); Parfitt (406)]. While many have assumed that osteoclast-mediated growth factor release accounts for coupling [Farley and Baylink (38); Mohan *et al.* (57−59); Pfeilschifter *et al.* (173−176)], there are serious arguments against such an interpretation. These arguments include the osteoclastic resorption mechanism, the time lag between resorption and osteoblastic proliferation, the presence of other macrophage-like cells in the freshly denuded resorption lacuna, and the response of osteoblasts and their precursors to the bare bone matrix.

The basic elements of the osteoclastic resorption mechanism include: 1) attachment to bone following permissive withdrawal by osteoblasts (possibly attended by collagenase dissolution of osteoid), 2) acidification of the subosteoclastic compartment, 3) release of lysosomal enzymes including acid proteinases, 4) demineralization and degradation of the underlying matrix, 5) secretion or release of matrix components, and 6) migration to a new site. [Baron *et al.* (394, 395); Blair *et al.* (396); Chambers and Fuller (398); Rodan and Martin (407); Sakamoto and Sakamoto (373); Shimizu *et al.* (408)]. Could matrix-bound growth factors survive such treatment and retain their activity? In principle, only a small fraction ($>1\%$) need survive to provide locally stimulatory growth factor levels (Table 2). The tightly disulfide crosslinked growth factors including EGF, TGF-alpha, IGFs, PDGF, and TGF-beta are stable to heat and low pH, but acid proteinase sensitivity is unclear. A bFGF-like activity in bone was found to be relatively resistant to tryptic digestion [Hauschka *et al.* (341)]. Acidic conditions *per se* can effect direct extraction of matrix growth factors [Hauschka *et al.* (341)] and may also strip factors such as IGF-I from specific binding proteins [Wilkins and D'Ercole (77)].

TGF-$\beta$ has unique precursor and latent forms which could actually be activated in the sub-osteoclastic compartment. In serum, TGF-$\beta$ is bound to $\alpha_2$-macroglobulin from which it can be released in active form by transient acidification to pH 3 [O'Connor-McCourt and Wakefield (167)]. Latent TGF-$\beta$ in platelets is a 220−235 kDa complex containing mature TGF-$\beta$ (25 kDa), the 74 kDa remainder of proTGF-$\beta$, and a 135 kDa protein in noncovalent association [Wakefield *et al.* (200)]. This latent complex can also be activated by transient acidification, and the released

TGF-β is then able to associate with $\alpha_2$-macroglobulin. Since $\alpha_2$-macroglobulin is a general trap for proteinases, it is of interest that plasmin and perhaps other proteinases can activate latent TGF-β [Keski-Oja et al. (404)]. The proportion of bone matrix TGF-β which is either latent or complexed with $\alpha_2$-macroglobulin is unknown, although acid enhancement of TGF-β activity in bone organ culture has been demonstrated [Pfeilschifter et al. (173, 174)]. However, whether this appealing mechanism is actually operative *in vivo* is uncertain. The observations that PTH induced resorption releases active TGF-β [Pfeilschifter et al. (173—175)] and SGF/IGF-II [Farley et al. (39, 39b); Mohan et al. (58); Wergedal et al. (75)] in bone organ cultures do not adequately address the origin of these factors. Osteoblasts produce TGF-β [Centrella and Canalis (136); Robey et al. (181)] as well as IGF-I and IGF-II [Canalis et al. (29); Frolik et al. (40); Wergedal et al. (75)]. PTH can directly enhance IGF-I production by osteoblastic cells [McCarthy et al. (56)]. PTH treatment of osteoblasts also elicits a *contact-mediated* mitogenic stimulation of periosteal fibroblasts (and putative pre-osteoblasts) [Van der Plas and Nijweide (409)]. Because this effect cannot be transmitted by conditioned medium, it raises the possibility of a new type of locally acting factor in the coupling phenomenon.

A final unanswered question concerning osteoclast action bears on the growth factor release mechanism. How are matrix components cleared from the sub-osteoclastic compartment? If the clear zone attachment remains tight for the duration of the resorption cycle, then extensive proteolysis by a combination of extracellular and endocytotic, lysosome-mediated digestion would be expected for all but the most resistant or specially protected proteins. However, if the osteoclast-bone matrix attachment is periodically broken during locomotion, spilling of the compartmental contents could perhaps release growth factors in active form.

## Osteoblast Cell-Mediated Phenomena

In addition to its importance as a primary producer of growth factors in bone, the osteoblast could effect the release of matrix-bound factors by several mechanisms. Proteinase activities of osteoblasts, particularly the osteoblastic collagenase [Sakamoto and Sakamoto (373)], could excise growth factors from osteoid and pericellular binding sites. In turn, the expression of collagenase and other proteinases is subject to regulation by hormones and growth factors in osteoblastic cells [Chikuma et al. (86); Partridge et al. (110)] and in fibroblasts [Chua et al. (88)]. Osteoblast-mediated exposure of hydroxyapatite has also been suggested as a prerequisite for osteoclastic degradation [Rodan and Martin (407); Chambers and Fuller (396)].

Baird and Ling (392) have demonstrated another potentially important release mechanism for heparin-binding growth factors such as aFGF and bFGF. Because these factors are apparently tightly bound to heparan sulfate-containing glycosaminoglycans in basement membranes [Folkman *et al.* (265)], local digestion of these glycosaminoglycans could effect FGF release and initiate a strong local mitogenic signal to capillary endothelial cells. By way of controlled secretion of heparinase or heparatinase activities, cells from tumors and perhaps normal tissues could trigger neovascularization without the specific requirement for *de novo* synthesis of angiogenic growth factors [Baird and Ling (392)]. Bone matrix is known to contain heparan sulfate-rich proteoglycans and high levels of FGFs, but the capacity for osteoblastic or osteoclastic expression of heparinase-like activity is unstudied. In principle, the secretion or activation of an osteoblastic proteinase or heparinase could initiate a cascade release of other growth factors into the local environment. Proliferation of osteoblasts and endothelial cells would be the likely consequence.

## Surface Phenomena

A layer of unmineralized osteoid typically separates osteoblasts from the true bone matrix [Jones *et al.* (359)]. Only when osteoblastic collagenase is activated, as perhaps in the initiation of bone resorption by PTH [Rodan and Martin (407); Sakamoto and Sakamoto (373)], is this osteoid layer lost and contact of osteoclasts with mineralized matrix achieved. Resorption lacunae produced by episodic osteoclast action apparently contain some residual fibrillar collagen [Shimizu *et al.* (408)] and may thus have a surface chemistry analogous to demineralized bone powder (DBP), a known osteo-inductive material.

Cellular response to mineralized bone particle surfaces *in vivo* is dominated by osteoclastic recruitment and resorption [Glowacki (300)]. *In vitro*, this particle resorption response is recapitulated with monocytes [Lian *et al.* (312)] and isolated osteoclasts [Blair *et al.* (396)], as well as on bone slices [Chambers and Fuller (398); Shimizu *et al.* (408)]. Bone matrix also increases osteoclast differentiation in a rabbit marrow culture system [Fuller and Chambers (402)]. The acid demineralization of bone surfaces, or the coating with extra collagen, reduces osteoclast attachment and excavation [Chambers and Fuller (398); Shimizu *et al.* (408)]. DBP *in vivo* elicits a totally different cellular response, namely a cascade of osteoinduction [see Section IX]. The collagenous surface of DBP is apparently mitogenic for mesenchymal cells [Landesman and Reddi (311); Kapur and Reddi (413); Rath and Reddi (413b)]. Another potentially important finding is the mitogenic effect of calcium phosphate powder [Barnes and Colowick (393)]. Could the direct contact of osteoblasts or osteoprogenitor cells with the mineralized bone surface trigger proliferation?

Colonization of the resorption lacuna is initiated after a "reversal phase"

LOCAL FACTORS AND BONE REMODELLING

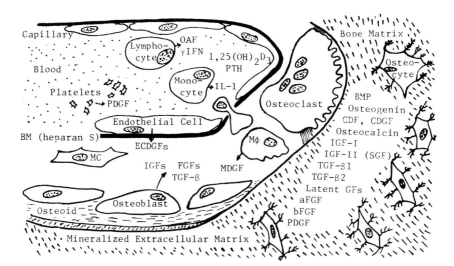

**Fig. 5** Complex topological relationship between the indigenous bone cell types and the various growth factors and other effector proteins of bone. An osteoclast leads a capillary into dense bone, forming a typical "cutting cone". Growth factors in plasma and those produced by blood-borne cells and capillary endothelial cells thereby gain intimate access to the bone matrix. Many growth factors are also produced by osteoblasts and macrophages. Factors trapped in the matrix may be released by the mining behavior of the osteoclast, or activated by the acidic pH of the sub-osteoclastic compartment, causing local stimulation of osteoblastic proliferation and bone formation (coupling). Alternately, macrophage-like cells and osteoblasts, the two early colonists of the resorption lacuna, can produce a spectrum of growth factors which could also explain the coupling phenomenon.

by macrophage-like cells, and the contact of these cells with bone matrix might be expected to elicit increased IL-1 secretion [Pacifici *et al.* (321)]. The chemotaxis of macrophages for TGF-β [Wahl *et al.* (390)] may also be involved in early colonization if chemotactically active bone matrix TGF-β is released in the resorption site. Macrophage production of PDGF-like factors [Kumar *et al.* (228), Shimokado *et al.* (240); Estes *et al.* (297); Peck *et al.* (322)], along with other factors mentioned above, could promote the subsequent proliferative invasion by osteoblasts and the "coupling" of new bone formation with resorption.

Figure 5 depicts the topology of the resorption lacuna in a "cutting cone", where capillary ingrowth into bone to form a new osteon is led by one or more osteoclasts. The coupling of new bone formation to resorption [Howard *et al.* (403), Parfitt (406)] has an analog in the coupling of neovascularization to resorption. These corollaries are governed by the same arguments regarding local production of new growth factors *vs.* osteoclastic mining and activation of bone matrix factors.

There is no compelling reason to expect all examples of bone growth to be equally dependent on the coupling phenomenon. In rapid growth of the developing skeleton, osteoblastic formation clearly dominates resorption, and appositional osteogenesis may persist locally in the virtual absence of osteoclasts. This contrasts with adult bone maintenance and remodeling, where osteoclastic action probably initiates each local remodeling cycle.

## IX. Osteoinduction as an *In Vivo* Model for Growth Factor Effects

One way to assess the multitude of possible interactions between the dozen osseous cell types and as many growth factors is to study the process *in vivo*. At first this might appear to be the incorrect approach, but its value lies in the more realistic modeling of all the competitive, antagonistic, and synergistic possibilities discussed above. A single growth factor acting on a single cell type *in vitro* may yield clear and interesting data, but such models are hopelessly simple and offer minimal predictive value for skeletal tissue *in vivo*.

The pioneering research of Urist, Huggins, and Reddi established useful models where osteoinduction could be studied *in vivo* in response to HCl-demineralized bone [Urist *et al.* (421, 422); Reddi (415)]. Careful study of the temporal response to DBP in rats has shown that the osteoinductive process essentially recapitulates the stages [Fig. 1] of endochondral bone formation to the endpoint of a remodelled ossicle filled with hematopoietic marrow [Reddi (415)]. Importantly, Reddi and Sampath were able to dissect the active factor from DBP and develop reconstituted implants which allowed assay and purification of the osteoinductive protein [Sampath *et al.* (417)]. Several forms of this protein which has been called "osteogenin", "osteoinductive protein", and "BMP" (bone morphogenetic protein, the original terminology of Urist), have been cloned and sequenced by biotechnology companies. The information to date suggests limited homology to TGF-β [Wozney *et al.* (416)], but biological activity of genetically engineered BMP is yet to be fully achieved.

Certain implanted tumors have osteogenic effects on surrounding soft tissues of the host [Forster *et al.* (411); Yoshikawa *et al.* (425, 426)] and on the periosteum [Wlodarski and Reddi (424)]. These and other potential sources of osteoinductive factors have been explored [Seyedin *et al.* (187−189); Tornberg and Bassett (420)].

The osteoinductive cascade may be triggered by a single osteoinductive protein, or there may be requirements for a progression of separate growth factors which must be provided at discrete times. The potential role of other growth factors in osteoinduction is accessible through manipulation of the reconstituted implant system [Sampath *et al.* (417)]. The total guanidine hydrochloride-extractable material from DBP, which contains the osteo-inductive protein as well as other growth factors [Hauschka *et al.* (341)], has been shown to produce dose-dependent acceleration and amplification of the osteoinductive response in rats [Spampata *et al.* (419); Werther *et al.* (423)]. Howes *et al.* (412) have incorporated 100 ng quantities of pure growth factors into osteoinductive DBP implants to examine the effect on host response. Interestingly, only PDGF (but not EGF, FGF, insulin, or TGF-β) was found to enhance osteoinduction compared to unsupplemented DBP, and this enhancement was observed only in mature (250g) rats in which osteoinduction is typically less robust than in young (70g) hosts. During the first few days of implantation, growth factors such as TGF-β which are present in DBP are normally lost, only to appear later as newly synthesized products of indigenous cells [Carrington *et al.* (134)]. Hence, before ruling out the participation of common growth factors in osteo-induction, they must be experimentally delivered at various times and doses.

## X. Future Directions for Bone Growth Factor Resarch

As growth factors become biochemically defined and accessible in large quantities, the exploration of their effects in the skeletal system will begin. Extrapolating from the information reviewed in this chapter, there will be many new testable hypotheses relevant to bone physiology and cell biology which involve growth factors. A major dilemma will be to design meaningful and effective delivery systems for growth factors. Where and when should they be delivered to an experimental model, and at what frequency and concentration? The complexities of synergy, antagonism, and biphasic re-sponse to growth factors are typical even with a well-defined and isolated model of cultured osteoblastic cells. One criticism which applies to most *in vitro* studies is the failure to characterize the endogenous background of autocrine factors throughout the experiment. Thus an effect produced by addition of factor A could be erroneously interpreted because it was actually produced by upregulation of receptors for endogenous factor B. An expanding panel of specific growth factor and receptor assays must be applied to culture systems to overcome these problems. There is a certain appeal to making empirical observations in animal models, but the mechanistic interpretation becomes virtually impossible.

While many growth factors act on target cells in a soluble form, others are probably presented in an adsorbed state on hydroxyapatite or organic matrix components. In distinction to endocrine, paracrine, and autocrine routes for growth factor stimulation, cellular interaction with matrix-adsorbed factors could be called "matricrine" [Hauschka *et al.* (342)]. The extracellular matrix apparently plays a critical role in controlling the distribution and presentation of growth factors. First, the matrix provides a temporally extended storage depot for local messages awaiting decipherment by cells which arrive on the scene long after the producing cell has departed or ceased to function. During bone remodeling, growth factors such as IGFs, FGFs, or TGF-β produced by chondrocytes and other cells during the endochondral phase of osteogenesis could be zonally concentrated and redistributed in bone matrix, only to be released at a later time by micro-fracture, gross fracture, or hormone-mediated osteoclastic remodeling. Second, the enhanced extracellular matrix biosynthesis in response to a local burst of growth factors could provide a sink for adsorption of these factors to new matrix; this feedback loop could prevent the triggering of a runaway response. The well characterized systemic responses of the skeleton to endocrine signals cannot explain the complex patterns of bone growth and remodelling which are exquisitely sensitive to local physical stresses (Wolff's Law). In a dense, labyrinthine mineralized tissue such as bone, with many barriers to the free diffusion of circulating hormones, it is provocative that these local responses may be regulated by the reservoir of specific growth factors in the matrix and by the local production of growth factors.

## Acknowledgements

Supported by grants AR38349 and DE08235 from the National Institutes of Health, DHHS.

## References

### I. Growth Factors and Their Relevance to Bone Growth

1. Canalis, E. (1985). Effect of growth factors on bone cell replication and differentiation. *Clin. Orthop.*, **193**: 246–63.
2. Canalis, E, McCarthy, T. and Centrella, M. (1988). Growth factors and the regulation of bone remodeling. *J. Clin. Invest.*, **81**: 277–81.
3. Glimcher, M. J. (1981). On the form and function of bone: from molecules to organs. Wolff's Law revisited. In *The Chemistry and Biology of Mineralized Connective Tissues*, A Veis, ed., Elsevier North Holland, New York, pp. 617–73.

### II. General Features of Receptor-Mediated Growth Factor Action

4. Ballard, F. J., Knowles, S. E., Wong, S. C., Bodner, J. B., Wood, C. M. and Gunn, J. M. (1980). Inhibition of protein breakdown is a consistent response to growth factors. *FEBS Lett.*, **114**: 209–12.
5. Barber, J. R., Sassone-Corsi, P. and Verma, I. M. (1987). Proto oncogene fos: factors

affecting expression and covalent modification of the gene product. *Ann. NY Acad. Sci.*, **511**: 117—30.

6. Berridge, M. J. (1987). Inositol triphosphate and diacylglycerol: two interacting second messengers. *Ann. Rev. Biochem.*, **56**: 159—93.

7. Bradshaw, R. A. and Prentis, S., eds. (1987). *Oncogenes and Growth Factors*, Elsevier, Amsterdam

8. Carpenter, G. (1987). Receptors for epidermal growth factor and other polypeptide mitogens. *Ann. Rev. Biochem.*, **56**: 881—914.

9. Clegg, C. H., Linkhart, T. A., Olwin, B. B. and Hauschka, S. D. (1987). Growth factor control of skeletal muscle differentiation: commitment to terminal differentiation occurs in $G_1$ phase and is repressed by fibroblast growth factor. *J. Cell. Biol.*, **105**: 949—56.

10. Clemmons, D. R., Van Wyk, J. J. and Pledger, W. J. (1980). Sequential addition of platelet factor and plasma to BALB/c 3T3 fibroblast cultures stimulates somatomedin-C binding early in cell cycle. *Proc. Natl. Acad. Sci. USA*, **77**: 6644—8.

11. Deuel, T. F. (1987). Polypeptide growth factors: roles in normal and abnormal cell growth. *Ann. Rev. Cell. Biol.*, **3**: 443—92.

12. Gilman, A. G. (1987). G proteins: transducers of receptor-generated signals. *Ann. Rev. Biochem.*, **56**: 615—49.

13. Limbird, L. (1988). Receptors linked to inhibition of adenylate cyclase: additional signaling mechanisms. *FASEB J.*, **2**: 2686—95.

14. Leof, E. B., Proper, J. A., Goustin, A. S., Shipley, G. D., DiCorletto P. E. and Moses, H. L. (1986). Induction of c-sis mRNA and activity similar to platelet-derived growth factor by transforming growth factor beta: a proposed model for indirect mitogenesis involving autocrine activity. *Proc. Natl. Acad. Sci. USA*, **83**: 2453—7.

15. Rollins, B. J. and Stiles, C. D. (1988). Regulation of c-myc and c-fos proto oncogene expression by animal cell growth factors. *In Vitro Cell Dev. Biol.*, **24**: 81—4.

16. Rosen, O. M. (1987). After insulin binds. *Science*, **237**: 1452—8.

17. Shipley, G. D., Tucker, R. F. and Moses, H. L. (1985). Type beta transforming growth factor/growth inhibitor stimulates entry of monolayer cultures of AKR-2B cells into S phase after a prolonged prereplicative interval. *Proc. Natl. Acad. Sci. USA*, **82**: 4147—51.

18. Singh, J. P., Chaikin, M. A., Pledger, W. J., Scher, C. D. and Stiles, C. D. Persistence of the mitogenic response to platelet-derived growth factor (competence) does not reflect a longterm interaction between the growth factor and the target cell. *J. Cell Biol.*, **96**: 1497—502.

19. Stiles, C. D., Capone, G. T. and Scher, C. D., Antoniades, H. N., Van Wyk, J. J. and Pledger, W. J. (1979). Dual control of cell growth by somatomedins and platelet-derived growth factor. *Proc. Natl. Acad. Sci. USA.*, **76**: 1279—83.

## III. Properties of Growth Factors (Including Individual GF Effects in Bone). Insulin, IGF-I, IGF-II(SGF).

20. Ashton, I. K., Zapf, J., Einschenk, I. and MacKenzie, I. Z. (1985). Insulin-like growth factors (IGF) 1 and 2 in human foetal plasma and relationship to gestational age and foetal size during mid-pregnancy. *Acta. Endocrinol.*, **110**: 558—63.

21. Adams, S. O., Nissley, S. P., Handwerger, S. and Rechler, M. M. (1983). Developmental patterns of insulin-like growth factor I and II synthesis and regulation in rat fibroblasts. *Nature*, **302**: 150—153.

22. Baumick, B. and Bala, R. M. (1987). Receptors for insulin-like growth factors I and II in developing embryonic mouse limb bud. *Biochim. Biophys. Acta.*, **927**: 117—128.

23. Barnes, D. and Sato, G. (1980). Methods for growth of cultured cells in serum-free

medium. *Anal. Biochem.*, **102**: 255–70.

24. Bennett, A., Chen, T., Feldman, D., Hintz, R. L. and Rosenfeld, R. G. (1984). Characterization of insulin-like growth factor I receptors on cultured rat bone cells: regulation of receptor concentration by glucocorticoids. *Endocrinology*, **115**: 1577–83.

25. Blatt, J., White, C., Dienes, S., Friedman, H. and Foley, T. P., Jr. (1984). Production of an insulin-like growth factor by osteosarcoma. *Biochem. Biophys. Res. Commun.*, **123**: 373–6.

26. Canalis, E. (1980). Effects of insulin-like growth factor I on DNA and protein synthesis in cultured rat calvaria. *J. Clin. Invest.*, **66**: 709–19.

27. Canalis, E., Peck, W. A. and Raisz, L. G. (1980). Stimulation of DNA and collagen synthesis by autologous growth factors in cultured fetal rat calvaria. *Science*, **210**: 1021–23.

28. Canalis, E. (1984). Effects of cartilage-derived factor on DNA and protein synthesis in cultured fetal rat calvaria. *Calcif. Tissue Int.*, **36**: 102–7.

29. Canalis, E., McCarthy, T. and Centrella, M. (1988). Isolation and characterization of insulin-like growth factor I (somatomedin-C) from cultures of fetal rat calvariae. *Endocrinology*, **122**: 22–7.

29a. Canalis, E. and Lian, J. B. (1988) Effects of bone associated growth factors on DNA, collagen, and osteocalcin synthesis in cultured fetal rat calvariae. *Bone* 9: 243–6.

30. Catherwood, B. D., Spanheimer, R., Phillips, L. S., Umpierrez, G., Arkin, D. and Dwelle, S. (1988). Relationship of serum bone gla protein to serum IGF-I and circulating somatomedin inhibitors in diabetic and fasting rats. *J. Bone Mineral Res.*, **3**: S179.

31. Centrella, M., McCarthy, T. L., Canalis, E. (1988). Beta$_2$ microglobulin enhances insulin-like growth factor I (IGF-I) mediated DNA synthesis, binding, and transcript levels in osteoblast-enriched parietal bone cell cultures. *J. Bone Mineral Res.*, **3**: S197.

32. Daughaday, W. H., Hall, K, Raben, M. S., Salman, W. D., van der Brande, L. J., Van Wyk, J. J. (1972). Somatomedin: proposed designation for sulfation factor. *Nature*, **235**: 107.

33. Daughaday, W. H., Kapadia, M. and Mariz, I. (1987). Serum somatomedin binding proteins: physiologic significance and interference in radioligand assay. *J. Lab. Clin. Med.*, **109**: 355–63.

34. D'Ercole, A. J. (1987). Somatomedins/insulin-like growth factors and fetal growth. *J. Dev. Physiol.*, **9**: 481–95.

35. Ernst, M. and Froesch, E. R. (1987). Osteoblastlike cells in a serum-free methylcellulose medium form colonies: effects of insulin and insulin-like growth factor I. *Calcif. Tissue Int.*, **40**: 27–34.

36. Ernst, M. and Froesch, E. R. (1988). Growth hormone dependent stimulation of osteoblast like cells in serum-free cultures via local synthesis of insulin-like growth factor I. *Biochem. Biophys. Res. Commun.*, **151**: 142–7.

37. Ernst, M., Schmid, C., Zapf, J. and Froesch, E. R. (1988). Osteoblasts synthesize specific carrier proteins for insulin-like growth factor in response to growth hormone and estradiol in vitro. *J. Bone Mineral Res.*, **3**: S206.

38. Farley, J. R. and Baylink, D. J. (1982). Purification of a skeletal growth factor from human bone. *Biochemistry*, **21**: 3502–7.

39. Farley, J. R. and Masuda, T., Wergedal, J. E. and Baylink, D. J. (1982). Human skeletal growth factor: characterization of the mitogenic effect on bone cells in vitro. *Biochemistry*, **21**: 3508–13.

39a Farley, J. R. and Baylink, D. J. (1985). *Fed. Proc.*, **44**: 1099a.

40. Frolik, G. A., Ellis, L. F. and Williams, D. C. (1988). Isolation and characterization of insulin-like growth factor-II from human bone. *Biochem. Biophys. Res. Commun.*, **151**: 1011–8.

41. Hayashi, I., Larner, J. and Sato, G. (1978). Hormonal growth control of cells in culture.

*In Vitro*, **14**: 23−30.

42. Hock, J. M., Centrella, M. and Canalis, E. (1988). Insulin-like growth factor I has independent effects on bone matrix formation and cell replication. *Endocrinology*, **122**: 22−7.
43. Hollenberg, M. D. (1987). Receptor for insulin and other growth factors: rationale for common and distinct mechanisms of cell activation. *Clin. Invest. Med.*, **10**: 475−9.
44. Hossenlopp, P., Seurin, D., Segovia-Quinson, B., Hardouin, S. and Binoux, M. (1986). Analysis of serum insulin-like growth factor binding proteins using western blotting: use of the method for titration of the binding proteins and competitive binding studies. *Anal. Biochem.*, **154**: 138−43.
45. Hylka, V. W., Teplow, D. B., Kent, S. B. and Straus, D. S. (1985). Identification of a peptide fragment from the carboxy-terminal extension region (E-domain) of rat proinsulin-like growth factor-II. *J. Biol. Chem.*, **260**: 14417−20.
46. Isaksson, O. G., Lindahl, A., Nilsson, A. and Isgaard, J. (1987). Mechanism of the stimulatory effect of growth hormone on longitudinal bone growth. *Endocr. Rev.*, **8**: 426−38.
47. Ituarte, E. A., Ituarte, H. G., Hahn, T. J. (1988). IGF-I binding in the UMR-106 osteoblastic osteosarcoma cell: down-regulation by PTH. *J. Bone Mineral Res.*, **3**: S219.
48. Kato, Y., Nomura, Y., Tsuji, M., Kinoshita, M., Ohmae, H., Suzuki, F. (1981). Somatomedin-like peptide(s) isolated from fetal bovine cartilage (cartilage-derived factor): isolation and some properties. *Proc. Natl. Acad. Sci.*, **78**: 6831−35.
49. King, G. L., Kahn, C. R. (1984). The growth-promoting effects of insulin. In *Growth and Maturation Factors* v 2, G. Guroff, ed, Wiley, New York, pp 223−265.
50. Kream, B., Smith M. D., Canalis E., Raisz L. G. (1985). Characterization of the effect of insulin on collagen synthesis in fetal rat bone. *Endocrinology*, **116**: 296−302.
51. LaTour, D. A., Merriman, H. L., Kasperk, C. H., Linkhart, T. A., Mohan, S., Strong, D. D., Baylink, D. J. (1988). The proto-oncogene c-fos − a potential regulator of bone cell proliferation − is induced by bone growth factors. *J. Bone Mineral Res.*, **3**: S207.
52. Levy, J. R., Murray, E., Manolagas, S., Olefsky, J. M. (1986). Demonstration of insulin receptors and modulation of alkaline phosphatase activity by insulin in rat osteoblastic cells. *Endocrinology*, **119**: 1786−92.
53. Linkhart, S., Mohan, S., Linkhart, T. A., Kumegawa, M., Baylink, D. J. (1986). Human skeletal growth factor stimulates collagen synthesis and inhibits proliferation in a clonal osteoblast cell line (MC3T3−E1). *J.Cell. Physiol.*, **128**: 307−12.
54. Marquardt, H., Todaro, G. J., Henderson, L. E., Oroszlan, S. (1981). Purification and primary structure of a polypeptide with multiplication-stimulating activity from rat liver cell cultures. *J. Biol. Chem.*, **256**: 6859−65.
55. Mathews, L. S., Norstedt, G., Palmiter, R. D. (1986). Regulation of insulin-like growth factor I gene expression by growth hormone. *Proc. Natl. Acad. Sci. USA*, **83**: 9343−7.
56. McCarthy, T. L., Centrella, M. and Canalis, E. (1988). The transcript and polypeptide levels of insulin-like growth factor I in osteoblast-enriched parietal bone cell cultures are stimulated by parathyroid hormone. *J. Bone Mineral Res.*, **3**: S218.
57. Mohan, S., Jennings, J. C., Linkhart, T. A. and Baylink, D. J. (1986). Isolation and purification of a low molecular weight skeletal growth factor from human bones. *Biochim. Biophys. Acta.*, **884**: 234−42.
58. Mohan, S., Linkhart, T., Jennings, J. and Baylink, D. J. (1986). Chemical and biological characterization of low-molecular-weight human skeletal growth factor. *Biochim. Biophys. Acta.*, **884**: 243−50.
59. Mohan, S., Jennings, J. C., Linkhart, T. A. and Baylink, D. J. (1988). Primary structure of human skeletal growth factor: homology with human insulin-like growth factor-II. *Biochim. Biophys. Acta.*, **966**: 44−55.

60. O'Hare, T. and Pilch, P. F. (1988). Separation and characterization of three insulin receptor species that differ in subunit composition. *Biochemistry*, **27**: 5693−5700.
61. Povoa, G., Roovete, A. and Hall, K. (1984). Cross-reaction of serum somatomedin-binding protein in a radioimmunoassay developed for somatomedin-binding protein isolated from human amniotic fluid. *Acta Endocrinol.*, **107**: 563−70.
62. Rinderknecht, E. and Humbel, R. E. (1978a). The amino acid sequence of human insulin-like growth factor I and its structural homology with proinsulin. *J. Biol. Chem.*, **253**: 2769−76.
63. Rinderknecht, E. and Humbel, R. E. (1978b). Primary structure of human insulin-like growth factor II. *FEBS Lett.*, **89**: 283−6.
64. Roth, R. A. (1988). Structure of the receptor for insulin-like growth factor II: the puzzle amplified. *Science*, **239**: 1269−71.
65. Schlechter, N. L., Russell, S. M., Spencer, E. M. and Nicoll, C. S. (1986). Evidence suggesting that the direct growth-promoting effect of growth hormone on cartilage in vivo is mediated by local production of somatomedin. *Proc. Natl. Acad. Sci. USA*, **83**: 7932−4.
66. Schmid, C., Steiner, T. and Froesch, E. R. (1982). Parathormone promotes glycogen formation from [$^{14}$C] glucose in cultured osteoblast-like cells. *FEBS Lett.*, **148**: 31−4.
67. Schmid, C., Steiner, T. and Froesch, E. R. (1984). Insulin-like growth factor I supports differentiation of cultured osteoblast-like cells. *FEBS Lett.*, **173**: 48−52.
68. Schoenle, E., Zapf, J. and Froesch, E. R. (1982). Insulin-like growth factor I stimulates growth in hypophysectomized rats. *Nature*, **296**: 252−3.
69. Shen, V., Rifas, L., Kohler, G. and Peck, W. A. (1985). Fetal rat chondrocytes sequentially elaborate separate growth- and differentiation-promoting peptides during their development in vitro. *Endocrinology*, **116**: 920−5.
70. Si, E. C. C., Spencer, E. M., Liu, C. C. and Howard, G. A. (1988). Synergism between insulin-like growth factor-I and parathyroid hormone on bone formation. *J. Bone Mineral Res.*, **3**: S113.
71. Sibonga, J. D., Mohan, S., Nishimoto, S. K., Holton, E. M., Linkhart, T. A., Wakley, G. K. and Baylink, D. J. (1988). Impairment of bone formation (BF) in response to skeletal unloading is associated with a skeletal growth factor (SGF) deficit. *J. Bone Mineral Res.*, **3**: S194.
72. Soares, M. B., Turken, A., Ishii, D., Mills, L., Episkopou, V., Cotter, S., Zeitlin, S. and Efstratiadis, A. (1986). Rat insulin-like growth factor II gene. *J. Mol. Biol.*, **192**: 737−52.
73. Stracke, H., Schulz, A., Moeller, D., Rossol, S. and Schatz, H. (1984). Effect of growth hormone on osteoblasts and demonstration of somatomedin-C/IGF I in bone organ culture. *Acta Endocrinol.*, **107**: 16−24.
74. Strong, D. D., Beachler, A. L., Mohan, S., Wergedal, J. E., Linkhart, T. A., Baylink, D. J. (1988). Multiple major skeletal growth factor (SGF) mRNA transcripts expressed in human bone cells. *J. Bone Mineral Res.*, **3**: S142.
75. Wergedal, J. E., Mohan, S., Taylor, A. K., Baylink, D. J. (1986). Skeletal growth factor is produced by human osteoblast-like cells in culture. *Biochim. Biophys. Acta*, **889**: 163−70.
76. Whitson, S. W., Schubkegel, S. R., Jenkins D. B., Whitson, M. A. (1988). Fetal bovine periosteum in organ culture: bone formation and dose response of alkaline phosphatase to insulin. *J. Bone Mineral Res.*, **3**: S103.
77. Wilkins, J. R., D'Ercole, A. J. (1985). Affinity-labeled plasma somatomedin-C/insulin-like growth factor I binding proteins. *J. Clin. Invest.*, **75**: 1350−58.
78. Zapf, J., Schoenle, E., Humbel, R. E., Froesch, E. R. (1978). Insulin-like growth factor I and II: some biological actions and receptor binding characteristics of two purified constituents of nonsuppressible insulin-like activity of human serum. *Eur. J. Biochem.*, **87**: 285−96.
79. Zapf, J., Schmid, C., Froesch, E. R. (1984). Biological and immunological properties of insulin-like-growth factors (IGF) I and II. *Clin. Endocrinol. Metab.*, **13**: 3−30.

## EGF and TGF-α

80. Adashi, E. Y., Resnick, C. E., Twardzik, D. R. (1987). Transforming growth factor-alpha attenuates the acquisition of aromatase activity by cultured rat granulosa cells. *J. Cell Biochem.*, **33**: 1−13.

81. Bell, G. I., Fong, N. M., Stempien, M. M., Wormsted, M. A., Caput, D., Ku, L., Urdea, M. S., Rall, L. B., Sanchez-Pescador, R. (1986). Human epidermal growth factor precursor: cDNA sequence, expression *in vitro*, and gene organization. *Nucl. Acids. Res.*, **14**: 8427−46.

82. Bernier, S. M., Goltzman, D. (1988). Influence of peptides acting through the EGF receptor on the action of synthetic human parathyroid hormone-like peptide of malignancy in renal and osseous cells in vitro. *J. Bone Mineral Res.*, **3**: S69.

83. Boland, C. J., Fried, R. M. and Tashjian, A. H., Jr. (1986). Measurement of cytosolic free $Ca^{2+}$ concentrations in human and rat osteosarcoma cells: actions of bone resorption-stimulating hormones. *Endocrinology*, **118**: 980−9.

84. Bringman, T. S., Lindquist, P. B. and Derynck, R. (1987). Different transforming growth factor-alpha species are derived from a glycosylated and palmitoylated transmembrane receptor. *Cell*, **48**: 429−440.

85. Carpentier, J. -L., White, M. F., Orci, L. and Kahn, R. C. (1987). Direct visualization of the phosphorylated epidermal growth factor receptor during its internalization in A-431 cells. *J. Cell Biol.*, **105**: 2751−62.

86. Chikuma, T., Kato, T., Hiramatsu, M., Kanayama, S. and Kumegawa, M. (1984). Effect of epidermal growth factor on dipeptidyl-aminopeptidase and collagenase-like peptidase activities in cloned osteoblastic cells. *J. Biochem. (Tokyo)*, **95**: 283−6.

87. Chinkers, M. and Garbers, D. L. (1986). Regulation of the phosphorylation state and function of the epidermal growth factor receptor by vitamin K-3. *Biochim. Biophys. Acta.*, **888**: 176−83.

88. Chua, C. C., Geiman, D. E., Keller, G. H. and Ladda, R. L. (1985). Induction of collagenase secretion in human fibroblast cultures by growth promoting factors. *J. Biol. Chem.*, **260**: 5213−6.

89. Cohen, S. (1962). Isolation of a mouse submaxillary gland protein accelerating incisor eruption and eyelid opening in the new-born animal. *J. Biol. Chem.*, **237**: 1555.

90. Cohen, S. and Carpenter, G. (1975). Human epidermal growth factor: isolation and chemical and biological properties. *Proc. Natl. Acad. Sci. USA*, **72**: 1317−21.

91. Gill, G. N., Santon, J. B. and Bertics, P. J. (1987). Regulatory features of the epidermal growth factor receptor. *J. Cell Physiol.*, Suppl **5**: 35−41.

92. Gutierrez, G. E., Mundy, G. R., Derynck, R., Hewlett, E. L. and Katz, M. S. (1987). Inhibition of parathyroid hormone-responsive adenylate cyclase in clonal osteoblast-like cells by transforming growth factor alpha and epidermal growth factor. *J. Biol. Chem.*, **262**: 15845−50.

93. Hata, R., Hori, H., Nagai, Y., Tanaka, S. and Kondo, M., Hiramatsu, M., Utsumi, N., Kumegawa, M. (1984). Selective inhibition of type I collagen synthesis in osteoblastic cells by epidermal growth factor. *Endocrinology*, **115**: 867−76.

94. Hiramatsu, M., Kumegawa, M., Hatakeyama, K., Yajima, T., Minami, N. and Kodama, H. (1982). Effect of epidermal growth factor on collagen synthesis in osteoblastic cells derived from newborn mouse calvaria. *Endocrinology*, **111**: 1810−6.

95. Hirata, Y., Uchihashi, M., Nakashima, H., Fujita, T., Matsukura, S. and Matsui K. (1984). Specific receptors for epidermal growth factor in human bone tumor cells and its effect on synthesis of prostaglandin E2 by cultured osteosarcoma cell line. *Acta Endocrinol.*, **107**: 125−30.

96. Hurley, M. M., Kream, B. E. and Raisz, L. G. (1988). Effects of recombinant transforming growth factor-alpha and interleukin-1 on collagen synthesis and prostaglandin $E_2$ produc-

tion in cultured fetal rat calvariae. *J. Bone Mineral. Res.*, **3**: S195.

97. Ibbotson, K. J., D'Souza, S. M., Ng, K. W., Osborne, C. K., Niall, M., Martin, T. J. and Mundy, G. R. (1983). Tumor-derived growth factor increases bone resorption in a tumor associated with humoral hypercalcemia of malignancy. *Science*, **221**: 1292.

98. Ibbotson, K. J., Harrod, J., Gowen, M., D'Souza, S., Smith, D. D., Winkler, M. E., Derynck, R. and Mundy, G. R. (1986). Human recombinant transforming growth factor alpha stimulates bone resorption and inhibits formation in vitro. *Proc. Natl. Acad. Sci. USA*, **83**: 2228−32.

99. Isackson, P. J., Dunbar, J. C. and Bradshaw, R. A. (1987). Role of glandular kallikreins as growth factor processing enzymes: structural and evolutionary considerations. *J. Cell Biochem.*, **33**: 65−75.

100. Kumegawa, M., Hiramatsu, M., Hatakeyama, K., Yajima, T., Kodama, H., Osaki, T. and Kurisu, K. (1983). Effects of epidermal growth factor on osteoblastic cells *in vitro*. *Calcif. Tissue Int.*, **35**: 542−8.

101. Lazar, E., Watanabe, S., Dalton, S. and Sporn, M. B. (1988). Transforming growth factor alpha: mutation of aspartic acid 47 and leucine 48 results in different biological activities. *Mol. Cell Biol.*, **8**: 1247−52.

102. Lian, J. B., Coutts, M. and Canalis, E. (1985). Studies of hormonal regulation of osteocalcin synthesis in cultured fetal rat calvariae. *J. Biol. Chem.*, **260**: 8706−10.

103. Madtes, D. K., Raines, E. W., Sakariassen, K. S., Assoian, R. K., Sporn, M. B., Bell, G. I. and Ross, R. (1988). Induction of transforming growth factor-alpha in activated human alveolar macrophages. *Cell*, **53**: 285−93.

104. Marquardt, H., Hunkapiller, M. W., Hood, L. E. and Todaro, G. J. (1984). Rat transforming growth factor type 1: structure and relation to epidermal growth factor. *Science*, **223**: 1079−81.

105. Moseley, J. M. and Suva, L. J. (1986). Molecular characterization of the EGF receptor and involvement of glycosyl moieties in the binding of EGF to its receptor on a clonal osteosarcoma line, UMR 106−06. *Calcif. Tissue Int.*, **38**: 109−14.

106. Mundy, G. R., Ibbotson, K. J., D'Souza, S. M., Simpson, E. L., Jacobs, J. W. and Martin, T. J. (1984). The hypercalcemia of cancer. *N. Eng. J. Med.*, **310**: 1718−27.

107. Ng, K. W., Partridge, N. C., Niall, M. and Martin, T. J. (1983). Stimulation of DNA synthesis by epidermal growth factor in osteoblast-like cells. *Calcif. Tissue Int.*, **35**: 624−8.

108. Ng, K. W., Partridge, N. C., Niall, M. and Martin, T. J. (1983). Epidermal growth factor receptors in clonal lines of a rat osteogenic sarcoma and in osteoblast-rich rat bone cells. *Calcif. Tissue Int.*, **35**: 298−303.

109. Osaki, Y., Tsunoi, M., Hakeda, Y., Kurisu, K. and Kumegawa, M. (1984). Immunocyto-chemical study of collagen in epidermal growth factor (EGF) treated osteoblastic cells. *J. Histochem. Cytochem.*, **32**: 1231−3.

110. Partridge, N. C., Jeffrey, J. J., Ehlich, L. S., Teitelbaum, S. L., Fliszar, C., Welgus, H. G. and Kahn, A. J. (1987). Hormonal regulation of the production of collagenase and a collagenase inhibitor activity by rat osteogenic sarcoma cells. *Endocrinology*, **120**: 1956−62.

111. Pierce, J. H., Ruggiero, M., Fleming, T. P., DiFiore, P. P., Greenberger, J. S., Varticovski, L., Schlessinger, J., Rovera, G. and Aaronson, S. A. (1988). Signal transduction through the EGF receptor transfected in IL-3dependent hematopoietic cells. *Science*, **239**: 628−30.

112. Popliker, M., Shatz, A., Avivi ,A., Ullrich, A., Schlessinger, J. and Webb, C. G. (1987). Onset of endogenous synthesis of epidermal growth factor in neonatal mice. *Develop. Biol.*, **119**: 38−44.

113. Rodan, S. B., Thiede, M., Wesolowski, G., Ianacone, J., Rosenblatt, M. and Rodan, G. A. (1988). Parathyroid hormone-like hypercalcemia factor is produced in a human osteosarcoma cell line, SAOS-2. *J. Bone Mineral Res.*, **3**: S71.

114. Schreiber, A. B., Winkler, M. E. and Derynck, R. (1986). Transforming growth factor-alpha: a more potent angiogenic mediator than epidermal growth factor. *Science*, **232**: 1250–3.

115. Shevrin, D. H., Lad, T. E. and Kukreja, S. C. (1987). Effect of epidermal growth factor infusion on serum urine and calcium in mice. *J. Bone Mineral Res.*, **2**: 297–301.

116. Shupnik, M. A. and Tashjian, A. H., Jr. (1982). Epidermal growth factor and phorbol ester actions on human osteosarcoma cells. Characterization of response and nonresponsive cell lines. *J. Biol. Chem.*, **257**: 12161–4.

117. Stern, P. H., Krieger, N. S., Nissenson, R. A., Williams, R. D., Winkler, M. E., Derynck, R. and Strewler, G. J. (1985). Human transforming growth factor-alpha stimulates bone resorption *in vitro*. *J. Clin. Invest.*, **76**: 2016–9.

118. Tashjian, A. H., Jr. and Levine, L. (1978). Epidermal growth factor stimulates prostaglandin production and bone resorption in cultured mouse calvaria. *Biochem. Biophys. Res. Commun.*, **85**: 966–75.

119. Tashjian, A. H., Jr. Voelkel, E. F., Lloyd, W., Rik, D., Winkler, M. E. and Levine, L. (1986). Actions of growth factors on plasma calcium. Epidermal growth factor and human transforming growth factor-alpha cause elevation of plasma calcium in mice. *J. Clin. Invest.*, **78**: 1405–9.

120. Todaro, G. F., Fryling, C. and DeLarco, J. E. (1980). Transforming growth factors produced by certain tumor cells: polypeptides that interact with epidermal growth factor receptors. *Proc. Natl. Acad. Sci. USA*, **77**: 5258–62.

121. Tsunoi, M. (1984). The effect of epidermal growth factor (EGF) on osteoblastic cells clone MC3T3E-1. *Josai Shika Daigaku Kivo* **13**: 331–49.

122. Twardzik, D. R., Ranchalis, J. E. and Todaro, G. J. (1982). Mouse embryonic transforming growth factors related to those isolated from tumor cells. *Cancer Res.*, **42**: 590–3.

123. Twardzik, D. R., Brown, J. P., Ranchalis, J. E., Todaro, G. J. and Moss, B. (1985). Vaccinia virus infected cells release a novel polypeptide functionally related to transforming and epidermal growth factors. *Proc. Natl. Acad. Sci. USA*, **82**: 5300–4.

124. Twardzik, D. R. (1985). Differential expression of transforming growth factor-alpha during prenatal development of the mouse. *Cancer Res.*, **45**: 5413–6.

125. Velu, T. J., Beguinot, L., Vass, W. C., Willingham, M. C., Merlino, G. T., Pastan, I. and Lowy, D. R. (1987). Epidermal growth factor-dependent transformation by a human EGF receptor proto-oncogene. *Science*, **238**: 1408–10.

126. Yokota, K., Kusaka, M., Ohshima, T., Yamamoto, S., Kurihara, N., Yoshino, T. and Kumegawa, M. (1986). Stimulation of prostaglanding E2 synthesis in cloned osteoblastic cells of mouse (MC3T3E1) by epidermal growth factor. *J. Biol. Chem.*, **261**: 15410–5.

127. Yoneda, T., Urade, M., Sakuda, M. and Miyazaki, T. (1986). Altered growth, differentiation, and responsiveness to epidermal growth factor of human embryonic mesenchymal cells of palate by persistent rubella virus infection. *J. Clin. Invest.*, **77**: 1613–21.

## TGF-β

128. Antosz, M. E. and Aubin, J. E. (1988). Differences in the temporal characteristics of EGF and TGF-beta effects on expression of the osteoblast phenotype in isolated rat calvaria cells *in vitro*. *J. Bone Mineral Res.*, **3**: S177.

129. Assoian, R. K., Komoriya, A., Meyers, C. A., Miller, D. M. and Sporn, M. B. (1983). Transforming growth factor-beta in human platelets: identification of a major storage site, purification, and characterization. *J. Biol. Chem.*, **258**: 7155–60.

130. Assoian, R. K. (1985). Biphasic effects of type beta transforming growth factor on epidermal growth factor receptors in NRK fibroblasts. *J. Biol. Chem.*, **260**: 9613–7.

131. Assoian, R. K., Fleurdelys, B. E., Stevenson, H. C., Miller, P. J., Madtes, D. K., Raines, E. W., Ross, R. and Sporn, M. B. (1987). Expression and secretion of type beta transforming growth factor by activated human macrophages. *Proc. Natl. Acad. Sci. USA*, **84**: 6020−4.

132. Brinckerhoff, C. E. (1983). Morphologic and mitogenic responses of rabbit synovial fibroblasts to transforming growth factor beta require transforming growth factor-alpha or epidermal growth factor. *Arth. Rheumatism*, **26**: 1370−9.

133. Burger, E. H., Klein Nulend, J., deJong M. and vanZoelen, J. (1988). Enhancement of DNA synthesis in calvaria by mechanical stimulation may be mediated by transforming growth factor-beta. *J. Bone Mineral Res.*, **3**: S178.

134. Carrington, J. L., Roberts, A., Flanders, K., Roche, N. and Reddi, A. H. (1988). Temporal appearance of transforming growth factor-beta during endochondral bone development and mineralization. *Third Int. Conf. Chem. and Biol. of Mineralized Tissues* Abst

135. Cate, R. L., Mattaliano, R. J., Hession, C., Tizard, R., Farber, N. M., Cheung, A., Ninfa, E. G., Frey, A. Z., Gash, D. J., Chow, E. P., Fisher, R. A., Bertonis, J. M., Torres, G., Wallner, B. P., Ramachandran, K. L., Ragin, R. C., Manganaro, T. F., MacLaughlin, D. T., Donahue, P. K. Isolation of the bovine and human genes for Mullerian inhibitory substance and expression of the human genes in animal cells. *Cell*, **45**: 685−698.

136. Centrella, M. and Canalis, E. (1985). Transforming and nontransforming growth factors are present in medium conditioned by fetal rat calvariae. *Proc. Natl. Acad. Sci. USA*, **82**: 7335−9.

137. Centrella, M., Massague, J. and Canalis, E. (1986). Human platelet derived transforming growth factor beta stimulates parameters of bone growth in fetal rat calvariae. *Endocrinology*, **119**: 2306−12.

138. Centrella, M., McCarthy, T. L. and Canalis, E. (1987). Transforming growth factor beta is a bifunctional regulator of replication and collagen synthesis in osteoblast-enriched cell cultures from fetal rat bone. *J. Biol. Chem.*, **262**: 2869−74.

139. Centrella, M. and Canalis, E. (1987). Isolation of EGF-dependent transforming growth factor (TGF-beta-like) activity from culture medium conditioned by fetal rat calvariae. *J. Bone Mineral Res.*, **2**: 29−36.

140. Centrella, M., McCarthy, T. L., and Canalis, E. (1987). Parathyroid hormone (PTH) modulates TGF-beta binding and mitogenesis in osteoblastic cells. *J. Cell. Biol.*, **105**: 21a

141. Centrella, M., McCarthy T. L. and Canalis E. (1988). TGF-beta effects on bone cells. *Third Int Conf. Chem. and Biol. of Mineralized Tissues*, Abst.

142. Centrella, M., Canalis, E., McCarthy, T. and Insogna, K. (1988). Synthetic parathyroid hormone-like protein regulates DNA and collagen synthesis by modulating transforming growth factor beta activity in fetal rat calvaria bone cells. *J. Bone Mineral Res.*, **3**: S223.

143. Cheifetz, S., Weatherbee, J. A., Tsang, M. L. S., Anderson, J. K., Mole, J. E., Lucas, R. and Massague, J. (1987). The transforming growth factor-beta system, a complex pattern of cross reactive ligands and receptors. *Cell*, **48**: 409−15.

144. Chenu, C., Pfeilschifter, J., Mundy, G. R. and Roodman, G. D. (1988). Transforming growth factor-beta inhibits formation of osteoclast-like cells in long-term human marrow cultures. *Proc. Natl. Acad. Sci. USA*, **85**: 5683−7.

145. Derynck, R., Jarrett, J. A., Chen, E. Y., Eaton, D. H., Bell, J. R., Assoian, R. K., Roberts, A. B., Sporn, M. B., Goeddel, D. V. (1985). Human transforming growth factor-beta complementary DNA sequence and expression in normal and transformed cells. *Nature*, **316**: 701−5.

146. Elford, P. R., Guenther, H. L., Felix, R., Cechini, M. G., Fleisch, H. (1987). Transforming growth factor-beta reduces the phenotypic expression of osteoblastic cells. *Bone*, **8**: 259−62.

147. Ellingsworth, L. R., Brennan, J. E., Fok, K., Rosen, D. M., Bentz, H., Piez, K. A., Seyedin, S. M. (1986). Antibodies to the N-terminal portion of cartilage-inducing factor A and transforming growth factor-beta. Immunohistochemical localization and association with differentiating cells. *J. Biol. Chem.*, **261**: 12362−7.
148. Frolik, C. A., Wakefield, L. M., Smith, D. M., Sporn, M. B. (1984). Characterization of a membrane receptor for transforming growth factor-beta in normal rat kidney fibroblasts. *J. Biol. Chem.*, **259**: 10995−11000.
149. Frolik, C. A., Dart, L. L., Meyers, C. A., Smith, D. M., Sporn, M. B. (1983). Purification and initial characterization of a type beta transforming growth factor from human placenta. *Proc. Natl. Acad. Sci. USA*. **80**: 3676−80.
150. Heine, U., Munoz, E. F., Flanders, K. C., Ellingsworth, L. R., Lam, H. Y., Thompson N. L., Roberts A. B., Sporn, M. B. (1987). Role of transforming growth factor-beta in the development of the mouse embryo. *J. Cell Biol.*, **105**: 2861−76.
151. Ibbotson, K. J., D'Souza, S. M., Mundy, G. R. (1986). Transforming growth factors and bone. *J. Cell Biochem.*, **10B (Suppl)**: 30.
152. Ignotz, R. A., Massague, J. (1985). Type beta transforming growth factor controls the adipogenic differentiation of 3T3 fibroblasts. *Proc. Natl. Acad. Sci. USA*, **82**: 8530−4.
153. Ignotz, R. A. and Massague, J. (1986). Transforming growth factor beta stimulates the expression of fibronectin and collagen and their incorporation into the extracellular matrix. *J. Biol. Chem.*, **261**: 4337−45.
154. Inman, W. H. and Colowick, S. P. (1985). Stimulation of glucose uptake by transforming growth factor beta: evidence for the requirement of epidermal growth factor-receptor activation. *Proc. Natl. Acad. Sci. USA*, **82**: 1346−9.
155. Komm, B. S., Terpening, C. M., Benz, D. J., Graeme, K. A., Gallegos, A., Korc, M., Greene, G. L., O'Malley, B. W. and Haussler, M. R. (1988). Estrogen binding, receptor mRNA, and biologic response in osteoblast-like osteosarcoma cells. *Science*, **241**: 81−84.
156. Kubota, T., Wrana, J. L., Butler, W. T., and Sodek, J. (1988). Stimulation of bone matrix phosphoproteins by transforming growth factor-beta. *Third Int. Conf. Chem. and Biol. of Mineralized Tissues, Abst.*
157. Like, B. and Massague, J. (1986). The antiproliferative effect of type beta transforming growth factor occurs at a level distal from receptors for growth-activating factors. *J. Biol. Chem.*, **261**: 13426−9.
158. Ling, N., Ying, S-Y, Ueno, N., Shimasaki, S., Esch, F., Hotta, M. and Guillemin, R. (1986). Pituitary FSH is released by a heterodimer of the beta-subunits from the two forms of inhibin. *Nature*, **321**: 779−782.
159. Massague, J. (1985). Transforming growth factor-beta modulates the high affinity receptors for epidermal growth factor and transforming growth factor-alpha. *J. Cell Biol.*, **100**: 1508−14.
160. Massague, J. (1985). Subunit structure of a high-affinity receptor for type beta-transforming growth factor. *J. Biol. Chem.*, **260**: 7059−66.
161. Moses, H. L., Coffey, R. J. Jr., Leof, E. B., Lyons, R. M., Keski-Oja, J. (1987). Transforming growth factor beta regulation of cell proliferation. *J. Cell Physiol.*, Suppl **5**: 1−7.
162. Mustoe, T. A., Pierce, G. F., Thomason, A., Gramates, P., Sporn, M. B., Deuel, T. F. (1987). Accelerated healing of incisional wounds in rats induced by transforming growth factor-beta. *Science*, **237**: 1333−6.
163. Noda, M. and Rodan, G. A. (1986). Type-beta transforming growth factor inhibits proliferation and expression of alkaline phosphatase in murine osteoblast-like cells. *Biochem. Biophys. Res. Commun.*, **140**: 56−65.
164. Noda, M. and Rodan, G. A. (1987). Type beta transforming growth factor (TGF beta) regulation of alkaline phosphatase expression and other phenotype-related mRNAs in

osteoblastic rat osteosarcoma cells. *J. Cell Physiol.*, **133**: 426—37.

165. Noda, M., Yoon, K., Rodan, G. A. (1988). Cyclic AMP-mediated stabilization of osteocalcin mRNA in rat osteoblast-like cells treated with parathyroid hormone. *J. Biol. Chem.* 263: 18574—7.

166. Noda, M., Yoon, K., Rodan, S. B., Prince, C. W., Butler, W. T. and Rodan, G. A. (1988). Transforming growth factor beta-1 stimulates and parathyroid hormone inhibits osteopontin gene expression in rat osteosarcoma (ROS 17/2.8) cells. *J. Bone Mineral Res.*, **3**: S218.

166a Noda, M. (1989). Transcriptional regulation of osteocalcin production by transforming growth factor-beta in rat osteoblast-like cells. *Endocrinology* 124: 612—7.

167. O'Connor-McCourt, M. D. and Wakefield, L. M. (1987). Latent transforming growth factor-beta in serum. A specific complex with alpha 2-macroglobulin. *J. Biol. Chem.*, **262**: 14090—9.

168. Ohta, M., Greenberger, J. S., Anklesaria, P., Bassols, A. and Massague, J. (1987). Two forms of transforming growth factor-beta distinguished by multipotential hematopoietic progenitor cells. *Nature*, **329**: 539—41.

169. Oreffo, R. O. C., Bonewald, L., Garrett, I. R., Seyedin, S. and Mundy, G. R. (1988). Transforming growth factors beta I and II inhibit osteoclast activity. *J. Bone Mineral Res.*, **3**: S178.

170. Overall, C. M., Wrana, J. L. and Sodek, J. (1988). Differential regulation of collagenase, 72 kDa-gelatinase, and metalloendoproteinase inhibitor (TIMP) expression in normal bone cell populations by transforming growth factor-beta and osteotropic hormones. *Third Int. Conf. Chem. and Biol. of Mineralized Tissues*, Abst.

171. Padgett, R. W., Johnson, R. D. and Gelbart, W. M. (1987). A transcript from a Drosophila pattern gene predicts a protein homologous to the transforming growth factor beta family. *Nature*, **325**: 81—84.

172. Petkovich, P. M., Wrana, J. L., Grigoriadis, A. E., Heersche, J. N. M. and Sodek, J. (1987). 1,25 Dihydroxyvitamin $D_3$ increases epidermal growth factor receptors and transforming growth factor beta-like activity in a bone-derived cell line. *J. Biol. Chem.*, **262**: 13424—8.

173. Pfeilschifter, J., D'Souza, S. and Mundy, G. R. (1986). Transforming growth factor beta is released from resorbing bone and stimulates osteoblast activity. *J. Bone Mineral Res.*, **1**: S51, a294.

174. Pfeilschifter, J., Bonewald, L. and Mundy, G. R. (1986). TGF-beta is released from bone with one or more binding proteins which regulate its activity. *J. Bone Mineral Res.*, **2**: S, a249.

175. Pfeilschifter, J. and Mundy, G. R. (1987). Modulation of transforming growth factor beta activity in bone cultures by osteotropic hormones. *Proc. Natl. Acad. Sci. USA*, **84**: 2024—28.

176. Pfeilschifter, J., D'Souza, S. M. and Mundy, G. R. (1987). Effects of transforming growth factor-beta on osteoblastic osteosarcoma cells. *Endocrinology*, **121**: 212—8.

177. Pfeilschifter, J., Schmidt, W., Naumann, A., Minne, H. W. and Ziegler, R. (1988). Interactions between the plasminogen system, transforming growth factor beta, and extracellular matrix in osteoblastlike cells. *J. Bone Mineral Res.*, **3**: S177.

178. Roberts, A. B., Anzano, M. A., Lamb, L. C., Smith, J. M. and Sporn, M. B. (1981). New class of transforming growth factors potentiated by epidermal growth factor: isolation from non-neoplastic tissues. *Proc. Natl. Acad. Sci. USA*, **78**: 5339—43.

179. Roberts, A. B., Anzano, M. A., Lamb, L. C., Smith, J. M. and Sporn, M. B. (1983). Purification and properties of a type beta transforming growth factor from bovine kidney. *Biochemistry*, **22**: 5692—8.

180. Roberts, A. B., Anzano, M. A., Wakefield, L. M., Roche, N. S., Stern, D. F. and Sporn,

M. B. (1985). Type beta transforming growth factor: a bifunctional regulator of cellular growth. *Proc. Natl. Acad. Sci. USA*, **82**: 119−123.

181. Robey, P. G., Young, M. F., Flanders, K. G., Roche, N. S., Kondaiah, P., Reddi, A. H., Termine, J. D., Sporn, M. B. and Roberts, A. B. (1987). Osteoblasts synthesize and respond to transforming growth factor-type beta (TGF-β) *in vitro*. *J. Cell Biol.*, **105**: 457−63.

182. Rosa, F., Roberts, A. B., Danielpour, D., Dart, L. L., Sporn, M.B. and Dawid, I. B. (1988). Mesoderm induction in amphibians: the role of TGF-β2-like factors. *Science*, **239**: 783−5.

183. Rosen, D. M., Stempien, S. A., Thompson, A. Y. and Seyedin, S. M. (1988). Transforming growth factor-beta modulates the expression of osteoblast and chondroblast phenotypes *in vitro*. *J. Cell Physiol.*, **134**: 337−46.

184. Rosier, R. N., O'Keefe, R. J., Crabb, I. D. and Puzas, J. E. (1988). Transforming growth factor beta: an autocrine regulator of chondrocytes. *Third Int. Conf. Chem. and Biol. of Mineralized Tissues*, Abst.

185. Rossi, P., Karsenty, G., Roberts, A. B., Roche, N. S., Sporn, M. B. and de Crombrugghe, B. (1988). A nuclear factor 1 binding site mediates the transcriptional activation of a type I collagen promoter by transforming growth factor beta. *Cell*, **52**: 405−14.

186. Segarini, P. R., Roberts, A. B., Rosen, D. M. and Seyedin, S. M. (1987). Membrane binding characteristics of two forms of transforming growth factor-beta. *J. Biol. Chem.*, **262**: 14655−62.

187. Seyedin, S. M., Thomas, T. C., Thompson, A. Y., Rosen, D. M. and Piez, K. A. (1985). Purification and characterization of two cartilage-inducing factors from bovine demineralized bone. *Proc. Natl. Acad. Sci. USA*, **82**: 2267−71.

188. Seyedin, S. M., Thompson, A. Y., Bentz, H., Rosen, D. M., McPherson, J. M., Conti, A., Siegel, N. R., Gallupi, J. R. and Piez, K.A. (1986). Cartilage-inducing factor -A; apparent identity to transforming growth factor-beta. *J. Biol. Chem.*, **261**: 5693−5.

189. Seyedin, S. M., Segarini, P. R., Rosen, D. M., Thompson, A. Y., Bentz, H. and Graycar, J. (1986). Cartilage-inducing factor-B is a unique protein structurally and functionally related to transforming growth factor-beta. *J. Biol. Chem.*, **262**: 1946−9.

190. Sporn, M. B., Roberts, A. B., Wakefield, L. M. and deCrombrugghe, B. (1987). Some recent advances in the chemistry and biology of transforming growth factor-beta. *J. Cell Biol.*, **105**: 1039−45.

191. Sporn, M. B. and Roberts, A. B. (1988). Peptide growth factors are multifunctional. *Nature*, **332**: 217−9.

192. Tashjian, A. H., Jr. Voelkel, E. F., Lazzaro, M., Singer, F. R., Roberts, A. B., Derynck, R., Winkler, M. E. and Levine, L. (1985). Alpha and beta human transforming growth factors stimulate prostaglandin production and bone resorption in cultured mouse calvaria. *Proc. Natl. Acad. Sci. USA*, **82**: 4543−8.

193. Ten Dijke, P., Hansen, P., Iwata, K., Pieler, C. and Foulkes, J. G. (1988). Identification of another member of the transforming growth factor type beta gene family. *Proc. Natl. Acad. Sci. USA*, **85**: 4715−9.

194. Tsunawaki, S., Sporn, M., Ding, A. and Nathan, C. (1988). Deactivation of macrophages by transforming growth factor-beta. *Nature*, **334**: 260−2.

195. Tucker, R. F., Shipley, G. D., Moses, H. L. and Holley, R. W. (1984). Growth inhibitor from BSC-1 cells closely related to platelet type beta transforming growth factor. *Science*, **226**: 705−7.

196. Tucker, R. F., Branum, E. L., Shipley, G. D., Ryan, R. J. and Moses, H. L. (1984). Specific binding to cultured cells of $^{125}$I-labeled type beta transforming growth factor from human platelets. *Proc. Natl. Acad. Sci. USA*, **81**: 6757−61.

197. VanObberghen-Schilling, E., Roche, N. S., Flanders, K. C., Sporn, M. B. and Roberts,

A. B. (1988). Transforming growth factor beta 1 positively regulates its own expression in normal and transformed cells. *J. Biol. Chem.*, **263**: 7741−6.

198. Wahl, S. M., Hunt, D. A., Wakefield, L. M., McCartney-Francis, N., Wahl, L. M., Roberts, A. B. and Sporn, M. B. (1987). Transforming growth factor type beta induces monocyte chemotaxis and growth factor production. *Proc. Natl. Acad. Sci. USA*, **84**: 5788−92.

199. Wakefield, L. M., Smith, D. M., Masui, T., Harris, C. C. and Sporn, M. B. (1987). Distribution and modulation of the cellular receptor for transforming growth factor-beta. *J. Cell Biol.*, **105**: 965−75.

200. Wakefield, L. M., Smith, D. M., Flanders, K. C. and Sporn, M. B. (1988). Latent transforming growth factor-beta from human platelets. A high molecular weight complex containing precursor sequences. *J. Biol. Chem.*, **263**: 7646−54.

201. Wrana, J. L., Maeno, M., Hawrylyshyn B., Yao, K. L., Domenicucci, C. and Sodek J. (1988). Differential effects of transforming growth factor-beta on the synthesis of extracellular matrix proteins by normal fetal rat calvarial bone cell populations. *J. Cell Biol.*, **106**: 915−24.

202. Wrana, J. L., Kubota, T. and Sodek, J. (1988). TGF-beta effects on the synthetic activity of bone cells derived from fetal rat calvaria. *Third Int. Conf. Chem. and Biol. of Mineralized Tissues, Abst.*

## PDGF

203. Antoniades, H. N. and Williams, L. T. (1983). Human platelet-derived growth factor: structure and function. *Fed. Proc.*, **42**: 2630−4.

204. Antoniades, H. N. (1984). Platelet-derived growth factor and malignant transformation. *Biochem. Pharmacol.*, **33**: 2823−8.

205. Bauer, E. A., Silverman, N., Busiek, D. F., Kronberger, A. and Deuel, T. F. (1986). Diminished response of Werner's syndrome fibroblasts to growth factors PDGF and FGF

206. Besmer, P., Murphy, J. E., George, P. C., Qiu, F., Bergold, P. J., Lederman L., Snyder H. W. Jr., Brodeur, D., Zuckerman, E. E. and Hardy, W. D. (1986). A new acute transforming feline retrovirus and relationship of its oncogene v-kit with the protein kinase gene family. *Nature*, **320**: 415−21.

207. Betsholtz, C., Westermark, B., Ek, B. and Heldin, C. H. (1984). Coexpression of a PDGF-like growth factor and PDGF receptors in a human osteosarcoma cell line: implications for autocrine receptor activation. *Cell*, **39**: 447−57.

208. Betsholtz, C., Johnsson, A., Heldin, C.-H., Westermark, B., Lind, P., Urdea M. S., Eddy R., Shows, T. B., Philpott, K., Mellor, A. L., Knott, T. J. and Scott, J. (1986). cDNA sequence and chromosomal location of human platelet-derived growth factor A-chain and its expression in tumor cell lines. *Nature*, **320**: 695−699 (1986)

209. Bonthron, D. T., Morton, C. C., Orkin, S. H. and Collins, T. (1988). Platelet-derived growth factor A chain: gene structure, chromosomal location, and basis for alternative mRNA splicing. *Proc. Natl. Acad. Sci. USA*, **85**: 1492−6.

210. Chan, C. P., Bowen-Pope, D. F., Ross, R. and Krebs, E. G. (1987). Regulation of glycogen synthase activity by growth factors. *J. Biol. Chem.*, **262**: 276−81.

211. Collins, T., Bonthron, D. T. and Orkin, S. H. (1987). Alternative RNA splicing affects function of encoded platelet-derived growth factor A chain. *Nature*, **328**: 621−4.

212. Deuel, T. F. and Huang, J. S. (1984). Platelet-derived growth factor: structure, function, and roles in normal and transformed cells. *J. Clin. Invest.*, **74**: 669−76 (1984).

213. Deuel, T. F. and Senior, R. M., Huang, J. S. and Griffin, G. L. (1982). Chemotaxis of monocytes and neutrophils to platelet-derived growth factor. *J. Clin. Invest.*, **69**: 1046−9.

214. Deuel, T. F., Huang, J. S., Huang, S. S., Stroobant, P. and Waterfield, M. D. (1983). Expression of a platelet-derived growth factor-like protein in simian sarcoma virus transformed cells. *Science*, **221**: 1348−50.
215. Doolittle, R. F., Hunkapiller, M. W., Hood, L. E., Devare, S. G., Robbins, K. C., Aaronson, S. A. and Antoniades, H. N. (1983). Simian sarcoma virus oncogene, v-sis, is derived from the gene (or genes) encoding a platelet-derived growth factor. *Science*, **221**: 275−7.
216. Graves, D. T., Owen, A. J. and Antoniades, H. N. (1983). Evidence that a human osteosarcoma cell line which secretes a mitogen similar to platelet-derived growth factor requires growth factors present in platelet-poor plasma. *Cancer Res.*, **43**: 83−7.
217. Graves, D. T., Owen, A. J., Barth, R. K., Tempst, P., Winoto, A., Fors, L., Hood, L. E. and Antoniades, H. N. (1984). Detection of c-sis transcripts and synthesis of PDGF-like proteins by human osteosarcoma cells. *Science*, **226**: 972−4.
218. Graves, D. T., Owen, A. J. and Antoniades, H. N. (1985). Demonstration of receptors for a PDGF-like mitogen on human osteosarcoma cells. *Biochem. Biophys. Res. Commun.*, **129**: 56−62
219. Graves, D. T., Owen, A. J., Williams, S. R. and Antoniades, H. N. (1986). Identification of processing events in the synthesis of platelet derived growth factor-like protein by human osteosarcoma cells. *Proc. Natl. Acad. Sci. USA*, **83**: 4636−40.
220. Hanks, C. T., Kim, J. S. and Edwards, C. A. (1986). Growth control of cultured rat calvarium cells by platelet-derived growth factor. *J. Oral. Pathol.*, **15**: 476−83.
221. Hart, C. E., Forstrom, J. W., Kelly, J. D., Seifert, R. A., Smith, R. A., Ross, R., Murray, M. J. and Bowen-Pope, D. F. (1988). Two classes of PDGF receptor recognize different isoforms of PDGF. *Science*, **240**: 1529−31.
222. Heldin, C. H , Johnsson, A., Wennergren, S., Wernstedt, C., Betsholtz, C., Westermark, B. (1986). A human osteosarcoma cell line secretes a growth factor structurally related to a homodimer of PDGF A-chains. *Nature*, **319**: 511−4.
223. Heldin, C. H. and Westermark, B. (1987). PDGF-like growth factors in autocrine stimulation of growth. *J. Cell Physiol.* Suppl. **5**: 31−4.
224. Heldin, C.-H., Backstrom, G., Ostman, A., Hammacher, A., Ronnstrand L., Rubin, K., Nister, M. and Westermark, B. (1988). Binding of different dimeric forms of PDGF to human fibroblasts: evidence for two different receptor types. *EMBO J.*, **7**: 1387−94.
225. Hoppe, J., Schumacher, L., Eichner, W., Weich, H. A. (1987). The long 3' untranslated regions of the PDGF-A and B mRNAs are only distantly related. *FEBS Lett.*, **223**: 243−6.
226. Huang, J. S., Huang, S. S. and Deuel, T. F. (1984). Specific covalent binding of platelet-derived growth factor to human plasma alpha-2macroglobulin. *Proc. Natl. Acad. Sci. USA*, **81**: 342−6.
227. Keating, M. T. and Williams, L. T. (1988). Autocrine stimulation of intracellular PDGF receptors in v-sis-transformed cells. *Science*, **239**: 914−6.
228. Kumar, R. K., Bennett, R. A. and Brody, A. R. (1988). A homologue of platelet-derived growth factor produced by rat alveolar macrophages. *FASEB J.*, **2**: 2272−7.
229. Leal, F., Williams, L. T., Robbins, K. C. and Aaronson, S. A. (1985). Evidence that the v-sis gene product transforms by interaction with the receptor for platelet-derived growth factor. *Science*, **230**: 327−30.
230. Martinet, Y., Bitterman, P. B., Mornex, J. F., Grotendorst, G. R., Martin, G. R. and Crystal, R. G. (1986). Activated human monocytes express the c-sis proto-oncogene and release a mediator showing PDGF-like activity. *Nature*, **319**: 158−60.
231. Matuoka, K., Fukami, K., Nakanishi, O., Kawai, S. and Takenawa, T. (1988). Mitogenesis in response to PDGF and bombesin abolished by microinjection of antibody to $PIP_2$. *Science*, **239**: 640−3.

232. Niman, H. L., Houghten, R. A. and Bowen-Pope, D. F. (1984). Detection of high molecular weight forms of platelet-derived growth factor by sequence-specific antisera. *Science*, **226**: 701−3.

233. Nister, M., Hammacher, A., Mellstrom, K., Siegbahn, A., Ronnstrand, L., Westermark, B. and Heldin, C. -H. (1988). A glioma-derived PDGF A chain homodimer has different functional activities from a PDGF AB heterodimer purified from human platelets. *Cell*, **52**: 791−9.

234. Pike, L. J., Bowen-Pope, D. F., Ross, R. and Krebs, E. G. (1983). Characterization of platelet-derived growth factor-stimulated phosphorylation of cell membranes. *J. Biol. Chem.*, **258**: 9383−90.

235. Raines, E. W. and Ross, R. (1982). Platelet-derived growth factor. I: high yield purification and evidence for multiple forms. *J. Biol. Chem.*, **257**: 5154−60.

236. Rao, C. D., Igarashi, H., Chiu, I.-M., Robbins, K. C. and Aaronson, S. A. (1986). Structure and sequence of the human c-sis/platelet-derived growth factor 2 (SIS/PDGF2) transcriptional unit. *Proc. Natl. Acad. Sci. USA*, **83**: 2392−6.

237. Robbins, K. C., Antoniades, H. N., Devare, S. G., Hunkapillar, M. W. and Aaronson, S. A. (1983). Structural and immunological similarities between simian sarcoma virus gene product(s) and human platelet-derived growth factor. *Nature*, **305**: 605−8.

238. Rollins, B. J., Morrison, E. D. and Stiles, C. D. (1987). A cell-cycle constraint on the regulation of gene expression by platelet-derived growth factor. *Science*, **238**: 1269−71.

239. Scher, C. D., Hendrickson, S. L., Whipple, A. P., Gottesman, M. M. and Pledger, W. J. (1982). Constitutive synthesis by a tumorigenic cell line of proteins modulated by platelet-derived growth factor. In *Growth of Cells in Hormonally Defined Media* Sato GH, Pardee AB, Sirbaske DA, eds. Cold Spring Harbor Laboratory, v. 9, pp. 280−303.

240. Shimokado, K., Raines, E. W., Madtes, D. K., Barrett, T. B., Benditt, E. P. and Ross, R. A. (1985). A significant part of macrophage-derived growth factor consists of at least two forms of PDGF. *Cell*, **43**: 277−86.

241. Shupnik, M. A., Antoniades, H. N. and Tashjian, A. H., Jr. (1982). Platelet-derived growth factor increases prostaglandin production and decreases epidermal growth factor receptors in human osteosarcoma cells. *Life Sci.*, **30**: 347.

242. Stroobant, P. and Waterfield, M. D. (1984). Purification and properties of porcine platelet-derived growth factor. *EMBO J.*, **12**: 2963−7.

243. Tashjian, A. H., Jr. Hohman, E. L., Antoniades, H. N. and Levine, L. (1982). Platelet-derived growth factor stimulates bone resorption via a prostaglandin mediated mechanism. *Endocrinology*, **111**: 118−24.

244. Tong, B. D., Auer, D. E., Jaye, M., Kaplow, J. M., Ricca, G., McConathy, E., Drohan, W. and Deuel, T. F. (1987). cDNA clones reveal differences between human glial and endothelial cell platelet-derived growth factor A-chains. *Nature*, **328**: 619−21.

245. Waterfield, M. D., Scrace, G. T., Whittle, N., Stroobant, P., Johnsson, A., Wasteson, A., Westermark, B., Heldin, C. H., Huang, J. S. and Deuel, T. F. (1983). Platelet-derived growth factor is structurally related to the putative transforming protein p28[sis] of simian sarcoma virus. *Nature*, **304**: 35−9.

246. Womer, R. B., Frick, K., Mitchell, C. D., Ross, A. H., Bishayes, S. and Scher, C. D. (1987). PDGF induces c-myc mRNA expression in MG-63 human osteosarcoma cells but does not stimulate cell replication. *J. Cell Physiol.*, **132**: 65−72.

247. Yarden, Y., Escobedo, J. A., Kuang, W.-J., Yang-Feng, T. L., Daniel, T. O., Tremble, P. M., Chen, E. Y., Ando, M. E., Harkins, R. N. and Francke, U. (1986). Structure of the receptor for platelet-derived growth factor helps define a family of closely related growth factor receptors. *Nature*, **323**: 226−32.

248. Zerwes, H. -G. and Risau, W. (1987). Polarized secretion of a platelet-derived growth factor-like chemotactic factor by endothelial cells in vitro. *J. Cell Biol.*, **105**: 2037−41.

## Acidic FGF

249. Esch, F., Ueno, N., Baird, A., Hill, F., Denoroy, L., Ling, N., Gospodarowicz, D. and Guillemin, R. (1985). Primary structure of bovine brain acidic fibroblast growth factor (FGF). *Biochem. Biophys. Res. Commun.*, **133**: 554–62.
250. Gautschi-Sova, P., Muller, T. and Bohlen, P. (1986). Amino acid sequence of human acidic fibroblast growth factor. *Biochem. Biophys. Res. Commun.*, **140**: 874–80.
251. Giminez-Gallego, G., Rodkey, J., Bennett, C., Rios-Candelore, M., DiSalvo, J. and Thomas, K. (1985). Brain-derived acidic fibroblast growth factor: complete amino acid sequence and homologies. *Science*, **230**: 1385–8.
252. Gospodarowicz, D., Neufeld, G. and Schweigerer, L. (1987). Fibroblast growth factor: structural and biological properties. *J. Cell Physiol.*, Suppl **5**: 15–26.
253. Guenther, H. L., Fleisch, H. and Sorgente, N. (1986). Endothelial cells in culture synthesize a potent bone cell active mitogen. *Endocrinology*, **119**: 193–201.
254. Lobb, R. R., Harper, J. W. and Fett, J. W. (1986). Purification of heparin-binding growth factors. *Anal. Biochem.*, **154**: 1–14.
255. Olwin, B. and Hauschka, S. D. (1986). Identification of the fibroblast growth factor receptor of Swiss 3T3 cells and mouse skeletal muscle myoblasts. *Biochemistry*, **25**: 3487–92.
256. Rodan, S. B., Wesolowski, G., Thomas, K. and Rodan, G. A. (1987). Growth stimulation of rat calvaria osteoblastic cells by acidic fibroblast growth factor. *Endocrinology*, **121**: 1917–23.
257. Schreiber, A. B., Kenney, J., Kowalski, J., Thomas, K. A., Giminez-Gallego, G., Rios-Candelore, M., DiSalvo, J., Barritault, D., Courty, J. and Courtois, Y. (1985) A unique family of endothelial cell polypeptide mitogens: the antigenic and receptor cross-reactivity of bovine endothelial cell growth factor, brain-derived acidic fibroblast growth factor, and eye-derived growth factor-II. *J. Cell Biol.*, **101**: 1623–6.
258. Thomas, K. A. and Gimenez-Gallego, G. (1986). Fibroblast growth factors — broad spectrum mitogens with potent angiogenic activity. *Trends Biochem. Sci.*, **11**: 81–4.
259. Thomas, K. A. (1987). Fibroblast growth factors. *FASEB J.*, **1**: 434–40.
260. Uhlrich, S., Lagente, O., Choay, J., Courtois, Y. and Lenfant, M. (1986). Structure activity relationship in heparin: stimulation of non-vascular cells by a synthetic heparin pentasaccharide in cooperation with human acidic fibroblast growth factors. *Biochem. Biophys. Res. Commun.*, **139**: 728–32.

## Basic FGF

261. Abraham, J. A., Whang, J. L., Tumolo, A., Mergia, A., Friedman, J., Gospodarowicz D. and Fiddes, J. C. (1986). Human basic fibroblast growth factor: nucleotide sequence and genomic organization. *EMBO J.*, **5**: 2523–8.
262. Baird, A., Schubert, D., Ling, N., Guillemin, R. (1988). Receptor- and heparin-binding domains of basic fibroblast growth factor. *Proc. Natl. Acad. Sci. USA*, **85**: 2324–8.
263. Coughlin, S. R., Barr, P. J., Cousens, L. S., Fretto, L. J. and Williams, L. T. (1988). Acidic and basic fibroblast growth factors stimulate tyrosine kinase activity in vivo. *J. Biol. Chem.*, **263**: 988–93.
264. Esch, F., Baird, A., Ling, N., Ueno, N., Hill, F., Denoroy, L., Klepper, R., Gospodarowicz, D. Bohlen, P. and Guillemin, R. (1985). Primary structure of bovine pituitary basic fibroblast growth factor (FGF) and comparison with the amino-terminal sequence of bovine brain acidic FGF. *Proc. Natl. Acad. Sci. USA*, **82**: 6507–11.
265. Folkman, J., Klagsbrun, M., Sasse J., Wadzinski, M., Ingber, D. and Vlodavsky, I.

(1988). A heparin-binding angiogenic protein — basic fibroblast growth factor — is stored within basement membrane. *Am. J. Pathol.*, **130**: 393−400.

266. Huang, J. S., Huang, S. S., and Kuo, M. D. (1986). Bovine brain-derived growth factor. Purification and characterization of its interaction with responsive cells. *J. Biol. Chem.*, **261**: 11600−7.

267. Kato, Y., Nakashima, K., Sato, K., Inoue, H., Suzuki, F. and Iwamoto, M. (1988). Fibroblast growth factor, at very low concentrations, stimulates proliferation of chondrocytes in the presence of transforming growth factor-beta. *Third Int. Conf. Chem. and Biol. of Mineralized Tissues* Abst.

268. Klagsbrun, M., Sasse, J., Sullivan, R. and Smith, J. A. (1986). Human tumor cells synthesize an endothelial cell growth factor that is structurally related to basic fibroblast growth factor. *Proc. Natl. Acad. Sci. USA*, **83**: 2448−52.

269. Klagsbrun, M., Smith, S., Sullivan, R., Shing, Y., Davidson, S., Smith, J. A. and Sasse, J. (1987). Multiple forms of basic fibroblast growth factor: amino-terminal cleavages by tumor cell-and brain cell-derived proteinases. *Proc. Natl. Acad. Sci. USA*, **84**: 1839−43.

270. Kurokawa, T., Sasada, R., Iwane M. and Igarashi K. (1987). Cloning and expression of cDNA encoding human basic fibroblast growth factor. *FEBS Lett.*, **213**: 189−94.

271. Magnaldo, I., L'Allemain, G., Chambard, J. C., Moenner, M., Barritault, D. and Pouyssegur, J. (1986). The mitogenic signalling pathway of fibroblast growth factor is not mediated through polyphosphoinositide hydrolysis and protein kinase C activation in hamster fibroblasts. *J. Biol. Chem.*, **261**: 16916−22.

272. Marx, J. (1987). Oncogene action probed (editorial). *Science*, **237**: 602−3.

273. Miller, M. D. and Puzas, J. E. (1988). Differential growth factor effects on normal and transformed rat bone cells. *J. Bone Mineral Res.*, **3**: S201.

274. Montesano, R., Vassalli, J. -D., Baird, A., Guillemin, R. and Orci, L. (1986). Basic fibroblast growth factor induces angiogenesis in vitro. *Proc. Natl. Acad. Sci. USA*, **83**: 7297−301.

275. Moscatelli, D., Presta, M., Joseph-Silverstein, J. and Rifkin, D. B. (1986). Both normal and tumor cells produce basic fibroblast growth factor. *J. Cell Physiol.*, **129**: 273−6.

276. Neufeld, G. and Gospodarowicz, D. (1985). The identification and partial characterization of the fibroblast growth factor receptor of baby hamster kidney cells. *J. Biol. Chem.*, **260**: 13860−8.

277. Phadke, K. (1987). Fibroblast growth factor enhances the interleukin-1-mediated chondrocytic protease release. *Biochem. Biophys. Res. Commun.*, **142**: 448−53.

278. Rodan, S. B., Yoon, K., Wesolowski, G. and Rodan, G. A. (1988). Opposing effects of basic fibroblast growth factor and pertussis toxin on the regulation of gene expression in ROS 17/2.8 cells. *Third Int. Conf. Chem. and Biol. of Mineralized Tissues*, Abst.

279. Saksela, O., Moscatelli, D. and Rifkin, D. B. (1987). The opposing effects of basic fibroblast growth factor and transforming growth factor beta on the regulation of plasminogen activator activity in capillary endothelial cells. *J. Cell Biol.*, **105**: 957−63.

280. Shing, Y., Folkman, J., Sullivan, R., Butterfield, C., Murray, J. and Klagsbrun, M. (1984). Heparin affinity: purification of a tumor-derived capillary endothelial cell growth factor. *Science*, **223**: 1296−9.

281. Slack, J. M. W., Darlington, B. G., Heath, J. K. and Godsave, S. F. (1987). Mesoderm induction in early Xenopus embryos by heparin-binding growth factors. *Nature*, **326**: 197−200.

282. Sommer, A., Brewer, M. T., Thompson, R. C., Moscatelli, D., Presta, M. and Rifkin, D. B. (1987). A form of human basic fibroblast growth factor with an extended amino terminus. *Biochem. Biophys. Res. Commun.*, **144**: 543−50.

283. Story, M. T., Esch, F., Shimasaki, S., Sasse, J., Jacobs, S. C. and Lawson, R. K. (1987). Amino-terminal sequence of a large form of basic fibroblast growth factor isolated from

human benign prostatic hyperplastic tissue. *Biochem. Biophys. Res. Commun.*, **142**: 702−9.

284. Sullivan, R. and Klagsbrun, M. (1985). Purification of cartilage-derived growth factor by heparin affinity chromatography. *J. Biol. Chem.*, **260**: 2399−403.


## Other Factors and Cytokines

285. Beresford, J. N., Gallagher, J. A., Gowen, M., Couch, M., Poser, J., Wood, D. D. and Russell, R. G. G. (1984). The effects of monocyte-conditioned medium and interleukin 1 on the synthesis of collagenous and non-collagenous proteins by mouse bone and human bone cells *in vitro*. *Biochim. Biophys. Acta*, **804**: 58−65.

286. Bertolini, D. R., Nedwin, G. E., Bringman, T. S., Smith, D. D. and Mundy, G. R. (1986). Stimulation of bone resorption and inhibition of bone formation *in vitro* by human tumor necrosis factors. *Nature*, **319**: 516−8.

287. Besedovsky, H., delRey, A., Sorkin, E. and Dinarello, C. A. (1986). Immunoregulatory feedback between interleukin-1 and glucocorticoid hormones. *Science*, **233**: 652−4.

288. Bosma, T., Levine, L. and Tashjian, A. H. Jr. (1988). Recombinant human interleukin-1-alpha and -1-beta: comparative activities and actions on neonatal mouse calvariae. *J. Bone Mineral Res.*, **3**: S196.

289. Boyce, B. F., Aufdemorte, T., Garrett, I. R., Yates, A. P. and Mundy, G. R. (1988). Stimulation of bone turnover in vivo by interleukin-1. *J. Bone Mineral Res.*, **3**: S204.

290. Broudy, V. C., Kaushansky, K., Segal, G. M., Harlan, J. M. and Adamson, J. W. (1986). Tumor necrosis factor type alpha stimulates endothelial cells to produce granulocyte/macrophage colony-stimulating factor. *Proc. Natl. Acad. Sci. USA*, **83**: 7467−71.

291. Canalis, E. (1986). Interleukin-1 has independent effects on DNA and collagen synthesis in cultures of rat calvariae. *Endocrinology*, **118**: 74−81.

292. Canalis, E., McCarthy, T. and Centrella, M. (1987). A bone-derived growth factor isolated from rat calvariae is beta$_2$ microglobulin. *Endocrinology*, **121**: 1198−1200.

293. Chan, S. H. and Metcalf, D. (1972). Local production of colony-stimulating factor within the bone marrow: role of nonhematopoietic cells. *Blood*, **40**: 646−53.

294. Dewhirst, F. E., Stashenko, P., Mole, J. E., Tsurumachi, T. (1985). Purification and partial sequence of human osteoclast-activating factor: identity with intrleukin-1-β. *J. Immunol.*, **135**: 2562.

295. Dinarello, C. A. (1988). Biology of interleukin-1. *FASEB J.*, **2**: 108−115.

296. Elford, P. R., Felix, R., Cecchini, M., Trechsel, U., Fleisch, H. (1987). Murine osteoblast-like cells and the osteogenic cell MC3T3-E1 release a macrophage colony-stimulating activity in culture. *Calcif. Tissue Int.*, **41**: 151−6.

297. Estes, J. E., Pledger, W. J., Gillespie, Y. (1984). Macrophage-derived growth factor for fibroblasts and interleukin-1 are distinct entities. *J. Leukocyte Biol.*, **35**: 115.

298. Gazit, D., Muhlrad, A., Shteyer, A., Bab, I. (1988). Osteogenic growth factor activity in healing bone marrow: separation by heparin-sepharose and ion exchange chromatographies. *Third Int. Conf. Chem. and Biol. of Mineralized Tissues* Abst.

299. Gowen, M., Wood, D. D., Ibrie, E. J., McGuire, M. K. B., Russell, R. G. G. (1983). An interleukin 1-like factor stimulates bone resorption *in vitro*. *Nature*, **306**: 378.

300. Glowacki, J. (1983). The effects of heparin and protamine on resorption of bone particles. *Life Sci.*, **33**: 1019−24.

301. Hanazawa, S., Ohmori, Y., Amano, S., Miyoshi, T., Kumegawa, M., Kitano, S. (1985). Spontaneous production of interleukin -1-like cytokine from a mouse osteoblastic cell line (MC3T3-E1). *Biochem. Biophys. Res. Commun.*, **131**: 774−9.

302. Hauschka, P. V. (1985). Osteocalcin and its functional domains. In: Butler WT, ed.,

*Chemistry and Biology of Mineralized Tissues*, EBSCO Media, Birmingham, 149−58.

303. Hughes, D. E., Gowen, M., Russell, R. G. G. (1988). Interleukin 1 as a paracrine factor in bone: effects on osteoclast-like cell formation and production by osteoblast-like cells. *J. Bone Mineral Res.*, **3**: S196.
304. Hurley, M. M., Kream, B. E., Raisz, L. G. (1988). Effects of recombinant transforming growth factor-alpha and interleukin-1 on collagen synthesis and prostaglandin $E_2$ production in cultured fetal rat calvariae. *J. Bone Mineral Res.*, **3**: S195.
305. Jennings, J. C., Mohan, S., Linkhart, T. A. and Baylink, D. J. (1988). $\beta_2$ microglobulin is not a bone cell mitogen. *J. Bone Mineral Res.*, **3**: S197.
306. Kirstein, M. and Baglioni, C. (1988). Tumor necrosis factor stimulates proliferation of human osteosarcoma cells and accumulation of c-myc messenger RNA. *J. Cell Physiol.*, **134**: 479−84.
307. Koutsilleris, M., Rabbani, S. A. and Goltzman, D. (1987). Effects of human prostatic mitogens on rat bone cells and fibroblasts. *Endocrinology*, **115**: 447−54.
308. Koutsilleris, M., Rabbani, S. A., Bennett, H. P. and Goltzman, D. (1987). Characteristics of prostate derived growth factors for cells of the osteoblast phenotype. *J. Clin. Invest.*, **80**: 941−6.
309. Koutsilleris, M., Rabbani, S. A. and Goltzman, D. (1986). Selective osteoblast mitogens can be extracted from prostatic tissue. *Prostate*, **9**: 109−15.
310. Krane, S. M., Goldring, M. B. and Goldring, S. R. (1988). Cytokines. In *Cell and Molecular Biology of Vertebrate Hard Tissues* CIBA Foundation Symposium 136, Wiley, New York, pp. 239−256.
311. Landesman, R. L. and Reddi, A. H. (1986). Chemotaxis of muscle-derived mesenchymal cells to bone-inductive proteins of rat. *Calcif. Tissue Int.*, **39**: 259−62.
312. Lian, J. B., Dunn, K. and Key, L. L. Jr. (1986). *In vitro* degradation of bone particles by human monocytes is decreased with the depletion of the vitamin K-dependent protein from the matrix. *Endocrinology*, **118**: 1636−42.
313. Liebovich, S. J., Polverini, P. J., Shepard, H. M., Wiseman, D. M., Shively, V. and Nuseir, N. (1987). Macrophage-induced angiogenesis is mediated by tumor necrosis factor-alpha. *Nature*, **329**: 630−2.
314. Linkhart, T. A., Mohan, S., Widstrom, R., Jennings, J. C., Peehl, D. M. and Baylink, D. J. (1988). Human prostatic cancer cells produce growth factors similar to those produced by osteoblasts. *J. Bone Mineral Res.*, **3**: S203.
315. Lucas, P. A., Syftestad, G. T. and Caplan, A. I. (1986). Partial isolation and characterization of chemotactic factor from adult bovine bone for mesenchymal cells. *Bone*, **7**: 365−71.
316. Malone, J. D., Teitelbaum, S. L., Griffin, G. L., Senior, R. M. and Kahn, A. J. (1982). Recruitment of osteoclast precursors by purified bone matrix components. *J. Cell Biol.*, **92**: 227−30.
317. McSheehy, P. M. and Chambers, T. J. (1986). Osteoblast-like cells in the presence of parathyroid hormone release soluble factor that stimulates osteoclastic bone resorption. *Endocrinology*, **119**: 1654−9.
318. Minkin, C., Bannon, D. J. Jr and Pokress, S. (1985). Bone-derived macrophage chemotactic factors: methods of extraction and further characterization. *Calcif. Tissue Int.*, **37**: 63−72.
319. Metcalf, D. (1986). The molecular biology and functions of the granulocyte-macrophage colony-stimulating factors. *Blood*, **67**: 257−67.
320. Mundy, G. R. and Poser, J. W. (1983). Chemotactic activity of the gamma-carboxyglutamic acid containing protein of bone. *Calcif. Tissue Int.*, **35**: 164−8.
321. Pacifici, R., Rifas, L., Blair, H., Konsek, J., McCracken, R., Halstead, L., Scott, M., Peck, W. A. and Avioli, L. V. (1988). Interleukin-1 secretion from human blood mono-

nuclear cells is increased by adherence to exposed bone matrix. *J. Bone Mineral Res.*, **3**: S195.

322. Peck, W. A., Rifas, L. and Shen, V. (1985). Macrophages release a peptide stimulator of osteoblast growth. *Ann. Biol. Clin. (Paris)* **43**: 751–4.

323. Pennica, D., Nedwin, G. E., Hayflick, J. S., Seeburg, P. H., Derynck, R., Palladino, M. A., Kohr, W. J. and Aggarwal, B. B. (1984). Human tumor necrosis factor: precursor structure, expression and homology to lymphotoxin. *Nature*, **312**: 724–9.

324. Povolny, B., Lee, M., Hauschka, P. and Clagett, J. (1987). Osteocalcin is a growth factor for bone marrow cells. *Fed. Proc.*, **46**: 988.

325. Rifas, L., Shen, V., Mitchell, K. and Peck, W. A. (1984). Macrophage derived growth factor for osteoblast like cells and chondrocytes. *Proc. Natl. Acad. Sci. USA*, **81**: 4558–62.

326. Rifas, L., Pacifici, R., Civitelli, R., Cheng, S. -L., Halstead, L., Scott, M., Hruska, K. and Avioli, L. V. (1988). Recombinant IL-1-beta has biphasic effects on normal rat osteoblast growth and stimulates TGF-beta secretion. *J. Bone Mineral Res.*, **3**: S195.

327. Sachs, L. (1987). The molecular control of blood cell development. *Science*, **238**: 1374–9.

328. Shiina-Ishimi, Y., Abe, E., Tanaka, H. and Suda, T. (1986). Synthesis of colony-stimulating factor (CSF) and differentiation-inducing factor (D-factor) by osteoblastic cells, clone MC3T3-E1. *Biochem. Biophys. Res. Commun.*, **134**: 400–6.

329. Somerman, M., Hewitt, A. T., Varner, H. H., Schiffman, E., Termine, J. and Reddi, A. H. (1983). Identification of a bone matrix-derived chemotactic factor. *Calcif. Tissue Int.*, **35**: 481–5.

330. Stashenko, P., Dewhirst, F. E., Peros, W. J., Kent, R. L. and Ago, J. M. (1987). Synergistic interactions between interleukin-1, tumor necrosis factor, and lymphotoxin in bone resorption. *J. Immunol.*, **138**: 1464.

331. Stashenko, P., Dewhirst, F. E., Rooney, M. L., Desjardins, L. A. and Heeley, J. D. (1987). Interleukin-1-beta is a potent inhibitor of bone formation. *J. Bone Mineral Res.*, **2**: 559.

332. Stashenko, P., Obernesser, M. S., Hauschka, P. V. and Dewhirst, F. E. (1988). Bone resorptive cytokines interleukin 1-alpha, interleukin 1-beta, and tumor necrosis factor inhibit bone formation. (Personal Communication)

333. Strewler, G. J., Price, P. A., Klein, R. F., Diep, D. and Nissenson, R. A. (1987). GTP-binding proteins may regulate alkaline phosphatase and BGP [osteocalcin] in ROS 17/2.8 cells. *J. Bone Mineral Res.*, **2**: Suppl 1, a121.

334. Thompson, B. M., Mundy, G. R. and Chambers, T. J. (1987). Tumor necrosis factors alpha and beta induce osteoblastic cells to stimulate osteoclastic bone resorption. *J. Immunol.*, **138**: 775–9.

335. Washington, L., Coleman, D. L., Einhorn, T. A. and Horowitz, M. (1988). Retinoids regulate murine osteoblast colony stimulating factor secretion. *J. Bone Mineral Res.*, **3**: S223.

336. Webber, D., Krukowski, M. and Osdoby, P. (1988). Osteoclast antigen expression is dependent on both mineral and non-collagenous components of bone matrix. *J. Bone Mineral Res.*, **3**: S99.

337. Yoshikawa, H. and Takaoka, K. (1988). Tumor necrosis factor inhibits ectopic bone formation induced by osteosarcoma-derived bone-inducing substance. *J. Bone Mineral Res.*, **3**: S198.

## IV. Growth Factors in Bone Matrix and Osseous Sources of Growth Factors

338. Canalis, E., McCarthy, T. and Centrella, M. (1988). Growth factors associated with adult bone matrix. *J. Bone Mineral Res.*, **3**: S202.

339. Finkelman, R. D., Mohan, S. and Baylink, D. J. (1988). Growth factor activity in extracts of human dentin. *Third Int. Conf. Chem. and Biol. of Mineralized Tissues* Abst.
340. Gospodarowicz, D. and Tauber, J. P. (1980). Growth factors and the extracellular matrix. *Endocr. Rev.*, **1**: 201–27.
341. Hauschka, P. V., Mavrakos, A. E., Iafrati, M. D., Doleman, S. E. and Klagsbrun, M. (1986). Growth factors in bone matrix. Isolation of multiple types by affinity chromatography on heparin-Sepharose. *J. Biol. Chem.*, **261**: 12665–74.
342. Hauschka, P. V., Chen, T. L. and Mavrakos, A. E. (1988). Polypeptide growth factors in bone matrix. In *Cell and Molecular Biology of Vertebrate Hard Tissues* CIBA Foundation Symposium 136, Wiley, New York, pp. 207–25.
343. Linkhart, T. A., Jennings, J. C., Mohan, S., Wakley, G. K. and Baylink, D. J. (1986). Characterization of mitogenic activities extracted from bovine bone matrix. *Bone*, **7**: 479–87.
344. Mallory, J. B., Norgard, E. M., Fiddes, J. C. and Chen, T. L. (1988). Identification of growth factors present in conditioned medium of rat osteoblast-like (ROB) cells using heparin sepharose chromatography. *J. Bone Mineral Res.*, **3**: S202.
345. Mohan, S., Linkhart, T. A., Jennings, J. C. and Baylink, D. J. (1987). Identification and quantitation of four distinct growth factors stored in human bone matrix. *J. Bone Mineral Res.*, **2**: S, a44.
346. Onizawa, K. (1987) Purification and characterization of bone cell proliferation factors from bovine bone matrix. *Kokubyo Gakkai Zasshi*, **54**: 349–64.

## V. Target Cells for Growth Factors within the Osteoblastic Lineage

347. Aubin, J. E., Heersche, J. N. M., Merrilees, M. J. and Sodek, J. (1982). Isolation of bone cell clones with differences in growth, hormone responses, and extracellular matrix production. *J. Cell Biol.*, **92**: 452–61.
348. Aufmkolk, B., Hauschka, P. V. and Schwartz, E. R. (1985). Characterization of human bone cells in culture. *Calcif. Tissue Int.*, **37**: 228–35.
349. Bellows, C. G., Aubin, J. E., Heersche, J. N. M. and Antosz, M. E. (1986). Mineralized bone nodules formed in vitro from enzymatically released rat calvarial cell populations. *Calcif. Tissue Int.*, **38**: 143–54.
350. Beresford, J. N., Gallagher, J. A., Poser, J. W. and Russell, R. G. (1984). Production of osteocalcin by human bone cells in vitro. Effects of $1,25(OH)_2D_3$, $24,25(OH)_2D_3$, parathyroid hormone, and glucocorticoids. *Metab. Bone Dis. Relat. Res.*, **5**: 229–34.
351. Catherwood, B. D. (1985). 1,25-Dihydroxycholecalciferol and glucocorticosteroid regulation of adenylate cyclase in an osteoblast-like cell line. *J. Biol. Chem.*, **260**: 736–43.
352. Chen, T. L., Cone, C. M. and Feldman, D. (1983). Glucocorticoid modulation of cell proliferation in cultured osteoblast-like bone cells: differences between rat and mouse. *Endocrinology*, **112**: 1739–45.
353. Chen, T. L. and Feldman, D. (1985). Retinoic acid modulation of $1,25(OH)_2$ vitamin $D_3$ receptors and bioresponse in bone cells: species differences between rat and mouse. *Biochem. Biophys. Res. Commun.*, **132**: 74–80.
354. Chen, T. L., Hauschka, P. V. and Feldman, D. (1986). Dexamethasone increases 1,25-dihydroxyvitamin $D_3$ receptor levels and augments bioresponses in rat osteoblast-like cells. *Endocrinology*, **118**: 1119–26.
355. Ecarot-Charrier, B., Glorieux, F. H., van der Rest, M. and Periera, G. (1983). Osteoblasts isolated from mouse calvaria initiate matrix mineralization in culture. *J. Cell Biol.*, **96**: 639–43.
356. Feyen J. H., van der Wilt G., Moonen P., Di-Bon A. and Nijweide P. J. (1984)

Stimulation of arachidonic acid metabolism in primary cultures of osteoblast-like cells by hormones and drugs. *Prostaglandins*, **28**: 769−81.

357. Gerstenfeld, L. C., Chipman, S. D., Glowacki, J. and Lian, J. B. (1987). Expression of differentiated function by mineralizing cultures of chicken osteoblasts. *Develop. Biol.*, **122**: 49−60.

358. Hamilton J. A., Lingelbach S. R., Partridge N. C. and Martin T. J. (1985). Regulation of plasminogen activator production by bone-resorbing hormones in normal and malignant osteoblasts. *Endocrinology*, **116**: 2186−91.

359. Jones, S. J., Boyde, A. and Ali, N. N. (1986). The interface of cells and their matrices in mineralized tissues: a review. *Scan. Electron. Microsc.*, **(Pt 4)**: 1555−69.

360. Kodama, H., Amagai, Y., Sudo, H., Kasai, S. and Yamamoto, S. (1981). Establishment of a clonal osteogenic cell line from newborn mouse calvaria. *Jpn. J. Oral Biol.*, **23**: 899−901.

361. Majeska, R. J., Nair, B. C. and Rodan, G. A. (1985). Glucocorticoid regulation of alkaline phosphatase in the osteoblastic osteosarcoma cell line ROS 17/2.8. *Endocrinology*, **116**: 170−9.

362. Manolagas, S. C., Spiess, Y. H., Burton, D. W. and Deftos, L. J. (1983). Mechanism of action of 1,25-dihydroxyvitamin $D_3$-induced stimulation of alkaline phophatase in cultured osteoblast-like cells. *Mol. Cell Endocrinol.*, **33**: 27−36.

363. Miller, S. C. and Jee, W. S. (1987). The bone lining cell: a distinct phenotype? *Calcif. Tissue Int.*, **41**: 1−5.

364. Nijweide, P. J., Burger, E. H. and Feyen, J. H. (1986). Cells of bone: proliferation, differentiation, and hormonal regulation. *Physiol. Rev.*, **66**: 855−86.

365. Owen M. E. and Friedenstein A. J. (1988). Stromal stem cells: marrow-derived osteogenic precursors. In *Cell and Molecular Biology of Vertebrate Hard Tissues* CIBA Foundation Symposium 136, Wiley, New York, pp. 42−60.

366. Partridge, N. C., Hillyard, C. J., Nolan, R. D. and Martin, T. J. (1985). Regulation of prostaglandin production by osteoblast-rich calvarial cells. *Prog. Clin. Biol. Res.*, **187**: 67−76.

367. Partridge, N. C., Jeffrey, J. J., Ehlich, L. S., Teitelbaum, S. L., Fliszar, C., Welgus, H. G. and Kahn, A. J. (1987). Hormonal regulation of the production of collagenase and a collagenase inhibitor activity by rat osteogenic sarcoma cells. *Endocrinology*, **120**: 1956−62.

368. Peck W. A. and Rifas L. (1982). Regulation of osteoblast activity and the osteoblast osteocyte transformation. *Adv. Exp. Med. Biol.*, **151**: 393−400.

369. Raisz, L. G. (1988). Hormonal regulation of bone growth and remodelling. In *Cell and Molecular Biology of Vertebrate Hard Tissues* CIBA Foundation Symposium 136, Wiley, New York, pp 226−238.

370. Robey, P. G. and Termine, J. D. (1985). Human bone cells *in vitro*. *Calcif. Tissue Int.*, **37**: 453−60.

371. Rodan, G. A., Heath, J. K., Yoon, K., Noda, M. and Rodan, S. B. (1988). Diversity of the osteoblastic phenotype. In *Cell and Molecular Biology of Vertebrate Hard Tissues* CIBA Foundation Symposium 136, Wiley, New York, pp. 78−91.

372. Rosen, D. M. and Luben, R. A. (1983). Multiple hormonal mechanisms for the control of collagen synthesis in an osteoblast like cell line, NMB-1. *Endocrinology*, **112**: 992−9.

373. Sakamoto, S. and Sakamoto, M. (1984). Osteoblast collagenase: collagenase synthesis by clonally derived mouse osteogenic (MC3T3-E1) cells. *Biochem. Int.*, **9**: 51−8.

374. Tenenbaum, H. C. (1988). Cellular origins and theories of differentiation of bone-forming cells. In *Bone. Vol. 1: The Osteoblast and Osteocyte*, BK Hall, ed. (this volume).

375. Wong, G. L. (1988). Isolation and behavior of bone-forming cells. In *Bone. Vol. 1: The Osteoblast and Osteocyte*, BK Hall, ed. (this volume).

376. Yoon, K., Buenaga, R. and Rodan, G. A. (1987). Tissue specificity and developmental expression of rat osteopontin. *Biochem. Biophys. Res. Commun.*, **148**: 1129−36.

## VI. Phenotypic Modulation of Osteoblasts by Growth Factors
(See individual references in Section III above)

## VII. Multiple Growth Factor Effects: Synergism/Antagonism

377. Baird, A. and Durkin, T. (1986). Inhibition of endothelial cell proliferation by type beta-transforming growth factor: interactions with acidic and basic fibroblast growth factors. *Biochem. Biophys. Res. Commun.*, **138**: 476−82.
378. Canalis, E. (1983). Effect of hormones and growth factors on alkaline phosphatase activity and collagen synthesis in cultured rat calvariae. *Metabolism*, **32**: 14−20.
379. Centrella, M., McCarthy, T. L. and Canalis, E. (1987). Mitogenesis in fetal rat bone cells simultaneously exposed to type beta transforming growth factor and other growth regulators. *FASEB J.*, **1**: 312−7.
380. Cheng, S. L., Shen, V., Wun, J. and Peck, W. A. (1988). Regulation of plasminogen activator production by growth factors. *J. Bone Mineral Res.*, **3**: S174.
381. Globus, R. K., Patterson-Buckendahl, P. and Gospodarowicz, D. (1988). Regulation of bovine bone cell proliferation by fibroblast growth factor and transforming growth factor beta. *Endocrinology*, **123**: 98−105.
382. Massague, J., Kelly, B. and Mottola, C. (1985). Stimulation by insulin-like growth factors is required for cellular transformation by type beta transforming growth factor. *J. Biol. Chem.*, **260**: 4551−4.
383. Mavrakos, A. and Hauschka, P. V. (1986). Effects of bone derived growth factors on rat osteoblasts. *J. Dent. Res.*, **65**: 832.
384. Mohan, S., Linkhart, T., Farley, J. and Baylink, D. (1984). Bone-derived factors active on bone cells. *Calcif. Tissue Int.*, **36(Suppl 1)**: S139−45.
385. O'Keefe, R. J., Crabb, I. D., Puzas, J. E., Hansen, L. A. and Rosier, R. N. (1988). TGF-beta, basic FGF, and IGF-I demonstrate interactive and synergistic effects on DNA synthesis in growth plate chondrocytes. *J. Bone Mineral Res.*, **3**: S176.
386. Simpson, E. (1987). Growth factors which affect bone. In *Oncogenes and Growth Factors* Bradshaw R. A., Prentis S. eds., Elsevier, Amsterdam, pp 183−8.
387. Sporn, M. B., Roberts, A. B., Roche, N. S., Kagechika, H. and Shudo, K. (1986). Mechanism of action of retinoids. *J. Am. Acad. Dermatol.*, **15**: 756−64.
388. Triffitt, J. T. (1987). Initiation and enhancement of bone formation-a review. *Acta. Orthop. Scand.*, **58**: 673−84.
389. Urist, M. R., DeLange, R. J. and Finerman, G. A. (1983). Bone cell differentiation and growth factors. *Science*, **220**: 680−6.
390. Wahl, S. M., Hunt, D. A., Wong, H. L., Dougherty, S., McCartney-Francis, N., Wahl, L. M., Ellingsworth, L., Schmidt, J. A., Hall, G., Roberts, A. B. and Sporn, M. B. (1988). Transforming growth factor-beta is a potent immunosuppressive agent that inhibits IL-1-dependent lymphocyte proliferation. *J. Immunol.*, **140**: 3026−32.
391. Wong, G. L., Roberts, R. and Miller, E. (1987). Production of and response to growth-stimulating activity in isolated bone cells. *J. Bone Mineral Res.*, **2**: 23−8.

## VIII.  Possible Mechanisms for Activation, Release, and Presentation of Growth Factors in Bone

392.  Baird, A. and Ling, N. (1987). Fibroblast growth factors are present in the extracellular matrix produced by endothelial cells *in vitro*: implications for a role of heparinase-like enzymes in the neovascular response. *Biochem. Biophys. Res. Commun.*, **142**: 428−35.

393.  Barnes D. W. and Colowick S. P. Stimulation of sugar uptake and thymidine incorporation in mouse 3T3 cells by calcium phosphate and other extracellular particles. *Proc. Natl. Acad. Sci. USA*, **74**: 5593−7 (1977)

394.  Baron, R., Neff, L., Louvard, D. and Courtoy, P. J. (1985). Cell-mediated extracellular acidification and bone resorption: evidence for a low pH in resorbing lacunae and localization of a 100−kD lysosomal membrane protein at the osteoclast ruffled border. *J. Cell Biol.*, **101**: 2210−22.

395.  Baron, R., Neff, L., Brown, W., Courtnoy, P. J., Louvard, D. and Farquhar, M. G. (1988). Polarized secretion of lysosomal enzymes: co-distribution of cation-independent mannose-6-phosphate receptors and lysosomal enzymes along the osteoclast exocytotic pathway. *J. Cell Biol.*, **106**: 1863−72.

396.  Blair, H. C., Kahn, A. J., Crouch, E. C., Jeffrey, J. J. and Teitelbaum, S. L. (1986). Isolated osteoclasts resorb the organic and inorganic components of bone. *J. Cell Biol.*, **102**: 1164−72.

397.  Burr, D. B., Martin, R. B., Schaffler, M. B. and Radin, E. L. (1985). Bone remodelling in response to *in vivo* fatigue microdamage. *J. Biomech.*, **18**: 189−200.

398.  Chambers, T. J. and Fuller, K. (1985). *Calcif. Tissue Int.*, **37**: 162a.

399.  Cheng, S. L., Shen, V., Wun, J. and Peck, W. A. (1988). Regulation of plasminogen activator production by growth factors. *J. Bone Mineral Res.*, **3**: S174.

400.  Ferrier, J., Ross, S. M., Kanehisa, J. and Aubin, J. E. (1986). Osteoclasts and osteoblasts migrate in opposite directions in response to a constant electrical field. *J. Cell Physiol.*, **129**: 283−8.

401.  Frost, H. M. (1987). Bone "mass" and the "mechanostat": a proposal. *Anat. Rec.*, **219**: 1−9.

402.  Fuller, K. and Chambers, T. J. (1988). Bone matrix stimulates osteoclastic differentiation in cultures of rabbit bone marrow cells. *J. Bone Mineral Res.*, **3**: S201.

403.  Howard, G. A., Bottemiller, B. L., Turner, R. T., Rader, R. I. and Baylink, D. J. (1981). Parathyroid hormone stimulates bone formation and resorption in organ culture: evidence for a coupling mechanism. *Proc. Natl. Acad. Sci. USA*, **78**: 3204−8.

404.  Keski-Oja, J., Leof, E. B., Lyons, R. M., Coffey, R. J. Jr., Moses, H. L. (1987) Transforming growth factors and control of neoplastic cell growth. *J. Cell Biochem.*, **33**: 95−107.

405.  Manishen, W. J., Sivananthan, K. and Orr, F. W. (1986). Resorbing bone stimulates tumor cell growth. A role for the host microenvironment in bone metastasis. *Am. J. Pathol.*, **123**: 39−45.

406.  Parfitt, A. M. (1982). The coupling of bone formation to bone resorption: a critical analysis of the concept and of its relevance to the pathogenesis of osteoporosis. *Metab. Bone Dis. Relat. Res.*, **4**: 1−6.

407.  Rodan, G. A. and Martin, T. J. (1981). Role of osteoblasts in hormonal control of bone resorption − a hypothesis. *Calcif. Tissue Int.*, **33**: 349−52.

408.  Shimizu, H., Sakamoto, S., Sakamoto, M. and Lee, D. D. (1989). The effect of substrate composition and condition on resorption by isolated osteoclasts. *Bone and Mineral*, **6**: 261−275.

409. Van der Plas, A. and Nijweide, P. J. (1988). Cell-cell interactions in the osteogenic compartment of bone. *Bone*, **9**: 107−111.

## IX. Osteoinduction as an In Vivo Model for Growth Factor Effects

410. Bolander, M. (1989). Growth factor effects in a healing fracture model. In Press.
411. Forster, S., Triffitt, J. T., Bauer, H. C. F., Brosjo, O., Nilsson, O. S., Smith, R. and Sykes, B. (1988). Interferon-inhibited human osteosarcoma xenografts induce host bone in nude mice. *J. Bone Min. Res.*, **3**: 199−202.
412. Howes, R., Bowness, J. M., Grotendorst, G. R., Martin, G. R. and Reddi, A. H. (1988). Platelet-derived growth factor enhances demineralized bone matrix-induced cartilage and bone formation. *Calcif. Tissue Int.*, **42**: 34−8.
413. Kapur, S. P. and Reddi, A. H. (1986). Chondrogenic potential of mesenchymal cells elicited by bone matrix *in vitro*. *Differentiation*, **32**: 252−9.
414. Rath, N. C. and Reddi, A. H. (1979). *Nature*, **278**: 855−857.
415. Reddi, A. H. (1981). Cell biology and biochemistry of endochondral bone development. *Collagen Res.*, **1**: 209−26.
416. Wozney, J. M., Rosen, V., Celeste, A. J., Mitsock, L. M., Whitters, M. J., Kriz, R. W., Hewick, R. M., Wang, E. A. (1988). Novel regulators of bone formation: molecular clones and activities. *Science*, **242**: 1528−34.
417. Sampath, T. K., Muthukumaran, N. and Reddi, A. H. (1987). Isolation of osteogenin, an extracellular matrix-associated, bone-inductive protein, by heparin affinity chromatography. *Proc. Natl. Acad. Sci. USA*, **84**: 7109−13.
418. Shimizu, N., Yoshikawa, H., Takaoka, K. and Ono, K. (1983). Extracts of cortical bone from adult rats stimulate DNA synthesis in osteoprogenitor cells from fetal rats. *Clin. Orthop.*, **178**: 252−7.
419. Spampata, R., Werther, J. R. and Hauschka, P. V. (1987). Accelerated osteoinduction in a rat bone implant model system. *J. Bone Min. Res.*, **2**: Suppl 1, 410A.
420. Tornberg, D. N. and Bassett, C. A. L. (1977). Activation of resting periosteum. *Clin. Orthop., Rel. Res.*, **129**: 305.
421. Urist, M. R., Huo, Y. K. and Brownell, A. G. (1984). Purification of bovine bone morphogenetic protein by hydroxyapatite chromatography. *Proc. Natl. Acad. Sci. USA*, **81**: 371−5.
422. Urist, M. R., Chang, J. J., Lietze, A., Huo, Y. K., Brownell, A. G. and DeLange, R. J. (1987). Preparation and bioassay of bone morphogenetic protein and polypeptide fragments. *Methods Enzymol.*, **146**: 294−312.
423. Werther, J. R., Spampata, R. and Hauschka, P. V. (1987). Enhanced osteoinduction in a rat bone implant model system. *J. Dent. Res.*, **66**: 220.
424. Wlodarski, K. H. and Reddi, A. H. (1987). Tumor cells stimulate *in vivo* periosteal bone formation. *Bone and Mineral*, **2**: 185−92.
425. Yoshikawa, H., Takaoka, K., Shimizu, N., Ono, K., Nakata, Y. and Amitani, K. (1982). Biochemical stability of a bone-inducing substance from murine osteosarcoma. *Clin. Orthop.*, **163**: 248−53.
426. Yoshikawa, H., Takaoka, K., Shimizu, N. and Ono, K. (1986). Acid solutions enhance bone-inducing activity of a murine osteosarcoma. *Bone*, **7**: 125−8.

# 5

# Isolation and Behavior of Isolated Bone-Forming Cells

**GLENDA WONG**
*Department of Biology,*
*University of Colorado at Colorado Springs,*
*Colorado Springs, Colorado*

## Introduction

Bone forming cells are mesenchymal in origin, normally reside in bone and are responsible for osteogenesis. This process is executed through the synthesis and secretion of an organic matrix which subsequently undergoes calcification by deposition of crystals of calcium and phosphate. The mechanism of biological calcification is still not understood.

More recently, the role of bone forming cells in bone metabolism has been expanded by evidence which demonstrates a possible stimulatory effect on bone resorbing cells, osteoclasts (Chambers *et al.*, 1985; McSheehy *et al.*, 1987; Perry *et al.*, 1987). These observations place bone forming cells in a pivotal role in both directing as well as maintaining a balance between the ongoing, dual processes of formation and resorption.

Heterogeneity exists *in situ* within bone forming cells. The evidence for this includes the morphological differences noted in bone sections. Developmental studies using pulse chase experiments with $^3$H thymidine confirm the presence of a rapidly dividing cell layer close to the bone surface. Biochemical evidence for heterogeneity has also been provided by more recent studies illustrating that many agents that stimulate bone formation do so by inducing proliferation and differentiation of osteoblast precursor cells, rather than through direct stimulation of mature osteoblasts (Canalis and Raisz, 1979; Hock *et al.*, 1987; Canalis, 1984).

These observations underscore the fact that bone forming cells consist of subpopulations with different biochemical characteristics and unique responses to physiological stimuli. An understanding of the functions, interactions and final contribution of each sub group to the complex reactions that culminate in bone deposition remains elusive in spite of the rapid progress achieved in recent years.

## Assessment of the Osteoblast Phenotype

The cellular heterogeneity of bone has been an impediment to understanding and tracking the cellular chain of events that are the basis of tissue response to hormones and drugs. In addition, the compositional heterogeneity of bone has made it difficult to obtain comparable tissue samples. These difficulties have led investigators to attempt characterization of bone forming cells using preparations of isolated, matrix-free cells (Wong *et al.*, 1974; Peck *et al.*, 1964; Chen *et al.*, 1977; Nijweidi *et al.*, 1987; Harrell *et al.*, 1973; Mills *et al.*, 1979). Although the ideal standard for assessment of such cell preparations would appear to be measurement of their immediate or eventual development of osteogenic capacity, *in vivo* and *in vitro* measurements of calcification are tedious and non-quantitative. As a result, indirect assessment of the bone forming phenotype has been most commonly used to date. Early attempts at *in vitro* cell characterization utilized the data derived from histochemical studies on bone slices and *in vivo* responses to parathyroid hormone. The former studies showed an abundance of alkaline phosphatase in the osteoblast layer, the latter an inhibition of bone formation by high levels of parathyroid hormone. Thus, even though alkaline phosphatase of bone is not unique to osteoblasts, being similar to that found in kidney, liver and placenta (Goldstein *et al.*, 1980) and even though the role of this enzyme in bone mineralization is still not understood, alkaline phosphatase has generally used as a characteristic marker for the osteoblast phenotype. Similarly, parathyroid hormone response has become synonymous with the osteoblast phenotype in bone derived cells. This characteristic was subsequently verified by the autoradiographical demonstration of PTH receptors on chick osteoblasts *in situ* in calvaria (Silve *et al.*, 1982) and on bone cells (Pliam *et al.*, 1982).

Additional markers for osteoblast cells became established when molecules secreted by bone organ cultures were subsequently shown to be also produced by mixtures of isolated osteoblastic bone-derived cells. Such molecules include $PGE_2$, a stimulator of bone resorption, (Voekel *et al.*, 1980; Feyen *et al.*, 1984; Rodan *et al.*, 1981) collagenase and collagenase inhibitor (Nagayama *et al.*, 1984; Otaska *et al.*, 1984; Sakamoto and Sakamoto, 1984), growth regulatory factors including transforming growth factor β (Centrella and Canalis, 1986), IGF-1 (Stracke *et al.*, 1984; Wong and Van de Pol, 1987) and IGF-II (Mohan *et al.*, 1988) and matrix components such as Type 1 collagen, osteonectin (Termine *et al.*, 1981) and osteocalcin (Price, 1983). Among these secreted products only osteocalcin appears to be bone specific, with all the others also being synthesized by other tissues. Taken together however, these products constitute a wide array of markers, the production of which can be used to both identify, as well as classify, osteoblasts into subgroups.

Similar comments can be made regarding the hormone receptors identified in bone tissue, in populations of isolated bone cells and in clones of bone cells. Osteoblastic cells contain receptors for bone active peptides including PTH (Silve *et al.*, 1982), $PGE_2$ (Partridge *et al.*, 1981), EGF (Ng *et al.*, 1983) and bone active steroids, including glucocorticoids (Feldman *et al.*, 1975; Chen *et al.*, 1978, 1979) and $1,25(OH)_2D_3$ (Chen *et al.*, 1983, 1979; Murray *et al.*, 1986).

To date, the most thorough comparison between hormone responsiveness and osteoblastic phenotype has been carried out for PTH and a direct correlation between these characteristics has been shown in calvarial cells (Luben *et al.*, 1976; Rao *et al.*, 1977) and in osteosarcoma cell lines (Majeska *et al.*, 1980; Partridge *et al.*, 1981, 1983; Rodan *et al.*, 1974).

Many other tissues respond to the hormones mentioned above, and so the presence of receptors for these agents cannot be used as specific osteoblast markers. Bone and osteoblast specific biological hormonal responses have been also identified however. The effects of glucocorticoids on osteoblasts include potentiation of PTH effects on citrate decarboxylation (Wong, 1979) and on cAMP production through stimulation of adenylate cyclase and inhibition of phosphodiesterase (Chen and Feldman, 1978, 1979). $1,25(OH)_2D_3$ has also been shown to stimulate the synthesis of the bone specific protein osteocalcin or bone gla protein by ROS17 osteosarcoma cells (Price *et al.*, 1980, 1981).

These various hormonal response studies were carried out primarily on mixtures of osteogenic cells and it remains to be seen if hormonal responses depend on, or are regulated by, the developmental stage of the osteogenic cells. Localization of bone-specific, hormonal responses within subgroups of osteogenic cells may allow us to map the communication and developmental pathways between mature and immature osteogenic cells. At present such studies are limited by preparative and isolation techniques that still do not provide a clear separation of subgroups of bone cells. Nevertheless, much progress in bone cell isolation and characterization has been achieved in the past decade, as is detailed below.

## Isolated Bone Cells — Models of Choice

To date, two general approaches have been used in the preparation of isolated matrix-free bone forming cells. One set of studies has utilized freshly-isolated, primary cultures of tissue-derived cells, while another has used permanent or immortal cell lines derived either from osteosarcoma tumors (Rodan and Rodan, 1983; Partridge *et al.*, 1981) or from bone cell clones selected from primary cultures (Kodama *et al.*, 1981; Aubin *et al.*, 1982). Each of these experimental models has unique advantages as well as limitations.

### Primary Cultures

One advantage of primary cultures or of freshly isolated bone cells is that studies are carried out on non-transformed cells; any possible contribution of the transformed phenotype to a measured response can be discounted. This is of particular relevance in studies on growth factors derived from bone since transformed cells may produce a different subset of growth regulators. Secondly, primary cultures have the potential to contain all the different classes of bone-forming cells known to be present in bone. If sufficient separation of these groups can be achieved and conditions are established for maintaining them in culture, studies on the unique characteristics of, as well as interactions between, these subpopulations can be carried out.

However the drawbacks associated with this system are many. Cell isolation is time consuming and optimum conditions for achieving high yields are still being developed. Enzymatic digestion of matrix is the most commonly used method but the cytotoxic effect of many proteases remains a problem and may result in low cell yield. Proteases may also remove many proteins on the cell surface, in which case studies such as the quantitation and characterization of hormone receptors cannot be carried out on freshly isolated cells.

Culture of isolated bone cells can also result in the alteration of phenotypic expression. Primary cultures of bone forming cells may retain their osteo-blastic phenotype for relatively short periods of time (Wong et al., 1974). Expression of osteoblastic features was reported to be decreased with each subculture of mouse bone cells, suggesting either dedifferentiation of mature cells or overgrowth by immature cells.

In contrast, transformed osteosarcoma cells that express osteoblastic characteristics can be maintained in permanent culture (Rodan and Rodan, 1983 for review) to provide large amounts of cells for biochemical studies. Unlike the heterogeneous populations present in cell preparations from bone, highly homogeneous populations can be obtained by cloning techniques that permit selection for cells expressing varying degrees of osteoblastic characteristics. However, it is not known whether differences between clones are due to the presence of cells fixed in various stages of development or arise from dedifferentiation in culture. Unique difference have been noted between UMR-6 (rat) ROS17-2 (rat) and MC3T3-$E_1$ (mouse) osteoblastic clones derived from different sources in several laboratories; UMR-6 cells exhibit EGF receptors (Ng et al., 1983) and do not synthesize $PGE_2$ (Nolan et al., 1983), both in contrast to ROS 17-2 cells. On the other hand, MC3T3-$E_1$ cells, described as immature bone cells, exhibit receptors for EGF (Hata et al., 1984) and $PGE_2$ (Hakeda, 1985) but not PTH, when tested in serum. It is not known if these clones represent osteoblastic phenotypes present in bone, or are aberrations induced by culture.

In addition to heterogeneity between clones, phenotypic variations exist between progeny cells within a single clone. These differences may arise as the cells cycle through different growth conditions such as high and low density. At low density osteoblast marker activities/cell are reduced. At high density, following several rounds of mitosis, osteoblastic expression is increased. These changes in osteoblastic expression are not unique to es-tablished cell lines however. Recent reports describe a tissue culture phenomenon in which confluency and high cell density are associated with expression of OB characteristics in both normal (Gerstenfeld et al., 1987) as well as transformed cells (Rodan and Majeska, 1982).

Against this background of changing osteoblast marker expression, changes of a more permanent kind also become apparent with time. Sister cells among the progeny from a single cloned osteosarcoma cell do not all retain the same characteristics; periodic subcloning and re-selection for the original phenotype is necessary (Murray and Manolagas, 1986; Limeback *et al.*, 1984). Finally, the contribution of the transformed phenotype to these variations between and within clones is not known.

From the above arguments it should be clear that the choice of an experimental model of bone forming cells will be dictated by the problem to be studied, based on utilizing the unique advantages of each system. Freshly isolated and/or primary cultures allow studies on developmental stages, differentiation, and cellular interactions among subpopulations of osteogenic cells. Markers established by these studies may permit and/or confirm the classification of transformed clones into several developmental stages. Transformed cloned cell lines on the other hand can provide large amounts of homogeneous material for large scale studies and biochemical purification of cellular products.

## Isolation of Bone-Forming Cells

Matrix-free, bone-forming cells have been isolated by two approaches; a) non-enzymatic procedures such as microdissection or tissue explant methods and b) by enzymatic dissolution of the bone matrix.

### Non Enzymatic Isolation Procedure

i) Microdissection of bone permits the investigator to separate the periosteum from the rest of the tissue (Nijweide *et al.*, 1981, 1982) but is of very limited use unless followed by a tissue explant procedure or by the enzymatic digestion of the remaining bone tissue.

ii) Tissue explant procedures allow cells to migrate from bone on to an adjoining solid substrate. This non-enzymatic isolation procedure has been used by investigators wishing to circumvent cytotoxicity and cell damage by proteases (Jones and Boyde, 1977; Beresford *et al.*, 1983).

The ability of osteoblasts to migrate out from bone after removal of the periosteum was described by Jones and Boyde in 1977 and has been adopted to human bone by others (Ecarot Charier *et al.*, 1983; Beresford *et al.*, 1983). This method appears to be highly suited to situations where tissue is very limiting and/or cell growth is slow, such as seen in adult bone, since cell survival may be enhanced by the close cell contact maintained during migration. The tissue explant method of cell preparation probably selects for the cells with the highest proliferative capacity in bone and, being a local phenomenon, may select for the bone cells adjoining the point of contact of tissue and solid substrate.

The cells obtained by tissue explant from adult bone (Auf'mkolk *et al.*, 1985) or newborn mouse calvaria (Ecarot-Charier *et al.*, 1983) appear to be primarily osteoblastic. In the latter studies the periosteum was removed and the osteoblast layer was exposed prior to cell migration. In cells so obtained (mouse calvarial explants) 11.2% of their total protein synthesis was devoted to collagen production which was greater than 90% type 1 collagen (Ecarot-Charier *et al.*, 1983). After 5–6 days in culture, cells grown in β glycerophosphate laid down mineral deposits in localized multilayered areas. Cells also stained intensely for alkaline phosphatase, in contrast to fibroblastic cultures.

Explants of adult human bone (Auf'mkolk *et al.*, 1985) were also shown to have the following osteoblastic characteristics — 1) a responsiveness to parathyroid hormone, as demonstrated by increased cyclic AMP 2) the production of the bone-specific protein osteocalcin 3) the enhancement of osteocalcin synthesis by $1,25(OH)_2D_3$ and 4) the lack of calcitonin response.

The net changes induced by either PTH or $1,25(OH)_2D_3$ varied widely between explants from different bones and no correlation was seen between absolute cAMP response to PTH and osteocalcin changes with $1,25(OH)_2D_3$ within the same explant.

The above data establish, however, that cells found in explants from bone tissue contain osteoblastic characteristics. Explants prepared from mouse calvaria were periosteum free and thus these cells are presumed to arise from the osteoblast layer of bone. Nevertheless, variability in terms of alkaline phosphatase and initiation of mineralization was clearly apparent within single cultures. Differentiated cells and osteocytes were apparent within multilayer cell clusters and less differentiated cells occurred on the periphery of the cell clusters. This phenomenon could occur if osteoblasts in culture dedifferentiate as they regain their proliferative capacity and then redifferentiate when growth is slowed within dense cell clusters. Another possibility is that precursor cells, with their high proliferative capacity, selectively migrate out of the tissue and undergo differentiation in dense cultures.

In summary, bone tissue explants consist of osteoblast-like cells, some of which undergo differentiation into matrix mineralizing centers as their cultures become dense and multilayered. This behavior is similar to that reported for cloned rat osteosarcoma cells, which show increasing osteoblastic characteristics when sparse cultures attain confluency (Majeska and Rodan, 1982). Similar induction of osteoblastic function in confluent monolayer cultures was reported in normal chicken cells obtained by enzymatic digestion of embryonic calvaria (Gerstenfeld *et al.*, 1987). In these latter experiments cells were selected by initial growth at low density.

In spite of being derived from cells prepared by 3 different methods of cell preparation the above data indicate that bone forming cells grown in monolayer culture in serum undergo proliferation and/or differentiation depending on cell density and time in culture. It is not known whether eventual differentiation in culture is a characteristic of osteoprogenitor cells. These experiments do further suggest however (Ecarot-Charier *et al.*, 1983) that mature osteoblasts also have the potential to re-initiate proliferation in culture.

## Enzymatic Isolation of Bone Cells

In contrast to tissue explant, enzymatic digestion of bone permits, in theory, recovery of all the cell types present in bone. Cell release from bone by proteolysis was reported as early as 1932 by Fitton-Jackson and Smith who used trypsin to obtain matrix degradation and cell release. The use of crude collagenase was introduced in 1964 by Peck *et al.*, Many laboratories studying primary cultures of bone cells presently use variations of the method introduced by Peck and his colleagues due to the rapidity of cell isolation, the relatively large yields of cells and completeness of cell extraction from bone.

A major disadvantage of enzymatic isolation is the presence of cytotoxic proteases in the crude collagenase preparation which may lead to decreased yields due to their cytoxic effects on cells. This phenomenon of enzymatic cytotoxicity has been studied in detail by Hefley *et al.*, (1983, 1987). Commercial preparations of crude bacterial collagenase were analyzed by ion exchange chromatography and found to contain varying proportions of at least 3 proteolytic activities in addition to collagenase. These include an amino peptidase, a neutral protease and clostripain. The latter activity was shown to be highly cytotoxic to bone cells. Blocking clostripain activity or removing clostripain from crude collagenase resulted in cell preparations that appeared relatively undamaged when assessed by equilibrium density. Cells prepared in the absence of clostripain averaged 1.074 g/ml in Ficoll gradients, in contrast to cells prepared with crude collagenase, which reached a median density of 1.063 g/ml with 16% of the cells failing to enter the gradient. These differences in equilibrium density profile suggest plasma membrane damage occurs in cells isolated in crude collagenase even though total cell yields and viability, as measured by trypan blue exclusion, were comparable.

More recently Hefley (1987) has demonstrated that two classes of collagenase (I and II) may be present in crude preparations of bacterial collagenase and decreased cell yield is associated with the class II ioszyme.

## Characteristics of Cells Obtained by Enzymatic Digestion of Bone.

Even though final cell yields from bone can vary widely between different commercial lots of crude collagenase, successful isolation of cells has been achieved with crude collagenase and/or trypsin in quantities sufficient to permit biochemical studies (Wong and Cohn, 1974, 1975).

Enzymatic digestion has been carried out on fetal, neonatal and adult calvaria and/or long bones from rat (Peck *et al.*, 1964; Dziak and Brand, 1974; Smith *et al.*, 1973; Partridge *et al.*, 1981), mouse (Wong and Cohn, 1974, 1975), chick (Nijweide *et al.*, 1981), rabbit (Yee, 1983) and man (Weigedal *et al.*, 1984; Auf'mkolk *et al.*, 1985).

Although a total digestion of bone would be expected to result in a cell mixture containing osteoblasts in various developmental stages, osteocytes and periosteal fibroblasts (the latter in cases where removal of periosteum was not performed) these cell preparations have consistently demonstrated hormonal responses and other activities regarded as characteristic of osteoblasts e.g. synthesis of bone matrix proteins such as collagen osteocalcin and osteonectin. These mixed cells also exhibit dose dependent sensitivity to and receptor-specific binding for parathyroid hormone (Pliam *et al.*, 1982; Auf'mkolk *et al.*, 1985). Furthermore, they contain alkaline phosphatase which appears to be the bone isoenzyme when tested by heat denaturation, enzyme inhibitor and immunochemical reactivity (Yee, 1983).

These data are not surprising since osteogenic cells are the most prevalent cell type in bone. However, a general mixture of bone cells remains inadequate for many types of current studies. There is at present much interest in autocrine and paracrine interaction between bone cells (see chapters 4 and 8 in this volume). Such interactions have been suggested by observations that bone resorbing agents including parathyroid hormone may induce the secretion of osteoclast activating cytokines by osteoblastic cells (Chambers *et al.*, 1985) and that osteoblastic cells synthesize several growth factors including TGFβ, IGF-I and IGF-II (Centrella and Canalis, 1986; Wong and VandePol, 1987; Mohan *et al.*, 1988) and bone active moieties such as $PGE_2$. Studies on the cellular origins and local targets for these bone derived biomolecules require separation of osteogenic cells into subclasses. Several isolation procedures have attempted to address this problem and these are described below.

### Free Flow Electrophoresis

Cells obtained by total digestion of fetal rat calvaria in crude collagenase were further separated into subgroups on the basis of their surface charge

(Puzas *et al.*, 1979, 1982). When the cells were passed through an electric field differential deflection towards the anode occurred. Three sets of cells were recovered which, when listed in order of decreasing electrophoretic mobility, were, Peaks I, II and III, representing 5%, 55—60% and 35% of the total cells respectively.

Peak II corresponded to the periosteal fibroblasts and loose connective tissue which was shown by histological examination of remaining tissue to be released within the first 20 minutes of digestion. These cells neither responded to PTH nor to calcitonin and synthesized large amounts of collagen. Peaks I and III were contained in the cells released from bone after removal of Peak II. Peak I exhibited specific binding of $^3$H acetazol-amide (a substrate for carbonic anhydrase) low collagen synthesis and high levels of acid phosphatase, an enzyme usually found in osteoclasts and shown to be present along the endocranial surface of calvaria. Peak I also responded with low but significant cAMP increases to PTH and calcitonin. Peak I cells were classified as osteoclast-related and endocranial surface-derived cells. Peak III cells were highly responsive to parathyroid hormone, and showed the highest DNA synthetic activity as well as substantial collagen synthesis, although no enrichment for alkaline phosphatase could be demonstrated. These cells were identified as a mixture of osteoprogenitor cells, osteoblasts from the endocranial bone surface, and suture line cells which could not be separated by differences in surface charge.

Free flow electrophoresis provided evidence that at least 3 cell groups could be partially separated from the cell mixture obtained following enzymatic digestion of rat calvaria. However, the method did not permit separation of osteoblasts from osteoprogenitor cells and other rapidly-dividing, mesenchymal cells.

## Microdissection and Enzymatic Digestion of Tissues

Four groups of cells were prepared by Nijweide *et al.* (1981) using microdissection of embryonic chick calvaria to remove the periosteum, followed by collagenase treatment to remove osteoblasts, leaving behind the osteocytes embedded in calcified matrix. Histological analysis of tissue after microdissection and after enzyme digestion was used to verify removal of periosteum by microdissection and of osteoblasts with collagenase. The isolated periosteum consisted mainly of fibroblasts in addition to blood and endothelial cells; no osteoblasts were apparent. Collagenase digestion of the periosteum provided a single cell suspension of periosteal fibroblasts. After microdissection, the surface of the periosteum-free bone was covered with osteoblasts in many areas. However, osteoblast loss was also often apparent, resulting in exposure of the uncalcified collagen matrix. Collagenase treatment led to the gradual removal of all uncalcified matrix and associated osteoblasts but cells in the lacuna remained associated with the bone and were subsequently studied *in situ* as osteocytes.

Cells from the periosteum and osteoblast layer underwent rapid proliferation after 3 days in culture in 10% cock serum and by day 9, cell numbers had increased 10−20 fold. Associated with this proliferation was a marked decrease in alkaline phosphatase in both cultures. Periosteal and osteoblastic culture both appeared fibroblastic; no distinguishing morphological features were noted. However, periosteum- and osteoblast layer-derived cells were found to differ in several respects. Osteoblasts contained up to a 10 fold higher alkaline phosphatase level than periosteal cells at the time of isolation, and continued to exhibit higher levels than periosteal cells during culture. In addition osteoblasts exhibited high basal rates of $6^{14}C$ citrate decarboxylation. The most definitive and striking differences between periosteal and osteoblastic cells became apparent when hormone responses and osteogenic capacity were measured. Osteoblasts demonstrated a large cyclic AMP response to parathyroid hormone. Responsiveness to parathyroid hormone increased during culture in osteoblasts, reaching a maximum on day 8, and declining thereafter. In contrast, periosteal cells exhibited only a small increase in cAMP upon PTH treatment (0.03 nmoles versus 2.0 nmoles/mg protein). In spite of this, both groups of cells responded to parathyroid hormone with increased lactate production. Unique responses to PTH were also seen in that citrate decarboxylation was stimulated in periosteal cells and inhibited in osteoblasts treated with PTH. These data point to the possibility that parathyroid hormone utilized second messengers other than cyclic AMP for its biological effects on periosteal cells.

In contrast to the situation with parathyroid hormone the maximum cyclic AMP elicited by $PGE_2$ was at least two fold higher in periosteal cells than in osteoblasts. $PGE_2$ also stimulated periosteal but not osteoblastic DNA synthesis, while the reverse was true for parathyroid hormone (VandePlas *et al.*, 1985). Proliferative effects of PTH and $PGE_2$ thus appeared to be correlated with the relative magnitude of cAMP increase that was induced. The lower response of osteoblasts to $PGE_2$ may however reflect endogenous desensitization of $PGE_2$ receptors since these chick osteoblast cultures appear to synthesize $PGE_2$ and other prostanoids (Feyen *et al.*, 1984).

Another major difference between osteoblastic and periosteal cells was noted in their osteogenic capacity. When cultured on the chorioallantoic membrane of 7 day old quail eggs osteoblasts produced calcified bone matrix, whereas periosteum-derived cells produced only fibrous tissue (Nijweide *et al.*, 1982).

The lack of osteogenic capacity in periosteal fibroblasts may indicate that they consist of highly immature cells not yet programmed to differentiate into osteoblasts. However, plasticity of the osteogenic developmental pathway has been shown in studies following the osteogenic potential of chick limb-bud mesenchymal cells (Osdoby and Caplan, 1980) and of chondroprogenitor cells (Silbermann et al., 1983). Thus, the possibility remains that periosteal fibroblasts may represent mesenchymal cells previously programmed to develop along a different pathway than those in the osteogenic cell pool.

## Special Enzymatic Digestion of Bone

The preparation of cells enriched for different phenotypes can be performed by using a series of timed digestions on bone. This method was first reported in 1974 by Wong and Cohn and involved the use of a mixture of crude collagenase and trypsin. The tissue source for this bone cell preparation was 0−1 day old newborn mice calvaria derived from about 10 different litters. Heterogeneity exists among these bones, and different rates of cell release from each may contribute to further heterogeneity among cells recovered at various times of digestion.

Using this procedure, it was found that the cells released late from bone were the most morphologically homogeneous. Biochemically, these later populations were consistently characterized by high basal levels of alkaline phosphatase and citrate decarboxylation, and were markedly responsive to PTH, expressing large, dose-dependent changes in cyclic AMP (increased) and citrate decarboxylation (decreased). Their demonstrated osteogenic capacity in vivo supported their identification as osteoblasts or cells that differentiated into osteoblasts in culture (Simmons et al., 1982).

The major problems related to heterogeneity have centered around the early released cells. This is probably to be expected since cells from the bone surface, the site of early released cells, would be expected to contain at least periosteum-derived cells, osteoclasts and preosteoclasts, and immature and mature osteoblasts in varying proportions. Thus, early released cells were found to be morphologically heterogeneous, characterized biochemically by low levels of alkaline phosphatase and PTH-inducible cyclic AMP and high levels of acid phosphatase and hyaluronate synthesis. These cells lacked osteogenic capability when cultured in vivo and, furthermore, contained cells that could resorb devitalized bone in response to PTH (Luben et al., 1976).

These early released cells were characterized further by examining their growth patterns, growth requirements, biochemical characteristics and hormonal responses during short term primary and secondary culture. By various methods, including growth selection procedures and cell surface characteristics, it was demonstrated that the subpopulations of cells present probably included periosteal fibroblasts, mature and immature osteoblasts and osteoclasts (Wong et al., 1979, 1983, 1986).

When early released cells were compared after growth for 6 days in 2% vs 10% fetal calf serum, major differences in both cell number and biochemical characteristics were noted (Wong and Kocour, 1983). Cells did not proliferate in 2% serum as rapidly as in 10% and total cell yield differed up to five fold. However, there appeared to have been a selection for osteoclastic cells in 2% serum since an enrichment for basal acid phosphatase and hyaluronate synthesis was seen (Wong and Kocour, 1983). Furthermore spindle shaped fibroblastic cells were absent and osteoblastic marker activities such as alkaline phosphatase and citrate decarboxylation were reduced three fold when compared to early cells grown in 10% serum. Culture conditions with high serum thus appeared to favor overgrowth of osteoclastic cells by osteoblasts. This conclusion is further supported by the absence of calcitonin responsiveness in 12 day old cultures (Wong et al., 1986).

Early populations were also divided into subgroups based on their ability or inability to adhere to polystyrene tissue culture surface in the absence of serum. Cells that required serum for attachment were found to also require high levels of serum (10% fetal calf serum) for initial growth proliferation (Wong et al., 1986). Hormonal responses to PTH and $PGE_2$ differed between early released cells that did or did not require serum for attachment. Serum dependent cells demonstrated neither a cAMP nor a proliferative response to PTH. Furthermore, they exhibited a greater increase in DNA synthesis after $PGE_2$ treatment (34% vs 16%). Preferential proliferative effects of $PGE_2$ on periosteal cells have been reported in human infants in vivo (Udea et al., 1980; Ringel et al., 1982) and in a chick model in vitro (Van de Plas et al., 1985). Thus, on the basis of their spindle shaped fibroblastic appearance, their lack of PTH response, and their proliferation in the presence of $PGE_2$, non-adherent early released cells appear to be enriched for periosteal fibroblasts.

Early released cells that attached in the absence of serum appeared to be related to osteoblasts since they showed a significant cAMP response to PTH that was about one-half that seen in late released cells previously characterized as highly osteoblastic. However, they differed from all other cell groups in their marked, dose-dependent, proliferative response to PTH, an effect that was not seen in serum-dependent adhering cells, and that was minimal (61% vs 22%) in late released osteoblasts. Hormonal stimulation of osteoblast proliferation has been reported to occur in bone in the layer of immature osteoblasts (Canalis and Raisz 1979; Hock et al. 1986). These data therefore suggested a similarity between adherent, early-released cells and immature osteoblasts.

To obtain more homogeneous cell populations this preparative procedure was modified to obtain periosteum removal by pure collagenase prior to enzymatic digestion of the matrix surrounding the cells below. This purification scheme utilized pretreatment of newborn mouse calvaria with pure collagenase, followed by digestion of bone in a clostripain-free mixture of collagenase and neutral protease (Hefley *et al.*, 1983) to obtain release of progenitor cells followed by osteoblasts.

Histological analysis of tissue after each digestion showed that preincubation of mouse bone in purified collagenase resulted in damage to the integrity of the periosteum. Subsequent, brief exposure to collagenase together with neutral protease rapidly completed the release of the periosteum from the bone. Sequential removal of the layer of immature bone cells, and the osteoblast layer, was then carried out in a series of timed digestions in collagenase and protease. Initial cell release was slow but proceeded rapidly once the first 20% of the total yield was released.

Using PTH as a probe, the biochemical profile again suggested no significant cAMP response in periosteal cells, and increasing cAMP response as digestion proceeded towards late released cells.

Immature osteoblasts constitute the proliferative zone of bone; tissue mitogenic response to EGF and IGF-1 is localized to this zone. When the effects of EGF and IGF-1 on $^3$H thymidine incorporation were compared in these groups of cells, all populations responded to IGF-1. However, the major stimulation of $^3$H thymidine incorporation occurred in intermediate populations, followed by periosteal enriched cells and lastly, by osteoblasts of late released populations. A similar response profile was seen with EGF, except that mature osteoblasts expressed almost no proliferative response. In keeping with these findings, intermediate cells also displayed the highest number of EGF receptors/cell. This difference encompassed both high and low affinity types of receptor (Wong *et al.*, in press).

These findings strongly suggested that intermediate released cells were enriched for cells with a high proliferative response to growth factors previously shown to induce mitosis in immature osteoblasts *in situ*. The localization of the major response to IGF-1 and EGF in these cells, and their high EGF receptor numbers suggest that they represent unique cells. Their low osteoblastic biochemical characteristics are not due to their being a mixture of periosteal fibroblasts and mature osteoblasts as has been suggested.

It has recently become apparent that non-systemic regulation of bone growth occurs through growth factors secreted locally by osteoblasts. (See chapter 4, this volume). The identification and hormonal regulation of these factors, and the elucidation of their autocrine and paracrine effects in bone is presently the topic of intense investigation. Transformed rat osteosarcoma cells and fetal rat calvaria (Centrella and Canalis 1986) have been shown to secrete TGFβ. Skeletal growth factor (IGF-II) has been isolated from bone tissue and from cultures of osteoblasts (Moham *et al.*, 1988) and rat bone and mouse bone cells synthesize and secrete IGF-1 (Stracke *et al.*, 1984; Wong *et al.*, 1986). Studies with sequentially derived populations of bone cells showed that extracts of highly osteoblastic cultures contained more growth stimulating activity than earlier released cells. Studies with these cell populations showed that all synthesized IGF-1 (Wong *et al.*, 1987). However, growth hormone-stimulated IGF-1 production was seen only in less mature osteoblastic populations released prior to the highly osteoblastic late populations (Kotliar *et al.*, 1988), again demonstrating the presence of a unique subclass of bone cells in earlier released cells.

Sequential enzymatic digestion of mouse calvaria thus has the potential to provide populations of bone cells enriched for different phenotypes. Further fractionation of these populations into different phenotypes may in the future permit isolation of, and studies on, periosteal fibroblasts, osteoblast precursor cells and osteoblasts.

## Cloning of Bone Cells

To circumvent the heterogeneity associated with bone cell preparations described above, many investigators have isolated clones of osteoblasts using limiting dilution to obtain single cells (Aubin *et al.*, 1982; Kodama *et al.*, 1981). Selection for osteoblastic clones was based on PTH responsive adenylate cyclase (Aubin *et al.*, 1982) high alkaline phosphatase activity (Kodama *et al.*, 1981) and extracellular mineralization of organic matrix. (Sudo *et al.*,) Although it was expected that cloned cells would provide homogeneous cell populations whose phenotype would reflect a specific cell type present in bone, studies with a clonal osteogenic cell line MC3T3-E$_1$ (Kodama *et al.*, 1981) showed that expression of osteoblastic activities is low in sparse cultures and increases as cells reach confluence. In contrast to the mixtures of cells obtained by tissue digestion, cloned cells arise from a single progenitor cell. Thus, variations that arise during later growth probably reflect changes in phenotypic expression rather than the heterogeneity found in cell mixtures. If so, then cloned osteogenic cells can undergo differentiation at high density and conversely, de-differentiation when re-established in culture at low density. Changes similar to those reported above with MC3T3-E$_1$ cells have been seen with transformed rat osteosarcoma clones (Rodan and Majeska, 1980) as well as nontransformed rat and chick osteoblasts. This behavior does not however typify that seen in bone *in situ*, in which osteoblasts and osteocytes generally appear as terminally differentiated. It is not known if these different *in situ* and *in vitro* patterns of behavior are due to the constraints of the surrounding matrix *in situ*, or to anomalies of tissue culture conditions *in vitro* e.g. cells grown in serum could be exposed to growth and differentiation factors not ordinarily present in their *in vivo* milieu.

Clonal cell lines of osteoblasts have been used to study hormonal regulation of osteoblast differentiation. Differentiation into osteoblasts has been defined as an increase in alkaline phosphatase activity and collagen synthesis. By these criteria, prostaglandin $E_2$ (Hakeda *et al.*, 1985a), forskolin (Hakeda *et al.*, 1985b), transferrin (Tsunoi *et al.*, 1984,), PTH and $1,25(OH)_2D_3$ (Kumegawa *et al.*, 1984) were found to induce differentiation of $MC3T3E_1$ osteogenic cells into osteoblasts.

EGF on the other hand, has opposing effects from the agents listed above, leading to a decrease in alkaline phosphatase and Type 1 collagen synthesis in confluent cultures of $MC3T3-E_1$ cells. These effects were accompanied by an increase in Type III collagen production and in DNA synthesis (Hata *et al.*, 1984). EGF effects thus appear to result in a decrease in osteoblastic characteristics accompanied by induction of proliferation.

In view of the above findings, experimental conditions can be adjusted to obtain $MC3T3-E_1$ cells expressing either low (sparse cultures) or high (dense cultures) basal levels of osteoblastic activity and these models can then be used to study developmental problems and hormonal regulation of phenotypic expression. Such studies must assume however that tissue culture manipulations that result in low levels of osteoblast activities also produce cells that are representative of immature osteoblasts.

There appears to be support for this in the temporal changes in gene expression reported by Gerstenfeld *et al.* (1987) in mineralizing second passage cultures of chick osteoblasts. In these cultures it was shown that as cell density increased and proliferation decreased, changes in gene expression occurred in a defined pattern — alkaline phosphatase and osteocalcin synthesis increased when cultures reached confluency and calcification began, and decreased as calcification proceeded. It is not known at present if the behavior of these cells mirrors the developmental stages of an osteoblast as it progresses from a proliferating to a matrix mineralizing entity.

These interesting studies have shown however that previously proliferating bone cells change their phenotype in culture. These findings point to the need to study bone cells under strictly defined culture conditions in order for comparison to be valid.

## Conclusion

Studies utilizing isolated bone cells have contributed to the rapid advance in our knowledge of bone physiology which has occurred in the last decade.

The dynamic nature of bone tissue has been underscored by the discovery of locally produced osteoblast-derived growth factors that probably are responsible for the autocrine and paracrine regulation of bone cell growth.

Intercellular communication, long hinted at by the phenomenon known as coupling, has been now shown to occur between osteoblasts and osteoclasts. The prevalence of PTH receptors on osteoblasts led to the hypothesis (Rodan and Martin, 1981) and eventual demonstration that the bone resorptive response to PTH in osteoclasts was channeled through the osteoblast. Studies with isolated bone cells have thus established bone as a fascinating model for local cellular interactions during tissue response to anabolic and catabolic stimuli.

## Future Directions

The hormonal response profile of bone forming cells has been well studied with isolated osteoblasts. These systems will continue to be used to identify target cells for various bone active agents. Methods in cell preparation are becoming increasingly sophisticated. Preparative procedures to obtain and quantitate highly purified subpopulations of freshly isolated bone forming cells that differ in developmental stage and/or phenotype may become available in the near future. Further characterization of transformed clones may indicate that they are appropriate models for various developmental phenotypes of bone forming cells. Highly purified populations of bone cells will be needed for future studies which will seek to identify the mediators of hormone action and to establish hormone regulated genes in bone forming cells. Methods for maintaining bone cells in culture with continued expression of their original phenotype will have to be developed. Future topics for research include the molecular basis of biological calcification and bone formation. For all such in depth studies isolated homogeneous cultures of bone forming cells will probably provide a suitable model system and cultures of isolated cells will thus continue to enhance and facilitate progress in bone metabolism.

## References

Aubin, J. E., Heersche, J. N. M., Merrilees, M. J., and Sodek J., (1982). Isolation of bone cell clones with differences in growth, hormone responses and extracellular matrix production. *J. Cell. Biol.*, **92**: 452–461.

Auf'mkolk, B., Hauschka, P., and Schwartz, E., (1985). Characterization of human bone cells in culture. *Calcif. Tiss. Int.*, **37**: 228–235.

Beresford, J. N., MacDonald, B. R., Gowen, M., Couch, M., Aked, D., Sharpe, P. T.,

Gallagher, J. A., Poser, J. W., Russell, R. G. G., (1983). Further characterization of a system for the culture of human bone cells. *Calcif. Tiss. Int.*, **35**: 637.

Canalis, E., (1984). Local bone growth factors. *Calcified Tiss. Int.*, **36**: 632−634.

Canalis, E. and Raisz, L. (1979). Effect of epidermal growth factor on bone formation in vitro. *Endocrinology*, **104**: 362−869.

Centrella, M. and Canalis, E. (1986). Transforming and non-transforming growth factors are present in medium conditioned by fetal rat calvaria. *Proc. Nat. Acad. Sci. USA*, **82**: 7335−7339.

Chambers, T. J., McSheehy, P. M. J., Thomson, B. M. and Fuller, K. (1985). The effect of calcium regulating hormones and prostaglandin $E_2$ on bone resorption by osteoclasts disaggregated from neonatal rabbit bones. *Endocrinology*, **116**: 234−239.

Chen, T. L., Aronow, L. and Feldman, D. (1977). Glucocorticoid receptors and inhibition of bone cell growth in primary culture. *Endocrinology*, **100**: 619−628.

Chen, T. L. and Feldman, D. (1978). Glucocorticoid potentiation of the adenosine 3'5' monophosphate response to parathyroid hormone in cultured rat bone cells. *Endocrinology*, **102**: 589−596.

Chen, T. L. and Feldman, D. (1979). Glucocorticoid receptors and actions in subpopulations of cultured rat bone cells: Mechanisms of dexamethasone potentiation of parathyroid hormone-stimulated cyclic AMP production. *J. Clin. Invest.*, **63**: 750−758.

Chen, T. L., Hirst, M. A. and Feldman, D. (1979). A receptor-like binding macromolecule for ,25 dihydroxycholecalciferol in cultured mouse bone cells. *J. Biol Chem.*, **254**: 7491−7494.

Chen, T. L., Cone, C. M., Morey-Holton, E. and Feldman, D. (1983). 1,25 dihydroxyvitamin $D_3$ receptors in cultured rat osteoblast-like cells. *J. Biol. Chem.*, **258**: 4350−4355.

Dziak, R. and Brand, J. S. (1974). Calcium transport in isolated bone cells I bone cell isolation procedure. *J. Cell. Physiol.*, **84**: 75−84.

Ecarot-Charrier, B., Glorieux, F., van der Rest, M. and Pereira, G. (1983). Osteoblasts isolated from mouse calvaria initiate matrix mineralization in culture. *J. Cell. Biol.*, **96**: 639−643.

Feldman, D., Dziak, R., Koehler, R. and Stern, P. (1975). Cytoplasmic glucocorticoid binding protein in bone cells. *Endocrinology*, **96**: 29−36.

Feyen, J. H. M., van der Wilt, G., Moonen, P., DiBon, A. and Nijweide, P. J. (1984). Stimulation of arachidonic acid metabolism in primary cultures of osteoblast-like cells by hormones and drugs. *Prostaglandins*, **28**: 769−781.

Fitton-Jackson, S. and Smith, R. H. (1957). Studies on the biosynthesis of collagen. *J. Biophys. Biochem. Cytol.*, **3**: 897−911.

Gerstenfeld, L. C., Chipman, S. D., Glowacki, J., and Lian J. B. (1987). Expression of differentiated function by mineralizing cultures of chicken osteoblasts. *Dev. Biol.*, **122**: 49−60.

Goldstein, D. J., Rogers, C. E. and Harris, H. (1960). Expression of alkaline phosphatase loci in mammalian tissues. *Proc. Nat. Acad. Sci. USA*, **77**: 2857−2860.

Hakeda, Y., Nakatani, Y., Hiramatsu, M., Kurihara, N., Tsunoi, M., Ikeda, E. and Kumegawa M. (1985a). Inductive effects of prostaglandins on alkaline phosphatase in osteoblastic cells, cone MC3T3-E1. *J. Biochem.*, **97**: 97−104.

Hakeda, Y., Ikeda, E., Kurihara, N., Nakatani, Y., Maeda, N., and Kumegawa, M. (1985a). Induction of osteoblastic cell differentiation by forskolin. Stimulation of cyclic AMP production and alkaline phosphatase activity. *Biochem. Biophys Acta*, **838**: 49−53.

Harrell, A., Binderman, I. and Rodan, G. A. (1973). The effect of calcium concentrations on calcium uptake by bone cells treated with thyrocalcitonin. *Endocrinology*, **92**: 550−555.

Hata, R., Hori, H., Nagai, Y., Tanaka, S., Kondo, M., Hiramatsu, M., Utsumi, N., and Kumegawa M. (1984). Selective inhibition of type 1 collagen synthesis in osteoblastic cells by epidermal growth factor. *Endocrinology*, **115**: 867−876.

Hefley, T. J. (1987) Utilization of FPLC-purified bacterial collagenase for the isolation of cells from bone. *J. Bone Min. Res.*, **2**: 505−516.

Hefley, T. J., Stern, P. H. and Brand, J. S. (1983) Enzymatic isolation of cells from neonatal calvaria using two purified enzymes from clostridium histolyticum. *Exp. Cell. Res.*, **149**: 227−236.

Hock, J. M., Centrella, M., and Canalis, E. (1986) Stimulation of bone matrix apposition and bone cell replication by insulin-like growth factor (IGF-1) in cultured rat calvaria. *J. Bone Min. Res. Suppl.*, **1**: 67.

Jones, J. J., and Boyde, A. (1977) The migration of osteoblasts. *Cell Tiss. Res.*, **184**: 179−193.

Kodama, H., Amagai, Y., Sudo, H., Kasai, S. and Yamamoto, S. (1981). Establishment of a clonal osteogenic cell line from newborn mouse calvaria. *Jpn. J. Oral. Biol.*, **23**: 899−901.

Kumegawa, M., Ikeda, E., Tanaka, S., Haneji, T., Yora, T., Sakagishi, Y., Minami, N. and Hiramatsu, M. (1984). The effects of prostaglandin E₂, parathyroid hormonef 1,25 dihydrocholecalciferol and cyclic nucleotide analogues on alkaline phosphatase activity in osteoblastic cells. *Calcif. Tiss. Int.*, **36**: 72.

Limeback, H., Otsuka, K., Yao, K. L., Augin, J. E., and Sodek, J. (1984). Change in phenotype in longterm cultures of clonal rat bone cell line: Switch to the synthesis of alpha₁ (I) − trimer collagen. *Canadian J. Biochem. Cell Biol.*, **62**: 462−469.

Luben, R. A., Wong, G. L., and Cohn, D. V. (1976). Biochemical characterization with parathormone and calcitonin of isolated bone cells: Provisional identification of osteoclasts and osteoblasts. *Endocrinol.*, **99**: 526−534.

Majeska, R. J. and Rodan, G. A. (1982). The effect of 1,25(OH)₂D₃ on alkaline phosphatase in osteoblastic osteosarcoma cells. *J. Biol. Chem.*, **257**: 3362−3365 (1982)

Majeska, R. J., Rodan, S. B. and Rodan, G. A. (1980) Parathyroid hormone responsive clonal cell lines from rat osteosarcoma. *Endocrinology*, **107**: 1494−1503.

McSheehy, P. J. and Chambers, T. J. 1,25 dihydroxyvitamin D₃ stimulates rat osteoblastic cells to release a soluble factor than increases osteoclastic bone resorption. *J. Clin. Invest.*, **80**: 425−429.

Mills, B. C., Singer, F. R., Weiner, L. P., and Holst, P. A. (1979). Long-term culture of cells from bone affected with Paget's disease. *Calcif. Tiss. Int.*, **29**: 79−87.

Mohan, S., Jennings, J. C., Linkhart, T. A., Wergedal, J. E. and Baylink, D. J. (1988). Primary structure of human skeletal growth factor (SGF) homology with IGF II. *J. Bone Min. Res.*, **3**: Suppl 1, 598.

Murray, E., Curran, D., Deftos, L., and Manolagas, S. (1986). Effects of 1,25 dihydroxyvitamin D₃ protein synthesis in phenotypically distinct clonal rat osteoblastic cell lines. *J. Bone Min. Res.* **1**: Suppl 1 149.

Nagayama, M., Sakamoto, S. and Sakamoto, M. (1984). Mouse bone collagenase inhibitor: Purification and partial characterization of the inhibitor from mouse calvaria cultures. *Arch. Biochem. Biophys.*, **228**: 653−659.

Ng, K. W., Partridge, N. C., Niall, M. and Martin, T. J. (1983). Epidermal growth factor receptors in clonal lines of a rat osteogenic sarcoma and in osteoblast-rich rat bone cells. *Calcif. Tiss. Int.*, **35**: 298−303.

Nijweide, P. J., van der Plas, A., and Scherft, J. P. (1981). Biochemical and histological studies on various bone cell preparations. *Calcif. Tiss. Int.*, **33**: 529−540.

Nijweide, P. J., van Iperen-van Gent, A. S., Kawilarang-de Hass, E. W. M., van der Plas, A. and, Wassenaar, A. M., Bone formation and calcification by isolated osteoblast-like cells. *J. Cell. Biol.*, **93**: 318−323.

Osdoby, P. and Caplan, A. I., A scanning electron microscopic investigation of in vitro osteogenesis. *Calcif. Tiss. Int.*, **30**: 43−50.

Otsuka, K., Sodek, J. and Limeback, H. F. (1984a). Collagenase synthesis by osteoblast-like cells. *Calcif. Tiss. Int.*, **36**: 722−724.

Otsuka, K., Sodek, J. and Limeback, H. (1984b). Synthesis of collagenase and collagenase inhibitors by osteoblast-like cells in culture. *Eur. J. Biochem.*, **145**: 123−129.

Partridge, N. C., Kemp, B. E., Veroni, M. C. and Martin, T. J. (1981). Activation of adenosine 3'5' monophosphate-dependent protein kinase in normal and malignant bone cells by parathyroid hormone, prostaglandin $E_2$ and prostacyclin. *Endocrinology*, **108**: 220−225.

Partridge, N. C., Alcorn, D., Michelangeli, V. P., Kemp, B. E., Ryan, G. B. and Martin, T. J. (1981). Functional properties of hormonally responsive cultured normal and malignant rat osteoblastic cells. *Endocrinology*, **108**: 213−219.

Partridge, N.C., Alcorn, D. and Michelangeli, V. P., Morphological and biochemical characterization of four clonal osteogenic sarcoma cell lines of rat origin. *Cancer Res.*, **43**: 4308−4314.

Peck, W. A., Birge, S. J., and Fedak, S. A. (1964) Bone cells: biochemical and biological studies after enzymative isolation. *Science*, **146**: 1476−1477.

Perry, H. M., Skogen, W., Chappel, J. C., Wilner, G. D., Kahn, A. J. and Teitelbaum, S. J. (1987). Conditioned medium from osteoblast-like cells mediate parathyroid hormone induced bone resorption. *Calcif. Tiss. Int.*, **40**: 298−300.

Pliam, N. B., Nyiredy, K. O., Arnaud, C. D. (1982). Parathyroid hormone receptors in avian bone cells. *Proc. Nat. Acad. Sci. USA*, **79**: 2061−2063.

Price, P. A. (1983). Non-collagen proteins of hard tissue. In: *Bone and Mineral Research*, Annual I, Editor W. A. Peck. Excerpta Medica, Amsterdam, 157−191.

Price, P. A., and Baukol, S. A. (1980). 1,25 dihydroxyvitamin $D_3$ increases synthesis of the vitamin K-dependent bone protein by osteosarcoma cells. *J. Biol. Chem.*, **255**: 11660−11663.

Price, P. A., and Baukol, S. A. (1981). 1,25 dihydroxyvitamin $D_3$ increases serum levels of the vitamin K-dependent bone protein. *Biochem. Biophys. Res. Comm.*, **202**: 235−241.

Puzas, J. E., and Jensen, J. A. (1982). Electrophoretically separated bone cell types from the foetal rat calvarium: a histochemical and biochemical study. *Histochemical Journal*, **14**: 561−571.

Puzas, J. E., Vignery, A., and Rasmussen, H. (1979). Isolation of specific bone cell types by free flow electrophoresis. *Calcif. Tiss. Int.*, **27**: 263−268.

Rao, L. G., Ng, B., Brunette, D. M., and Heersche, J. N. M. (1977). Parathyroid hormone and prostaglandin $E_1$ response in a selected population of bone cells after repeated sub culture and storage at −80°C. *Endocrinol*, **100**: 1233−1241.

Ringel, R. E., Brenner, J. I., Haney, P. J., Burns, J. E., Moulton, A. L. and Berman, M. A. (1982). Prostaglandin-induced periostitis: a complication of long term $PGE_1$ infusion in an infant with congenital heart disease. *Radiology*, **142**: 657−658.

Rodan, S. B., and Rodan, G. A. (1974). The effect of parathyroid hormone and thyrocalcitonin on the accumulation of cyclic adenosine 3'5' monophosphate in freshly isolated bone cells. *J. Biol. Chem*, **249**: 3068−3074.

Rodan, G. A., and Martin, T. J. (1981). Role of osteoblasts in hormonal control of bone resorption − a hypothesis. *Calcif. Tiss. Int.*, **33**: 349−351.

Rodan, G. A. and Majeska, R. J. (1982). Phenotypic maturation of osteoblastic osteosarcoma cells in culture In: Kelley R. O., Goetnick P. F., MacCabe J A (eds): *Limb Development and Regeneration Part B.* New York, Alan R. Liss, 249−259.

Rodan, G. A., and Rodan, S. B. (1983). Expression of the osteoblastic phenotype. In: *Bone and Mineral Research Annual 2* Editor: W. A. Peck. Elsevier, Amsterdam, 244−285.

Rodan, S. B., Rodan, G. A., Simmons, H. A., Walenga, R. W., Feinstein, M. B., and Raisz, L. G. (1981). Bone resorptive factor produced by osteosarcoma cells with osteoblastic features is PGE$_2$. *Biochem Biophys Res. Commun.*, **102**: 1358−1365.

Sakamoto, S., and Sakamoto, M. (1984). Osteoblast collagenase: Collagenase synthesis by clonally derived mouse osteogenic (MC373-E1) cells. *Biochem. Int.*, **9**: 51−58.

Silbermann, M., Lewinson, D., *Gonen Hedra*, Lizarbe, M. A. ,and von der Mark K. (1983). In vitro transformation of chondroprogenitor cells into osteoblasts and the formation of new membrane bone. *Anatomical Record*, **206**: 373−383.

Silve, C. M., Hradek, G. T., Jones, A. L. and Arnaud, C. D. (1982). Parathyroid hormone receptor in intact embryonic chicken bone: Characterization and cellular localization. *J. Cell Biol.*, **94**: 379−386.

Simmons, D. J., Kent, G. N., Jilka, R. L., Scott, D. M., Fallon, M. and Cohn, D. V. (1982). Formation of bone by isolated cultured osteoblasts in Millipore diffusion chambers. *Calcif. Tiss. Int.*, **34**: 291−294.

Smith, D. M., Johnston, C. C., and Severson, A. R. (1973). Studies of the metabolism of separated bone cells. *Calcif. Tiss. Res.*, **11**: 56−69.

Stracke, H., Schulz, A., Moeller, D., Rossol, S. and, Schatz H. (1984). Effect of growth hormone on osteoblasts and demonstration of somatomedin C/IGF-1 in bone organ culture. *Acta Endocrinology*, **107**: 16−24.

Termine, J. D., Kleinmann, H. K., Whitson, S. W., Conn, K. M., McGarvey, M. L. and Martin, G. R. (1981). Osteonectin, a bone specific protein linking mineral to collagen. *Cell*, **26**: 99−105.

Tsunoi, M., Hakeda, Y., Kurihara, N., Maeda, N., Utsumi, N. and Kumegawa, M. (1984). Effect of transferrin on alkaline phosphatase activity and collagen synthesis in osteoblastic cells derived from newborn mouse calvaria. *Exp. Cell. Res.*, **153**: 240−244.

Ueda, K., Saito, A., Nakano, H., Aoshima, M., Yokota, M., Muraoka, R., and Iwaya, T. (1980). Cortical hyperostosis following long term administration of protaglandin E$_1$ in infants with cyanotic congenital heart disease. *J. Pediatrics*, **97**: 834−836.

van der Plas, A., Feyen, J. H. M., and Nijweide, P. J. (1985). Direct effect of parathyroid hormone on the proliferation of osteoblast-like cells: a possible involvement of cyclic AMP. *Biochem Biophys Res. Comm.*, **129**: 918−925.

Voelkel, E. F., Tashjian, A. H., and Levine, L. (1980). Cyclooxygenase products of arachidonic acid metabolism by mouse bone in organ culture. *Biochem. Biophys. Acta*, **620**: 418.

Wergedal, J. E., and Baylink, D. J. (1984). Characterization of cells isolated and cultured from human bone. *Proc. Soc. Exp. Biol. Med.*, **176**: 27−31.

Wong, G. L. (1979). Basal Activities and hormone responsiveness of osteoclast-like and osteoblast-like bone cells are regulated by glucocorticoids. *J. Biol. Chem.*, **254**: 6337−6340.

Wong, G. L., and Cohn, D. V. (1974). Separation of parathyroid hormone and calcitonin-sensitive cells from non responsive bone cells. *Nature*, **252**: 713−715.

Wong, G. L., and Cohn, D. V. (1975). Target cells in bone for parathormone and calcitonin are different: enrichment for each cell type by sequential digestion of mouse calvaria and selective adhesion to polymeric surfaces. *Proc. Nat. Acad. Sci. USA*, **72**: 3167−3171.

Wong, G. L. and Kocom, B. A. (1983) Differential serum dependence of cultured osteoclastic and osteoblastic bone cells. *Calcif. Tiss Int.*, **35**: 778−782.

Wong, G., and VandePol, C. (1987). Osteoblasts as a source of bone-growth factors. In: *Calcium Regulation and Bone Metabolism-basic and clinical aspects*, Vol 9, Eds D V Cohn, T J Martin and P J Meunier, Excerpta Medica, Amsterdam, N.Y. Oxford 288−294.

Wong, G. L., Frantz, K., and Lam, C. (1986). Isolation and characterization of highly serum-dependent cells released early from collagenase digested calvaria. *J. Bone Min. Res.*, **1**: 417−424.

Wong, G. L. Kotliar, D., Schlager, D. and Vande Pol, C. (1986). Somatomedin C-like and somatomedin C binding activity are present in, and secreted by mouse osteoblasts. *J. Bone*

*Min. Res.*, **2**: Suppl 1, 54.

Wong, G. L., Roberts, R., and Miller, E. (1987). Production of and response to growth stimulating activity in isolated bone cells. *J. Bone Min. Res.*, **2**: 23–28.

Yee, J. A. (1983). Properties of osteoblast-like cells isolated from the cortical endosteal bone surface of adult rabbits. *Calcif. Tiss. Int.*, **35**: 571–577.

# 6

# Mechanisms of Bone Formation *in Vivo*

**DAVID J. SIMMONS**
*University of Texas Medical Branch*
*Dept. Surgery, Division Orthopedic Surgery*
*Galveston, Texas*


*AND*


**MARC D. GRYNPAS**
*University of Toronto*
*Mt. Sinai Hospital*
*Department of Pathology*
*Toronto, Ontario*
*Canada*

## Introduction

The osteoblast is a cell which was recognized on bone surfaces by microscopists in the late-19th Century. Gegenbauer, Goodsir, De Morgan and Muller all described its morphology in much the same terms that we employ today: flat, elongated, polygonal, or having degrees of plumpness (see reviews by Enlow, 1963; Pritchard, 1972), and they speculated that they were important in the economy of bone. It is long since Leriche and Policard (1928) suggested that osteoblasts were "banal, reactionary fibro-blasts", cells whose variety of shapes seemed to preclude an important function in bone formation. It was James Pritchard's lucid perspective that an appreciation of the cell's osteogenic role was not fully realized until there had been a "marriage between morphology and histochemistry...and bio-chemistry" (Pritchard 1972). While the mysteries about how these cells function really began to be clarified 30−40 years ago, it seemed obvious to the Goodsir's in 1845 that these cells, by virtue of their proximity to "all the morbid changes of bone...could not be overlooked in any question regarding the economy of bone in health and disease". We now know that osteoblasts have a very large repertoire. They are known to produce Type I collagen as well as a wide variety of matrix components which have been implicated importantly in the autocrine and paracrine regulation of cell division, collagen production, collagen turnover, bone mineralization and even bone resorption.

## Organization of the Skeleton

The bone matrix deposited by osteoblasts takes several forms. We are accustomed to dividing the tissue on the basis of its gross appearance:

**Compact bone:** a thick well-vascularized and mineralized tissue comprising the cortex of the long bones, a tissue overlain with the musculature which dissipates the mechanical forces generated by motility.

**Trabecular Bone:** thin flattened elements of well-mineralized bone which form during endochondral ossification along lines of stress, and subserve this supporting function throughout adulthood. Trabeculae comprise the bulk of the the vertebral bodies in man.

**Chondroid Bone (CB):** a term reserved for tissues which sit astride the histotypic definitions of bone and cartilage. Such a tissue has large cells, an absence of cell processes, a high collagen content, and a somewhat higher content of proteoglycans than 'mature bone' (Beresford 1981): CB-I-tumors and fracture callus; CB-II (mineralized fibrocartilage) — ossifying avian tendons and tracheal cartilage; CB-III piscine chondroid bone. The change in the expression of the collagen matrix produced by maturing chondrocytes is a prime example of this form of ossification. This category would exclude the areas of cortical and trabecular bone in small mammals and avian species which exhibit persistent rests of epiphyseal cartilage (Ruth 1961).

*Osteoid* has not been included in these definitions because it is a surface component normally present on some fraction of cortical and trabecular bone surfaces. In fact, this tissue is seldom completely devoid of mineral, except in some pathological states such as uremia ($\pm$ aluminum in the dialysate); in situations characterized by rapid bone formation such as fracture healing (Sela *et al.*, 1987; Anderson, 1985; Bab *et al.*, 1983; Muhlrad *et al.*, 1981), it is usual to find apatite crystals nucleating within extracellular matrix vesicles within the larger mass of osteoid which, in man, may represent as much as 20−30% of trabecular bone volume.

## The Origin of the Osteoblast

Osteoblasts are derived from two sources: undifferentiated primitive mesenchymal cells and differentiated chondrocytes. Mesenchyme cells are capable of different routes of differentiation which, it has been demonstrated convincingly in vitro, are dependent upon the density of explants of cells from prechondrogenic Stage 14 embryonic chick limb buds. Following the formation of the anlage of the cartilaginous long bone models, there is a stage at which cells in the multilayered perichondrium convert to a periosteum, and several laboratories have determined that the primitive bony collar forms under the aegis of a 76 kDa paracrine growth factor produced by the hypertrophying chondrocytes of the cartilaginous model. This is also the stage at which the model is invaded by the nutrient vessel, an observation which correlates with information that developmentally and functionally, oxygen tensions need to be higher for osteoblast differentiation and function than for chondroblast-cartilage formation. Such distinctions have been reported in fracture healing models as well. A number of cell lineage studies in other embryonic systems, and in young, growing and mature animals have also emphasized the osteoblast-generating potential of the mesenchymal cell and its mature derivatives, among which are bone marrow pericytes and connective tissue cells within muscle. Marrow cells exhibit both osteogenic and chondrogenic functions when implanted into muscle or enclosed within Millipore diffusion chambers (Owen, 1985). Radiothymidine labeling has been used to show that mature chondrocytes contained within bone-free epiphyseal cartilage tissue grafts can transform to osteoblasts; similar findings have been reported in the quail-chick chimeric system, a model in which the cells from the chick host and quail graft tissues can be differentiated by the presence or absence of a distinct nuclear marker (Kahn and Simmons, 1977). Many other lines of evidence indicate that chondrocytes can assume an osteoblast-like function. Collagen typing studies indicate that the youngest hypertrophic chondrocytes in growth cartilage begin to form typical Type I bone collagen prior to vascular invasion, and it is common to find thickly banded and immunologically distinct Type I collagen in other cartilaginous tissues such as the trachea and normal or diseased articular cartilages. These evidences support the concept that osteoblasts belong to a monophyletic lineage which takes its origin from primitive mesenchymal elements.

## Characterization of Osteoblasts

Issues as simple as cell shape — whether conventional or not, are critical to histomorphometrists who seek to understand metabolic bone disease in terms of the percent occupancy of osteoblasts (and osteoclasts) on mineralized and unmineralized bone surfaces. This matter is now dealt with operationally or functionally (see chapter 9). By convention, active osteoblasts are identified as cells which overlie forming bone tissue as defined by the uptake and incorporation of non-radioactive and radioactive markers. The 'tracers' most often employed for this purpose are the tetracyclines which mark surfaces undergoing *de novo* mineralization. More flattened cells apposed to bone surfaces which do not incorporate the markers have been classed as 'inactive osteoblasts' or bone lining cells. The problem, then, of what an osteoblast is has been resolved in a kinetic sense, but the knowledge that the osteoblast has transitional forms is several hundred years old. The different cellular signatures prevail and define certain metabolic bone diseases. The predominence of one another or of these cells types speaks to the mechanisms by which steroids, for instance, operate to diminish or enhance osteogenesis. Function, then, is an important determinant of osteoblast morphology.

*Microscopy*

There is not a considerable species variation in osteoblast size, but the appearance of the cells can differ according to their functional state:

| Type | Species Age | Range | Reference |
| --- | --- | --- | --- |
| Fiber Bone | Chick 13d | 19−51 µm | Volpi *et al.*, 1981 |
| Compact Bone | Man   Adult | 15−80 µm | Pritchard, 1972 |
| Compact Bone | Dog   3mos | 23−62 µm | Volpi *et al.*, 1981 |

The higher their rate of matrix formation, the greater their volume and density, and the smaller their secretory territory.

Whether located on periosteal or endosteal/trabecular surfaces, scanning electron micrographs show that osteoblasts are arrayed as though they were a monolayer of hexagonal roofing tiles with concave-convex edges (Fig. 1, and see chapter 1). They usually have a long axis which is oriented parallel to the underlying collagen fibers (Jones *et al.*, 1975). Projections of the typically trilaminar outer plasma membrane make limited contact with their more fibroblast-like progenitor cell elements and with adjacent osteoblasts. On the endosteum where the lining cells are separated from the marrow by an epithelioid sac of pericyte-like cells, there is controversy whether, at least in mammals osteoblasts directly contact myeloid cells (Menton *et al.*, 1982; Matthews, 1982). Direct osteoblast-to-osteoblast contact appears to be via gap junctions (in rats:Doty, 1981; Miller *et al.*, 1980; in rabbits: Whitson, 1972). Because the injection of a fluoroscein dye into one osteoblast rapidly labels adjacent cells (Jeansonne *et al.*, 1979), it has been proposed that the activities of osteoblasts are coordinated via the exchange of electrochemical information (Ferrier *et al.*, 1986).

At the transmission electron microscopic level, the nucleus is normally smooth contoured and limited by two membranes, but in tangential section one may observe sires of membrane fusion creating pores. The distribution of heterochromatin is somewhat variable across species lines. In most cells, it is disposed marginally at the inner nuclear membrane and

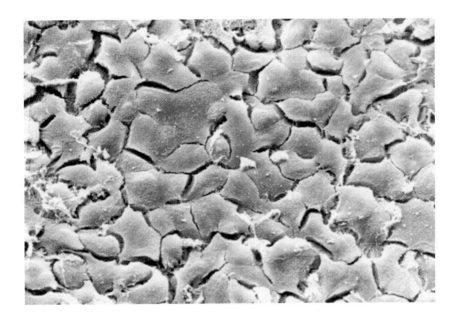

**Fig. 1**  Scanning electron micrograph of osteoblasts on rat parietal bone.

there is a small nucleolus. Quail osteoblasts have multiple, very conspicuous, centrally located nucleoli. Scattered within the cytoplasm are
mitochondria, which may contain calcium-phosphate granules bound to
their cristae, some free ribosomes, primary lysosomes, a (cilia) cytocentrum
which consists of 2 centrioles, satellite bodies, microtubules (Luk *et al.*,
1974; Matthews 1980; Miller *et al.*, 1980; Shapiro, 1988), and some lipid
inclusions. Presecretory, protein secreting granules per se are not evident.
Cytoplasmic microtubules and microfilaments course within the interstitial
spaces between these elements, and these structures are thought to be
important to the cells protein secretory activities and motility (Lomri *et al.*,
1987; Weiniger and Holtrop 1974). Additional filament systems surround

the nucleus, and radiate from the nucleus to the plasma membrane where they occasionally terminate at the inner membrane. These contact 'points' appear arrow headed after heavy meromycin staining (King and Holtrop, 1975) while the filaments stain with fluorescein conjugated antiactin immunoglobulins. The presence of such contractile microfilament systems is important to the cell not only in terms of its competence as a secretor of extracellular products. In their osteoprogenitor state, the ability to migrate would appear to be important. As mature cells, they undergo conformational changes when inactive or following challenge with calciotrophic hormone, and migrate within electric fields *in vitro* (Ferrier *et al.*, 1986). Cytocalasin-mediated disruption of microfilament bundles operates within minutes to transform osteoblasts to a spheroidal shape, an effect which is reversible after the agent is removed.

The bone-side or inner surface of a cell which is actively producing collagen is separated from mineralized bone by a meshwork of unmineralized collagen fibers (osteoid). Cilia, with the distinctive eucaryotic 9+2 arrangement of microtubules, (a core of nine doublets of tubules surrounding 2 central tubules) more often project from this surface; because they connect with the contractile microfibrillar network, they may operate as swizzle sticks to equilibrate ion concentrations in the extracellular fluid (Matthews, 1982). More conspicuous are the branching cytoplasmic processes which project through the osteoid into the canaliculi of the mineralized bone and contact but do not fuse with osteocytic processes. The richly syncytial arrangement of cell processes is established early in the differentiation of the cells from their mesenchymal-like progenitors, long before the matrices they produce begin to calcify (Menton *et al.*, 1984). These processes are richly supplied with microtubules which have a 7µm cross sectional diameter, and are presumed to function in the transport of water, electrolytes, and organics (Federman and Nichols, 1974). The tubules consist of tubulin subunits, and while they might be depolymerized by colchicine/colcemid, such experiments have not yet been recorded. These processes are of course short in the acellular boned species of teleost fish which lack osteocytes.

In special situations, the plasma membranes of very active osteoblasts may bleb and pinch off, releasing membrane bound vesicles which associate with the newly synthesized collagen to form sites of nascent mineralization.

## Histochemistry

Osteoblasts clearly have a distinct morphology when they are fully differentiated, but the spectrum of precursor types is sufficiently broad to make it difficult to know when such cells become functionally competent bone-builders. It was early recognized that 'progenitor mesenchymal cells' were richer in glycogen than osteoblasts and that osteoblasts were richer in alkaline phosphatase than acid phosphatase (see review by Cabrini, 1961; also Hanker et al., 1973; Henrichsen, 1958; Nakamura et al., 1984; Yoshikawa, 1971). Osteoblasts and their progenitors could also be defined by their positive cytoplasmic staining with periodic acid-Schiff reaction as well as by the propensity of osteoid to stain PAS-positive, even though this property was shared with osteoclasts (Heller-Steinberg, 1951). This problem extended to the identity of the osteoclast; bone resorbing cells, whether uninucleate or multinucleate, were found to be particularly rich in acid phosphatase, carbonic anhydrase, succinic dehydrogenase, cytochrome oxidase, and mucoprotein, but osteoblasts also stained, albeit to a lesser degree (Fischer, 1975, and see Chapter 3 and Volume 2, Chapter 3).

## Cytochemical Characterization

While tissue level studies present relatively few barriers to osteoblast identity-they can be defined by their association with morphotypic extra-cellular matrices, modern osteoblast studies are usually pursued in isolated cell preparations in which other criteria need to be employed (see chapter 3). The fetal/neonatal rodent or chick calvarium is most commonly employed because the cell layers in its thick, well-organized periosteum can be stripped away by serial 20−30 min digestions in solutions of trypsin, trypsin-collagenase, or collagenase-neutral protease (review by Cohn and Wong, 1979, and see chapter 5). Ideally, fibroblasts will concentrate in the first digestate, osteoblasts in the 2nd−3rd, osteoclasts and their mononuclear progenitors in the 4th, and osteocytes in a 5th. Studies with cells digested from the periosteal and long bone endosteal bone surfaces of 'young adult' animals are less common (100 g rat, Smith and Johnston, 1974; Williams et al., 1980; 50−80d rabbit, Yee, 1983; smaller mammals, Bitz et al. 1981; human, Uchida et al. 1988). In practice, the populations are never entirely unitypic. Subsequent 'purification' procedures can involve density gradient separation (Wong, 1982) or the preferential growth of osteoblasts vs osteo-clasts in 5−10% fetal calf serum. Alternatively, some laboratories work almost exclusively with transformed osteoblast-like cell lines derived from osteogenic sarcomas [Man; MG63, Saos-l, Saos-2, Rat; Ros 17/2.8, UMR and mouse calvaria (MC3T3-E1)], with the awareness that long-term mainten-ance/serial passage can affect the characteristics of all cells (Aubin et al., 1988; Heersche et al., 1985; Kurihara et al., 1984; Ng et al., 1988; Raisz and

Martin 1984; Sodek *et al.*, 1985; Williams *et al.*, 1980). Alkaline phosphatase is still a useful parameter to test whether a population is osteoblastrich, but the compendium which defines an osteoblast has expanded with the increase in information about the biochemistry of calcifying matrices. To qualify convincingly as an osteoblast, cells are required to display some part of their complete synthetic repertoire (Table I): Type I collagen, alkaline phosphatase, osteocalcin (with $1,25(OH)_2D_3$ enhancement), osteonectin, osteopontin, specific growth factors (bone derived growth factor/bone growth factor= b-microglobulin), cAMP-responsivity to PTH stimulation and enhancement following pretreatment with glucocorticoids (Aubin *et al.*, 1982; Majeska and Rodan 1982ab; Majeska *et al.*, 1985; Rodan and Rodan 1984; Schmid *et al.*, 1983; Spiess *et al.*, 1986; Wrana *et al.*, 1988), and receptors for PTH, $1,25(OH)_2D_3$, and β-adrenergic substances such as iso-proterenol (Rodan and Rodan, 1986). The cell lines are not all equal in these respects:

a) *Vitamin-D metabolism*: The cell lines vary in their capacities to metabolize Vitamin D (UMR 106-Lohnes and Jones, 1987). Most ROS cells express 1,25-dihydroxyvitamin $D_3$ receptors (Kream *et al.*, 1977; Chen *et al.*, 979, Rodan *et al.*, 1987), but 1,25-dihydroxyvitamin D3 stimulates less cAMP activity in 24/1 cells than in 17/2.8 cells (Majeska and Rodan, 1981). The rat osteosarcoma OS-2/3 and ROS 24/1 lines have no vitamin D-receptors and fail to produce alkaline phosphatase when appropriately stimulated (Manolagos *et al.*, 1980, 1981).

b) *Prostaglandin production*: Bradykinin stimulated $PGE_2$ production is more easily elicited in MC3T3-E1 cells than in UMR-106 cells, and is such a normal product of ROS 17/2.8 cells that a bradykinin effect cannot be easily shown (Lerner *et al.*, 1989). ROS cell cAMP activity is not stimulated by prostaglandins (Rodan and Rodan, 1983). Rat UMR cells [Lines 194,105, 106,108,201] show variable degrees of PTH and $PGE_2$ stimulated alkaline phosphatase (Partridge *et al.*, 1983).

c) *Interleukin Action*: MC3T3-E1 cells produce little or no IL-1 (Horowitz *et al.*, 1988). Other lines differ with respect to expression of high affinity receptors for IL-1 [Saos-2/B-1O & Saos-2/E-1O vs rat RCT-3] (Rodan *et al.*, 1988).

d) *Alkaline Phosphatase*: Human Saos and Saos-2 alkaline phosphatase activity is only latently stimulated by glucocorticoids *et al.*, 1983; Rodan *et al.*, 1987).

e) *Osteocalcin*: Saos-2 UMR 106 and ROS 25/1 cells fail to produce osteocalcin (Nishimoto and Price, 1980; Yoon *et al.* 1988).

f) *PTH-mediated cAMP*: Zinc inhibits this mechanism in UMR 4-7 cell line derived from UMR 106—01 clones (Bringhurst *et al.*, 1989).

**Table I**

Survey of Properties of Osteoblasts and Osteoblast-like Cells

| | Type I | BGP | OP | ON | ALP | FN | D3 | PTH | CT | Adren. Ster. | E2 | D3 | Dex | Tox.* | NaF | PTH | IP | PGE2 | CT | |
|---|---|---|---|---|---|---|---|---|---|---|---|---|---|---|---|---|---|---|---|---|
| | | | | | | | \<-- Receptors --\> | | | | | \<-- cAMP Stimulation --\> | | | | | | | |
| **Chick Embryo Calvarium** | | | | | | | | | | | | | | | | | | | | |
| | – | – | – | – | G | – | – | – | – | – | – | – | – | – | – | – | – | – | – | Wergedal & Baylink 1984 |
| | – | – | – | – | – | – | – | X | – | – | – | – | – | – | – | – | – | – | – | Silve et al., 1982 |
| | – | – | – | – | – | – | X | – | – | – | – | – | – | – | – | – | – | – | – | Kodicek & Thompson 1964 |
| **Mouse Calvarium** | | | | | | | | | | | | | | | | | | | | |
| Fetal | @ | – | – | @ | – | – | – | – | – | – | $ | – | – | – | – | – | – | – | – | Wong et al., 1977 |
| | – | – | – | – | – | – | – | – | – | – | – | – | – | $+E | – | – | – | – | – | Ransjo & Lerner 1987 |
| Postnatal | | | | | | | | | | | | | | | | | | | | |
| | – | – | – | – | – | – | X | – | – | – | – | – | – | – | – | – | – | – | – | Boivin et al., 1987a |
| | + | – | – | – | – | – | G | – | – | – | – | – | – | – | – | – | – | – | – | Chen and Feldman 1981 |
| | @ | – | – | – | @ | – | – | – | NE | – | – | – | – | – | – | $ | – | – | – | Luben et al., 1976 |
| | – | – | – | – | – | – | – | X | X | – | – | – | – | – | – | – | – | – | – | Morel et al., 1975 |
| | – | – | – | – | – | – | – | – | – | – | – | AD | – | * | – | $ | – | – | – | Chen and Feldman 1984 |
| | B | – | – | – | – | – | – | – | – | – | – | – | – | – | – | $ | – | – | – | Simmons et al., 1982 |
| **MCST3–E1** | | | | | | | | | | | | | | | | | | | | |
| | – | – | $10^{-10}$ | – | $ | – | – | – | – | – | – | – | – | – | – | $ | – | – | – | Haneji et al., 1983 |
| | – | – | – | – | $ | – | – | – | – | – | – | – | – | – | – | $ | – | – | – | Nakatani et al., 1984 |
| | +GP | – | +GP | – | – | – | – | – | – | – | – | +GP | – | – | – | – | – | – | – | Haneji et al., 1983 |
| | +GP | – | +GP | – | – | – | – | – | – | – | – | +GP | – | – | – | – | – | – | – | Kurihara et al., 1986 |
| | % | – | G | – | – | – | – | – | – | – | – | – | – | – | – | – | GH | – | – | Sudo et al., 1983 |
| | – | – | – | – | – | + | – | – | – | – | – | – | – | – | – | – | – | – | – | Hakeda et al., 1987 |
| | X | – | – | – | – | – | – | – | – | – | – | – | – | – | – | – | – | – | – | Hata et al., 1984 |
| | E | – | – | – | – | – | – | – | – | – | – | – | – | – | – | – | – | – | – | Hakeda et al., 1985 |
| | – | – | – | – | E+P | – | – | – | – | – | – | – | – | – | – | NE | – | – | X | Kumegawa et al., 1984 |

| Reference | | | | | | | | | | | | | | | | |
|---|---|---|---|---|---|---|---|---|---|---|---|---|---|---|---|---|
| Neuman et al., 1975 | — | — | — | — | — | — | — | — | — | X | — | — | — | — | — | — |
| Rouleau et al., 1986 | — | — | — | — | — | — | — | X | — | — | — | — | — | — | — | — |
| Boivin et al., 1987a | — | — | — | — | — | — | X | — | — | — | — | — | — | — | — | — |
| Boivin et al., 1984, 1987b | — | — | — | — | — | X | — | — | — | — | — | — | — | — | — | — |
| Ernst et al., 1988 | — | — | — | — | — | — | — | — | — | — | — | — | — | — | — | — |
| Chen and Feldman 1984 | — | $ | — | — | * | * | — | — | — | — | — | — | — | @# | %*C | G |
| Dietrich et al., 1976 | — | — | — | — | — | — | — | — | — | — | — | — | — | % | X |
| Antosz et al., 1987 | — | — | — | — | — | — | — | — | — | — | — | — | — |
| Binderman et al., 1984 | — | — | — | — | — | — | — | — | — | — | — | — | — |
| Bellows et al., 1986 | — | — | — | — | — | — | — | — | — | X | X | X | X | — | %*C | I |
| Chen et al., 1986 | — | — | — | — | — | — | — | — | — | * | — | — | — | G | X | — |
| Wrana et al., 1988 | — | — | — | — | — | — | — | — | I | I | I | I | — | I |
| Yee 1985 | — | — | — | — | — | — | — | — | — | $ | — | — | — |
| Liberman et al., 1983 | — | $ | — | — | — | — | — | — | — | X | X | X | — | + | X |
| Wergedal & Baylink 1984 | — | — | — | — | — | — | — | — | — | G | — | — | — |
| Crisp et al., 1984 | ± | E | — | ± | — | — | — | — | — | G | — | — | — | +L |
| Beresford et al., 1984 | — | — | — | — | — | — | — | — | — | — | — | — | — | + |
| NE Aufmkolk et al., 1985 | NE | — | — | — | — | — | — | — | — | — | — | — | X | X |
| Nishimoto et al., 1987 | — | — | — | — | — | — | — | — | — | X | X | — | — | % | X |
| Majeska et al., 1980 | — | — | — | — | — | — | — | — | — | — | — | — | — | OS | X |
| Nishimoto & Price 1980 | — | — | — | — | — | — | — | — | — | — | — | — | — |
| Shteyer et al., 1986 | — | — | — | — | — | — | — | — | — | — | — | — | — | B |
| Price and Baukol 1980 | — | — | — | — | — | — | — | — | — | — | — | — | — | X+ |
| Manolagos et al., 1981 | — | — | — | — | — | — | — | — | — | — | +P | — | — |
| Majeska & Rodan 1982ab | — | — | — | — | — | — | — | — | — | GJ | — | — | — |

Rat Cavarium

Human Tibia
Iliac Crest &
Femoral head
Trabec. Bone
Trabec. Bone
Trabec. Bone
Osteosarcoma
Rat Ros 17/2

**Table 1 (continued)**

| Cell Line | Type I | BGP | OP | ON | ALP | FN | D3 | PTH | CT | Adren. Ster. | E2 | D3 | Dex | Tox.* | NaF | PTH | IP | PGE2 | CT | Reference |
|---|---|---|---|---|---|---|---|---|---|---|---|---|---|---|---|---|---|---|---|---|
| Rat ROS 17/2.8 | – | – | – | – | – | – | – | – | – | *A | – | A | A | A | A | – | – | – | – | Catherwood 1985 |
| | $ | – | – | – | +G | – | – | – | – | – | – | A | – | – | – | – | – | – | – | Majeska & Rodan 1982b |
| | $ | – | – | – | $GP:e | T+G | – | – | – | – | – | – | * | – | – | $ | A | – | – | Majeska et al., 1985 |
| | – | – | + | – | – | – | – | – | – | – | – | – | – | o | – | $ | X | – | – | Pines et al., 1986 |
| | – | – | – | – | – | – | X | – | – | – | – | – | – | – | – | – | – | – | – | Prince and Butler 1987 |
| | A | – | – | – | – | – | – | – | – | – | – | – | – | – | – | – | – | – | – | Manolagos et al., 1980 |
| | – | + | – | – | – | – | – | – | – | – | – | – | – | – | – | – | – | – | – | Kream et al., 1986 |
| | – | – | – | – | – | – | – | – | – | – | – | – | – | – | – | – | – | – | – | Price and Baukol 1980 |
| | – | – | – | – | – | – | – | – | – | – | – | – | *P | X*$P | X*P | $*P | – | – | – | Rodan et al., 1984 |
| | C+ | – | – | – | – | – | – | – | – | – | – | – | – | – | – | – | – | – | – | Yamoaka et al., 1986 |
| RatUMR 104/105 | – | – | – | – | X | – | – | – | – | – | – | – | – | – | – | $ | – | E | – | Partridge et al., 1983 |
| RatUMR–106–06 | – | – | – | – | R– | – | – | – | – | – | – | – | – | – | – | – | – | – | – | -- |
| RatUMR–108 | – | – | – | – | X | – | – | – | – | – | – | – | – | – | – | $ | – | E | – | Partridge et al., 1983 |
| Rat UMR–201 | X%R– | – | – | – | X | – | – | – | – | – | – | – | – | – | – | $ | – | E | – | Partridge et al., 1983 |
| Ros 17/2.8G12 | – | – | – | – | RPG | – | – | – | – | – | – | – | – | – | – | – | – | – | – | Ng et al., 1988 |
| Ros 17/2.8C2 | – | – | – | – | – | + | – | – | – | – | – | – | – | – | – | – | – | – | – | Franchesci et al., 1987 |
| Rat ROS 24/1 | – | – | – | – | – | – | – | – | – | – | – | – | H | – | – | – | – | – | – | Pines et al., 1986 |
| | C | – | – | – | – | N | – | – | – | – | – | – | – | – | – | – | – | – | – | Yamaoka et al., 1986 |
| Rat OS–12 | – | – | – | – | +P | – | – | – | – | – | – | – | – | – | – | – | – | – | – | Manolagos et al., 1981 |
| Rat OS–2/3 | – | – | – | N | – | N | – | – | – | – | – | – | – | – | – | – | – | – | – | Manolagos et al., 1980, 1981 |

Human
Osteosarcoma Cells

| | | | | | | +GP | | | | | | | | | | | | | | | — | Mulkins et al., 1983 |
| Saos | | | | | | | | | | | | | | | | | | | | | | |
| TE85 | — | — | — | — | +GP | — | — | — | — | — | — | — | — | — | — | — | — | — | — | — | — | Mulkins et al., 1983 |

ALP—alkaline phosphatase
BGP—osteocalcin
FN—fibronectin
ON—osteonectin
OP—osteopontin

D3—1,25 (OH)$_2$D$_3$
CT—Calcitonin
PTH—Parathyroid hormone
Ster—Glucocorticoids
Dex—Dexamethasone

Tox—Toxins
NaF—sodium fluoride
IP—isoproteronol
PGE$_2$—Prostaglandin
Type I—collagen

B  Bone formed in millipore diffusion chambers
OS Sarcoma formed in millipore diffusion chambers
%  In vitro calcification.
O  PTH required as an agonist
G  Growth phase dependent (mature cells)
N  No response to 1,25 (OH)$_2$D$_3$
NE No stimulation of cAMP
R− Not stimulated by retinoic acid

**Stimulated by:**
E  Prostagladin E$_2$
I  TGF−b
L  Interleukin−1
R  Retinoic Acid
*  Glucocorticoids
+  1,25 (OH)$_2$D$_3$
$  PTH
:  Progesterone

**Decreased/Inhibited by:**
A  1,25-dihydroxyvitamin D$_3$
D  Dexamethasone
E  Estrogen
J  Isoproteronol
L  Interleukin−1
P  Cycloheximide/Actinomycin D
T  Testosterone
#  Calcitonin
@  PTH

Synthesis of the Extracellular Matrices of Bone (Fig. 2)

## Collagen

Collagen synthesis initially involves the translation and transcription of specific mRNA on osteoblast ribosomes. Moreover, there is such a close relationship between the levels of osteoblastic mRNA and the generation of the specific $\alpha 1$ (I) and $\alpha 2$ (I) chains of nascent bone Type I pro-collagen that the gene activity must be coordinately regulated. The subsequent steps in the intracellular processing of procollagen occur in the golgi apparatus, and they entail the hydroxylation of lysine and proline residues, chain inter-twining via the formation of disulfide bridges, glycosylation reactions (proteoglycans), and the enzymatic removal of the amino- and carboxy terminal pro-peptides. The latter occurs as the penultimate event before the fibrils are extruded from the cell. Electron microscopic immunocytochemistry has identified procollagen rich granules in the golgi apparatus (Doty, 1985).

The collagen fibrils which accumulate in the extracellular space (osteoid) mature by non-enzymatic mechanisms, steps which involve self-assembly involving their linear and lateral growth. There is some evidence that the limits to lateral growth are set by the association with the clipped procollagen carboxyterminal pro-peptide (Fleischmajer, 1987). The fibrils ultimately pack in the typical 1/4 stagger array by the formation of intermolecular links. In the process of collagen assembly, gaps or "hole zones" are produced which are sites of nascent mineralization. A useful *in vitro* model with the potential to test the regulatory steps for each of the events occurring during gene transcription, translation, and posttranslational, as well as collagen fiber mineralization, has been developed by Gerstenfeld (1987, 1988). The crystalline structure of collagen provided by the high degree of fiber orien-tation can be disrupted by agents such as lathyrogens. These interfere not only with lysyl oxidase- mediated synthesis of intramolecular and thereby intermolecular crosslinking (Piez, 1968; Siegel, 1976) leading to impairments in tensile strength, but also with the synthesis of non-collagen matrix components (Ponseti and Aleu, 1958) and mineralization (Simmons *et al.*, 1965). Thus, preservation of the three dimensional relationships within collagen is required for calcification, and may well be important in deter-mining the rate of collagen catabolism by collagenase (Harris & Farrell, 1972; Vater *et al.*, 1979).

While mature bone consists entirely of Type I collagen, osteoblast-like cells derived from the calvariae of mice (MC3T3-E1 cells: Hata *et al.*, 1984; Kumegawa *et al.*, 1983; Scott *et al.*, 1980) and fetal rats (Aubin *et al.*, 1982; Bellows *et al.*, 1986) produce Type III collagen. Such cells isolated from

# Bone Matrix Synthesis

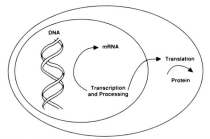

| | | | Proteoglycan Synthesis | Collagen Synthesis |
|---|---|---|---|---|
| **Stage** | **Subcellular Compartment** | **Event** | | |
| Transcription | Nucleus | Core Protein Gene | | Collagen Gene |
| Translation | Nucleus | Core Protein mRNA Synthesis | | Procollagen mRNA Synthesis |
| Post-translation | RER/Ribosome | Core Protein Processing & Modification | | Procollagen Processing & Modification |
| Glycoprotein Synthesis | Golgi Zone | Enzymes for:<br>• Nucleotide Diphosphate Sugars<br>• Linkage Regions<br>• Glycosyltransferases for the Repeating Disaccharides of Chondroitin & Keratan Sulfates<br>• Activation and Transfer of the Sulfate to an Acceptor | | Enzymes for:<br>• Hydroxylation of lysine residues<br>Interchain Disulfide Bridge Formation Packaging of Procollagen in Secretory Vesicles<br><br>Enzymes:<br>Clipping of NH₂ and COOH terminal Pro-peptides of Procollagen |
| | | — Cell Wall — | | |
| Extracellular Processing | | Aggregation | | Aggregation of Collagen Fibrils in Their 1/4-Stagger Array |

**Fig. 2** Synthesis of extracellular matrices of bone.

chick embryos (Wiestner *et al.*, 1981) and mouse MC3T3-E1 cells (Hata *et al.*, 1984) have been reported also to synthesize small quantities of (pericellular) Type V collagen, but these moieties may reflect contamination of the cultures by fibroblasts.

There is little definitive information about the actual volume of osteoid produced by single active osteoblasts. The values derived from autoradiographic and histomorphometric studies are widely variant, ranging from a low of $470\mu m^3/d$ in the rat (Jones, 1974), $220\mu m^3/d$ in man (Schen *et al.*, 1965), $2.9 \times 10^{-5} mm^2/d$ in postmenopausal women (Gruber *et al.*, 1986), and $2860\mu m^3/d$ in the rabbit (Owen, 1963). These differences are certain to reflect the age and metabolic status of the cells rather than what appears to be unimportant differences in cell size (see below and chapter 9).

*Osteoblast-mediated Mineralization of Bone*

Osteoblast-generated alkaline phosphatase was implicated early as an important mediator of collagen mineralization. Robison (1923) believed that calcification could be explained by its role in hydrolysis of soluble calcium salt-phosphoric acid ester to produce a local excess of phosphate ions. The assumption was that because blood is normally in equilibrium with the inorganic constituents of bone, supersaturation was required for the precipitation of calcium and phosphorus in osteoid. An unidentified local factor seemed necessary since kidney cells and uncalcified embryonic avian cartilage were also rich in alkaline phosphatase. This story is developed more completely elsewhere [Volume 4, Chapter I], but osteoblasts do appear to play a central role in maintaining environments favorable for mineralization.

*The Osteoblastic Milieu*

Because osteoblasts are loosely arrayed on bone surfaces and have few intercellular junctions, there might appear to be little reason to anticipate impedance to the free movement of solutes between the extracellular spaces and bone surface. This expectation was met when an injected rare earth such as $^{140}$La found its way to bone surfaces without difficulty (Neuman, 1964). Subsequently, electron microscopy determined that parenterally administered electron dense markers such as thorotrast (Seliger, 1970), lanthanum nitrate, ferritin (Dillaman, 1984) and horseradish peroxidase (Doty and Schofield, 1972; Lorenz and Plenk, 1977; Norimatsu, 1980) easily passed between adjacent osteoblasts. The canalicular network (Johnson and Highison, 1983) potentially exposes a wide surface area which, if osteocytes are included, has been estimated to be 5−6% of bone volume in most mammals (Jowsey, 1964). Robinson (1960) set this figure as high as 10−15% in the dog radius, and estimated further that when fully hydrated, unmineralized osteoidal water could be as high as 162% of its dry volume.

Because the osteoblasts microfilament system permits it to alter its shape (Jones and Boyd, 1976ab; Jones and Ness, 1977; Matthews *et al.*, 1975; Krempien *et al.*, 1978, membrane flow can either constrict or expand the dimensions of intercellular channels. The morphologic response to pharmacologic challenges of hormones such as PTH (not calcitonin) and to growth factors such as TGF-β, involves both cell contraction/elongation and development of pinocytotic/endocytotic vesicles on the bone fluid side of the cell (Jones and Boyd, 1976; Lindskog *et al.*, 1987; Lomri and Marie, 1988; Matthews and Talmage, 1981; Norimatsu *et al.*, 1979; Wrana *et al.*, 1988).

Such changes must have profound consequences for the electrical properties of cell membranes, and the composition of that fluid compartment. In this regard, Talmage (1969, 1970) proposed that osteoblasts form a physiological bone membrane, an entity which is passive in terms of the entry of calcium ions into the bone fluid compartment — calcium ions could pass through and around cells, but one which closely supervised the egress of calcium, thereby exerting (a global) control via cAMP on the rapidity with which serum calcium levels can be adjusted following hormone stimulation. Bone potassium provides a critical proof for this thesis since it is an exchangeable ion which is 25-times more concentrated in bone water than in extracellular fluids, and is conserved when blood potassium levels fall following hypophysectomy and in the vitamin D deficient state. Moreover, it is neither incorporated into bone mineral, nor concentrated or bound by proteoglycans and collagen. In their summary of this evidence, Neuman and Ramp (1971) projected that only 20% of the bone potassium could be ascribed to the intracellular fluid; the remaining 80% had to be partitioned in the extracellular fluid within the confines of the bone membrane. They also reported that iodoacetate poisoning impaired the integrity of the bone lining cells in chick tibial organ cultures, permitting bone potassium to accumulate in the culture medium. Other disequilibria between serum and bone levels of magnesium in mammals and carbonate in teleosts exist which indirectly support the concept that the uniqueness of the bone fluid environment is controlled by osteoblasts. Hormones appear to influence the transport mechanisms at a number of levels (cAMP, calmodulin) including aerobic glycolysis and how this may be controlled by external bone fluid compartment lactate and $K^+$ and intracellular/bone fluid pH (Brand *et al.*, 1979; Felix *et al.*, 1978; Norimatsu *et al.*, 1979; Redhead and Baker, 1988; Talmage, 1976). PTH treatment provokes intracellular acidification and decreases DNA synthesis in UMR-106 osteoblast-like cells by selectively inhibiting sodium-hydrogen exchange by amiloride (Reid *et al.*, 1987). Other studies directed at inhibiting acid production show that lactate production is diminished by a shift in pH from 7.4 to 6.8 and inhibited in cell cultures at pH 6.1, indicating that the pH of the fluid compartment could vary from 6.8–7.1 (Felix *et al.*, 1978; Redhead and Baker, 1988). Lactate/intracellular acidification is also auto-regulated by a negative feedback mechanism, and high external $K^+$ concentrations also inhibit lactate production (Brand *et al.*, 1979; Felix *et al.*, 1978). If there is an extracellular local factor which controls the initial mineralization of the matrix, current evidence indicates that it must be sought at the molecular level of the association between the collagenous and non-collagenous components of the osteoid. While osteoblasts do not appear to influence the rate at which the matrical and mineral moieties mature (see below), it seems clear that they can limit the access of mineral ions to the larger bone mineral volume and thereby control the apparent rate of exchange at bone crystal surfaces which is so necessary for the moment-to-moment control of blood ion levels.

### Non-collagenous Components of Bone (Table II)

Approximately 10% of bone matrix produced by osteoblasts consists of non-collagenous components. Of these, 5−7% represent the glycosamino-glycans (hexosamines, uronic acid) while 2% represent plasma proteins (albumin, globulin, transferrin). The remainder consist of phosphoprotein, and the anionic glycoproteins and sialoprotein (Leaver, 1979; Triffitt, 1987). Following *in vivo* and *in vitro* pulse radiosulfate labeling, the predominant bone cell glycosaminoglycan products associated with fetal and neonatal osteogenesis are small chondroitin sulfate moieties with a molecular weight range between 40−50K (Beresford *et al.*, 1987). While the inverse relation-ship between the glycosaminoglycans, their important proteoglycan elements, and mineralization has long been appreciated, it is only within the last decade that the roles the other moieties play in ossification and mineralization have been defined. Some of these have been characterized as growth factors which mediate the proliferation of osteoprogenitor cells, their association with bone matrix, and their maturation into bone-forming cells (Somerman *et al.*, 1982, 1983; Lucas *et al.*, 1988a,b).

*Osteocalcin* Otherwise known as the bone-Gla protein (bGP), osteo-calcin has a molecular weight of 6,500, and its distribution is restricted to the cells of calcified tissues, including dentin and subcutaneous calcifications in rats (Bianco *et al.*, 1985; Bronckers *et al.*, 1985; Mark *et al.*, 1987b). The molecule has 2-to-3 residues of gamma-carboxyglutamic acid which make it a calcium-phospholipid-binding amino acid (Vermeer, 1984), and it therefore concentrates in bone, increasing with age (Macek *et al.*, 1980; Price *et al.*, 1980a). It's concentration in bovine bone is 2mg/g (Price, 1985). Studies in the rat with the Vitamin K antagonist Warfarin have shown that serum osteocalcin levels arise from bone cell synthesis rather than from the turnover of bone matrix (Price and Williamson, 1981; Price *et al.*, 1981; Nishimoto and Price, 1979, 1985), and there is now ample evidence that, in health and in a variety of disease states, serum levels correlate with the extent of bone surface osteoid coverage, the volume of fibrosis and the mineralization rate (Delmas *et al.*, 1983; Garcia-Carrasco *et al.*, 1988; Malluche *et al.*, 1983; Price and Williamson, 1981; Price *et al.*, 1980b, 1981) (Table III). The serum half life is short, on the order of minutes, being cleared by the renal glomeruli. Uremia appears to be one

**TABLE II**

| Approximate Composition of Mineralized Bone | |
|---|---|
| Collagen & Non-collagen Protein Fraction | Bone Mineral Fraction |

| Collagen & Non-collagen Protein Fraction | | Bone Mineral Fraction | |
|---|---|---|---|
| Soluble Collagen | 25% | | |
| Blood-derived Proteins | 25% | | |
|   Albumin | | | |
|   Fibronectin | | | |
| Cellular Components | 15% | Phosphoglycoprotein. (62kD) | 10% |
|   Nucleic Acids | | | |
|   Glycogen | | | |
|   Cell Protein | | | |
| Matrix/Cell Components | | | |
|   Proteoglycans | 10% | Proteoglycans | 7% |
|     Protein core (38 kD) | O.1% | | |
|   Alpha$_2$ HS-Glycoprotein | | Alpha$_2$ HS-Glycoprotein | 25% |
|   Osteocalcin (57 kD) | ? | Osteocalcin.(57kD) | 15−20% |
|   Osteonectin (32 kD) | ? | Osteonectin (32 kD) | 8% |
|   Phosphoprotein | | Phosphoprotein. (24kD) | 8% |
|   Sialoprotein (70−80 kD) | 24% | Sialoprotein. (25kD) | 8% |
|   Unidentified | 10% | Unidentified | 5% |
|   Glycoprotein (ex. BMP) | ? | | |

condition in which this relationship may falter; osteocalcin levels are disproportionately high in uremic patients due to failure of renal metabolism on the one hand and on the other the increased pace of bone formation due to secondary hyperparathyroidism. Deficits in osteocalcin production cannot be produced alone, for in the presence of warfarin, embryonic chick osteo-blasts grow poorly, producing only 30−40% of their normal protein and collagen, and this tissue fails to accumulate normal amounts of mineral (Chipman *et al.*, 1987). Models of heterotopic ossification (osteoinduction) have shown that osteocalcin-deficient matrices are less chemoattractive to osteoclastic precursor cells than normal, and are not very actively resorbed (Lian, 1984).

Osteocalcin production and secretion appears to be regulated by 1,25(0H)$_2$D$_3$ (osteosarcoma cells: Price and Baukol, 1980, 1981; embryonic chick calvaria: Tsutsumi *et al.*, 1987). Serum levels of osteocalcin have generally been found to be better correlate with bone formation than alkaline phosphatase (de la Piedra *et al.*, 1987; Stepan *et al.*, 1987).

**TABLE III**

Changes in Serum and Bone Osteocalcin Levels in Metabolic Bone Disease

| | |
|---|---|
| Normal serum levels | |
| Senile osteoporosis | Gundberg et al., 1983a |
| Indomethacin-Rx (Rat) | Boiskin et al., 1988 |
| | |
| Decreased Serum Osteocalcin/Bone Formation | |
| Spaceflight (rat) | Patterson-Buckendahl et al., 1985 |
| | Patterson-Buckendahl et al., 1987 |
| Hypokinesia (primate) | Grynpas et al., 1986 |
| Chloropromazine treatment (rat) | Komoda et al., 1988 |
| Age (rat) | Kiebzak et al., 1988 |
| | Price et al., 1980b |
| Age (bovine) | Price and Nishimoto 1980 |
| Age(man) | Gundberg et al., 1983a |
| Hypoparathyroidism | Delmas et al., 1983 |
| Tetracycline treatment | Deyl et al., 1981 |
| Osteoporosis | Hyldstrup et al., 1988 |
| | Diamond et al., 1989 |
| Cobalamin deficiency | Carmel et al., 1988 |
| | |
| Increased Bone Formation | |
| Postmenopausal osteoporosis | Brown et al., 1984 |
| | Delmas et al., 1983 |
| | Delmas et al., 1985 |
| Paget's disease | Price et al., 1980 |
| | Melick et al., 1985 |
| | Delmas 1986ab |
| | Gundberg et al., 1983 |
| Primary hyperparathyroidism | Price et al., 1980 |
| | Deftos et al., 1982 |
| | Delmas et al., 1983 |
| | Delmas et al., 1985 |
| | Delmas 1986a |
| | Delmas et al., 1986c |
| | de la Piedra et al., 1987 |
| | Hyldstrup et al., 1988 |
| Hyperthyroidism | Garrell et al., 1986 |
| | Delmas et al., 1985 |
| | Hasling et al., 1987 |
| | Hyldstrup et al., 1988 |
| Glucocorticoid-treatment | Godschalk and Downs 1988 |
| | Nielsen et al., 1988 |
| Osteomalacia | Hyldstrup et al., 1988 |

Pachydermoperiostosis                                      Venencie *et al.*, 1988
Increased osteoprogenitor cell proliferation
   1,25(0H)₂D₃ stimulation                                 Price 1985
                                                           Price and Baukol 1980
                                                           Price and Baukol 1981

                                                           Lian *et al.*, 1982
   (rat osteosarcoma cells)                                Nishimoto and Price 1980b
   (human osteosarcoma cells)                              Kaplan *et al.*, 1985
   (human, normal bone cells)                              Beresford *et al.*, 1984b

   1,25(0H)₂D₃ treatment in vitro
   (rat osteoblasts)                                       Groot *et al.*, 1985
                                                           Stronski *et al.*, 1988

   Vitamin D-deficiency                                    Lian *et al.*, 1982

   X-linked Hypophosphatemic
      Rickets                                              Gundberg *et al.*, 1983b

   1,25(0H)₂D₃-resistant rickets                           Silve *et al.*, 1986
   Hyperphosphatasia                                       Silve *et al.*, 1986
   Acroosteolysis/Osteoporosis                             Silve *et al.*, 1986

Exceptions, showing higher/lower bGP values
   Malignant hypercalcemia                                 Delmas *et al.*, 1986c*
                                                           de la Piedra *et al.*, 1987

---

* attributed to uncoupling


   There is some thought that osteocalcin is important for the recruitment of osteoprogenitor cells in regions of bone resorption. Osteocalcin mediated chemotaxis has been described (Lucas *et al.*, 1988) for undifferentiated Stage 24 chick limb bud mesenchyme and muscle-derived fibroblasts, as well as for transformed osteoblast-like ROS 17/2.8 and 25/1 cells. This property does not appear to depend upon the presence of the molecule's L-glutamic acid moeity. Yet, the effect on muscle derived fibroblasts has not always been observed (Malone *et al.*, 1986), so the issue remains unresolved.

   *Matrix-Gla Protein.*   Matrix Gla-protein (MGP) is a moiety unrelated to osteocalcin, and it makes its appearance in developing bone at an earlier stage of development (Price *et al.*, 1983). This glycoprotein was isolated from a preparation of demineralized bovine cortical bone; it's molecular weight is 15000 daltons, and it represents only 0.2−0.5 mg/g of dry bovine bone. MGP appears to be strongly associated with the osteo-inductive bone morphogenetic protein (BMP), but unlike BMP, which is water soluble, denaturants are required to prepare MGP. Price proposed that MGP might either serve as a carrier for BMP, or be involved in the anomalous patterns of calcification observed when warfarin-treated rats are treated with calcitriol.

*Sialoprotein.* The acidic nature of this phosphorylated glycoprotein moiety confers on it a high capacity to bind calcium which interestingly is not altered by acid hydrolysis.

*Sialoprotein I (44 kDal Phosphoprotein, Osteopontin)* The 44 kD phosphoprotein has been identified immunohistochemically in the golgi apparatus of osteoprogenitor cells, osteoblasts, and osteocytes from newborn rat endochondral and membranous bones prior to their mineralization (Mark *et al.*, 1987bc; Yoon *et al.*, 1987). It accumulates at the mineralization front and at several sites where ectopic calcification is known to occur, making likely an essential role in mineralization and crystal growth (Glimcher, 1984). Osteopontin has also been recorded in rat osteoblast-like osteosarcoma cells (Prince *et al.*, 1987), as well as in a number of soft tissues such as the kidney, anlage of ear cartilage, and nerve tissue (Mark *et al.*, 1988). This bone-specific phosphoprotein has not been detected in odontoblasts or in non-osteogenic mesenchyme. It's function may be fibronectin-like, that of a cell attachment protein, but osteopontin's action is the more protracted (Somerman *et al.*, 1987).

A $M_r$ 24,000 phosphoprotein isolated from bovine and human bone has recently been identified as the $NH_2$-terminal propeptide of the αl chain of Type I collagen (Fisher *et al.*, 1987). While it's precise function is unknown, the possibilities include the regulation of collagen fibrillogenesis and mineralization, the latter by temporarily blocking reactions within the collagen hole zones

*Osteonectin.* Osteonectin, a 32 kD glycoprotein, has been heralded as another differentiation marker for bone cells. Immunocytochemical studies have localized this bone-specific protein to the cytoplasm of endosteal osteoprogenitor cells, osteoblasts, the youngest newly buried osteocytes and mineralized bone (Fisher and Termine, 1985; Jundt *et al.*, 1987; Whitson *et al.*, 1984). It is likely that chondroid bone cells would also qualify as osteoblasts since it is present also in fracture callus chondrocytes just prior to endochondral ossification. Several roles for osteonectin have been proposed due to its high affinity for calcium and Type I collagen. It has been identified by immunocytochemistry in osteoblasts (odontoblasts, ameloblasts) and at points of association between proteoglycans and collagen fibers (Termine *et al.*, 1981), suggesting that its major role is to confer stability on the extracellular matrix. By extension, osteonectin is presumed to exert some control over the orientation and growth of mineral crystals in osteoid.

*Bone Morphogenetic Protein*[BMP]    BMP is a low molecular weight (19KD) cyto-differentiating growth factor (Urist *et al.*, 1983) which has been partially purified from proteoglycan extracts of demineralized bone, dentin, and osteogenic sarcoma (DBM). The identity of the cells which produce BMP has not been firmly established. The cytokine is diffusible and acts to stimulate the proliferation of mesenchymal cells; it does not affect their subsequent differentiation into cartilage and thence to bone. The ossicle which forms becomes populated with hemopoietic marrow. Purified bovine BMP contains 14K, 17.5K, 24K and 32K proteins; the 17.5K form predominates, but the partially purified 'whole' has the greater osteoinductive potential. Murine osteosarcoma BMP contains $12.5-30K$ protein fractions, with predominant $22K-30K$ subunits. The integrity of BMP is maintained in collagenase digests, but it can be degraded by proteolysis and reducing agents (Harakas, 1984). Irradiation ($>$5Mrad:Buring and Urist, 1967; Weintroub and Reddi, 1988) or autoclaving, as devices for intraoperative sterilization of DBM, reduce its competency as a osteoinductive graft material (Amler, 1987; Kohler, 1986; Van Winkle and Neustein, 1987).

*Fibronectin.*    As part of the extracellular matrix, fibronectin serves as an attachment protein for osteoblasts. However, mouse calvarial cells have a greater requirement for this moiety than 16 day embryonic chick calvarial celks which readily attach to fibronectin-depleted Type I collagen films (Royce and Barnes, 1988; Somerman *et al.*, 1982).

*Tenascin.*    Tenascin is a component of the glycoproteinacious extracellular matrix produced by perichondrium and chondrocytes during chondrogenesis, endochondral and membranous ossification. In the neonatal rat skull and mandibular condyle, tenascin has been localized to the periosteum and endosteum (Thesleff *et al.*, 1988), but it seems not to be present in 'mature' bone and is less effective than fibronectin in promoting cell attachment.

*Thrombospondin.*    Thrombospondin, a disulfide-linked trimeric molecule with an Mr=450,000 (subunits=150kD) is produced by osteoblasts. Its calcium binding domains localize it to the mineralization front. Like osteonectin, its apparent role is that of an attachment protein. Its synthesis is increased by a number of cytokines which stimulate mitogenesis and collagen formation (PDGF, TGF-b, EGF) (Gehron-Robey *et al.*, 1989).

*Alpha 2Hs-Glycoprotein.* This 50 kD proteoglycan is synthesized in the liver, appears in serum, and 40% of the liver production concentrates in the mineral phase of dentin and bone matrix formed in the fetus (Triffitt *et al.*, 1978) and adult (Ashton *et al.*, 1976; Dickson *et al.*, 1974, 1983; Triffitt *et al.*, 1976). The moiety has a high affinity for calcium ions (40X that for albumin, Triffitt, 1987). The variability of αHS-glycoprotein in the serum and urine of patients with widely varying bone formation rates is so great as to negate its importance as an osteoblast activity marker. It does however play a role in bone resorption. In bone matrix, α2HS is a low affinity matrix chemoattractant for the putative monocytic-macrophagic precursors of osteoclasts, and enhances macrophage phagocytosis (Triffitt, 1987). A 52 kD α2HS isolated from human cancer ascites fluid will mobilize bone-bound radiocalcium from cultured murine calvaria (Colclasure *et al.*, 1988).

Bone also contains a number of non-collagenous low molecular weight peptides (cytokines) which are either produced locally by mesenchymal cells and osteoblasts or which are removed from the systemic circulation by adsorbance onto bone mineral crystals. However, these growth factors should not properly be considered to be constituents of the bone mineral fraction. Unlike the cytodifferentiation-promoting peptide BMP, most of the generic substances classed as bone-derived growth factors do not re-program the genome of mesenchymal cells so that they can differentiate into chondroblasts and osteoblasts.

## Mineral Metabolism and Calcification.

It is implicit in the cellular partitioning of the bone fluid from the extracellular fluid that osteoblasts mediate the operation of the local factor which supports mineralization (see volume 4). Electron microscopy has provided evidence that mineralization processes may involve the mobilization and translocation of insoluble mitochondrial calcium-phosphate to the plasma membrane. According to this scheme, ions are 'packaged' and pinched off within trilaminar membrane bound vesicles ($0.09-0.17\mu m$: average$= 0.1\mu m$) which are enriched and complexed with acidic phospholipid and contain alkaline phosphatase and non-collagenous protein/proteolipid (Gilder and Boskey, 1989; Peress *et al.*, 1974). The phosphate-concentrating alkaline phosphatase within these now extracellular matrix vesicles is a species which is electrophoretically distinct from the form of the enzyme which is restricted to intracellular sites (Arsenis *et al.*, 1976; Kahn and Arsenis, 1979). Calcification occurs within this environment with the nucleation of the first calcium-phosphate crystals. While this process has been detailed largely in epiphyseal cartilage cells, there is little reason to doubt that the mechanism is similar for osteoblasts or for cells in any calcifying tissue (Anderson, 1969; Bab *et al.*, 1983; Boothroyd, 1975; Brighton and Hunt, 1974, 1978; Cecil and Anderson, 1978; Gay and Schraer, 1975; Matthews *et al.*, 1978; Reinholt *et al.*, 1983; Wuthier *et al.*, 1978).

The nature of the incipient mineral phase which is formed within the special ionic milieu of the bone extracellular space is known to some degree. While the concentration of potassium is higher and calcium lower than that in the serum or the general extracellular fluid, other ions such as Cl, $HCO_3$, $PO_4$ and Mg were essentially the same (Triffit *et al.*, 1968). But the bone extracellular fluid also contains large quantities of citrate and pyrophosphate which are potent inhibitors of mineralization.

There are essentially five solid phases of calcium phosphate which have been linked to biological mineralization (Table IV). Of these, hydroxyapatite (HAP) is universally recognized as the final solid mineral phase of bone. All others have been implicated as minor or precursor phases; they are acid stable and will convert to the thermodynamically stable and very insoluble HAP at a high pH. HAP alone is stable at neutral or basic pH. Whitlockite (TCP) requires the presence of Mg for its formation at room temperature. Both Brushite (DCDP) and Octacalcium phosphate (OCP) have acid phosphate groups ($HPO_4$) and a structural plane on which HAP can be grown epitaxially (Neuman and Neuman, 1958). Amorphous calcium phosphate (ACP), by definition, does not possess a definite crystal structure, but it is believed by Posner and Betts (1975) to be formed of small clusters of $CaXPO_4$ ions which have a structure similar to a fraction of the unit cell of HAP into which it transforms spontaneously and rapidly under physiological conditions. There is an abundant literature regarding the thermodynamics of these various phases, their kinetics of growth and dissolution in aqueous media, and their solubilities. But it is extremely difficult to extrapolate from the *in vitro* studies of these systems to bone mineral because bone crystals are formed on a solid matrix of macromolecules in an imperfectly known milieu where the kinetics of ion diffusion are so different from aqueous solutions.

*Bone Mineral.* The chemical constituents of the mineral phase of bone are calcium ions (Ca), inorganic orthophosphate ions ($PO_4$) and hydroxyl ions (OH) which form the apatite lattice. However, many substitutions can occur such as sodium (Na), magnesium (Mg) and strontium (Sr) for Ca,

**TABLE IV**

|                       | Biological Calcium-Phosphate (CaXPO$_4$) Phases* | | |
| --------------------- | --------------------------------- | ------------ | ----------- |
| Name                  | Formula                           | Abbreviation | Molar Ratio |
| Hydroxyapatite        | Ca$_{10}$(PO$_4$)$_6$(OH)$_2$     | HAP          | 1.66        |
| Whitlockite           | (Ca,Mg)$_3$ (PO$_4$)$_2$          | TCP          | 1.50        |
| Amorphous CaXPO$_4$   | Ca$_9$ (PO$_4$)$_6$ (variable)    | ACP          | 1.30–1.50   |
| Octacalcium phosphate | Ca$_8$H$_2$ (PO$_4$).5H$_2$O      | OCP          | 1.33        |
| Brushite              | CaHPO$_4$.2H$_2$O                 | DCDP         | 1.00        |

\* Listed in order of increasing acidity and increasing solubility.

carbonate (CO$_3$) for PO$_4$ and fluoride (F) and chloride (Cl) for OH. In addition, large ions like citrate and trace elements such as iron, zinc, lead, potassium, bromine and barium reside on the surface of the crystals or in their hydration shell. One of the salient characteristics of bone mineral is its changing mineral chemistry with maturation. Newly formed bone mineral has a low Ca/P ratio, low CO$_3$ and high HPO$_4$ content, together with a high content of bound water and a very poor X-ray diffraction pattern which reveals its extremely small crystal size (Glimcher, 1976). With maturation, the Ca/P ratio increases to reach that of hydroxyapatite, the CO$_3$ content increases while HPO$_4$ decreases, and the X-ray diffraction improves, indicating an increase in crystal size and perfection (Bonar et al., 1983). The literature notes considerable variation in bone crystal size, and this reflects the methods used for its determination. By X-ray diffraction, crystal size in its long dimension (c-axis) ranges from 10–25 nm (Bonar et al., 1983; Boskey and Marks, 1985; Grynpas et al., 1986). By electron microscopy, bone crystal length varies from 30–70 nm (Landis and Glimcherr 1978; Stev-Bocciarelli, 1970; Weiner and Price, 1986). Many theories of bone mineral development have been proposed to explain these changes:

(a) Precursor phase theories state that bone crystals are deposited as a calcium phosphate phase distinct from apatite with a lower Ca/P ratio and that, with time, these crystals convert to poorly crystalline hydroxyapatite (PCHA) which is the final form. Of these precursor phases, the most prominent is the octacalcium (OCP) concept first proposed by Brown (1966). OCP has a low Ca/P molar ratio of 1.33 and a structure consisting of calcium and phosphate-rich layers similar to HA alternating with water-rich layers (Brown and Chow, 1976). Its X-ray diffraction pattern is similar to HA with a few additional lines and its plate-like morphology makes it similar to the biological crystals see in the electron microscope. Based on seeded growth experiments *in vitro* and solubility considerations, Tomson and Nancollas (1978) also suggested that OCP must occur as an intermediate in the deposition of the mineral phase of bone, but no OCP has ever been convincingly demonstrated in bone mineral.

(*b*) The Amorphous Calcium Phosphate (ACP) theory states that bone is first formed as an amorphous compound which slowly transforms into crystalline HA. This concept, first proposed by Termine and Posner, (1967), is based on the fact that an amorphous phase does not diffract X-rays, and as such, the structural and chemical changes in bone mineral could occur by a changing ratio of ACP and HA. However, this theory has evolved from the assumptions that ACP has a role equivalent to a precursor phase in newly formed bone (Posner and Betts, 1975), and that it plays a major role in bone mineral throughout life (Harper and Posner, 1966). Yet, Grynpas *et al.*, (1984) were not able to detect ACP by radial distribution function analysis of X-ray diffraction data from newly forming bone in 17 day old chick embryos.

(*c*) Bone mineral formation represents a single apatitic phase of variable chemical composition which gradually becomes more crystalline such that the Ca/P molar ratio approaches that of stoichiometric HA [1.66]. This is the most likely theory. The changes in molar ratio can be explained by the changing size of the crystals alone. Whereas the surface layers comprise 50% of the volume of newly formed crystals, these layers represent only 25% of fully mature crystals (assuming a doubling in size). Due to the heterogeneous nature of bone mineral and to the technical difficulties in studying the structure and chemistry of bone crystals, the debate about the true nature of bone mineral remains open and will be considered at length in Volume 5.

## Measurement of Osteoblastic Function

The attributes of the osteoblast in collagen formation and mineralization, and its role in resorptive processes present a complicated picture. However, the cell is specialized to perform one major function, that of collagen formation, and this is something which can be measured directly by microscopic methods with their adjunctive techniques of autoradiography and histomorphometry, and by biochemical analysis of the rates at which radioactive precursors of matrical proteins are utilized for the synthesis of matrical components such as the proteoglycans and collagen digestible protein.

The osteoblast's functional lifespan appears to range from days-to-weeks, the time being dependent upon the specific surface:

| | | |
|---|---|---|
| Rabbit femoral periosteum | 3d | Owen 1963 |
| Rat metaphysis | 2–5d | Kember 1960; Young 1962 |
| Mouse periodontium | 10d | McCulloch and Heersche 1988 |
| Mouse metaphysis (E2-Rx) | 12h | Simmons 1963 |
| Dog haversian canal | 2 wks | Jaworski and Hooper 1980 |

## Histomorphometry of Bone Formation

### Cell Aging

Our most complete information about aging in bone osteoblasts is derived from a long series of morphometric, autoradiographic and histochemical studies performed by Tonna in the rapidly aging BNL mouse (see review by Tonna, 1985). The cells in the fibrous and osteogenic layers of the femoral periosteum develop pycnotic nuclei, reduce their golgi and RER zones, lose Janus Green stainable mitochondria which become restricted to the peripheral cytoplasm, and exhibit degenerative changes in all residual organelles (microfilaments etc., Tonna 1975, 1985). Lipid content increases in year-old animals [and probably represents accumulations of triglycerides even though total lipid synthesis decreases. (rat: Dirksen et al., 1972)].

While this is the general pattern, osteoblastic mitochondrial numbers and their enzymes such as succinic dehydrogenase and cytochrome oxidase, as well as ATP, are thought to increase from the 1st to the 5th weeks of life (Tonna, 1958, 1971; Tonna and Pillsbury, 1959; Tonna and Severson, 1971). Cilia are retained (7–8 wks of age).

### Bone Formation

Aging is associated with a global decrease in the numbers of histotypic osteoprogenitor cells and osteoblasts on cortical and endosteal/trabecular bone surfaces [mice:−90% (Tonna and Lampen, 1972; Tonna 1975) dog: Miller et al., 1980]. If however, data are expressed from the standpoint of the numbers of osteoblasts on actively forming surfaces, this decline may not be obvious: (Average for 0–94y human rib= 4550/mm$^2$: Schen et al., 1965). Osteoblast packing is even higher on rat calvarial surfaces (Jones,

1974), so that if a comparison can be made, the secretory territories of human osteoblasts is the larger ($220\mu m^2$ vs $160\mu m^2$). On the basis of early data which defined formation surfaces in human bone on the basis of their microradiographic appearance, i.e. smooth contours and relatively low mineral density, osteoblasts were thought to occupy approximately 3−4% of intracortical femoral space from 10−25yrs and about half that value after 50 yrs (Jowsey, 1960). This technique would tend to overestimate the surfaces of actively growing bone. Even so, it did provide the first quantitative information about the strong site and 'sex' specificity of such measurements (Amprino and Marotti, 1964; Marotti, 1976; Schulz and Delling, 1976). Definitive/histotypic osteoblasts do not usually occupy more than 10% of trabecular bone surfaces in the adult human iliac crest (Merz and Schenk, 1970). Parfitt (1983 and chapter 9) cites values of 3% for cortical bone, 6% for trabecular bone overall, and 12% for the iliac crest. In the 2 yr old beagle, osteoblasts cover 7−8% of trabecular surfaces in the anterior iliac crest (Quarles *et al.*, 1988). Their relative paucity in adult human bone led Jaffee (1972) to propose that aging produced naked bone surfaces. Whether one deals with an embryonic chick model (Volpi *et al.*, 1981) or a postnatal subject, we now appreciate that osteoblasts dedifferentiate, becoming transformed to the thinner bone lining cells which retain their capacity to become chondrogenic and osteogenic elements. However, the responsivity of these dedifferentiated mesenchymal-like cells, and their counterparts in soft tissues, declines with age. This has been demonstrated in terms of the periosteal response to fracture (*Rat*: Ekeland *et al.*, 1982; *BNL Mouse*: Tonna, 1961; Tonna and Cronkite, 1962) and the competency of connective tissue cells to respond to the osteoinductive stimulus provided by the bone morphogenetic protein (Irving *et al.*, 1981; Nishimoto *et al.*, 1985; Syftestad and Urist, 1982). The 18 month mouse heals its fractures slower than a 1−8 week mouse. Two year rabbits produce 25−30% less new bone around and within DBM implants than 3 week old animals.

The iliac crest has furnished most of normative values for the daily production of bone volumes. Some of these data are reported in Tables V & VI.

Discernment of local microscopic rates of bone formation is made possible by techniques which tag either newly forming matrix or the mineral which deposits when the matrix calcifies (mineralization front, Tonna, 1979; Ibsen and Urist, 1964, and see chapter 9). Localization of newly forming collagen is afforded by injecting radioactive precursors for collagen such as $^3$H- or $^{14}$C-proline and glycine; the sites of bone formation are identified by autoradiography. Procion (black, red, green, orange: Goland, 1968) and the chlorazol dyes (Weatherell, 1960) represent non-radioactive options for

**TABLE V**

Histomorphometry of Bone Formation in Skeletal Pathology[1] (Melsen *et al.*, 1983)

|  | Bone Formation ($um^3/um^2$/d | | Fractional active Formation Surface ($um^2/um^2$) | |
|---|---|---|---|---|
|  | Male | Female | Male | Females |
| Normal | 0.58±0.06 (13) | 0.48±0.03 (29) | 0.183±0.021 (13) | 0.115±0.008 (29) |
| Normal Avg | 0.36 ±0.06 | (10) | 0.077±0.014 (10) | |
| Hypothyroid | 0.12 ±0.05 | (10) | 0.042±0.014 (12) | |
| Normal Avg | 0.076±0.008 | (20) | 0.135±0.013 (10) | |
| Hyperthyroid | 0.137±0.017 | (20) | 0.189±0.019 (19) | |
| Normal Avg | 0.076±0.008 | (20) | 0.135±0.013 (10) | |
| Hyperparathyroid | 0.113±0.011 | (19) | 0.204±0.019 (19) | |
| Normal Avg | 0.067±0.011 | (9) | 0.112±0.019 (9) | |
| Acromegaly | 0.198±0.038 | (9) | 0.231±0.026 (9) | |

1 Average normal values will be seen to differ on the basis of the distributions of sex and age within diagnostic categories.

histologic analyses in demineralized sections. There is a similar range of options to localize the sites of newly depositing mineral. The most widely employed non-radioactive materials include a large number of the tetracycline antibiotics which chelate calcium and can be localized by their characteristic fluorescent colors under UV light (yellow-to-green).

|  | Fluorescence |
|---|---|
| Tetracycline | yellow-orange |
| Oxytetracycline | yellow-orange |
| Chlortetracycline | green |
| Demethylchlortetracycline | green |

Other fluorescent compounds such as quecertin (Ribelin, 1960), minicytline (Benitz, 1967), chlorazol fast pink, calcein blue (Rahn, 1970) xylenol orange, and alizarin red-S are less widely used, as are the radioactive alkaline earth elements such as $^{45}Ca$ and $^{85}Sr$. Except for the procion dyes, the non-radioactive substances have a half-life in the circulation which is usually short, on the order of hours, or at most 24h; they deposit in a fairly narrow sharp band, and the thickness of the labeled band serves as a tissue time

**TABLE VI**

6. Mechanisms of Bone Formation *In Vivo* — 223

Reconstruction of Bone Morphogenic Units in Skeletal Pathology (Eriksen 1986)

| Phase | Sequential Activity | Control (Days) | Control (% of Cycle) | Hyperthyroid[1] (Days) | Hyperthyroid[1] (% of Cycle) | Control (Days) | Control (% of Cycle) | Hypothyroid[2] (Days) | Hypothyroid[2] (% of Cycle) | Control (Days) | Control (% of Cycle) | PHP[3] (Days) | PHP[3] (% of Cycle) |
|---|---|---|---|---|---|---|---|---|---|---|---|---|---|
| **I** | **Resorption** | | | | | | | | | | | | |
| | Osteoclasts | 7 | 3.35 | 3 | 2.6 | 5 | 2.7 | 13 | 1.9 | 8 | 4.0 | 8 | 4.6 |
| II | Mononuclear cells | 44 | 21.0 | 14 | 12.4 | 13 | 7.1 | 39 | 5.6 | 11 | 5.5 | 21 | 12.3 |
| III | **Reversal** | | | | | | | | | | | | |
| | Preosteoblasts | 7 | 3.4 | 6 | 5.3 | 14 | 7.6 | 22 | 3.2 | 8 | 4.0 | 8 | 4.7 |
| IV | **Bone Formation** [=Mineralization lag time] | | | | | | | | | | | | |
| | Osteoblasts | 15 | 7.2 | 5 | 4.4 | 16 | 8.7 | 62 | 8.9 | 12 | 6.0 | 12 | 7.0 |
| V | **Bone Mineralization** | 136 | 65.1 | 85 | 75.2 | 135 | 73.7 | 558 | 80.4 | 160 | 80.4 | 122 | 71.3 |
| | Completion BMU | 209 | — | 113 | — | 183 | — | 694 | — | 199 | — | 171 | — |

*Summation of Effects*

| | Bone Resorption (Rate) | Bone Resorption (Period) | Bone Resorption (Depth) | Bone Formation (Rate) | Bone Formation (Period) | Mineralization Lag time (Rate) | Mineralization Lag time (Period) | Mineral Apposition (Rate) | Mineral Apposition (Period) | Mean Wall Thickness |
|---|---|---|---|---|---|---|---|---|---|---|
| 1 Hyperthyroidism: | I | D | U | I | D | D | D | U | D | D |
| 2 Hypothyroidism: | D | I | D | D | I | U | U | D | D | I |
| 3 1° Hyper-parathyroidism | I | U | D | D | U | U | U | D | D | D |

I— Increased    D— Decreased    U— Unchanged

marker. When tetracycline is administered to individuals or animals at 2 time points, growing surfaces are multiply labeled and record time-dependent rates of appositional growth/mineralization. Stained bone section planimetry yields information about the percentage of surface labeled, the census of cells on those surfaces, the distances between successive bands, and the volume of bone formed between bands. The radioactive markers are less useful for these purposes because the photographic emulsion required to record their position in tissue decreases resolution; in experiments of long duration, the resorption of bone affords reutilization of label in processes of secondary mineralization. Tritiated tetracycline is not reutilized to any great extent (Klein, 1981), but its potential in autoradiographic studies to record site-specific changes in osteoblastic activity has not been exploited to the degree it deserves.

Table VII compiles some typical mammalian data for local rates of appositional bone formation/mineralization observed at the microscopic level. We have already noted that osteoblast size is fairly similar across species lines. So too are rates of matrix production at different skeletal sites within species, although the rates do tend to be higher, on average, in regions which are better-vascularized (red marrow>yellow marrow; Wronski et al., 1981). Lozupone (1988) even reports secular differences—that the more proximally located trabeculae in the long bones of dogs (2−8 mos) show the higher mineralization rates. There may also be racial differences in the sense the black Afro-Americans tend to have somewhat lower rates of bone formation than white Americans (iliac crest; Weinstein and Bell, 1988). This overview indicates that osteoblastic activity decreases with age at all locations, with rates approximating 1-1.5µm/day in the young to <1.0µm/day in maturity. Values much higher than 1.5µm/day in double digits, are typical for actively growing periosteal surfaces in small animals. The most complete skeletal-wide data have been reported for the short-lived BNL mouse (Tonna, 1985) and the rat (Raman, 1969; Tam et al., 1978), and indicate that an age dependent decline in the rates of postcranial bone formation also reflect a decrease in the more global specific surfaces of formation and mineralization, and, as well, a decease in the rate of bone turnover. In modern parlance, aging without incident from metabolic bone disease is associated with a decrease in the number of activation (=remodeling) centers. It is of interest that some biochemical parameters of osteoblast activity are not sensitive markers of aging. Alkaline phosphatase values in murine vertebrae do not decline during the period of trabecular bone atrophy (Bar-Shiva-Maymon et al., 1989).

As noted above, histomorphometrists most frequently express bone formation in terms of its volume, i.e., a linear length of forming surfaces per

**TABLE VII**

Appositional Rates of Bone Formation-mineralization

| Animal | Area | Age | Change (μm/d) | Reference |
|---|---|---|---|---|
| **Mouse** | | | | |
| BNL: JAW | | | | |
| | Paradontal Bone | | | |
| | Alveolar bone-crestal | 5–104 wk | 4.19–0.0 | Tonna 1976 |
| | Alveolar bone-subgingival | 5–104 wk | 2.99–0.19 | Tonna 1976 |
| | Alveolar bone-endosteal | 5–104 wk | 3.21–0.00 | Tonna 1976 |
| | Basal bone-mesial | 5–104 wk | 2.13–0.42 | Tonna 1976 |
| | Basal bone-distal | 5–104 wk | 4.56–0.43 | Tonna 1976 |
| | Interradicular bone | | | |
| | –mesial | 5–104 wk | 3.05–0.00 | Tonna 1976 |
| | –coronal | 5–104 wk | 4.38–0.26 | Tonna 1976 |
| | | 4–24 wks | 6.00–0.20 | Baumhammmers 1965 |
| | –distal | 5–104 wk | 3.8–0.00 | Tonna 1976 |
| | –endosteal | 5–104 wk | 3.01–0.87 | Tonna 1976 |
| BNL: FEMUR | Shaft | 7 wks | 0.9–1.4 | Tonna 1966 |
| **Guinea Pig** | | | | |
| Femur | | | | |
| | –Condylar Trabeculae | — | 2.0–5.0 | Oberg *et al.*, 1969 |
| Maxilla | | | | |
| | –Distal | 20d, 50d | 3.8–0.00 | Soni 1969 |
| | –Endosteal | 20d, 50d | 3.01–0.87 | Soni 1969 |

**TABLE VII** (Continued)

Appositional Rates of Bone Formation-mineralization

| Animal | Area | Age | Change (µm/d) | Reference |
|---|---|---|---|---|
| **Rat** (Sprague Dawley & Wistar) | | | | |
| | Skull | — | — | Vilmann 1968, 1969 |
| | Femur | | | |
| | −Osteocytic | 1.4−18.4d | 0.2−0.006 | Baylink & Wergedal 1971 |
| | −Periosteal | 38d | 11.1 | Baylink & Wergedal 1971 |
| | −Periosteum-midshaft | 4−16wks | 10.5−2.4 | Raman 1969 |
| | −Periosteum-midshaft | 214−339g | 3.2 | Hammond & Storey 1970 |
| | −Distal Metaphysis | 250−300g (1−8d) | 1.13 1.54−0.79 | Tam et al., 1978 |
| | Tibia | | | |
| | −Periosteum-midshaft (SD) | 91−156g | 10.3 | Baylink et al., 1970 |
| | −Periosteum-midshaft (W) | 170−220g | 6.0 | Stauffer et al., 1972 |
| | −Periosteum-midshaft | 4−16wks | 8.3−1.9 | Raman 1969 |
| | Humerus | | | |
| | −Prox. Metaphysis | 250−300g (1−8d) | 1.104 1.39−0.89 | Tam et al., 1978 |
| | Ilium | 250−300g (1−8d) | 1.176 **1.56-0.91** | Tam et al., 1978 |
| | Vertebra | | | |
| | L1-trabeculae | **250-300g (1-8d)** | 1.176 1.51−0.91 | Tam et al., 1978 |
| | Caudal-1 | | | |
| | −periosteum (W) | 26g | 10.0 | Hammond & Storey 1974 |

**RABBIT**

| Skull: Cranial Sutures | | | |
|---|---|---|---|
| —Interfrontal | 31–141d | 9.8–1.8 | Alberius 1986 |
| —Interparietal | | 6.9–1.8 | |
| —Temporal (left) | | 11.1–2.1 | |
| —Temporal (right) | | 11.9–3.1 | |
| Mandible (NZ) | 2.5–3.0kg | 1.52 | Tam et al., 1978 |
| Postcranial Skeleton (NZ) | 2.5–3.0kg | 1.94–1.46 | Tam et al., 1978 |
| Femur | | | |
| —Distal Metaphysis | 2.5–3.0kg | 1.68 | Tam et al., 1978 |
| Humerus | | | |
| —Prox. Metaphysis | 2.5–3.0kg | 1.68 | Tam et al., 1978 |
| Ilium | 2.5–3.0kg | 1.68 | Tam et al., 1978 |
| Vertebra | | | |
| —T6 | 2.5–3.0kg | 1.632 | Tam et al., 1978 |

**DOG**

| Parietal-trabeculae | 3 mos | 2.7 | Lee 1964 |
|---|---|---|---|
| Auditory Ossicles | | | |
| —Malleus | 10–46d | 1.38/0.54 | Roberto 1978 |
| :Head | | 1.47 | Roberto 1978 |
| —Neck | | 2.46 | Roberto 1978 |
| —Incus | | 1.37/0.57 | Roberto 1978 |
| —Stapes | | 1.76 | Roberto 1978 |
| —Tibia | | 2.20/0.70 | Roberto 1978 |
| Femur[B] | | | |
| —Head Trabeculae (T) | 3mo/1–2y | 2.5/1.3 | Lee 1964 |
| —Head Trabeculae (A) | 8mo/2y | 2.3/1.0 | Lozupone 1988 |
| —Proximal Metaphysis | 12(M)/14mo(F) | 1.0/0.8 | Kimmel and Jee 1982 |
| —Proximal Shaft (Trabeculae) | 3mo/1–2y | 2.7/1.6 | Lee 1964 |

**TABLE VII** (Continued)

**DOG**

| | | | |
|---|---|---|---|
| —Midshaft (Trabeculae) | 1–2y | 1.2 | Lee 1964 |
| —Midshaft (Cortical) | 19–35mos. | 1.11±0.09(M) 0.95±0.12(F) | High 1988 |
| —Distal Shaft (T) | 3mo/1–2y | 1.9/1.3 | Lee 1964 |
| —Distal Metaphysis (T) | 12(M)/14mo(F) | 1.4/0.7 | Kimmel and Jee 1982 |
| —Distal Condyle (T) | 3mo/1–2+y | 2.3/1.9 | Lee 1964 |
| Tibia | | | |
| —Proximal Metaphysis (T) | 14mo(F) | 0.7 | Kimmel and Jee 1982 |
| Proximal Metaphysis (A) | | | |
| —Prox. endosteal | 5mo/2y/3y | 2.5/1.1/0.85 | Lozupone 1988 |
| —Dist. Endosteal | 5mo/2y/3y | 1.9/0.8/0.8 | Lozupone 1988 |
| —Prox. central | 5mo/2y/3y | Avg.=1.6 | Lozupone 1988 |
| —Dist. central | 5mo/2y/3y | Avg.=1.1 | Lozupone 1988 |
| Proximal Metaphysis (T) | 14mo(F) | 0.7 | Kimmel and Jee 1982 |
| Humerus | | | |
| —Proximal Metaphysis (T) | 14mo(F) | 0.8 | Kimmel and Jee 1982 |
| —Proximal Metaphysis[+] | 18–30mo | 0.97–1.82(1.23) | Wronski et al., 1981 |
| —Distal Metaphysis* | 18–30mo | 0.60–1.35(0.97) | Wronski et al., 1981 |
| Radius | | | |
| Proximal Metaphysis (A) | 8mo/2y | 2.8/1.0 | Lozupone 1988 |
| Proximal Metaphysis (T) | 14mo(F) | 0.6 | Wronski et al., 1981 |
| —Proximal Metaphysis (T) | 14mo(F) | 0.6 | Wronski et al., 1981 |
| —Midshaft Trabeculae | 3mo | 2.7 | Lee 1964 |
| Ulna | | | |
| —Proximal Metaphysis | 14mo(F) | 0.5 | Kimmel and Jee 1982 |
| —Proximal Metaphysis* | 18–30mo | 0.85–1.22(0.90) | Wronski et al., 1981 |

**DOG**

Rib

| | | | |
|---|---|---|---|
| −5th-Trabeculae | 3mo | 2.3 | Lee 1964 |
| −9th-Cortical | 19−35mos | 0.88±0.15(M) | High 1988 |
| | | 0.87±0.06(F) | |
| Pelvis[+] | 18−30mo | 1.10−1.37 | Wronski et al., 1981 |

Vertebrae

| | | | |
|---|---|---|---|
| −Body-trabeculae | 3mo/1−2y | 2.9/1.1 | Lee 1964 |
| −1T (T) | 14(F)mo | 0.8 | Kimmel and Jee 1982 |
| −1L | 12(M)−14(F)mo | 0.8 | Kimmel and Jee 1982 |
| −1L | 18−30mo (MF) | 1.10−1.35[+] | Wronski et al., 1981 |
| Iliac Crest-trabeculae | 3mo/1−2y | 2.9/1.5 | Lee 1964 |
| | 2y | 0.69±0.08 | Quarles et al., 1988. |

**PRIMATE** (Rhesus Monkey)

Mandible

| | | | |
|---|---|---|---|
| −Lingula (O) | 6.4kg | 1.47±0.2 | Simmons et al., 1986 |
| −Periosteum | | 1.21±0.29 | Simmons et al., 1986 |
| −Endosteum | | 1.28±0.05 | Simmons et al., 1986 |

**MAN**

| | | | |
|---|---|---|---|
| Rib-osteonal | 9−73y | 1.5−0.26 | Pirok et al., 1966 |
| | | | Frost 1966a |

Pelvis-Iliac Crest

| | | | |
|---|---|---|---|
| Trabecular Bone | 19−46y | 0.630 (Blacks) | Weinstein & Bell 1988 |
| | 19−46y | 0.904 (Whites) | Weinstein & Bell 1988 |
| Trabecular Bone | 18−90y | 0.63* | Klagstrup et al., 1983 |
| Trabecular Bone | 19−56y | 0.65* | Melsen & Mosekilde 1978 |
| | 19−60y | 0.56* | Eriksen et al., 1984a |
| | 19−80y | 0.67−0.53 | Vedi et al., 1983 |

* no age or sex differences
+ Area of redmarrow/richly vascular
* Area of yellowmarrow/lowly vascularized
T Tetracycline
A Alizarin Red S

unit volume of trabecular or cortical bone ($\mu m/mm^3$), the fraction of available surface ($\mu m^2/\mu m^2$) (*Human*: Eriksen *et al.*, 1984ab; Melsen and Mosekilde, 1978; Vedi *et al.*, 1983; *Rat*: Baylink and Wergedal, 1971), or the mean wall thickness of new bone packets (Lips *et al.*, 1978; Melsen *et al.*, 1978). Yet, it is now rare to find bone formation analyzed as an event isolated from the pace of the activation/resorptive event which is responsible for the creation of bone remodeling foci. Modern microscopists reconstruct in 3-dimensions the geometry of these foci, using tetracycline labeling to estimate the rates and depth of bone resorption (osteoclasts and mononuclear cells) and the rates and duration of the subsequent phases of bone formation and calcification. In Eriksen's (1986) series of 20 normal individuals, 19—60 years (mean 32 years: 10 females & 10 males), the phases of cellular activity within a typical trabecular bone remodeling center were distributed as follows:

| Phase | Sequential Activity | Duration Activity | Percent of the Remodeling Cycle |
|-------|---------------------|-------------------|---------------------------------|
| I | Resorption | | |
| | Osteoclasts | 8 days | 4.0 |
| II | Mononuclear cells | 34 days | 17.3 |
| | Reversal | | |
| III | Preosteoblasts | 9 days | 4.6 |
| | Bone Formation | | |
| IV | [=Mineralization lag time] | | |
| | Osteoblasts | 15 days | 7.6 |
| V | Bone Mineralization | 130 days | 66.3 |

The normal values presented in Tables V & VI for humans used as controls in different studies of metabolic bone disease will differ somewhat from these data owing to age and sex. Eriksen's series of hypo/hyperthyroid and hyperparathyroid patients demonstrate significant changes in the timing with which certain phases of the remodeling cycle are completed (Table VI). Hypothyroidism is associated with a diminution in depth of osteoclastic resorption and bone formation. The timing of these aspects is accelerated nearly 2-fold in hyperthyroidism, without change in the depth of resorption. In hyperparathyroidism, the depth of resorption is also subnormal but the duration of the mononuclear phase of bone resorption is somewhat protracted. The major change is a diminution in bone volume (mean wall thickness: 51.1 μm vs 55.9 μm) due to a lower rate of appositional bone formation [0.32 vs 0.46 $\mu m^3/\mu m^2/d$]. The outcome in these two instances is a negative bone balance.

A relationship has been long been sought between the site-specific rates of bone formation and bone-blood flow. The evidence is [1] that global bone-blood flow rates decrease with age (*Rabbit*: Kita et al., 1987; *Rat*: Hruza and Wachtlova, 1969; MacPherson and Tothill, 1978; *Man*: Lahtinen, 1981)[2] that marrow vasculature is richer in the regions of high bone formation (*Dog*: Tondevold and Eliasen, 1982; Wronski et al., 1981), [3] that the temporal conversion of richly vascular red marrow to yellow marrow in the long bones is associated with a decrease in the appositional bone formation rate (Tothill et al., 1985), and [4] that trauma causes neovascularization and higher rates of repair bone formation (Barron et al., 1977; Daum et al., 1985, 1987; Martin, 1987; Paradis & Kelly, 1975; Rhinelander, 1968; Rhinelander and Baragry, 1962; Rhinelander et al., 1968; Stromqvist, 1985; Vanderhoeft et al., 1963) and [5] that the effect of altered bone formation rates in endocrinopathies or in Paget's disease are mirrored by increases or decreases in bone blood flow (Green et al., 1987; Schoenecker et al., 1978; Wang et al., 1983). However, none of this evidence is clear cut since the richly anastomotic and compensating system of peri-osteal, metaphyseal and nutrient artery vessels make it impossible to attribute local changes in bone formation to a particular change in local blood supply (Trueta and Caladias, 1984; Rhinelander, 1968; Rhinelander and Baragry, 1962; Rhinelander et al., 1968; Whiteside and Lesker, 1978; Whiteside et al., 1978).

The decrease in both site specific osteoblastic activity and specific surfaces of formation is implicit in the developmental patterns of bone, which show decreases in allometric modeling and remodeling (formation and resorption, osteon formation; Epker and Frost, 1964; Kerley, 1965; Ortner, 1975; Simmons, 1985)(Tables VII, VIII, IX). The reduction in cell membranes and organelles presages the decline in the synthesis of all cytochemical and tissue biochemical markers of osteoblast vigor. Most of our detailed knowledge derives from animal studies. In rats, serum (osteoblastic) osteocalcin declines 60% within the first 3 months of life and is only 30% of its highest value at 9 months (Nishimoto et al., 1985). Femoral soluble collagen and its hexosamine content decline 60% between 5 weeks and 2.5 years (Hughs and Tanner, 1970b), and it is appreciated that indices such as these in part reflect an age dependent decline in collagen/proteoglycan synthesis (modeling) and tissue turnover (Mohan and Radha, 1980). Qualitative changes, notably the higher than normal sialic acid, uronic acid and hydroxyproline concentrations which appear in soluble collagenase resistant fractions in the

**TABLE VIII**
Cortical Bone Involution

| | | Cortical Bone | | Marrow Cavity Diameter | |
|---|---|---|---|---|---|
| | | Diameter | Thickness | | |
| **MOUSE** | | | | | |
| Femur (midshaft) | 26 vs 70wk | I | — | — | Hooper 1983 |
| Femur (midshaft) | | I | D | I | Matsushita et al., 1986 |
| Tibia (midshaft) | | I | — | — | Hooper 1983 |
| Humerus (midshaft) | | I | — | — | Hooper 1983 |
| Radius (midshaft) | | NC | — | — | Hooper 1983 |
| Femur | Adult | I | I | — | Rao and Draper 1969 |
| Femur (midshaft) | | I | D | I | Matsushita et al., 1986 |
| Tibia | | NC | NC | — | Rao and Draper 1969 |
| **RAT** | | | | | |
| Femur | 20—400d | I(4.25X) | — | — | Keller et al., 1986 |
| **PRIMATES** | | | | | |
| Macaques | | | | | |
| Metacarpal | 14,10,20y | — | D | — | Bowden et al., 1979 |
| Femur | 1—6y | I** | — | — | DeRousseau 1985 |
| Humerus | 6+y | D(10%) | — | — | DeRousseau 1985 |

**MAN**

| Bone | Age | | | | Reference |
|---|---|---|---|---|---|
| Humerus | 20–85+y | D* | — | — | Bergot and Boquet 1976 |
| Humerus | 15–89y | D* | — | — | Lindahl and Lindgren 1967 |
| Femur | 1–90y | D* | D | I | Arnold *et al.*, 1966 |
| Femur | 20–90y | D(12%)* | — | — | Bartley and Arnold 1967 |
| Femur | 20–85+y | D(25%)* | — | — | Bergot and Boquet 1976 |
| Femur | | — | D(20–25%)*+ | — | Carlson *et al.*, 1976 |
| Femur | | — | D(24%)*+° | — | Dewey *et al.*, 1969 |
| Femur | | — | D(11–23%)*+° | — | Martin and Armelagos 1979 |
| Femur | to 55+y | — | D(16–36%)*+r | — | Ericksen 1976, 1982 |
| Femur | 20–98y | — | D(14%)*+° | — | Ericksen 1982 |
| Femur | 20–50+y | I | — | — | Martin and Armelagos 1979 |
| Femur/Tibia | 20–35y | I° | — | I | Ruff and Hayes 1982 |
| | 30–55y | NC | — | I* | VanGerven *et al.*, 1969 |
| Femur | | — | D(30%)*° | — | VanGerven and Armelagos 1970 |
| Femur | 15–89y | — | D | — | Lindahl and Lindgren 1967 |
| Metacarpal | 20–90+y | D | D | I | Plato and Norris 1980 |
| Clavicle | | — | D | — | Aoyagi *et al.*, 1988 |

\* sexual dimorphism (= females>males, males show no change or non-statistical losses —
   about 4–14%

\*\* sexual dimorphism: males only

+ site specific: 8–9cm below the greater trochanter

° Archaeological populations.

r Racial (black vs white population)

**TABLE IX**

Survey of Allometric Changes in Bone Growth and Maturation which Reveal an a Age-wise Decrease in Bone Formation

| | Sutural Growth | Ash | Ca,P | Allometry/Remodeling | Reference |
|---|---|---|---|---|---|
| **RAT** | | | | | |
| Skull | X | X | X | | Murthy et al 1986 |
| | | | X | | Baer, 1954 |
| | | | X | | Diamond et al 1965 |
| | | | X | | Furtwangler et al., 1985 |
| | | | X | | Massler and Schour 1951 |
| | | | X | | Moss 1954 |
| | | | X | | Moss and Baer 1956 |
| | | | X | | Vilmann 1972 |
| Parietal Bone | | | X | X | Vilmann 1968 |
| Nasal Bone | | | X | X | Vilmann 1976 |
| Femur | | | X | | Murthy et al 1986 |
| | | | X | X | Sontag 1986 |
| | | X | X | | Saville and Smith 1966 |
| | | X | | | Riesenfeld 1981 |
| Pelvis | | | X | | Bernstein and Crelin 1967* |
| | | | | | Hughs & Tanner 1970ab, 1973* |
| | | | | | Riesenfeld 1972* |
| **MOUSE** | | | | | |
| Pelvis | | | X | | Harrison 1968 |
| Vertebrae | | | X | | Hooper 1983* |
| | | | X(Ca,P) | | Bar-Shira-Maymon 1989 |

| | | | | Reference |
|---|---|---|---|---|
| **GUINEA PIG** | | | | |
| Maxilla | X | | | Soni and Messer 1970 |
| Mandible | X | X | | Soni 1969, 1970 |
| **RABBIT** | | | | |
| Skull | X | X | | Alberius 1986 |
| **DOG** | | | | |
| Skull | X | | | Masoud et al., 1986 |
| Occipital Bone | | X | | Amprino and Marotti 1964 |
| Sutural Growth | | X | | Babler et al., 1987 |
| Jaw | X | | | Masoud et al., 1986 |
| Tibia | | | X | Martin et al., 1981 |
| **MAN** | | | | |
| Vertebrae | | X | X | Arnold et al., 1966 |
| Rib | | X | X | Arnold et al., 1966 |

femoral head trabeculae of osteoporotic individuals (Mbuyi-Muamba *et al.*, 1987), are perhaps indicative of the (temporarily) increased bone formation which occurs at the onset of osteoporosis in certain populations (Brown *et al.*, 1987; Stepan *et al.*, 1987; Thomsen *et al.*, 1986). Perturbations of this nature are associated with an increase in both formation and resorption which occurs shortly after ovariectomy in rats (Aitken *et al.*, 1972; Tabuchi *et al.*, 1986; Turner *et al.*, 1987; Wronski *et al.*, 1986, 1987ab).

Global bone resorption rates may not decrease with age; instead, osteoclast numbers may achieve stability, but erode shorter and shorter intracortical channels (osteons):

Human Metacarpal Osteons
(Filogamo, 1946a)

| Age (yrs) | Maximum Length (mm) | Average Length (mm) |
|---|---|---|
| 14 | 9.6 | 5.0 |
| 23 | 8.9 | 5.5 |
| 68 | 7.0 | 3.2 |

Osteon length in the metacarpals of other large vertebrate species range from 3.0–6.0 mm. The proposition that osteoblasts regulate the optimal activity of osteoclasts provides a rationale for observations of an association between osteoblast numbers, activity, and the decreasing diameters of osteons; at least in some bones. Jowsey (1966, 1968) and Currey (1970) reported that the diameters of rib osteons decrease by 25% in the 6th–7th decades of life. Support for this relationship is meagre since it could not be confirmed by a second laboratory (Takahashi *et al.*, 1965; Wu *et al.*, 1970), and Jowsey did not find that it pertained to femoral midshaft osteons. There is a similar level of confusion in terms of data regarding osteon geometry, particularly the length of their cement lines (Jowsey, 1966, 1968).

On the other hand, osteoclastic resorption involves an increasing area of human trabecular surface with age, in females more than males. In the absence of pathology (eg. hyperthyroidism, hyperparathyroidism), the cells do not individually appear more aggressive in males, but they erode deeper Howship's Lacunae in females (Eriksen *et al.*, 1985ab, 1986). This has not been confirmed for cortical bone, but the patterns are likely to be similar. Thus, the imbalance struck between cortical-trabecular bone formation and resorption leads to osteopenia and/or osteoporosis which is defined as a global loss of bone mass. Cortical bone loss and thinning (involution) is observed in both small laboratory species (rats etc.), in primates and man (Table VIII). In the latter, there may be a notable increase in osteoprogenitor cell production and maturation at the onset of menopause, producing a transitory spurt in the number of remodeling foci. The time course will be different for different bones; in the Rhesus monkey metacarpal, bone loss begins to occur before the age of 12 years even though the greatest changes in physiology and morphology do not become apparent in Rhesus and Macaques until the reproductive decline in their third decade of life (de Rousseau, 1985).

## Osteoblasts and Bone Resorption

Histomorphometric analyses of cortical and trabecular bone from metabolically normal human subjects in the first 5 decades of life usually show a proportional relationship between the percent of bone surfaces undergoing formation and resorption (Jowsey, 1960), between the numbers of osteoblasts and osteoclasts, or between the numbers of osteoblasts and the numbers of nuclei per osteoclast (Gruber et al., 1986; Holtrop et al., 1978). The term devised for these relationships is "coupling". The relationships become "uncoupled" beyond the fifth decade when the osteoblast census stabilizes and some parameter such as osteoclast number or activity increases. Iliac crest biopsies from Gruber et al's (1986) population of postmenopausal women showed an increase in the resorptive capacity of individual acid phosphatase-positive osteoclasts relative to the volume of bone deposited by the numerically superior osteoblasts. The development of this concept depended heavily upon the results of histomorphometric studies in metabolically disturbed animals during their period of active skeletal growth and (pharmacologic) studies in neonatal bone organ cultures (Stern and Raisz, 1979). A form of uncoupling typified by reduced periosteal and endosteal osteoblastic activity and exaggerated osteoclastic surfaces and linear rate of resorption occurs in the tibial cortex of intact and thyroparathyroidectomized hypophosphatemic rats (Baylink et al., 1971). Vitamin-D deficiency depressed periosteal ($-20\%$) but not endosteal bone formation, and increased endosteal osteoclastic ($+80\%$) activity (Baylink et al., 1970). Such studies are instructive because they emphasize that the cellular basis for homeostatic deregulation is site-specific, that osteopenia/osteoporosis in itself needs to be interpreted in terms of changes in resorption-formation activation at different "bone envelopes" (Frost, 1966b).

There is growing appreciation that the complex of collagen and calcium-binding proteins (sialoproteins, osteocalcin etc.) and phospholipids which favor calcification also endows bone with a suite of chemoattractants for the precursors of osteoclasts. However, while these moieties are ubiquitous, osteoclastic resorption tends to occur with more site-selectivity. Osteoclasts appear to require better defined local 'traffic signals'. Recent studies have shown that osteoblasts excercize other mechanisms which are autoregulatory in the local control of matrix production and degradation. The degradation issue is central to a current hypothesis that osteoblasts predispose bone surfaces to resorption by exposure of bone mineral (Chambers and Fuller, 1985) and that osteoclastic activity can be optimized by growth factors produced by osteoblasts (see below). This attractive scenario is continually being fine-tuned by discoveries about how these relationships are maintained (Figs 3, 4; Table XII).

## Osteoblast Collagenase

Collagenolytic activity can be detected in growing rat bone (Walker *et al.*, 1968), regenerating newt limbs (Grillo *et al.*, 1967), and in cultured mouse bone cells (Sakamoto and Sakamoto, 1984ab). The enzyme was localized immunocytochemically to the perinuclear regions of the cell. In the absence

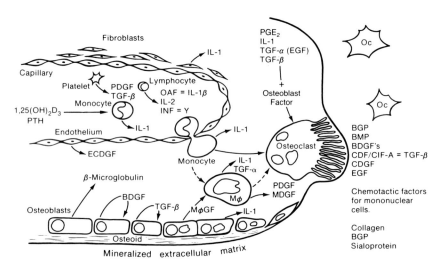

**Fig. 3** Schematic of bone remodeling site to illustrate the nature of some of the cellular interactions thought to play a role in (*a*) angiogenesis, (*b*) the mobilization of the mononuclear precursors of osteoclasts (monocytes and macrophages), and (*c*) osteoblastic proliferation, matrix formation and production of growth factors which mediate osteoclastic performance. In its turn, bone resorption is believed to liberate apatite-bound growth factors, thereby creating microenvironmental changes in cytokine abundance which further influences the processes of cytologic differentiation and function (see Fig. 4).

# Model of Bone Resorption

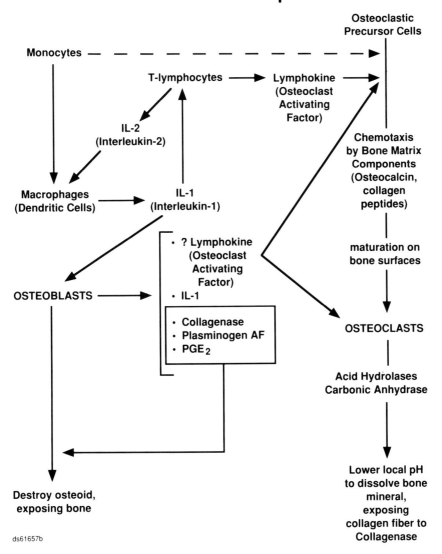

**Fig. 4** Schematic model of bone resorption, illustrating (*a*) the putative roles of the immune system and osteoblasts in the mobilization of osteoclast precursor cells, (*b*) how skeletal matrical components influence their movement and occupany of mineralized bone surfaces, and (*c*) the function of mature osteoclasts.

**TABLE X**

| | |
|---|---|
| Ultrastructural Evidence for Cell Mediated Collagen Turnover | |
| Cells Competent to Phagocytose Collagen Fibrils (TEM) | |

| | |
|---|---|
| *Teeth* (Periodontal Ligament) | |
| — PDL | Garant 1976 |
| — Fibroblasts | Ten Cate & Deporter 1974 |
| — Odontoblasts | Sasaki *et al.*, 1984 |
| | |
| *Cartilage* | |
| — Chondrocytes | *Takagi et al.*, 1981 |
| *Bone* | |
| — Osteoblasts* | Sasaki *et al.*, 1985 |
| :Calvaria | Takahashi *et al.*, 1986 |

of serum blockers, it is capable of degrading tissue collagen fibrils at 37°C and at neutral pH (Sodek and Heersche, 1981). *In vivo*, it may operate with other proteolytic enzymes such as pronase, which removes collagen terminal telopeptides, (Shulman *et al.*, 1972). An early report that an endogenous collagenase was present in isolated rat calvarial bone cells cultures indicated that enzyme levels were diminished by pretreating the cells with PTH (Puzas and Brand, 1976), but PTH was stimulatory in murine cultures (Sakamoto and Sakamoto, 1984a). More recent studies indicate that cultured, untransformed murine and rat calvarial osteoblast-like cells and transformed UMR−106−01 osteoblast-like cells synthesize a bone-specific *neutral collagenase* (Heath *et al.*, 1984; Otsuka, 1984; Partridge *et al.*, 1987; Shen *et al.*, 1989) as well as a neutral protease plasminogen activator (Hamilton *et al.*, 1984; Vaes *et al.*, 1976), and that their production can be stimulated by the bone resorptive agents PTH, EGF, calcitriol, IL-1, TNF-$\alpha$, and prostaglandin $E_2$. Collagenase production in the UMR cells was unaffected by other cytokines such as interleukin-1 and heparin which otherwise stimulate osteoclast progenitor cells (Partridge *et al.*, 1987). Partridge believes that in serum the collagenase is activated by the conversion of plasminogen to plasmin. Notably, the same cells concomitantly and coordinately synthesize a collagenase inhibitor (Otsuka, 1984; Partridge *et al.*, 1985). The data take their significance from numerous ultrastructural observations that calvarial cells, as well as a wide variety of other skeletal cells, phagocytose and 'turnover' collagen fibrils (Table X).

## Prostaglandin

Prostaglandin(s) is a derivative of fatty acid (arachnidonic) metabolism. These agents have different concentration dependent actions, regulating both bone formation and bone resorption. The effects of $PGE_2$ and other prostaglandins on stimulating bone resorption *in vivo* (Goodson *et al.*, 1974), in bone organ culture (Hirata *et al.*, 1983; Holtrop and Raisz, 1978; Klein and Raisz, 1970; Santoro *et al.*, 1977; Voekel and Tashjian, 1972; Yonaga and Morimoto, 1979) and osteoclast cultures (Chambers and Dunn, 1983) were so striking that the consequences for bone formation were little studied. This was due, in part, to evidence that there were many cells within bone (fibroblast, endothelial cells, osteoblasts, osteocytes) competent to produce prostaglandins, that it would be difficult to interpret the results from organ culture experiments, and in part to the long standing concept that, if there was an *in vivo* effect on bone formation, it would be determined by the rate of bone resorption. In fact, most of the early evidence from calvarial cultures was that these agents inhibited collagen and non-collagen protein synthesis. In organ cultures of fetal rat calvaria, $PGE_2$ and other prostaglandins ($PGE_1$, $PGF_1a$, $PGA_1$ and $PGA_2$: $10^{-7}M - 10^{-4}M$), inhibited the incorporation of radioproline into newly formed collagen without affecting the synthesis of non-collagen proteins (Harvey, 1988a). The effect was latent, not acute, and occurred only at the higher end of the dose range. However, cell culture systems have shown that prostaglandins have a direct effect on osteoblasts and osteoblast-like cells (Table XI).

Despite the limitation of organ culture systems, Blumenkrantz and Sondergaard (1972) found that $PGE_1$ and $PGF_{1a}$ stimulated proline and lysine hydroxylation in chick tibial explants. Osteoblast-like cells grown in culture produce prostaglandins of the E series when stimulated by tensile

**TABLE XI**

| Prostaglandin | |
|---|---|
| Clinical Evidence for a Biological Role in Bone Formation. | |
| Promotes | Circumstance |
| Lamellar Periosteal Bone Formation and Cortical Hyperostosis. | Long term PGE1-Rx in an infant with ductus dependent cyanotic congenital cardiac defects.[1] |
| Cortical Bone Hypertrophy | Elevated endogenous $PGE_2$ levels in burn injuries.[2] |
| Fracture Healing[3] | Early Post-fx= PGE production. 2 wks Post-fx= PGF increased. |
| Bone Remodeling | Osteomyelitic bone has high PGE levels.[4] |

1. Ueda *et al.*, 1980
2. Stern et al. 1985
3. Dekel *et al.*, 1981
4. Dekel *et al.*, 1981

mechanical forces (Binderman *et al.*, 1984; Davidovitch *et al.*, 1984; Yeh and Rodan 1984), followed by increased activities of cAMP, ornithine decarboxylase and DNA synthesis (Binderman *et al.*, 1988). Prostaglandin production is, on the other hand, suppressed by PTH (McDonald *et al.*, 1984), adrenalectomy, and by glucocorticoids (Danon and Assouline, 1978; Sandberg *et al.*, 1982; Tashjian *et al.*, 1975) and other non-inflammatory agents such as indomethacin which interferes with the enzyme cyclooxygenase required for PGE synthesis (Flower 1974; Nuki *et al.*, 1981; Raisz and Martin, 1983; Weaks-Dybvig *et al.*, 1982). PGE synthesis also appears to be regulated by positive feedback mechanisms because tissue content is enhanced in PGE-treated animals. Bone mass is actually increased in growing rats injected chronically with small doses of $PGE_2$ and 16,16-dimethyl $PGE_2$; the effect is restricted largely to metaphyseal trabecular bone and cortico-endosteal surfaces (Furuta and Jee, 1986; Jee *et al.*, 1985, 1987; Ueno *et al.*, 1985). A local periosteal reaction followed chronic infusion of $PGE_1$ to the jaws of beagles (Miller and Marks, 1988). Mature dogs [19−35 months] treated orally with $PGE_2$ responded with increased serum alkaline phosphatase, higher rates of bone turnover on femoral/rib periosteal and intracortical sites, but without a change in the activities of individual osteoblasts (High, 1988). It is not unusual to expect site-specific effects. Chyun and Raisz (1984) also reported differential effects of low concentrations of $PGE_2$ ($10^{-10}$ M) on DNA and collagen synthesis in rat calvarial cultures. Periosteal cell DNA synthesis was increased, but the osteoprogenitor cells which lay within the intracortical spaces did not respond; intracortical collagen formation increased, but periosteal collagen formation was unaffected. In this sense, prostaglandin's anabolic effect is expressed in much the same fashion as the effect of ch.onic PTH-treatment, and both agents independently have the capacity to increase bone cell cAMP levels (Chase and Aurbach, 1970; Dziak *et al.*, 1979; Marcus and Orner, 1977; Yu *et al.*, 1976) and elevate plasma calcium levels (Franklin and Tashjian, 1975). The cAMP response is observed in osteoblasts in response to a number of prostanoids besides $PGE_2$ [$PGI_2$, 13,14 dihydro $PGE_2$, 6 keto $F_1a$ (Partridge *et al.*, 1981). The parallel extends also to, and may be causal for, the malignant hypercalcemia observed in patients with osseous and extraosseous tumors (see review by Jaffe and Santoro, 1977; Harvey, 1988b).

## Presumptive Bone Resorptive Factors Unrelated to PGE, IL-1, TNF, TGF-b

Osteoblasts appear to produce small (Mr<2000) and large (Mr=50,000−60,000) molecular weight factors unrelated to Il-1 or PGE that effect resorption in cultured murine calvaria (Sandy *et al.*, 1989). A 50kD Differentiation Inducing Factor (DIF) has been isolated from MC3T3-E1 cells which Abe *et al* (1988) believe operates via $PGE_2$ to promote osteoclast precursor cells maturation. The detailed characterization of DIF will be important for the development of the thesis that osteoblasts control the intensity of osteoclastic bone resorption via the production of short-range soluble mediators.

## Cell-Cell and Cell-Matrix Interactions

Because trabecular bone resorption and osteon formation involves activation/recruitment of osteoclast precursor cells, their maturation and subsequent erosion of bone surfaces, the concept developed early that osteoblasts were relatively passive cells. Their task was to refill cavities, and it was the resorptive event which dictated the intensity of bone formation. There was little appreciation that osteoblasts and osteoclasts actively interacted. A decade ago, scanning electron microscopy generated the hypothesis that (PTH-mediated) osteoblast contraction could be the mechanism which exposed mineralized surfaces to osteoclast-precursor cells and osteoclasts (Rodan and Martin, 1981). The coordinate development of culture systems which maintain isolated populations of active osteoblasts and osteoclasts provided the required 'test materials'. To summarize and expand some parts of the story we have already evolved, we now know that:

1. Osteoblasts in culture secrete a macrophage growth factor which could activate the granulocytic cell lineage which produces osteoclastic precursor cells.

2. Certain products secreted by the osteoblast such as fibronectin, sialoprotein, $\alpha_2$HS-glycoprotein, Gla protein/osteocalcin and collagen are chemotactic for osteoclast precursor cells (Bar-Shavit *et al.*, 1983b; Kahn *et al.*, 1981; Malone *et al.*, 1982; Mundy *et al.*, 1978; Polla *et al.*, 1987; Postlewaite and Kang, 1976). Such cells failed to mature and resorb osteocalcin depleted matrices or fragments of bone from which the sialoprotein had been enzymatically stripped (Bar-Shavit *et al.*, 1983b; Malone *et al.*, 1982). One or more matrix components may be required to stimulate the monocytes and macrophages present in areas of bone formation to produce lysosomal enzymes and the collagenase required for the uptake and degradation of collagen fibers of osteoid origin and those released by bone resorption (Okimura *et al.*, 1979; Rifkin *et al.*, 1980). Macrophages grown on devitalized particles of rat bone (0.115 mg/500,000 cells) were stimulated to produce aryl sulfatase which is required for the hydrolysis of the sulfated glycosaminoglycans released from bone during calcification and in areas of resorption (Gics and Dorey, 1981). As noted above, this function is also

shared by osteoblasts (Lindskog *et al.*, 1987; Sasaki *et al.*, 1985; Takahashi *et al.*, 1986) and may be stimulated by macrophagic IL-1. Osteoblasts are also capable of metabolizing $25(OH)D_3$ to 1,25-dihydroxyvitamin $D_3$ which is a factor which indirectly increases osteoclast formation (Roodman *et al.*, 1985) and function (Bar-Shavit *et al.*, 1983a).

3. Co-cultures of osteoblasts/osteoblast-like cells with osteoclasts enhance the capacity of the osteoclasts to resorb calcified bone and dentin matrices.

4. Tissue culture medium from osteoblast cultures stimulate osteoclast formation (mice: Burger *et al.*, 1987; Klein-Nulend *et al.*, 1987a; chicks: Oursler and Osdoby, 1988), isolated osteoclast motility and their capacity to resorb calcified bone and dentin matrices.

5. Agents such as the PTH, 1,25-dihydroxyvitamin $D_3$, prostaglandins and interleukins which enhance osteoclastic resorption in mixed osteoblast-osteoclast cell system have no effect on osteoclast maturation (chicks: Oursler and Osdoby, 1988) or on osteoclastic motility and resorption when osteoblasts are absent (Chambers *et al.*, 1984, 1985; Chambers and Dunn, 1983). IL-1 stimulated osteoblasts do, however, produce $PGE_2$ and plasminogen activating factor required to activate collagenase (Tatakis *et al.*, 1988). Collectively, the evidence suggests that osteoblasts operate on several different levels to regulate the traffic of putative osteoclastic precursor cells to sites of resorption, perhaps influence their maturation, and police the activities of the differentiated cells. It is also conceivable that osteoblast-generated neutral collagenase and neutral proteases could serve to degrade collagen fragments exposed by mineralysis and thereby prepare a suitable table upon which osteoclasts can dine (Chambers and Fuller, 1985). There is no evidence, however, that osteoclasts perform a reciprocal function. Osteoblasts in culture are not stimulated when grown in medium conditioned by mature osteoclasts. A cell-tissue interactive system needs to be invoked to satisfy the requirement to maintain proliferative and functional osteoblast populations. The coupling mechanism appears to be driven by the resorptive-release of bone-bound growth factors that had originally been synthesized by osteoblasts, and operates mainly to increase cell proliferation rather than cell maturation (Farley *et al.*, 1987).

There is a maze of interlocking systems which maintain osteoblast vigor which are related to the proliferative potential of osteoprogenitor cells (Figs. 3,4; Table XII). The monocytic cell line helps maintain the capacity of the osteogenic precursor stromal cell complex in marrow and within intracortical bone spaces, but their production of a factor which stimulates calvarial osteoblasts and ROS cells to proliferate (Bal *et al.*, 1988; Gazit, 1988; Tabuchi and Simmons, 1986; Seitz and Simmons, unpublished 1988) is not associated with other stromal cell products such as the colony stimulating factor (CSF-1) which, while stimulating granulopoiesis, may inhibit the growth of osteoclastic precursor cells (Wijngaert *et al.*, 1987). It is clear that

**TABLE XII**

Local Regulators of Bone Growth
(Adapted from Centrella and Canalis Endocrine Rev. 6: 544, 1985)

| | | Synthesis of | | |
|---|---|---|---|---|
| | Mr | DNA | Collagen | Noncollagen Protein |
| *Growth Factors from Skeletal Cells* Transforming Growth Factor TGF-b | 25,000 | D | I | I |
| Non-transforming Growth Factors BDGF ($\beta_2$ microglobulin) | 11,000 | I | I | I |
| IGF-I | 7,500 | I | I | I |
| SGF (=IGF-II) | 83,000 | I | I | N/A |
| *Bone/Cartilage Inducing Factors from Bone Matrix* | | | | |
| BMP | 19,000 | I | NE | NE |
| TGF-$\beta$ | 26,000 | N/A | N/A | N/A |
| *Monokines* IL−1 | Multiple forms | I | I/D[a] | I/D[a] |
| MDGF/M-CSA | 15−43,000[+] | I | N/A | N/A |
| *TNFa | 17,000 | I | D | I-NE |
| *TNFb | 18,600 | N/A | N/A | N/A |
| *Prostaglandin* PGE$_2$ | <1,000 | I/D[a] | I/D[a] | I/D[a] |

a = Stimulatory & inhibitory effects which are dose and time related.
I = Increased
D = Decreased
N/A = data not available
NE = no effect
+ = species differences
* Production of osteoblastic resorptive factor(s)

these same factors are pertinent to a role for the osteoprogenitor cells and osteoblast in repair and regeneration.

## Bone Cell-Derived Growth Factors

Cultured osteoblast-like cells produce a number of peptides with diverse roles in the autoregulation of proliferation and matrix building activity (modeling) (Fig. 3; Table XII and see chapter 4). They also feed-back to regulate the proliferation of their forebears, the fibroblast-like periosteal osteoprogenitor cells (Plas and Nijweide, 1988). In turn, these activities are moderated by systemic factors. This family of autologous growth factors isolated from bone differs from the bone morphogenetic protein (BMP) in the sense that BMP has no direct action on the stimulation of bone cell alkaline phosphatase and collagen production. About a decade ago, several laboratories reported that medium conditioned by bone cells stimulatated osteoblast growth and collagen formation (Peck *et al.*, 1979; Canalis *et al.*, 1980). The factor or factors has variously been called bone growth factor (BGF), bone-derived growth factor (BDGF), or skeletal growth factor (SGF). As will be noted below, BDGF has recently been identified as $b_2$-microglobulin (Canalis et al 1987), SGF as IGF-II, and some fractions of BMP with Mr's about 13kD or >20kD as belonging to the TGF-b family. However, the literature about these factors is important in terms of their history.

### Insulin-like Growth Factor

While first defined in cartilage, IGF-I, an insulin-like peptide mitogen, is produced as a local autocrine and perhaps paracrine growth factor synthesized by osteoblasts (D'Ercole *et al.*, 1980, 1984; Slootweg *et al.*, 1988). It is immunologically identical to Somatomedin-C/IGF-1/IGF-II, the systemic, pituitary-dependent liver metabolite of growth hormone and the IGF-I's produced by other mesenchymal derived cells such as W138 fibroblasts (Atkinson *et al.*, 1980), human fibroblasts (Clemmons, 1981, 1985), and muscle cells (Clemmons *et al.*, 1985, Hill *et al.*, 1984). The levels of serum SmC/IGF-1 increase with gestational age and during the period of somatic growth, decreasing thereafter during adult life (Hammerman, 1987). This parameter is tied to nutrition and food intake, and not so closely tied to the rate of body growth in rats that it can be considered a growth mediator. The growth promoting effect of 1,25-dihydroxyvitamin $D_3$ can occur in vitamin D-deficient rats without a concomitant increase in blood SmC/IGF (Clark *et al.*, 1986). Nor do serum SmC values reflect the circadian change in the rates of endochondral bone growth or bone collagen formation in rats (Simmons *et al.*, 1986b).

The administration of purified IGF-1 stimulates *in vivo* endochondral bone growth in hypophysectomized rats (Schoenle *et al.*, 1982). *In vitro* it stimulates DNA, collagen and non-collagen protein, glycogen and alkaline phosphatase synthesis in chick (Canalis, 1980) and newborn rat calvarial cells (Schmid *et al.*, 1983), and can reverse glucocorticoid suppression of collagen mRNA synthesis (Schmid *et al.*, 1988). The DNA and glycogen effects of IGF are specific (serum-independent) and of equal magnitude in cells procured from intact and hypophysectomized rats. It also enhances

PTH-mediated cAMP production some 100-fold while challenges with calcitonin produce only a 1.2X increase. Bone cell IGF-1 synthesis is regulated by a number of hormones other than growth hormone (*thyroid, cortisol, and insulin*) (Canalis, 1980). It may also be regulated by testosterone since serum IGF-I levels are increased during antlerogenesis (Suttie *et al.*, 1988). IGF-1 is now thought to be a second effector in growth hormone action, growth hormone increasing the receptor sensitivity of cells to IGF-1. Thus, IGF-1 carries $G_0$ cells into the $G_1$ stage of the cell cycle, but is sufficient in-and-of itself to initiate mitosis and clonal growth in chondrocytes (Lindahl *et al.*, 1987) and bone cells (Canalis 1980; Ernst and Froesch, 1988). IGF appears to be required for estrogen stimulated growth of bone cells *in vitro* (Ernst *et al.*, 1988a).

## BDGF

It was early observed that tissue culture medium conditioned by fetal rat calvaria contained a factor which stimulated DNA and protein (collagen and non-collagen protein) synthesis (Canalis *et al.*, 1980). Initially, two autologous factors which had a low molecular weight (<35Kd) were identified (Canalis *et al.*, 1980; Peck and Rifas, 1982). Purification indicated that the two factors were: BDGF-I which stimulated DNA synthesis and was similar to platelet derived growth factor (PDGF), and BDGF-II which, like IGF-I, stimulated both DNA and collagen (see review by Canalis, 1985). BDGF is, however, a distinctly different polypeptide. It's production was stimulated by pre-culturing calvarial-derived osteoblast-like cells with glucocorticoids at physiologic concentrations (see also Wong *et al.*, 1987). Nevertheless, it has since been identified $\beta_2$ microglobulin (Centrella and Canalis, 1985).

## SGF (=IGF-II)

Early publications reported that cultures of human bone (Farley and Baylink, 1982; Farley *et al.*, 1982; Mohan *et al.*, 1986), fetal rat (Wergedal and Baylink, 1984) and check bone (Drivdahl *et al.*, 1981, 1982; Lau *et al.*, 1988) contained a high molecular weight peptide (60K−80K) which stimulates DNA and protein synthesis in chick tibiae and in serum free calvarial cell cultures. It was originally called the Skeletal Growth Factor, and because it failed to stimulate proliferation in MC3T3-E1 and BalbC 3T3 cells, it was thought to be unlike other growth factors such as EGF, FGF, IGF-I and PDGF (Farley *et al.*, 1988; Mohan *et al.*, 1987). A similar 83kDk human SGF did not increase DNA synthesis in the clonal mouse MC3T3-E1 cells, or inhibit the growth promoting effect of serum, but it did stimulate collagen and NCP synthesis (Linkart *et al.*, 1986). However, because PTH stimulated SGF production, SGF was called the "coupling factor" (Howard *et al.*, 1981)—meaning that it was *the* factor which provided the local mechanism for the internal remodeling of bone. It's concentration is human femoral head trabecular bone matrix was on the order of 0.00024% (Mohan *et al.*, 1986).

We now appreciate the SGF is homologous with IGF-II (Mohan *et al.*, 1988) and that it is most likely produced by osteoblasts since IGF-II levels fall in situations which impair bone formation (Sibonga *et al.*, 1989). Local conditions, those created by osteoclastic resorption, are thought to provide direction by the release and creation of locally high concentrations of factors which, while they may originate from bone cells (autocrine), have then a paracine role.

*Transforming Growth Factor*

*In vivo*, TGF-β may promote adhesion of osteoblasts to extracellular matrix components such as fibronectin, collagen and proteoglycans (Ignotz and Massague, 1987). In fact, it promotes fibronectin and osteopontin production (Centrella, 1988a; Noda *et al.*, 1988a; Oldberg *et al.*, 1986). As noted, the cytokine is produced by (mixed) fetal rat calvarial cells (Gehron Robey *et al.*, 1987; Petkovich *et al.*, 1987), and is present in fetal human calvarial osteoblasts and osteoclasts—osteoblasts being the more numerous cell type (Sandberg *et al.*, 1988). Its concentration in bone matrix is low (200ug/kg; Sandberg *et al.*, 1988; Seyedin *et al.*, 1986), and during culture, the cytokine can be released into the medium (Centrella and Canalis 1985, 1987).

TGF-b is considered to be both a mitogen and a maturation factor. With increasing levels of TGF-b, calvarial osteoprogenitor cells and fetal bovine osteoblasts—as well as ROS 17/2.8 and MC3T3-E1 cells—respond by first increasing and then decreasing DNA synthesis (Gehron Robey *et al.*, 1987; Hock *et al.*, 1988), and by increasing collagen and alkaline phosphatase synthesis as cell proliferation wanes (Elford *et al.*, 1987b; Hock *et al.*, 1988; Noda and Rodan, 1986). Osteoblasts from rat parietal bone appear to have 3 discrete TGF-b receptors—2 with low affinity ($Mr < 20,000 = 85,000$) and one with high affinity ($Mr = 65,000$) (Centrella *et al.*, 1988b).

These differentiated cell functions can be inhibited in serum free media by agents such as actinomycin D and cyloheximide which interfere with RNA and protein synthesis (Noda and Rodan, 1987; Pfeilshifter *et al.*, 1987). TGF-β derived from platelets (Centrella *et al.*, 1986, 1988b) has been reported to have similar effects, increasing cell division and collagen and non-collagen protein synthesis and alkaline phosphatase in calvarial cultures as well as in less differentiated cells in incisional wounds (Cromack *et al.*, 1987; Mustoe *et al.*, 1987). Mixed results, a cell density-independent decrease in DNA synthesis, alkaline phosphatase and collagen synthesis, with no change in NCP synthesis, have been observed in osteoblasts derived from neonatal rat calvaria and ROS 17/2.8 cells (Guenther *et al.*, 1988).

While the results are controversial, perhaps due to differences in cell lines and experimental conditions, the most conservative interpretation of the results is that TGF-β's action is bidirectional depending upon the state of maturation (Centrella *et al.*, 1986; Centrella *et al.*, 1987) and inter-action with locally high concentrations of other (paracrine) cytokines and hormones. Thus, while physiologic concentrations of PTH (0.2−2.0mM) might have no direct action on osteoblast alkaline phosphatase production *in vitro*, it does oppose TGF-β's enhancement of the enzyme and its other skeletally anabolic effects (Centrella *et al.*, 1988b). In some studies, TGF-β augments (Pfeilschifter *et al.*, 1986) or diminishes (Guenther *et al.*, 1988) PTH responses such as alkaline phosphatase and cAMP. $1,25(OH)_2D_3$ potentiates EGF/TGF-α receptors to which TGF-β does not bind (Petkovich *et al.*, 1987), but EGF in combination with TGF-β inhibits the normal EGF-mediated increase in bone cell proliferation within semisolid media (Guenther *et al.*, 1988). It is believed that EGF is required for the full expression of TGF-β's activity.

TGF-β like activity is also found in canine apocrine cell adenocarcinoma of the anal sac and in tumor tissue associated with malignant hypercalcemia and bone resorption. Tumor extracts have also proven to promote bone resorption (Weir *et al.*, 1988). TGF-b, like EGF and TNF, stimulate bone resorption *in vitro* (Raisz *et al.*, 1980; Tashjian *et al.*, 1985).

## Beta-2 Microglobulin

Its effects are similar to IGF-1. It may not be a growth factor by strict criteria, but it seems to act by modulating the binding of hormones and growth factors such as IGF-1 to their receptor (Centrella, cited by Canalis *et al.*, 1988a).

## Interleukin-1

Osteoblast-like cells isolated from murine calvariae produce the monokine IL-1 (Hanazawa *et al.*, 1987) which is a more characteristic product of macrophages stimulated by endotoxin, silica, immune complexes etc. IL-1 stimulates bone resorption in osteoblast-osteoclast co-cultures (Thomson *et al.*, 1986), probably by mediating osteoblast prostaglandin synthesis

(Gowen, 1988; Gowen et al., 1985; Sato et al., 1987; Tatakis et al., 1988) and quite possibly tumor necrosis factor (TNF, Gowen et al., 1988). The issue addresses the mechanism(s) by which the coupling of bone formation and resorption occur. The effects of IL-1 are dose dependent. In calvariae, human trabecular bone cells and UMR-106 cells, low concentrations of IL-1 ($10^{-12}-10^{-13}$M) efficiently stimulate DNA and collagen/non-collagen protein synthesis, alkaline phosphatase as well as prostaglandin synthesis (Pacifici et al., 1988; Yajima et al., 1988), while higher doses ($10^{-11}$M) and indomethacin inhibit bone protein synthesis (Beresford et al., 1984a). The indomethacin effect indicates that the resorptive effects of IL-1 may be prostaglandin mediated.

Osteoblasts exposed to macrophagic IL-1$\beta$ respond in an 'opposite direction' via a non-PGE$_2$ mechanism, indicating that the cytokine does not fulfill the requirements of a coupling factor (Stashenko et al., 1987). Any osteogenic response to IL-1 is, then, difficult to interpret. Recent work shows that mice implanted i.m. with BMP-rich matrix produced an excesses of heterotopic bone following IL-1 injection, but that anti-IL-1 injections were only partially inhibitory (Mahy and Urist, 1988).

### Macrophage-Colony Stimulating Activity

Peritoneal macrophages and the murine J774A.1 macrophage cell line appear to produce factor(s) unrelated to prostaglandin and IL-1 which stimulate DNA synthesis and alkaline phosphatase in cultures of fetal rat calvarial-derived osteoblast-like cells (Cheng et al., 1987; Rifas et al., 1984). In turn, osteoblasts seem able to potentiate hematopoiesis by their ability to produce M-CSF and GM-CSF (Elford et al., 1987a; Horowitz et al., 1988, 1989a). The general rule is that cloned osteoblast lineages constitutively produce both of these CSF's, but primary osteoblast which produce only GM-CSF cultures require some stimulation (Lipolysaccharide, PTH) to produce M-CSF (Horowitz et al., 1989).

### Bone Derived Growth Factors

Because hydroxyapatite has a high affinity for locally and systemically derived growth factors, resorption can effect high local concentrations of BMP, IGF-1, IGF-II, TGF-b, and b$_2$-microglobulin. The process also releases PDGF, epidermal growth factor (EGF), and fibroblast growth factor (FGF), moieties which operate alone or syngergistically to promote or inhibit DNA and bone protein synthesis and to stimulate one or more of the events which regulate bone resorption. (Canalis et al., 1988; Hauschka et *al.*, 1986; Urist *et al.*, 1983).

## Epidermal Growth Factor

The little extant *in vivo* experience has shown that a 7 day course of daily s.c. injections in mice will increase bone formation (periosteum +45% > endosteum +20%) and the number of osteoclasts (+65%) in caudal vertebrae (Marie *et al.*, 1988). It is likely that this is due to the stimulation of osteoprogenitor cell proliferation, their subsequent maturation and increased bone turnover (viz marrow stromal cells (Owen *et al.*, 1987)). EGF receptors have been characterized for murine calvarial cultures (Shupnik *et al.*, 1980), clonal osteogenic sarcoma cell lines (Ng *et al.*, 1983a), and in the mesenchymal cells responsible for craniofacial development (Pisano and Greene, 1986). In *in vitro* murine (MC3T3-E1) and rat cell/organ cultures, EGF promotes osteoblast cell proliferation (Canalis and Raisz, 1979; Guenther *et al.*, 1988; Ng *et al.*, 1983b), inhibits collagen formation turnover without affecting NCP synthesis (Canalis and Raisz 1979; Hata *et al.*, 1984; Osaki *et al.*, 1984) and stimulates bone resorption (Ibbotson *et al.*, 1985; Tashjian *et al.*, 1978; Voelkel *et al.*, 1980). The "system" differenes in effect on collagen synthesis may mean that EGF also mediates collagen degradation. There is controversy as to whether the cytokine significantly increases intracellular collagen degradation via a collagenase-peptidase in MC3T3-E1 cells (Chikuma *et al.*, 1984; Hata *et al.*, 1984) but this appears not to occur in rat calvarial organ cultures (Canalis and Raisz, 1979). The EGF-target cell has not been identified *in vivo*, but it seems likely from Type I collagen immunocytochemical studies (Osaki *et al.*, 1984) and EGF receptor binding studies in UMR-108 and calvarial cells (Lorenzo and Raisz, 1982; Ng *et al.*, 1983ab) that the cytokine's resorptive effect reflects an aspect of the coupling mechanism, possibly via indomethacin-blocked/osteoblast-mediated prostaglandin synthesis. Indomethacin does not block EGF-mediated DNA and alkaline phosphatase synthesis [MC3T3 cells: Yokota *et al.*, 1986].

With respect to bone turnover, there is no evidence that the ability of EGF to promote bone resorption depends upon other agents. EGF receptor numbers or affinity in calvarial cultures was not altered by other calcitropic hormones such as PTH, $1,25(OH)_2D_3$, calcitonin, or $PGE_2$ (Shupnik *et al.*, 1980) and the time course of EGF and PTH-mediated resorption of cultured calvaria is identical (Tashjian and Levine, 1978). Only cortisol and other glucocorticoids will block mitogenesis (fibroblasts: Kohase *et al.*, 1987), the mechanisms of EGF-mediated collagen synthesis (Canalis and Raisz, 1979) and resorption (Tashjian and Levine, 1978). The stimulating effects of insulin on bone formation are unaltered (Canalis and Raisz, 1979).

*Platelet-Derived Growth Factor*

PDGF, a 'wound hormone' which is produced by macrophages and stored in platelets, is chemotactic and mitogenic for fibroblasts (Seppa *et al.*, 1982; Senior *et al.*, 1983) and stimulates the proliferation of calvarial bone cells (periosteal fibroblasts and non-periosteal osteoblasts: Canalis, 1985). PDGF is not a normal bone cell product, but certain human osteosarcoma cell lines (2T: Graves *et al.*, 1983; U-2 OS: Graves *et al.*, 1984) synthesize PDGF-like proteins. The cytokine has little influence *per se* on collagen and non-collagen protein synthesis although this occurs as a consequence of the maturation of the increased population of osteoprogenitor cells in osteo-inductive models (Howes *et al.*, 1988). Since PDGF also activates monocytes and promotes bone resorption (Kay *et al.*, 1983; Key *et al.*, 1983; Williams *et al.*, 1983), the stimulus for bone protein synthesis is mediated via prostaglandin(s). Human platelets are also a source of TGF$\beta$ (Centrella *et al.*, 1986).

*Fibroblast Growth Factor*

FGF is a mitogen for fibroblasts (Wellmitz *et al.*, 1980), chondrocytes (Adolphe *et al.*, 1984), periosteal fibroblasts and cavarial osteoblasts (Canalis and Raisz, 1980; Canalis *et al.*, 1988). Its effect on differentiated bone cells is largely to decrease protein synthesis, but collagen formation is affected to a much greater degree than non-collagen protein (NCP). On the other hand, collagen formation alone may be stimulated slightly after short-term exposure to basic FGF, but this is a specific effect not mediated by prostaglandin. The effect of FGF on DNA and NCP synthesis is blunted by cortisol. It's suppressive effect on collagen synthesis is also exerted in calvarial cultures stimulated by insulin (Canalis and Raisz, 1980).

*Bone Cell Stimulating Substance*: A BCSS isolated from an acid extract of cancellous calf bone has been shown to stimulate tetracycline incorporation into rat bones *in vivo*, and stimulate DNA-collagen synthesis in various embryonic chick bones *in vitro* (Clark *et al.*, 1988). The material doubtless contains a mixture of factors, but it has some interesting properties. When injected near the periostea of rat forelimb elements, BCSS produced a remarkably intense periosteal reaction in 7 days (a bone-within-a-bone) — whereas less specific noxious agents elicited only a local periostitis. The response in whole bone was unlike that produced by BMP (TGF-$\beta$ family), and much less responsive to purified TGF-$\beta$ over the time of *in vitro* studies (3d). The target cell for BCSS has not been defined, but it is probably operates on both the osteoblast and the osteoprogenitor cell, affecting their proliferative capacities differently. The extract inhibits marrow free calvarial cell proliferation while stimulating cells from intact tibiae. Removal of marrow abolishes the inhibitory effect. BCSS's effects on collagen synthesis, on the other hand, are always stimulatory and are not influenced by marrow cells. Partial purification has yielded an active fraction which seems unlike PDGF and has an $Mr < 20,000$ (Clark, 1989).

## Endocrine Effects on Bone Formation

We have already considered some of the actions of hormones in terms of their capacity to alter the local production and 'resorptive-release' of growth factors. An entry into the early literature on what are often species-specific cell and tissue responses has been provided by Simmons (1976). Herein, the main focus will be on the hormones which have been demonstrated to exert clearly defined matrical and calciotrophic effects. Chapter 8 deals with hormonal effects in detail.

### Adrenal Glucocorticoids

There have been occasional reports that small doses of, or short-term exposure to, glucocorticoids enhance bone formation in explants of long bones and calvariae (Canalis, 1980). These suggest that under physiological conditions, steroids can promote osteoprogenitor cell proliferation. However, the effect of protracted exposure to small doses or to high levels of glucocorticoids are *generally* antianabolic *in vivo* and *in vitro*, inhibiting-osteoprogenitor cell proliferation, osteoblast maturation, and bone formation, as well as bone turnover by the suppression of osteoclastic activity. On balance, resorptive activity predominates, resulting in osteopenia/osteoporosis.

The mechanism of glucocorticoid action depends on the presence of specific cytoplasmic receptors in both osteoblasts (Chen *et al.*, 1977; Feldman *et al.*, 1975; Yoshioka *et al.*, 1980) and osteoclasts (Chen and Feldman, 1979), and upon an intact adrenal-parathyroid axis (Jee *et al.*, 1970). In culture, dexamethasone coordinately increases the number of vitamin D receptors and cell proliferation (Chen and Feldman, 1981; Chen *et al.*, 1986; Manolagas *et al.*, 1979), but decreases collagen formation. Dexamethasone also potentiated the sensitivity of osteoblast cell lines to PTH, increasing cAMP production by suppressing a phosphodiesterase inhibitor. Such interactions would tend to increase the sensitivity of osteoblasts to 1,25-dihydroxyvitamin $D_3$, β-adrenergic agents, prostaglandin, toxins, and EGF and fluoride which also operate via a cAMP mechanism. One would anticipate a similar potentiation: of PTH-mediated cAMP and osteoclastic resorption *in vivo*, and Gennari (1985) has affirmed the relationship in patients treated with either prednisone or deflazacort, a less active prednisolone-derivative.

Glucocorticoids, then, are uncoupling agents which most significantly impair osteoblastic bone formation. Osteopenia and osteoporosis are the major consequence of high doses and/or protracted exposure. The clinical severity of bone wasting can be ameliorated by dose-scheduling [alternate-day treatment and chronopharmacologic protocols (Eratalay *et al.*, 1981; Ogata and Simmons 1976, 1981; Rosenberg *et al.*, 1981).

## Calcitonin

With the exception of some early reports that bone formation/mass and alkaline phosphatase were stimulated in a number of species by chronically administered calcitonin, conventional wisdom suggests that the hormone does not directly affect this process. The tendency has been to ascribe the effects of the PTH- and $1,25(OH)_2D_3$ -rebound to intermittantly imposed hypocalcemia and phosphaturia respectively (Talmage *et al.*, 1983). Rodent osteoblasts neither express calcitonin receptors nor exhibit a marked alkaline phosphatase-cAMP response after calcitonin injection (Auf'mkolk *et al.*, 1985; Luben *et al.*, 1976; Partridge *et al.*, 1983; Wong, 1986), despite immunocytochemical localization of endogenous hormone to the osteoblast's cytoplasm and nuclear and plasma membranes (Boivin *et al.*, 1984, 1987b; Morel *et al.*, 1985; Rao *et al.*, 1981). Nevertheless, such unusual biochemical effects were recorded in 'mature' bone cell cultures derived from human trabecular bone chips (Crisp *et al.*, 1984). Recent cell and organ culture data support a mitogenic and osteogenic effect at certain dose levels which in mouse tissue also decrease bone resorption (Farley *et al.*, 1988a)

Because calcitonin has receptors on osteoclasts (Rao *et al.*, 1981) and suppresses their mobility and resorptive capacity, it has become an effective therapeutic tool in the treatment of high turnover states (Paget's disease, hyperparathyroidism, and malignant hypercalcemia).

## Estrogen

Estrogens have long been thought to exert their effects on bone indirectly via a number of axes such as the pituitary, adrenal and parathyroid (Morel *et al.*, 1985). Only recently have estrogen receptors been demonstrated in rat calvarial osteoblasts, and, in culture, estradiol stimulated both proliferation and the synthesis of Type I collagen mRNA and collagen (Ernst *et al.*, 1988ab). There is much evidence from human and animal studies that cortical and trabecular bone formation decreases with long-term estrogen lack.

The early literature dealt largely with estrogen's pharmacologic effects. Osteoblastic differentiation accelerated in birds, guinea pigs, and mice, but probably without affecting the rate at which individual cells form collagen (Simmons, 1966). The opposite side of the coin was that a pattern of decreased cell proliferation and maturation and *bone resorption* typified the outcome of estrogen therapy in man and other mammals. Recently, however, therapy has been reported to increase serum osteocalcin concentrations in postmenopausal osteoporotic patients (Stepan, 1987; Civitelli *et al.*, 1988), suggesting that osteoblast activity might have been increased. Estradiol also stimulates IGF-I production from the cultured rat osteosarcoma cell line UMR-106 (Gray *et al.*, 1989). There has been no assurance that in altered estrogen states the matrices deposited will be normal. Estrogen administered to rats (Henneman, 1972) decreases hexosamine: collagen ratios. The matrix formed in estrogen deficient osteoporotic women appears richer than normal in hexoses, sialic and uronic acids (Mbuyi-Muamba *et al.*, 1987), and it may be that the attraction of osteoclast-precursor cells to hexosamine-rich matrices is greater than normal (Bar-Shavit *et al.*, 1983b; Malone *et al.*, 1982). In this expression of uncoupling, peri-postmenopausal, serum monocytic IL-1 levels are higher than normal, but it is not known whether there is an increase in osteoblastic interleukin production to provide a local resorptive stimulus. Circulating estrogen levels do not appear to influence the concentrations of serum prostaglandin (Saksena *et al.*, 1973).

## Growth Hormone

At the cellular level, growth hormone stimulates collagen synthesis via somatomedin-C and its capacity to mediate the synthesis of [osteoblastic] insulin growth factor. Osteoblasts are target cells. Small molecular weight inhibitors of Sm-C [<50,000 MW] are present in serum from diabetic, starved, and uremic rats, circumstances in which bone formation is impaired, and these moieties also have been isolated from liver as well as cartilage (Vassilopoulou-Sellin, 1986).

## Insulin

Insulin is required for protein, lipid and nucleic acid synthesis and cell growth, and these effects are expressed within a matter of hours (Rosen, 1987). The hormone influences 'coupling' by stimulating *in vivo* and *in vitro* osteoblastic RNA and collagen synthesis (Canalis, 1980; Canalis and Raisz, 1980; Hahn *et al.*, 1969; Ituarte *et al.*, 1988; Peck and Messinger, 1970;

Schwartz *et al.*, 1970; Wettenhall *et al.*, 1970) and bone resorption (Puche *et al.*, 1973). The diabetic insulin and IGF-deficit are implicated in the uncoupling between bone formation and resorption which produces osteopenia/osteoporosis in laboratory animals and man (Simmons, 1976).

## Parathyroid Hormone

Autoradiography, immunocytochemical, and radioligand receptor studies have shown that osteoblasts and bone-lining cells have PTH-plasma/nuclear and cytoplasmic receptors (*rat*: Neuman *et al.*, 1975; Rouleau *et al.* 1988; mouse: Morel *et al.*, 1985; *chick*: Silve *et al.*, 1982). Depending upon the species, dose, and duration of treatment, PTH has been reported to either stimulate or depress the rate of *in vivo* collagen synthesis/bone formation. An osteopetrotic-like condition has developed in rats treated chronically with parathyroid extract (see review by Simmons, 1976; Guiness-Hey and Hock, 1984), signaling PTH-mediated mobilization of osteoprogenitor cells and their maturation to osteoblasts. This situation has been approximated *in vitro* by the demonstration that PTH enhances the capacity of osteoblasts to produce a non-$PGE_2$ cytokine which stimulates the proliferation of osteoprogenitor cells (Plas and Nijweide, 1988). Cell-to-cell contact is required to achieve that response. That condition is not frequently met in less heterogeneous cell cultures where PTH suppresses osteoprogenitor cell DNA synthesis (Reid *et al.*, 1987), and is antianabolic in osteoblast cultures. Due at least in part to the heterogeneity of different cell lines, the hormone has variable growth phase-dependent effects on alkaline phosphatase and osteocalcin production (Table III). PTH more uniformly stimulates cAMP synthesis.

All these observations have led to the concept that small doses, frequently applied [with 1,25-dihydroxyvitamin $D_3$ as a mitogen], might be of use in the treatment of osteoporosis in man. The results of such clinical trials have generally been favorable over the short term (Slovik *et al.*, 1986). These records have also contributed to the thesis that PTH-related stimulation of osteoblast maturation-collagen synthesis is secondary to its capacity to induce bone resorption by enhancing [osteoblastic] prostaglandin-collagenase synthesis, the release of osteoclastic calciolytic lysosomal enzymes, and changes in osteoblastic conformation to expose bone surfaces to osteoclastic precursor cells. Guiness-Hey *et al.* (1988) did not find that rat's bone mass was increased by 4–8ug hPTH and 5mg 1,25$(OH)_2D_3$ *vs* 4–8 ug PTH. PTH alone provided the maximal response seen by an increase in the mineral apposition rate. Other studies have also shown the benefit of PTH (Rats: Guiness-Hey and Hock 1984/Dog: Podbesek *et al.*, 1983; Malluche *et al.*, 1986/Man: Reeve *et al.*, 1981). In Malluche's study, the decrease in the bone formation rate which occurs in vitamin D deficiency could be corrected only by combining repletion doses of $1,25(OH)_2D_3$ with PTH. As noted above, it is unlikely that PTH operates via EGF, although systemic and bone-bound EGF released by resorption probably stimulates the production of the osteoblast protease required for collagenase activation. The recent thinking is that PTH could serve to increase bone formation via the TGF-$\beta$ mediated transcriptional regulation of IGF-I (Canalis *et al.*, 1989; McCarthy *et al.*, 1989), osteocalcin (Noda 1989) and collagen formation (Centrella *et al.*, 1988b). This would be its anabolic role. Conversely, PTH's antianabolic role could operate in-part through regulation of synthesis of important non-collagenous protein moieties such as osteopontin, decreasing the capacity of the cells to cooperate by sharing of electrochemical information.

## Testosterone

Testosterone binding proteins have been localized immunohistochemically in perichondrial fibroblasts of growing antlers (Bubenik *et al.*, 1974) and in human osteoblast-like cells (Colvard *et al.*, 1989), but not unequivocably in growth plate cartilage cells (Ackerman and Hamilton, 1976). Androgens promote DNA and bone collagen/alkaline phosphatase synthesis secondary to the effect on proliferation. Their effect in mouse and human osteoblasts (and transformed human osteosarcoma cells (TE89) is antagonized by antiandrogens steroids in pharmacological concentrations (Kasperk *et al.*, 1989). Clinically, their principle benefit is as a tool to reduce bone resorption (Lafferty *et al.*, 1964; Ede and Burr, 1973; Exner, 1980).

## Thyroid Hormone

In man and animals, thyroid hormone enhances while hypothyroidism depresses bone formation, presumably via opposing effects on systemic and osteoblastic Sm-C/IGF-I production (Canalis, 1980). The systemic effects are probably of greater significance. The hormone is incapable of sustaining normal bone growth in hypophysectomized animals or stimulating RNA-protein synthesis *in vitro* (Vaes and Nichols, 1962). Exposure of murine radius cultures to thyroxine diminishes their metaphyseal and diaphyseal osteoblast populations (Simmons, 1976). In man, the bone balance (coupling) becomes positive early in a treatment schedule, as indicated by increased serum alkaline phosphatase and osteocalcin levels (Hasling *et al.*, 1987), but it tilts toward bone resorption with excessively large 'challenges' of thyroxine or triiodothyronine (see below) (Eriksen *et al.*, 1975b; Hasling *et al.*, 1987; Melsen and Mosekilde, 1977).

Vitamin D

Autoradiography and immunocytochemistry have localized the major metabolites of vitamin D to cartilage and bone cells in regions of calcification (see volume 4). Osteoclasts have no D-receptors.

$25(OH)D_3$: Hypertrophic chondrocytes and osteoblasts [$25(OH)D_3$ (Wezeman, 1976)]

$1\alpha(OH)D_3$: Chondrocytes, osteoblasts and osteocytes (Kodicek and Thompson, 1964).

$1,25(OH)_2D_3$: Osteoblastic and osteocytic cytoplasmic/nuclear receptors (Boivin et al., 1987a.)

Vitamin D receptor numbers are augmented by physiological levels of PTH (Chen and Feldman, 1984; Pols et al., 1988) and diminished by gluco-corticoids (Wong et al., 1977), although these effects are dependent upon the growth phase of osteoblast-like cells in culture (Chen and Feldman, 1984; Kurihara et al., 1986).

While differences in the responsivity of different osteoblastic cell lines to $1,25(OH)_2D_3$ exist [see above], it's role is three-fold, to promote intestinal calcium absorption, proliferation and maturation of osteoprogenitor cells, and mineralization. The vitamin has no independent action on collagen formation per se, but the other effects work toward maintaining a positive calcium balance. We have previously noted that vitamin D could have an adjunctive effect on the coupling mechanism, primarily by stimulating osteoblast-mediated bone resorption. In vivo, the mechanism requires the presence of PTH, with its ability to directly stimulate neutral collagenase. The osteoblast involvement extends to $1,25(OH)_2D_3$ stimulation of M-CSA production (Elford et al., 1987a; Horowitz et al., 1988), EGF sensitivity (Shupnik et al., 1980), and potentiation of PTH-EGF interactions (Petkovich et al., 1987). Other growth factors such as IGF-I and SGF/BDGF seem not to be involved in such mechanisms (Clark et al., 1986).

## Chronobiology of Bone Formation/Mineralization

Circadian Relationships

Cartilage and bone cells in the appendicular skeleton of rats and mice exhibit well-defined and reproducible circadian rhythms for all of the elements that contribute to the pace of bone turnover. In man, Valk's studies (1983) indicate that children 'grow' most actively at night. Similarly, day-night measurements of alkaline phosphatase, β-glucuronidase and acid phenylphosphatase in alveolar bone biopsies indicated that human bone turnover was more rapid at night (Petrovic *et al.*, 1981). In this regard, there is a notable nocturnal increase in serum osteocalcin (Colle *et al.*, 1988; Gundberg *et al.*, 1985; Markowitz *et al.*, 1987; Nielsen *et al.*, 1988a) and other calciotrophic hormones (Jubiz *et al.*, 1972) which regulate osteo-progenitor cell proliferation and maturation.

The documented rhythmic spectra are most complete for fetal (Barr 1973) and young growing rats and rabbits. Because of their nocturnal activity period, these species have rhythms 12 hours out of phase from that of man. They encompass the major metabolic activities for cartilage and bone cells [DNA, collagen, NCP, proteoglycan, osteoclastic bone resorption (see, for a review, Simmons, 1979; also Oudet and Petrovic, 1982; Russell *et al.*, 1983, 1984ac). These activities usually show single time-dissociated peaks during a 24h day, indicating that in an operational sense, the different classes of bone cells operate as single physiological populations (Simmons *et al.*, 1981, 1988). Growth cartilage and osteoprogenitor cell proliferation everywhere is $3-4X$ more active during the early nighttime than during the day, while matrical synthetic activities and osteoclastic resorption peak during the middle of the daytime. Mineralization of newly formed bone matrix occurs most rapidly at night, such that the maturational lag-time is on the order of 12h (Russell *et al.*, 1984b). The same temporal patterns of cellular activity have also been observed in fracture healing (Simmons *et al.*, 1977) and the osteoinductive responses to intramuscular grafts of demineralized bone (Simmons *et al.*, 1976). A somewhat more complex pattern of cell division and osteoblast differentiation obtains on rat and mouse periodontal bone surfaces due to the presence of two populations of mitotic osteoprogenitor-preosteoblast cells. In this specialized tissue, one population proliferates most actively during the day, the other during the night (Roberts *et al.*, 1982; Tonna *et al.*, 1987).

The persistence of these rhythms and their normal phase relationships to mediators of calcium metabolism are dictated by the rhythmical nutritional and endocrine variables (adrenal, PTH, calcitonin, Vitamin D). Adrenal-ectomized rats lack a distinct DNA synthetic rhythm while parathyroid-ectomy selectively abolishes the collagen synthetic rhythm (Russell *et al.*, 1984a). The mineralization rhythm is lost in Vitamin D deficient rats (Russell *et al.*, 1984b). Meal-scheduling and the stress this imposes (Russell *et al.*, 1983), as well as the time of day when animals are injected with steroids (Rosenberg *et al.*, 1981; Walker *et al.*, 1985), are all capable of shifting the timing of the peaks of DNA and collagen synthesis.

There is a growing awareness that these biorhythms are not only intrinsi-cally interesting, but can have practical import for the biomedical com-munity. Disease processes can be defined not only by changes in the 'shape' of a circadian rhythmic curve, but also by the absence of normal bio-rhythmicity [ex. cortisol in Cushing's disease; circulating PTH in osteo-porosis (see Simmons, 1979) and Paget's disease (Nuti *et al.*, 1983); hydroxyproline excretion in postmenopausal osteoporosis (Eastell *et al.*, 1988; Radom *et al.*, 1972); nephrectomy and gut calcium transport (Wrobel, 1983); $1,25(OH)_2D_3$-Rx on calcemia (Markowitz *et al.*, 1985)].

### Seasonal Rhythms

The season is also a source of variation in the rates of cartilage and bone growth. In man, this is reflected in the spring-summer maxima for the appearance of ossification centers (Reynolds and Sontag, 1944), preadolescent human bone linear growth (Gindhart, 1972; Marshall, 1975), and the distal forearm bone mineral content of adult males (Hyldstrup *et al.*, 1986). The pace of rat epiphyseal/condylar cartilage growth also shows a spring maxima (Oudet and Petrovic, 1982). The environmental factors most closely related to these phenomena in man and free-ranging animals are daylength, the seasonal serum vitamin D level and calciotrophic hormone rhythms (Cecchettin *et al.*, 1983). In deer, seasonal antlerogenesis is accompanied by increases in circulating levels of PTH, calcitonin, thyroid hormones and alkaline phosphatase (Bubenik *et al.*, 1987; Chao *et al.*, 1984).

## Nutritional Influences

Ensuring a nutritive intake which will maximize bone formation and the biomechanical competence of the skeleton throughout the age span has always received attention, particularly with respect to minerals and trace elements, their capacity to be absorbed at the level of the gut, their utilization in bone, as well as the metabolic and endocrine consequences dietary protein, carbohydrates and lipids have on these processes. One of the central issues is that of the dietary calcium intake recommended for osteoporotic individuals; it has not been firmly established that the level, *per se*, makes a difference. In these individuals, the coexistence of "responders and non-responders" to vitamin D metabolite therapy makes it difficult to establish a universal therapeutic rationale.

### Protein

Low levels of dietary protein and essential amino acids (lysine, leucine, histidine, phenylalanine and tryptophan) all have negative effects on linear and radial bone growth even when there is compensation for the caloric energy deficiency. The general effect is to impair osteoblastic activity, and the result is osteopenia/osteoporosis without significant rickets or osteomalacia in growing and mature animals and man respectively (Einhorn, 1989; Garn and Kangas, 1981; Hammond and Storey, 1970). Osteoporosis/osteopenia may also result from high dietary protein levels; this is associated with decreased gut calcium absorption, decreased osteoid formation and increased bone resorption-presumably an attempt to use skeletal $CaHCO_3$ stores to buffer the protein-acid load-and reduced retention of the renal filtered calcium load. These issues, including the protective effect of high levels of meat and phosphorus and calcium supplements, and the appropriateness of animal models are discussed comprehensively by Einhorn (1989).

## Carbohydrates

Complex sugars (glucose, lactose, sucrose, cellobiose) enhance the absorption and thereby increase the skeletal bioavailability of calcium and phosphorus. Carbohydrates, then, are essential for the general maintenance of skeletal integrity. The inability to absorb lactose in certain individuals is associated with bone loss and osteoporosis (see review by Armbrecht, 1989).

## Lipid

Essential fatty acids must be supplied in the diet since they cannot be synthesized *in vivo*. Certain classes of lipids such as cholesterol and phospholipids play a role in cell membrane integrity, and tissue proteolipids and the calcium-binding acidic phospholipids contained within matrix vesicles are significant for the calcification of extracellular cartilage and bone matrices (Gilder and Boskey, 1989). Fatty acids are required for the synthesis of prostaglandin mediators of bone formation and resorption. Recent evidence indicates that alkaline phosphatase rich, osteoblast-like cells isolated enzymatically from neonatal 4-day rat calvaria have a lower capacity to facilitate fatty acid (FA: palmitate) oxidation than osteoprogenitor or mature osteocyte-like cells (Adamek *et al.*, 1987). While 1,25-dihydroxyvitamin $D_3$ stimulated FA-metabolism, insulin was inhibitory, while PTH and calcitonin were without effect.

## Trace Elements

An overview of the contributions trace elements make to skeletal integrity indicates that there are few which exert any local effects on bone which are independent of the endocrine system. Many have only a low order of skeletal toxicity, but their expression is usually associated with poor body growth, bone formation and mineralization [ex. Ag, Ge, Rb, V](Hudson, 1964; Nielsen, 1986). Some elements which are of primary nutritional importance are as follows:

## Aluminum

Aluminum is a bone volume seeker which interferes locally with osteoblast maturation; bone formation and bone mineralization. The mineralization deficit is associated with an inhibition of the formation and maturation of hydroxapatite crystals. The usual histologic outcome is osteomalacia in all species tested. This effect is pronounced in renal failure patients who receive parenteral dialysis with aluminum-containing solutions, or who receive oral aluminum containing, phosphate binding antacids to control their secondary hyperparathyroidism (see review by Goodman, 1989). An exceptional pattern of Al-enhanced osteogenesis has been described recently in beagles following long-term therapy with low and high doses which did not alter serum Ca, PTH or creatinine levels (Quarles *et al.*, 1988). However, even in this study, which showed an increased osteoblastic surfaces and woven-trabecular bone volume, there was increased osteoid/decreased resorptive surface and a protracted mineralization lag time.

With respect to bone mineral, aluminum appears to rapidly bind to the surface of apatite crystals, thereby slowing their subsequent growth (Blumenthal, 1985). This would explain the localization of Al at the mineral front of patients with Al-associated osteomalacia.

## Boron

Boron deficiency (BD) impairs body growth and produces osteopenia in rats and man. It may be a valuable therapeutic adjunct to dietary calcium in the treatment of osteoporosis, especially when the diet is adequate in magnesium because it benefits PTH, estrogen and testosterone production. For this reason, the benefit accrued to boron is thought to involve a primary interaction with magnesium metabolism and its capacity to regulate PTH secretion. However, the evidence is indirect and largely based on the observation that the hyperparathyroid state of Mg deficiency in rats is more readily achieved in a boron-deficient animal [$0.3-0.4\mu g/g$ diet (Nielsen, 1986)]. It is the endocrine relationships in boron deficiency which seem most important. Osteopenia and low estrogen levels are expressed in both BD and ovariectomized rats, but ovariectomized rats alone tend to gain body weight and have normal serum PTH levels (Tabuchi *et al.*, 1986).

## Fluoride

Fluoride is now used as an adjunctive therapy in osteoporosis for its capacity to stimulate bone formation and reduce the incidence of fractures (see review by Mariano-Menez *et al.*, 1989). The mechanism is not entirely known, but it may involve suppression of PTH and its negative effects on osteoblast maturation and bone collagen formation (Chase *et al.*, 1969; Chambers *et al.*, 1985; Wergedal *et al.*, 1984; Lundy *et al.*, 1986). The evidence is based on work in chick embryonic models where it (*a*) permits the initiation of osteogenesis from mesenchyme [mandibular anlage (Hall, 1987)]. (*b*) potentiates the proliferation of osteoprogenitor cells, osteoblast alkaline phosphatase (Farley *et al.*, 1983) and cAMP concentrations (Chase *et al.*, 1969; Ophaug *et al.*, 1979) in calvarial cultures, and (*c*) increases bone forming surfaces in 14 day postnatal animals (Lundy *et al.*, 1986). Cytokines may not be involved in the mechanism since fluoride does not alter the alkaline phosphatase response to the skeletal growth factor moiety (Wergedal *et al.*, 1984).

Fluoride has profound physico-chemical effects on bone apatite since nearly all dietary F is built into the crystals, where it substitutes for the hydroxyl lattice sites (Eanes and Reddi, 1979), thereby altering magnesium carbonate and citrate levels. Such effects decrease crystal surface area and increase crystallinity. The change in the rate of mineral formation is reflected histomorphometrically as an increase in the mineralization lag time (Vigorita and Suda, 1983). Such changes make fluorapatite more stable and less soluble than hydroxyapatite, and such tissues exhibit a decreased rate of resorption.

## Strontium

Strontium is an alkaline earth element which, like calcium, behaves as a bone mineral volume seeker. It competes with calcium for position in the hydroxyapatite lattice of forming crystals. With dietary excess, Sr produces "strontium rickets" and osteomalacia in growing rats fed adequate levels of vitamin D (Shipley *et al.*, 1922; Storey, 1961) due presumably to an impairment of the renal $1,25(OH)_2D_3$ formation [chicks (Omdahl and DeLuca, 1971)]. On the other hand, there may be some benefit to lower levels of exposure. Rats fed 0.16−0.34% SrCl for 9 weeks exhibit a 10% increase in trabecular calcified bone volumes, without deleterious effects on body growth, mineral homeostasis, or change in the rate of bone resorption (Marie *et al.*, 1985).

## Tin

Tin is relatively non-toxic, but it can be growth-inhibitory when the level of intake in man is >500µg/g. Some of the adverse changes in man and other animals (eg. rats at intakes of 100−200µg/g) involve anemia, decreased intestinal absorption of Zn-Se-Ca, decreases in serum-bone alkaline phosphatase and lactic dehydrogenase levels, collagen synthesis, and decreased skeletal utilization of calcium and other trace metals (see review by Greger, 1989). It's metabolism at the skeletal level involves interactions with calcium, zinc, copper, iron and selenium.

## Zinc

Zinc status is significant for the coupling-uncoupling of skeletal remodelling (see review by Wallwork and Sandstead, 1989) via local and systemic effects on bone cell metabolism. Zn appears to stimulate differentiated cell function in cultures of calvaria isolated from 3-wk old rats. Zn ($10^{-3}$−$10^{-6}$) promoted collagen synthesis, but not DNA (Yamaguchi *et al.*, 1987). The systemic effects of Zn have been expressed in terms of linear growth and radial and intracortical bone formation. Poor zinc nutrition is associated with decreased circulating levels of plasma [and perhaps also osteoblast-generated] Sm-C/IGF-I (Cossack, 1984), as well as with impaired synthesis of DNA, alkaline phosphatase, collagen and NCP, prostaglandin, and mineralization. In terms of bone resorption, zinc deficiency [ZnD] compromizes immune responsiveness and the activity of Zn-containing collagenase, with the result that collagen turnover is decreased in ZnD-chicks (Starcher *et al.*, 1980). PTH-mediated bone carbonic anhydrase levels do not appear to be affected by zinc deficiency in rats (Waite, 1972). In general, the Z-skeletal content of zinc is reflective of the growth-promoting effects of dietary levels of calcium, phytic acid, vitamin D, and protein (Wallwork and Sandstead, 1989).

## Biomechanical Influences

The skeleton is normally engaged in the transmittal of mechanical forces and the energies they generate. With a reduction in loading, a situation met by inactivity (bed rest), immobilization (paraplegia) and fixation of stress-shielding plates in fracture fixation, bone loss ensues. The association between exercize and the maintenance of bone mass (Margulies *et al.*, 1986; Mazess *et al.*, 1985; Simkin *et al.*, 1986; Talmage *et al.*, 1986) is now more firmly entrenched in the literature than the benefit that has been accrued to osteoporotic individuals by calcium or vitamin-rich dietary regimens (Schaafsma *et al.*, 1987).

Cyclical loading regimens in a number of experimental systems (Carter *et al.*, 1987), including the *in vivo*, isolated turkey ulna (Rubin and Lanyon, 1984), is effective in promoting new endosteal, periosteal, and intracortical bone formation. This subject; the adaptive value of mechanical forces, is considered at length elsewhere in these volumes (Vol. 5, Chapter 6). We note that these results express the proliferative and functional response of osteoprogenitor and osteoblast populations to *in vitro* loads. Intermittant [hydrostatic] compressive forces enhance proteoglycan synthesis and ossification in embryonic long bone rudiments. When murine calvaria were cultured under similar conditions, autocrine growth factor(s) released into the [conditioned] media enhanced DNA and bone protein [collagen & NCP] synthesis, and decreased resorption by inhibiting the differentiation and function of osteoclasts [$^{45}$Ca release](Klein-Nulend 1987ab). The nature of the 'factor(s)' has not been clarified; it could be an IGF or a prostaglandin, such as that released by cultured osteoblasts subjected to tensile forces (Binderman *et al.*, 1984, 1988; Davidovitch *et al.*, 1984; Yeh and Rodan, 1984).

**Summary**

In the 1960–1970's, histomorphometry provided the basic evidence that the processes of bone formation and bone resorption were linked or "coupled". It became understood that individual bones normally had different rates of remodeling, and that the 'arithmetic' involved a balance between the number of developing, resorptive foci and the vigor with which osteoblasts are able to sustain their populations and refill resorptive "Howship's Lacunae". The dynamics of the system in animal models, in normal patients and patients with bone disease were accessed by the use of flurochrome labeling so that the local rates and volumes of bone formed and resorbed could be measured accurately. This time period was one in which 'coupling' appeared driven by bone resorption and it was hypothesized that osteoblastic bone formation occurred in response to the chemistry of the bone matrix released at resorptive foci.

The last decade has been witness to an burgeoning of information about the origin and fate of osteoblasts and osteoclasts, the kinetics of (osteoprogenitor) cell proliferation, the biochemistry of bone formation/

mineralization/resorption and the role of the immune system. The rapid development of organ and cell culture systems has begun to clarify the physiologic and endocrine mechanisms which mediate those events. The outcomes have forced an awareness of the centrality of the osteoblast in all phases of bone remodeling. In fact, it has been necessary to redefine the osteoblasts and the coupling phenomenon. Not only do osteoblasts synthesize Type I collagen. They also produce growth factors which autoregulate their population (IGF-1, SGF, BDGF), factors shared with the immune system which mobilize osteoclast precursor cells (IL-1, $PGE_2$, M-CSF), and less-well characterized factors which optimize the activities of mature osteoclasts. Moreover, the non-collagenous matrices osteoblast produce are chemo-attractacts for osteoclast precursors, while their neutral collagenases and motility help expose previously calcified bone matrix for resorption. The "coupling" phenomenon has, then, been significantly restructured.

As predicted by the Goodsirs (1895), the cell fails the requirements of a banal reactionary fibroblast and emerges an active agent in the economy of bone in health and disease.


## References

Abe, E., Y. Ishimi, N. Takahashi, T. Akatsu, H. Ozawa, H. Yamana, S. Yoshiki and T. Suda. (1989) A differentiation-inducing factor produced by the osteoblastic cell line MC3T3-E1 stimulates bone resorption by promoting osteoclast formation. *J. Bone Min. Res.* **3**: 635–645, 1989.

Ackerman, R. J. Jr., and Hamilton, D. W. (1976). Testosterone metabolism in male rat epiphysis. *Calif. Tissue Res.*, **20**: 31.

Adamek, G., Felix, R. Guenther, H. and Fleisch, H. (1987). Fatty acid oxidation in bone tissue and bone cells in culture. Characterization and hormonal influences. *Biochem. J.*, **248**: 129.

Adolphe, M., Froger, B., Ronot, X., Corvol, M. T. and Forest, N. (1984). Cell multiplication and Type II collagen production by rabbit articular chondrocytes cultivated in defined medium. *Exp. Cell Res.*, **155**: 527.

Aitken, J. M., Armstrong, E. and Anderson, J. B. (1972). Osteoporosis after ovariectomy in the mature female rat and the effect of oestrogen and/or progestogen replacement therapy in its prevention. *J. Endocr. (London)*, **55**: 79.

Alberius, P. (1986). Growth of calvarial width. An experimental investigation in rabbits. *Acta Anat.*, **125**: 263.

Amler, M. H. (1987). Osteogenic potential of nonvital tissues and synthetic implant materials. *J. Periodontol.*, **58**: 758.

Amprino, R. R., and Marotti, G. (1964). A topographic quantitative study of bone formation and reconstruction. In: Blackwood, H. J. J. (ed). *Bone and Tooth.* MacMillan Co., N.Y., 21.

Anderson, H. C. (1969). Vesicles associated with calcification in the matrix of epiphyseal cartilage. *J. Cell Biol.*, **41**: 59.

Anderson, H. C. (1985). Matrix vesicle calcification: review and update. In: Peck, W. A. (ed).

*Bone and Mineral Research*, Vol. 3, Elsevier Science, N.Y., 109.

Antosz, M. E., Bellows, C. G., and Aubin, J. E. (1987). Biphasic effects of epidermal growth factor on bone nodule formation by isolated rat calvarial cells *in vitro. J. Bone Min. Res.*, **2**: 385.

Aoyagi, K., T. Takemoto and K. Moji (1988) Changes in cortical thickness of the clavicle and serum gamma-carboxyglutamic acid-containing protein in the elderly in an island community in western Japan. Tohoku *J. Exp. Med.* **156**: 251.

Armbrecht, H. J. (1989). Stimulation of intestinal calcium and phosphorus absorption by carbohydrates. In: Simmons, D. J. (ed.). *Nutrition and Bone Development.* Oxford University Press, N.Y. In press.

Arnold, J. S., Bartley, M. H., Tont, S. A., and Jenkins, D. P. (1966). Skeletal changes in aging and disease. *Clin. Orthop. & Rel. Res.*, **49**: 17.

Arsenis, C., Hackett, M. H., and Huang, S. M. (1976). Resolution, specificity and transphosphorylase activity of calcifying cartilage alkaline phosphatases. *Calcif. Tissue Res.*, **20**: 159.

Ashton, B. A., Hohling, H.-J., and Triffitt, J. T. (1976). Plasma proteins present in human cortical bone: enrichment of the $a_2$HS-glycoprotein. *Calif. Tissue Res.*, **22**: 27.

Atkinson, P. R., Weirman, E. R., Bhaumick, B., and Bala, R. M. (1980). Release of somatomedin-like activity by cultured WI-38 human fibroblasts. *Endocrinol.*, **106**: 2006.

Aubin, J. E., Heersche, J. N. M., Merrilees, M. J., and Sodek, J. (1982). Isolation of bone cell clones with differences in growth, hormone responses and extracellular matrix production. *J. Cell Biol.*, **92**: 452.

Aubin, J. E., Tertinegg, I., Ber, R., and Heersche, J. N. M. (1988). Consistent patterns of changing hormone responsiveness during continuous culture of cloned rat calvarial cells. *J. Bone Min. Res.*, **3**: 333.

Auf'mkolk, B., Hauschka, P. V., and Schwartz, E. R. (1985). Characterization of bone cells in culture. *Calcif. Tissue Int.*, **37**: 228.

Bab, I., Schwartz, Z., Deutsch, D., Mulhrad, A., and Sela, J. (1983). Correlative morphometric and biochemical analysis of purified extracellular matrix vesicles from rat alveolar bone. *Calcif. Tissue Int.*, **35**: 320.

Bab, I., D. Gazit, A. Muhlrad and A. Shteyer (1988) Regenerating bone marrow produces a potent growth-promoting activity to osteogenic cells. *Endocrinology* **123**: 345.

Babler, W. J., Persing, J. A., Nagorsky, M. J., and Jane, J. A. (1987). Restricted growth at the frontonasal suture: alterations in craniofacial growth in rabbits. *Am. J. Anat.*, **178**: 90.

Baer, M. J. (1954). Patterns of growth of the skull as revealed by vital staining.; *Human Biol.*, **26**: 80.

Bar-Shavit, Z., Teitelbaum, S. L., Reitsma, P., Hall, A., Pegg, L. E., Trial, J., and Kahn, A. J. (1983a). Induction of monocyte differentiation and bone resorption by 1,25-dihydroxyvitamin $D_3$. *Proc. Natl. Acad. Sci. U.S.A.*, **80**: 5907, (1983a).

Bar-Shavit, Z., Teitelbaum, S. L. and Kahn, A. J. (1983b). Saccharides mediate the attachment of rat macrophages to bone *in vitro. J. Clin. Invest.*, **72**: 516.

Bar-Shira-Maymon, B., R. Coleman, E. Steinhagen-Thiessen and M. Silbermann. (1989) Correlation between alkaline and acid phosphatase activities and age-related osteopenia in murine vertebrae. *Calcif. Tissue Int.* **44**: 99.

Barr Jr., M. (1973). Prenatal growth of Wistar rats: circadian periodicity of fetal growth late in gestation. *Teratology*, **7**: 283.

Barron, S. E., Robb, R. A., Taylor, W. F., and Kelly, P. J. (1977). The effect of fixation with intramedullary rods and plates on fracture-site blood flow and bone remodeling in dogs. *J. Bone Joint Surg.* **59A**: 376.

Bartley, M. H., and Arnold, J. S. (1967). Sex differences in human skeletal involution. *Nature*, **214**: 908.

Baumhamnmers, A. R., Stallard, E., and Zander, H. A. (1965). Remodeling of alveolar bone. *J. Periodont.*, **36**: 439.

Baylink, D., Stauffer, M., Wergedal, J., and C. Rich. (1970). Formation, mineralization and resorption of bone in vitamin D-deficient rats. *J. Clin. Invest.*, **49**: 1122.

Baylink, D., and Wergedal, J. (1971). Bone formation and resorption by osteocytes. In: Nichols, G.Jr and R. H. Wasserman (eds). *Cellular Mechanisms for Calcium Transfer and Homeostasis.* Academic Press Inc., N.Y., p. 257.

Baylink, D., Wergedal, J., and Stauffer, M. (1971). Formation, mineralization, and resorption of bone in hypophosphatemic rats. *J. Clin. Invest.*, **50**: 2519.

Bellows, C. G., Aubin, J. E., Heersche, J. N. M., and Antosz, M. E. (1986). Mineralized bone nodules formed *in vitro* from enzymatically released calvaria cell populations. *Calcif. Tissue Int.*, **38**: 143.

Benitz, K. F., Roberts, G. K. S., and Yusa, A. (1967). Morphological effects of minocycline in laboratory animals. *Toxicol. Appl. Pharm.*, **11**: 150.

Beresford, J. N., Gallagher, J. A., Poser, J. W. and Russell, R. G. G. (1984). Production of osteocalcin by human bone cells *in vitro*. Effects of $1,25(OH)_2D_3$, parathyroid hormone, and glucocorticoids. *Metab. Bone Dis. & Rel. Res.*, **5**: 229.

Beresford, J. N., Gallagher, J. A., Gowen, M., Couch, M., Poser, J., Wood, D. D., and Russell, R. G. G. (1984a). The effects of monocyte-conditioned medium and interleukin 1 on the synthesis of collagenous and non-collagenous proteins by mouse bone and human bone cells *in vitro*. *Biochim. Biophys. Acta*, **801**: 58.

Beresford, J. N., Fedarko, N. S., Fisher, L. W., Midura, R. J., Yanagashita, M., Termine, J. D., and Robey, P. G. (1987). Analysis of the proteoglycans synthesized by human bone cells *in vitro*. J. Biol. Chem., **262**: 17164.

Beresford, W. A. (1981). *Chondroid Bone, Secondary Cartilage and Metaplasia*. Urban & Schwarzenberg, Baltimore.

Bergot, C., and Boquet, J.-P. (1976). Etude systematique en fonction de l'age de l'os spongieux et de l'os cortical de l'humerus et du femur. *Bull. Mem. Soc. d'Anthrop., Paris 3* (**XIII**): 215.

Bernstein, P., and Crelin, E. S. (1967). Bony pelvic sexual dimorphism in the rat. *Anat. Rec.*, **157**: 517.

Bianco, P., Hayashi, V., Silvestrini, G., Termine, J. D., and Bonucci, E. (1985). Osteonectin and Gla protein in cow bone: ultrastructural immunohistochemical localization using the protein A-gold method. *Calcif. Tissue Int.*, **37**: 684.

Binderman, I., Shimshoni, Z., and Somjen, D. (1984). Biochemical pathways involved in the translation of physical stimulus into biological message. *Calcif. Tissue Int.*, **36**: S82.

Binderman, I., Zor, U., Kaye, A. M., Shimshoni, Z., Harell, A., and Somjen, D. (1988). The transduction of mechanical force into biochemical events in bone cells may involve activation of phospholipase $A_2$. *Calif. Tissue Int.*, **42**: 261.

Bitz, D. M., L. A. Whiteside, J. E. Russell, D. J. Simmons, and K. Loeffelman. (1981). Derivation, culture, and osteogenic capacity of rabbit periosteal cells. *Orthopedic Trans.* **5**: 372.

Blumenkrantz, N., and Sondergaard, J. (1972). Effect of porostaglandins $E_1$ and $E_1\alpha$ on biosynthesis of collagen. *Nature New Biology*, **239**: 246.

Blumenthal, N. C. (1985). Binding of aluminum to hydroxyapatite and amorphous calcium phosphate as a model for aluminum-associated osteomalacia. In. Butler, W. T. (ed). *The Chemistry and Biology of Mineralized Tissues*. EBSCO Media, Birmingham, Ala, p. 385.

Bocciarelli, D. S. (1970). Morphology of crystallites in bone. *Calcif. Tissue Res.* **5**: 261.

Boiskin, I., Epstein, S., Ismail, F., Fallon, M. D., and Levy, W. (1988). Long term administration of prostaglandin inhibitors *in vivo* fail to influence cartilage and bone mineral metabolism in the rat. *Bone and Mineral* **4**: 27.

Boivin, G., Morel, G., Mesguich, P., Pike, J. W., Chapuy, M. C., Bouillon, R., Haussler, M. R., Dubois, P. M., and Meunier, P. J. (1984). Ultrastructural-immunocytochemical localization of endogenous steroid and peptide hormones and of steroid receptors in osteoblasts of neonatal mice calvaria. *Calcif. Tissue Int.*, **36**: 452.

Boivin, G., Mesguich, P., Pike, J. W., Bouillon, R., Meunier, P. J., Haussler, M. R., Dubois, P. M., and Morel, G. (1987a). Ultrastructural immunocytochemical localization of endogenous 1,25-dihydroxyvitamin $D_3$ and its receptors in osteoblasts and osteocytes from neonatal mouse and rat calvaria. *Bone and Mineral* **3**: 125.

Boivin, G., Morel, G., Charnot, Y., Meunier, P. J., and Dubois, P. M. (1987b). Ultrastructural-immunocytochemical localization of endogenous calcitonin in osteoblasts of silicon-treated rats. *Ann. d'Endocrinologie* **48**: 481.

Bonar, L. C., Roufosse, A. H., Sabine, W. K., Grynpas, M. D., and Glimcher, M. J. (1983). X-ray diffraction studies of the crystallinity of bone mineral in newly synthesized and density fractionated bone. *Calcif. Tissue Int.*, **35**: 202.

Boothroyd, B. (1975). Observations on embryonic chick-bone crystals by high resolution transmission electron microscopy. *Clin. Orthop. & Rel. Res.*, **106**: 290.

Boskey, A. L., and Mark, S. C. (1985). Mineral and matrix alterations in the bones of incisor absent (ia ia) osteopetrotic rats. *Calcif. Tissue Int.*, **37**: 287.

Bowden, D. M., Teets, C., Witkins, J., and Young, D. M. (1979). Long bone calcification and morphology. In: Bowden, D. M. (ed). *Aging in Nonhuman Primates.* Van Nostrand Reinhold Co., N.Y., 335.

Brand, J. S., Cushing, J., and Hefley, T. (1979). Potassium, sodium, and the intracellular fluid space of cells from bone. *Calcif. Tissue Int.*, **29**: 119.

Brighton, C. T., and Hunt, R. M. (1974). Mitochondrial calcium and its role in calcification. *Clin. Orthop. & Rel. Res.*, **100**: 406.

Bringhurst, F. R., J. D. Zajec, A. S. Daggett, R. N. Skurat and H. M. Kronenberg. (1989) Inhibition of parathyroid hormone responsiveness in clonal osteoblastic cells expressing a mutant form of 3′, 5′-cyclic adenosine monophosphate-dependent protein kinase. Molec. Endocrinol. 3: 60.

Bronckers, A. L. J. J., Gay, S., Dimuzio, M. T., and Butler, W. T., (1985). Immunolocalization of y-carboxyglutamic acid containing proteins in developing molar tooth germs of the rat. *Collagen and Rel. Res.*, **5**: 17.

Brown, W. E. (1966). Crystal growth of bone mineral. *Clin. Orthop. & Rel. Res.*, **44**: 205.

Brown, W. E., and Chow, L. C. (1976). Chemical preparation of bone mineral. *Ann. Rev. Mater. Sci.*, **6**: 213.

Brown, J. P., Delmas, P. D., Malaval, L., Edouard, C., Chapug, M. C., and Meunier, P. J. (1984). Serum bone Gla-protein: a specific marker for bone formation in postmenopausal osteoporosis. *Lancet*, i. 1091.

Brown, J. P., Delmas, P. D., Arlot, M., and Meunier, P. J. (1987). Active bone turnover of the cortico-endosteal envelope in postmenopausal osteoporosis. *J. Clin. Endocrinol. Metab.*, **64**: 954.

Bubenik, G. A., Brown, G. M., Bubenik, A. B., and Grota, L. J. (1974). Immunohistological localization of testosterone in the growing antler of the white tailed deer (*Odocoileus virginianus*). *Calcif. Tissue Res.*, **14**: 121.

Bubenik, G. A., Sempere, A. J., and Hamr, J. (1987). Developing antler, a model for endocrine regulation of bone growth. Concentration gradients of $T_3$, $T_4$, and alkaline phosphatase in the antler, jugular and the saphenous veins. *Calcif. Tissue Int.*, **41**: 38.

Burger, E. H., van de Wijngaert, F. P., Tas, M. C., and Van der Meer, J. W. M. (1987) Fetal bone conditioned medium stimulates osteoclast precursor cell growth but has no effect on macrophages. In: Cohn, D., J. T. Martin and P. J. Meunier (eds.). *Calcium regulation and bone Metabolism*. Exerpta Medica, Elsevier Sci. Publ., Amsterdam, p. 308.

Buring, K., and Urist, M. R. (1967). Effects of ionizing radiation on the bone induction principle in the matrix of bone implants. *Clin. Orthop. & Rel. Res.*, **44**: 225.

Cabrini, R. L. (1961). The histochemistry of ossification. In: Bourne, G. H. and Danielli, J. F. (eds). *International Review of Cytology*, Vol. 11, Academic Press Inc., N.Y., 283.

Canalis, E. (1980). Effect of insulinlike growth factor I on DNA and protein synthesis in cultured rat calvaria. *J. Clin. Invest.*, **66**: 709.

Canalis, E. (1985). Effect of growth factors on bone cell replication and differentiation. *Clin. Orthop. & Rel. Res.*, **193**: 246.

Canalis, E., and Raisz, L. G. (1979). Effect of epidermal growth factor on bone formation *in vitro. Endocrinol.*, **104**: 862.

Canalis, E., and Raisz, L. G. (1980). Effect of fibroblast growth factor on cultured fetal rat calvaria. *Metabolism*, **29**: 108.

Canalis, E., Peck, W. A., and Raisz, L. G., (1980). Stimulation of DNA and collagen synthesis by autologous growth factor in cultured fetal rat calvaria. *Science*, **210**: 1021.

Canalis, E., McCarthy, T., and Centrella, M. (1987b). A bone-derived growth factor isolated from rat calvariae is beta$_2$-microglobulin. *Endocrinol.*, **121**: 1198.

Canalis, E., Centrella, M., and McCarthy, T. (1988). Effects of basic fibroblast growth factor on bone formation *in vitro. J. Clin. Invest.* **81**: 1572.

Canalis, E., T. McCarthy and M. Centrella. (1988a). Isolation of growth factors from adult bovine bone. *Calcif. Tissue Int.* **43**: 346−351.

Canalis, E., M. Centrella, W. Burch and T. L. McCarthy (1989) Insulin-like growth factor I mediates selective anabolic effects of parathyroid hormone in bone cultures. J. Clin. Invest. 83: 60.

Carlson, D. S., Armelagos, G. J., and VanGerven, D. P. (1976). Patterns of age-related cortical bone loss (osteoporosis) within the femoral diaphysis. *Human Biol.*, **48**: 295.

Carmel, R., K.-H. W. Lau, D. J. Baylink, S. Saxena and F. R. Singer. (1988). Cobalamin and osteoblast-specific proteins. *New Engl. J. Med.* **319**: 70−75.

Carter, D. R., Fyhrie, D. P., and Whalen, R. T. (1987). Trabecular bone density and loading history regulation of connective tissue biology of mechanical energy. *J. Biomech.*, **8**: 785.

Catherwood, B.D. (1985). 1,25-dihydroxycholecalciferol and glucocorticosteroid regulation of adenylate cyclase in an osteoblast-like cell line. *J. Biol. Chem.*, **260**: 736.

Cecchettin, M., Albertini, A., and Tarquini, B. (1983). Evidence for a low frequency (circannual) rhythm in some circulating hormones of calcium metabolism. *Calcif. Tissue Int.*, **35** (Suppl.): **A44**.

Cecil, R. N. A., and Anderson, H. C. (1978). Freeze fracture studies of matrix vesicle calcification in epiphyseal growth plate. *Metab. Bone Dis. & Rel. Res.* **1**: 89.

Centrella, M., and Canalis, E. (1985). Transforming and nontransforming growth factors are present in medium conditioned by fetal rat calvariae. *Proc. Natl. Acad. Sci., U.S.A.*, **82**: 7335.

Centrella, M., and Canalis, E. (1985a). Local regulators of skeletal growth: a perspective. *Endocrine Rev.*, **6**: 544.

Centrella, M., and Canalis, E. (1987). Isolation of EGF-dependent transforming growth factor (TGFb-like) activity from culture medium conditioned by fetal rat calvariae. *J. Bone Min. Res.*, **2**: 29.

Centrella, M., Massague, J., and Canalis, E. (1986). Human platelet derived transforming growth factor-β stimulates parameters of growth in fetal rat calvariae. *Endocrinology,* **119**: 2306.

Centrella, M., McCarthy, T. L., and Canalis, E. (1987). Transforming growth factor β is a bifunctional regulator of replication and collagen synthesis in osteoblast-enriched cell cultures from fetal rat bone. *J. Biol. Chem.*, **262**: 2869.

Centrella, M., T. L. McCarthy and E. Canalis. (1988a.) Skeletal tissue and transforming growth factor b. *FASEB J.* **2**: 3066–3073.

Centrella, M., T. L. McCarthy and E. Canalis. (1988b.) Pasrathyroid hormone modulates transforming growth factor b activity and binding in osteoblast-enriched cell cultures from fetal rat parietal bone. *Proc. Natl. Acad. Sci. U.S.A.* **85**: 5889–5893.

Chambers, T. J., and Dunn, C. J. (1983). Pharmacologic control of osteoclastic motility. *Calcif. Tissue Int.*, **35**: 566.

Chambers, T. J., and Fuller, K. (1985). Bone cells predispose bone surfaces to resorption by exposure of mineral to osteoclastic contact. *J. Cell Sci.*, **76**: 155.

Chambers, T. J., Athanasou, N. A., and Fuller, K. (1984). Effect of parathyroid hormone and calcitonin on the cytoplasmic spreading of isolated osteoclasts. *J. Endocr.(London)*, **102**: 281.

Chambers T. J., McSheehy, P. M. J., Thomson, B. M., and Fuller, K. (1985). The effect of calcium-regulating hormones and prostaglandins on bone resorption by osteoclasts disaggregated from neonatal rabbit bones. *Endocrinology*, **116**: 234.

Chao, C. C., Brown, R. D., and Deftos, L. J. (1984). Seasonal levels of serum parathyroid hormone, calcitonin and alkaline phosphatase in relation to antler cycles in white-tailed deer. *Acta Endocrinologica*, **106**: 234.

Chase, L. R., Fedak, S. A., and Aurbach, G. D. (1969). Activation of skeletal adenyl cyclase by parathyroid hormone *in vitro*. *Endocrinol.*, **84**: 761.

Chase, L. R., and Aurbach, G. D. (1970). The effect of parathyroid hormone on the concentration of adenosine 3',5'-monophosphate in skeletal tissue *in vitro*. *J. Biol. Chem.*, **245**: 1520.

Chen, T. L. and D. Feldman, D. (1979). Glucocorticoid receptors and actions in subpopulations of parathyroid hormone stimulated cyclic AMP production. *J. Clin. Invest.*, **63**: 750.

Chen, T. L. and Feldman, D. (1981). Regulation of 1,25-dihydroxyvitamin D$_3$ receptors in cultured mouse bone cells. Correlation of receptor concentration with the rate of cell division. *J. Biol. Chem.*, **256**: 5561.

Chen, T. L. and Feldman, D. (1984). Modulation of PTH-stimulated cyclic AMP in cultured rodent bone cells: the effects of 1,25(OH)$_2$ vitamin D$_3$ and its interaction with glucocorticoids. *Calcif. Tissue Int.*, **36**: 580.

Chen, T. L., Aranow, L., and Feldman, D. (1977). Glucocorticoid receptors and inhibition of bone cell growth in primary culture. *Endocrinol.*, **100**: 619.

Chen, T. L., Hirst, M. A., and Feldman, D. (1979). Receptor-like binding macromolecule for l-alpha-dihydroxycholecalciferol in cultured mouse bone cells. *J. Biol. Chem.*, **254**: 7491.

Chen, T. L., Hauschka, P. V., and Feldman, D. (1986). Dexamethasone increases 1,25-dihydroxyvitamin D$_3$ receptor levels and augments bioresponses in rat osteoblast-like cells. *Endocrinol.*, **118**: 1119.

Cheng, S.-L., Rifas, L., Shen, V., Tong, B., Pierce, G., Deuel, T., and Peck, W. A. (1987). J774.1 macrophage cell line produced PDGF-like and non-PDGF-like growth factors for bone cells. *J. Bone Min. Res.*, **2**: 467.

Chikuma, T., Kato, T., Hiramatsu, M., Kanayama, S., and Kumegawa, M. (1984). Effect of epidermal growth factor on dipeptidyl-aminopeptidase and collagenase-like peptidase activities in cloned osteoblastic cells. *J. Biochem.*, **95**: 283.

Chipman, S. D., Gerstenfeld, L. C., and Lian, J. B. (1987). The effect of warfarin on the differentiation and mineralization of cultured chick embryo osteoblasts. *Trans. Orthop. Res. Soc.*, **12**: 310.

Chyun, Y. S. and Raisz, L. G. (1984). Stimulation of bone formation by prostaglandin $E_2$. *Prostaglandins*, **27**: 97.

Civitelli, R., Agnusdei, D., Nardi, P., Zacchei, F., Avioli, L. V., and Gennari, C. (1988). Effects of one-year treatment with estrogens on bone mass, intestinal calcium absorption, and 25-hydroxyvitamin D-1a-hydroxylase reserve in postmenopausal osteoporosis. *Calif. Tissue Int.*, **42**: 77.

Clark, I., J. P. Zawadsky, W. Lin and P. A. Berg. (1988). Bone cell stimulating substance. *Clin. Orthop. & Rel. Res.* **237**: 226−235.

Clark I. Personnal Communication 1989

Clark, S. A., D'Ercole, A. J., and Toverud, S. U. (1986). Somatomedin-C/insulin-like growth factor I and vitamin D-induced growth. *Endocrinology*, **119**: 1660.

Clemmons, D. R., Underwood, L. E., and Van Wyk, J. J. (1981). Hormonal control of immunoreactive somatomedin production by cultured human fibroblasts. *J. Clin. Invest.*, **67**: 10.

Clemmons, D. R., and Van Wyk, J. J. (1985). Evidence for a functional role of endogenously produced somatomedin-like peptides in the regulation of DNA synthesis in cultured human fibroblasts and porcine smooth muscle cells. *J. Clin. Invest.*, **85**: 1914.

Cohn, D. V., and Wong, G. L. (1979). Isolated bone cells. In: Simmons, D. J. and A. S. Kunin (eds.). *Skeletal Research — An Experimental Approach*. Academic Press Inc. N.Y., 3.

Colclasure, G. C., Lloyd, W. S., Lamkin, M., Gonnerman, W., Troxler, R. F., Offner, G. D., Burgi, W., Schmid, K., and Nimberg, R. B. (1988). Human serum αlHS-glycoprotein modules *in vitro* bone resorption. *J. Clin. Endocrinol. Metab.*, **66**: 187.

Colle, M., A. Ruffie and E. Ruedas (1988). Osteocalcin in children with short stature. In: Acta Pediatr. Scand. (Suppl.). *Growth and Growth Disorders* (P. Chatelain and R. Gunnarsson (eds). **343**: 196−197.

Colvard, D. S. Eriksen, E. F., Keeting P. E., Wilson, E. M., Lubahn, D. B., French, F. S., Riggs, B. L. and Spelsberg, T.C. (1989). Identification of andgrogen receptors in normal human osteoblast-like cells. *Proc. Natl. Acad. Sci. USA* **86**: 854.

Cossack, Z. T. (1984). Somatomedin-C in zinc deficiency. *Experientia*, **40**: 498.

Crisp. A. J., McGuire-Goldring, M. B., and Goldring, S. R. (1984). A system for culture of human trabecular bone and hormone response profiles of derived cells. *Br. J. Exp. Path.*, **65**: 645.

Cromach, D. T., Sporn, M. B., Roberts, A. B., Merino, M. J., Dart, L. L., and Norton, J. A. (1987). Transforming growth factor β levels in rat wound chambers. *J. Surg. Res.*, **42**: 622.

Currey, J. D. (1964). Some effects of aging in human haversian systems. *J. Anat.* **98**: 69.

D'Ercole, A. J., Applewhite, G. T., and Underwood, L. E. (1980). Evidence that somatomedin is synthesized by multiple tissues in the fetus. *Develop. Biol.*, **75**: 315.

D'Ercole, A. J., Stiles, A. D., and Underwood, L. E. (1984). Tissue concentrations of somatomedin-C. Further evidence for multiple sites of synthesis and paracrine or autocrine mechanisms of action. *Proc. Natl. Acad. Sci. U.S.A.*, **81**: 935.

Danon, A. and Assouline, G. (1978). Inhibition of prostaglandin biosynthesis by corticosteroids requires RNA and protein synthesis. *Nature*, **273**: 552.

Daum, W. J., Simmons. D. J., Chang, S.-L., Lehman, R. C., and Webster, D. (1985). Effect of fixation devices on radiostrontium clearance in the intact canine femur. *Clin. Orthop. & Rel. Res.*, **194**: 306.

Daum, W. J., Simmons, D. J., Fenster, R., and Shively, R. A. (1987). Radiostrontium clearance on bone formation in response to simulated internal screw fixation. *Clin. Orthop. & Rel. Res.*, **219**: 283.

Davidovitch Z., Shanfeld, J. L., Montgomery, P. C., Lally, E., Laster, L., Furst, L., and Korostoff, E. (1984). Biochemical mediators of the effects of mechanical forces and electric currents on mineralized tissues. *Calcif. Tissue Int.*, **36**: S86.

de la Piedra, C., Toural, V., and Rapado, A. (1987). Osteocalcin and urinary hydroxyproline/creatinine ratio in the differential diagnosis of primary hyperparathyroidism and hypercalcemia of malignancy. *Scand. J. Lab. Clin. Invest.*, **47**: 587.

DeRousseau, C. J. (1985). Aging in the musculoskeletal system of Rhesus monkeys. III. Bone loss. *Am. J. Phys. Anthrop.*, **68**: 157.

Deftos, L. J., Parthemore, J. G., and Price, P. A. (1982). Changes in plasma bone Gla protein during treatment of bone disease. *Calcif. Tissue Int.*, **34**: 121.

Dekel, S. F., Lenthall, F., and Francis, M. J. O. (1981). Release of prostaglandins from bone and muscle after tibial fracture. *J. Bone Joint Surg.*, **63-B**: 185.

Dekel, S. F., and Francis, M. J. (1981). Cortical hyperostosis after administration of prostaglandin E. *J. Pediatrics*, **99**: 3.

Delmas, P. D., Wahner, H. W., Mann, K. G., and Riggs, B. L. (1983). Assessment of bone turnover in postmenopausal osteoporosis by measurement of serum bone Gla-protein. *J. Lab. Clin. Med.*, **102**: 470.

Delmas, P. D., Malaval, L., Arlot, M. E., and Meunier, P. J. (1985). Serum bone Gla-protein compared tol bone histomorphometry in endocrine diseases. *Bone* **6**: 339.

Delmas, P. D. (1986a). Bone Gla-protein (osteocalcin): a specific marker for the study of metabolic bone diseases. In: Cecchetiin, M. and G. Segre (eds.): *Calciotropic Hormones and Calcium Metabolism*. Int. Congress Ser. no. 679, Excerpta Medica Fnd., Amsterdam, Netherlands, p. 19.

Delmas, P. D., Demiaux, B., Malaval, L., Chapug, M. C., and Meunier, P. J. (1986b). Serum bone Gla-protein is not a sensitive marker of bone turnover in Paget's Disease of bone. *Calcif. Tissue Int.*, **38**: 60.

Delmas, P. D., Demiaux, B., Malaval, L., Chapug, M. C., Edouard, C., and Meunier, P. J. (1986c). Serum bone gamma carboxyglutamic acid-containing protein of primary hyperparathyroidism and in malignant hypercalcemia. *J. Clin. Invest.*, **77**: 985.

Dewey, J. R., Armelagos, G. J., and Bartley, M. H. (1969). Rates of femoral cortical bone loss in two Nubian populations. *Clin. Orthop. & Rel. Res.*, **65**: 61.

Deyl, Z., Vancikova, O., and Macek, K. (1981). The effect of oxytetracycline and some related antibiotics upon the γ-carboxyglutamic acid level in bone and kidney cortex. *Biochem. Biophys. Res. Commun.*, **100**: 79.

Diamond, M. C., Rosenzweig, M. R., and Krech, D. (1965). Relationships between body weight and skull development of rats raised in enriched and impoverished conditions. *J. Exp. Zool.*, **160**: 29.

Diamond, T. H., D. Stiel, M. Lunzer, D. McDonald, R. P. Eckstcin and S. Posen. (1989). Hepatic osteodystrophy. Static and dynamic bone histomorphometry and serum Gla-protein in 80 patients with chronic liver disease. *Gastroenterology* **86**: 213−221.

Dickson, I. R., Poole, A. R., and Veis, A. (1974). Localization of plasma $\alpha_2$HS-glycoprotein in mineralizing human bone. *Nature*, **256**: 430.

Dickson, I. R., Bagga, M., and Paterson, C. R. (1983). Variations in the serum concentrations and urine excretion of $\alpha_2$HS-glycoprotein, a bone related protein, in normal individuals and in patients with osteogenesis imperfecta. *Calcif. Tissue Res.*, **35**: 16.

Dietrich, J. W., Canalis, E. M., Maina, D. M., and Raisz, L. G. (1976). Hormonal control of bone collagen synthesis *in vitro*: effects of parathyroid hormone and calcitonin. *Endocrinol.*, **98**: 943.

Dillaman, R. M. (1984). Movement of ferritin in the 20 day-old chick femur. *Anat. Rec.*, **209**: 445.

Dirksen, T. R., and O'Dell, N. L. (1972). *In vitro* lipid biosynthesis from [$^{14}$C]acetate by *Rattus norvegicus* calvaria of different ages. *Int. J. Biochem.*, **3**: 151.

Doty, S. B. (1981). Morphological evidence of gap junctions between bone cells. *Calcif. Tissue Int.*, **33**: 509.

Doty, S. B. (1985). Morphologic and histochemical studies of bone cells from SL-3 rats. *The Physiologist*, **28**: 379.

Doty, S. B., and Schofield, B. H. (1972). Metabolic and structural changes within osteocytes of rat bone. In: Talmage, R. V. and P. L. Munson (eds.). *Calcium, Parathyroid Hormone and the Calcitonins*. Exerpta Medica, Amsterdam, p. 353.

Doty, S. B., Robinson, R. A., and Schofield, B. (1976). Morphology of bone and histochemical staining characteristics of bone cells. In: Greep, R. O. and E. B. Atwood (eds). *Handbook of Physiology*. Am. Physiol. Soc., Washington, D.C., 3.

Drivdahl, R. H., Puzas, J. E., Howard, G. A., and Baylink, D. J. (1981). Regulation of DNA synthesis in chick calvaria cells by factors from bone organ culture. *Proc. Soc. Exp. Biol. Med.*, **168**: 143.

Drivdahl, R. H., Howard, G. A., and Baylink, D. J. (1982). Extracts of bone contain a potent regulator of bone formation. *Biochim. Biophys. Acta*, **714**: 26.

Dziak R., Hausmann, E., and Chang, Y. W. (1979). Effects of lipopolysaccharide and prostaglandins on rat bone cell calcium and cyclic AMP. *Arch. Oral Biol.* **24**: 347.

Eanes, E. D., and Reddi, A. H. (1979). The effect of fluoride on bone mineral apatite. *Metab. Bone Dis.*, **2**: 3.

Eastell, R., Calvo, M., Mann, K. G., Offord, K. P., Burritt, M. F., and Riggs, B. L. (1988). Abnormal day/night pattern of bone turnover in Type I osteoporosis. *J. Bone Min. Res.*, **3** (Suppl. 1): S203 (Abstr. 539).

Ede, M. C., and Burr, R. G. (1973). Circadian rhythm of therapeutic effectiveness of oxymethalone in paraplegic patients. *Clin. Pharm. & Therapeutics.*, **14**: 448.

Einhorn, T. A. (1989). Dietary protein and bone calcium metabolism. In: Simmons, D. J. (ed). *Nutrition and Bone Development*. Oxford University Press (in Press).

Ekeland, A., Engesaet, L. S., and Langelan, N. (1982). Influence of age on mechanical properties of healing fractures and intact bones in rats. *Acta Orthop. Scand.*, **53**: 527.

Elford, P. R., Felix, R., Cecchini, M., Trechsel, U., and Fleisch, H. (1987). Murine osteoblast-like cells and the osteogenic cell MC3T3-E1 release a macrophage colony-stimulating activity in culture. *Calcif. Tissue Int.*, **41**: 151.

Elford, P. R., Guenther, H. L., Felix, R., Cecchini, M. G., and Fleisch, H. (1987b). Transforming growth factor-β reduces the phenotypic expression of osteoblastic MC3T3-El cells in monolayer culture. *Bone* **8**: 259.

Enlow, D. H. (1964). *Principles of Bone Remodeling*. C. C. Thomas Publ., Springfield, IL, (1963).

Epker, B. N. and H. M. Frost. Aging and the kinetics of human osteon formation. *J. Am. Geriat. Soc.*, **12**: 401.

Eratalay, Y. K., Simmons, D. J., El-Mofty, S. K., Rosenberg, G. D., Nelson, W., Haus, E., and Halberg, F. (1981). Bone growth in the rat mandible following every-day or alternate-day methylprednisolone treatment schedules. *Arch. Oral Biol.* **26**: 769.

Ericksen, M. F. (1976). Cortical bone loss with age in three native American populations. *Am. J. Phys. Anthrop.*, **45**: 443.

Ericksen, M. F. (1982). Aging changes in thickness of the proximal femoral cortex. *Am. J. Phys. Anthrop.*, **59**: 121.

Eriksen, E. F. (1986). Normal and pathological remodeling of human trabecular bone: three dimensional reconstruction of the remodeling sequence in normals and in metabolic bone disease. *Endocrine Rev.*, **7**: 379.

Eriksen, E. F., Melsen, F., and Mosekilde, L. (1984a). Reconstruction of the resorptive site in iliac trabecular bone: a kinetic model for bone resorption in 20 normal individuals. *Metab. Bone Dis. & Rel. Res.*, **5**: 235.

Eriksen, E. F., Gundersen, H. J. G., Melsen, F., and Mosekilde, L. (1984b). Reconstruction of the formative site in iliac trabecular bone in 20 normal individuals employing a kinetic model for matrix and mineral apposition. *Metab. Bone Dis. & Rel. Res.*, **5**: 243.

Eriksen, E. F., Mosekilde, L., and Melsen, F. (1985a). Trabecular bone resorption depth decreases with age: differences between normal males and females. *Bone* **6**: 141.

Eriksen, E. F., Mosekilde, L., and Melsen, F. (1985b). Trabecular bone remodeling and bone balance in hyperthyroidism. *Bone* **6**: 421.

Eriksen, E. F., Mosekilde, L., and Melsen, F. (1986). Trabecular bone remodeling and balance in primary hyperparathyroidism. *Bone* **7**: 213.

Ernst, M., and Froesch, E. R. (1988). Growth hormone-dependent stimulation of osteoblast-like cells in serum-free cultures via local synthesis of insulin-like growth factor I. *Biochem. Biophys. Res. Commun.*, **151**: 142.

Ernst, M., Schmid, C., Frankenfeldt, C., and Froesch, E. R. (1988a). Estradiol stimulation of osteoblast proliferation *in vitro*: mediator roles for TGFβ, $PGE_2$, insulin-like growth factor (IGF) I? *Calcif Tissue Int.*, **42** (suppl.): A30 (Abstr. 117).

Ernst, M., Schmid, Ch., and Froesch, E. R. (1988b). Enhanced osteoblast proliferation and collagen gene expression by estradiol. *Proc. Natl. Acad. Sci.*, **85**: 2307.

Exner, G. U., Prader, A., Elsasser, U., and Ankiker, M. (1980). Effects of high dose oestrogen and testosterone treatment in adolescents upon trabecular and compact bone measured by $^{125}I$ computed tomography. A preliminary study. *Acta Endocrinologica*, **94**: 126.

Farley, J. R., and Baylink, D. J. (1982). Purification of a skeletal growth factor from human bone. *Biochemistry*, **21**: 3502.

Farley, J. R., Masuda, T., Wergedal, J. E., and Baylink, D. J. (1982). Human skeletal growth factor. Characterization of the mitogenic effect on bone cells *in vitro*. *Biochemistry*, **21**: 3508.

Farley, J. R., Wergedal, J. E., and Baylink, D. J. (1983). Fluoride acts directly on bone cells *in vitro* and interacts with a putative human skeletal coupling factor. *Trans. Orthop. Res. Soc.*, **8**: 48.

Farley, J. R., Tarbaux, N., Murphy, L. A., Masuda, T., and Baylink, D. J. (1987). *In vitro* evidence that bone formation may be coupled to resorption by release of mitogen(s) from resorbing bone. *Metabolism*, **36**: 314.

Farley, J. R., Tarbaux, N. M., Vermeiden, J. P. W., and Baylink, D. J. (1988). *In vitro* evidence that local and systemic skeletal factors can regulate $^3[H]$-thymidine incorporation in chick calvarial cell cultures and modulate the stimulatory action(s) of embryonic chick bone extract. *Calcif. Tissue Int.*, **42**: 23.

Farley, J. R., N. M. Tarbaux, S. L. Hall, T. A. Linkhart, and D. J. Baylink. (1988a) The anti-bone-resorptive agent calcitonin also acts *in vitro* to directly increase bone formation and bone cell proliferation. *Endocrinol.* **123**: 159–167.

Federman, M., and Nichols Jr. G. (1974). Bone cell cilia: vesigial or functional organelles. *Calcif. Tissue Res.*, **17**: 81.

Feldman, D., Dziak, R., Koehler, R., and Stern, P. (1975). Cytoplasmic glucocorticoid binding proteins in bone cells. *Endocrinol.*, **96**: 29.

Felix, R., Neuman, W. F., and Fleisch, H. (1978). Aerobic glycolysis in bone: lactic acid production by rat calvaria cells in culture. *Am. J. Physiol.*, **234**: C51.

Ferrier, J., Ross, S. M., Kanesha, J., and Aubin, J. E. (1986). Osteoblasts and osteoclasts migrate in opposite directions in response to a constant electrical field. *J. Cellular Physiol.*, **129**: 283.

Filogamo, G. (1946). Forma e lunghuzza degli osteoni della compatta ossa lunghe nell'homo. *Ric. Morph.*, **22**: 1.

Fischer, G. (1975). Untersuchungen zur Verteilung der Glycogenphosphorylase und der Succinat-dehydrogenase in der Humerusepiphyse von Ratten verschiedenen Alters. *Acta Anat.*, **92**: 321.

Fisher, L. W., and Termine, J. D. (1985). Noncollagenous proteins influencing the local mechanisms of calcification. *Clin. Orthop. & Rel. Res.,* **200**: 362.

Fisher, L. W., Robey, P. G., Tuross, N., Otsuka, A. S., Tepen, D. A., Esch, F. S., Shimasaki, S.,and Termine, J. D. (1987). The $M_r$ phosphoprotein from developing bone is the $NH_2$-terminal propeptide of the al chain of Type I collagen. *J. Biol. Chem.,* **262**: 13457.

Fleischmajer, R., Perlish, J. S., and Olsen, B. R. (1987). Amino and carboxyl propeptides in bone collagen fibrils during embryogenesis. *Cell Tissue Res.,* **247**: 105.

Flower, R. J. (1974). Drugs which inhibit prostaglandin biosynthesis. *Pharmacol. Rev.,* **26**: 33.

Franceschi, R. T., Romano, P. R., and Park, K.-Y. (1988). Regulation of collagen synthesis by 1,25-dihydroxyvitamin $D_3$. *J. Bone Min. Res.,* **3** (Suppl. 1): S83 (Abstract 57).

Franklin, R. B., and Tashjian Jr. A. H. (1975). Intravenous infusion of prostaglandin $E_2$ raises plasma calcium concentration in the rat. *Endocrinol.,* **97**: 240.

Frost, H. M. (1966a). Relation between bone tissue and cell population dynamics, histology and tetracycline labeling. *Clin. Orthop. & Rel. Res.,* **49**: 65.

Frost, H. M. (1966b). Bone dynamics in metabolic bone disease. *J. Bone Joint Surg.* **48A**: 1192.

Furtwangler, J. A., Hall, S. H., and Koskinen-Moffett, L. K. (1985). Sutural morphogenesis in the mouse calvaria: the role of apoptosis. *Acta Anat.* **124**: 74.

Furuta, Y., and Jee, W. S. S. (1966). Effect of 16,16-dimethyl prostaglandin $E_2$ methyl ester on weanling rat skeleton: daily and systemic administration. *Anat. Rec.,* **215**: 305.

Garant, P. R. (1976). Collagen resorption by fibroblast. A theory of fibroblastic maintenance of the periodontal ligament. *J. Periodont.,* **47**: 380.

Garcia-Carrasco, M., Gruson, M., deVernejoul, C., Denne, M. A., and Miravet, L. (1988). Osteocalcin and bone morphometric parameters in adults without bone disease. *Calcif. Tissue Int.,* **42**: 13.

Garn, S. M., and Kangas, J. (1981). Protein intake, bone mass, and bone loss. In: DeLuca, H. F., H. M. Frost, W. S. S. Jee, C. C. Johnston Jr and A. M. Parfitt (eds). *Osteoporosis. Recent Advances in Pathogenesis and Treatment.,* University Park Press, Baltimore, 257.

Garrel, D. R., Delmas, P. D., Malaval, L., and Tournaire, J. (1986). Serum bone Gla-protein: a marker of bone turnover in hyperthyroidism. *J. Clin. Endocrinol.,* Metab. **62**: 1052.

Gay, C., and Schraer, H. (1975). Frozen thin-sections of rapidly forming bone: bone cell ultrastructure. *Calcif. Tissue Res.,* **19**: 39.

Gazit, D., Shteyer, A., Muhlrad, A., and Bab, I. (1988). Partial purification and biological activity of an osteogenic growth factor derived from healing bone marrow. *Calcif. Tissue Int.,* **42** (Suppl.): A30 (Abstr. 119).

Gehron-Robey, P., M. F. Young, K. C. Flanders, N. S. Roche, P. Kondaiah, A. H. Reddi, J. D. Termine, M. B. Sporn and A. B Roberts. (1987). Osteoblasts synthesize and respond to transforming growth factor type β (TGF-β) *in vitro. J. Cell Biol.* **105**: 457−463.

Gehron-Robey, P. M. F. Young, L. W. Fisher and T. D. McClain (1989). Thrombospondin is an osteoblast-derived component of mineralized extracellular matrix. *J. Cell Biol.* **108**: 719.

Gennari, C. (1985). Glucocorticoids and bone. In: Peck, W. A. (ed). *Bone and Mineral Research,* Vol. 3, p. 213.

Gerstenfeld, L. C., Chipman, S. D., Glowacki, J., and Lian, J. B. (1987). Expression of differentiated function by mineralizing cultures of chicken embryo osteoblasts. *Develop. Biol.,* **122**: 49.

Gerstenfeld, L. C., Chipman, S. D., Kelly, C. M., Hodgens, K. J., Lee, D. D., and Landis, W. J. (1988). Collagen expression, ultrastructural assembly, and mineralization in cultures of chicken embryo osteoblasts. *J. Cell Biol.,* **106**: 979.

Gies, J. P. and Dorey, C. K. (1981). Stimulation of aryl sulfatase in rat peritoneal macrophages exposed to bone *in vitro. Calcif. Tissue Int.,* **33**: 181.

Gilder, H., and Boskey, A. (1989). In: Simmons, D. J. (ed): *Nutrition and Bone Development.*

Oxford University Press, N.Y., (In press).

Gindhart, P. S. (1972). The effect of seasonal variation on long bone growth. *Human Biol.*, **44**: 335.

Glimcher, M. J. (1976). Composition, structure and organization of bone and other mineralized tissues and the mechanism of calcification. In: Greep, R. O. and E. B. Astwood (eds). *Handbook of Physiology: Endocrinology*, Vol. 7, 25.

Glimcher, M. J. (1984). Recent studies of the mineral phase in bone and its possible linkage to the organic matrix by protein-bound phosphate bonds. *Phil. Trans. R. Soc. London B. Biol. Sci.*, **304**: 479.

Godschalk, M. F., and Downs, R. W. (1988). Effect of short-term glucocorticoids on serum osteocalcin in healthy young men. *J. Bone Min. Res.*, **3**: 113.

Goland, P. P., and Grand, N. G. (1968). Chloro-s-triazines as markers and fixatives for the study of growth in teeth and bones. Am. J. Phys. Anthrop., **29**: 201.

Goodman, W. G. (1989). Aluminum metabolism and the uremic patient. In: Simmons, D. J. (ed). *Nutrition and Skeletal Development*. Oxford University Press, N.Y., (In press).

Goodson, J., McClathy, M. K., and Revell, C. (1974). Prostaglandin-induced resorption of the adult rat calvarium. *J. Dent. Res.*, **53**: 670.

Gowen, M. (1988). Actions of IL-1 and TNF on human osteoblast-like cells: similarities and synergism. In: *Monokines and Other Non-Lymphocyte Cytokines*. A. R. Liss Inc., N. Y., p. 261.

Gowen, M., Wood, D. D., and Russell, R. G. G. (1985). Stimulation of the proliferation of human bone cells *in vitro* by human monocyte products with interleukin activity. *J. Clin. Invest.*, **75**: 1223.

Gowen, M., Hughes, D. E., and Russell, R. G. G. (1988). Tumor necrosis factor alpha (TNF): an autocrine and paracrine regulator of human bone metabolism. *Calcif. Tissue Int.*, **42** (Suppl.): A31 (Abstr. 122).

Graves, E. T., Owen, A. J., and Antoniades, H. N. (1983). Evidence that a human osteosarcoma cell line which secretes a mitogen similar to platelet-derived growth factor requires growth factors present in platelet-poor plasma. *Cancer Res.*, **43**: 83.

Graves, D. T., Owen, A. J., Barth, R. K., Tempst, P., Winoto, A., Fors, L., and Hood, L. E. (1984). Detection of c-sis transcripts and synthesis of PDGF-like proteins by human osteosarcoma cells. *Science*, **226**: 972.

Gray, T. K., S. Mohan, T. A. Linkhart and D. J. Baylink (1989) Estradiol stimulates *in vitro* the secretion of insulin-like growth factors by the clonal osteoblastic cell line, UMR106. *Biochem. Biophys. Res. Commun.* **158**: 407.

Green, J. R., Reeve, J., Tellez, M., Veall, N., and Wootton, R. (1987). Skeletal blood flow in metabolic disorders of the skeleton. *Bone*, **8**: 293.

Greger, J. (1989). Tin. In: Simmons, D. J. (ed). *Nutrition and Bone Development*. Oxford University Press, N.Y., (in press).

Grillo, H. C., Lapiere, C. M., Dresden, M. H., and Gross, J. (1968). Collagenolytic activity in regenerating forelimbs of the adult newt (*Triturus viridescens*). *Develop. Biol.*, **17**: 571.

Groot, C. G., Danes, J. K., van der Meer, J. M., and Herrmann-Erlee, M. P. M. (1985). Osteocalcin antigenicity in cultured osteoblast-like cells after stimulation with 1,25-vitamin D3. *Cell Biol. Int. Rept.*, **9**: 528.

Grynpas, M. D., Bonar, L. C., and Glimcher, M. J. (1984). Failure to detect an amorphous calcium phosphate solid phase in bone mineral — a radial distribution function study. *Calcif. Tissue Int.*, **36**: 291.

Grynpas, M. D., Patterson-Allen, P., and Simmons, D. J. (1986). The changes in quality of mandibular bone mineral in otherwise totally immobilized Rhesus monkeys. *Calcif. Tissue Int.*, **39**: 57.

Gruber, H. E., Ivey, J. L., Thompson, E. R., Chestnut III, C. H., and Baylink, D. J. (1986).

Osteoblast and osteoclast cell number and activity in postmenopausal osteoporosis. *Min. Electrolyte Metab.*, **12**: 246.

Guenther, H. L., Cecchiunbi, M. G., Elford, P. R., and Fleisch, H. (1988). Effects of transforming growth factor type beta upon bone cell populations grown either in a monolayer or semisolid medium. *J. Bone Min. Res.*, **3**: 269.

Guiness-Hey, M. and Hock, J. M. (1984). Increased trabecular bone mass in rats treated with synthetic parathyroid hormone. *Metab. Bone Dis. & Rel. Res.*, **5**: 177.

Guiness-Hey, M., I Gera, K. Fonesca, L. G. Raisz and J. M. Hock. (1988). 1,25-dihydroxy-vitamin $D_3$ alone or in combination with parathyroid hormone does not increase bone mass in young rats. *Calcif. Tissue Int.* **43**: 284−288.

Gundberg, C. M., Lian, J. B., and Gallop, P. M. (1983a). Measurements of y-carboxyglutamate and circulating osteocalcin in normal children and adults. *Clin. Chim. Acta*, **128**: 1.

Gundberg, C. M., Cole, D. E. C., Lian, J. B., Reade, T. M., and Gallop, P. M. (1983b). Serum osteocalcin in the treatment of inherited rickets with 1,25-dihydroxyvitamin $D_3$. *J. Clin. Endocrinol. Metab.*, **56**: 1063.

Gundberg, C. M., M. E. Markowitz, M. Mizruchi and J. F. Rosen. Osteocalcin in human serum. A circadian rhythm. *J. Clin. Endocrinol. Metab.* **60**: 736−739, 1985.

Hahn, T. J., Downing, S. J., and Phang, J. M. (1969). Insulin effect on amino acid transport in bone. *Biochim. Biophys. Acta*, **184**: 675.

Hakeda, Y., Nakatani, Y., Kurihara, N., Ikeda, E., Maeda, N., and Kumegawa, M. (1985). Prostaglandin $E_2$ stimulates collagen and non-collagen protein synthesis and prolyl hydro-xylase activity in osteoblastic clone MC3T3-E1 cells. *Biochem. Biophys. Res. Commun.*, **126**: 340.

Hakeda, Y., Hotta, T., Kurihara, N., Ikeda, E., Maeda, N., Yagyu, Y., and Kumegawa, M. (1987). Prostaglandin $E_1$ and $F_2\alpha$ stimulate differentiation and proliferation, respectively, of clonal osteoblastic MC3T3-E1 cells by different second messengers *in vitro*. *Endocrinol.*, **121**: 1966.

Hall, B. K. (1987). Sodium fluoride as an initiator of osteogenesis from embryonic mesenchyme *in vitro*. *Bone*, **8**: 111.

Hamilton, J. A., Lingelbach, S., Partridge, N. C., and Martin, T. J. (1985). Regulation of plasminogen activator production by bone-resorbing hormones in normal and malignant osteoblasts. *Endocrinol.*, **116**: 2186.

Hammerman, M. R. (1987). Insulin-like growth factors and aging. *Endocrinol. Metabol. Clinics*, **16**: 995.

Hammond, R. H. and Storey, E. (1970). Measurement of growth and resorption of bone in rats fed meat diet. *Calcif. Tissue Res.*, **4**: 291.

Hammond, R. H., and Storey, E. (1974). Measurement of growth and resorption of bone in the seventh caudal vertebra of the rat. *Calc. Tissue Res.*, **15**: 11.

Hanazawa, S., Asmano, S., Nakada, K., Ohmori, Y., Miyoshi, T., Hirose, K., and Kitano, S. (1987). Biological characterization of interleukin-1-like cytokine produced by cultured bone cells from newborn mouse calvaria. *Calcif. Tissue Int.*, **41**: 31.

Haneji, T., Kurihara, N., Ikeda, K., and Kumegawa, M. (1983). 1α,25-dihydroxyvitamin $D_3$ induce alkaline phosphatase activity in osteoblastic cells derived from newborn mouse calvaria. *J. Biochem.*, **94**: 1127.

Hanker, J. S., Dixon, A. D., and Smiley, G. R. (1973). Acid phosphatase in the golgi apparatus of cells forming the extracellular matrix of hard tissues. *Histochemie*, **35**: 39.

Harakas, N. K. (1984). Demineralized bone matrix-induced osteogenesis. *Clin. Orthop. & Rel. Res.*, **188**: 239.

Harper, R. S., and Posner, A. S. (1966). Measurement of non-crystalline calcium phosphate in bone mineral. *Proc. Soc. Exp. Biol. Med.*, **122**: 137.

Harris, E. D. Jr., and Farrell, M. E. (1972). Resistance to collagenase: a characteristic of collagen fibrils cross-linked by formaldehyde. *Biochim, Biophys. Acta*, **278**: 133.

Harrison, T. J. (1968). The growth of the caudal part of the pelvis in the rat. *J. Anat.*, **103**: 155.

Harvey, W. (1988a). Source of prostaglandins and their influence on bone resorption and formation. In: Harvey, W and A. Bennett (eds.). *Prostaglandins and Bone Resorption*. CRC Press, Boca Raton, FL, 27.

Harvey, W. (1988b). Prostaglandins and bone resorption in cancer. In: Harvey, W. and A. Bennett (eds). *Prostaglandins and Bone Resorption*. CRC Press, Boca Raton, FL, 115.

Hasling, C., Eriksen, E. F., Charles, P., and Mosekilde, L. (1987). Exogenous triiodothyronine activates bone remodeling. *Bone*, **8**: 65.

Hata, R.-I., Hori, H., Nagai, Y., Tanaka, S., Kondo, M., Hiramatsu, M., Utsumi, N., and Kumegawa, M. (1984). Selective inhibition of Type I collagen synthesis in osteoblastic cells by epidermal growth factor. *Endocrinol.*, **115**: 867.

Hauschka, P. V., A. E. Mavrakos, M. D. Iafrati, S. E. Doleman and M. Klagsbrun. Growth factors in bone matrix. *Proc. Natl. Acad. Sci, U.S.A.* **21**: 12665–12674, 1986.

Heath, J. K., Atkinson, S. J., Meikle, M. C., and Reynolds, J. J. (1984). Mouse osteoblasts synthesize collagenase in response to bone resorbing agents. *Biochim. Biophys. Acta*, **802**: 151.

Heersche, J. N. M., Aubin, J. E., Grigoriadis, A. E., and Moriya, Y. (1985). Hormone responsiveness of bone cell populations. Searching for answers *in vivo* and *in vitro*. In: Butler, W. T. (ed). *The Chemistry and Biology of Mineralized Tissues*. Ebsco Media Inc., Birmingham. 286.

Heller-Steinberg, M., McLean, F. C., and Bloom, W. (1950). Cellular transformations in mammalian bones induced by parathyroid extract. *Am. J. Anat.*, **87**: 315.

Henneman, D. H. (1972). Inhibition by β-estadiol-17β of the lathyritic effect of β-aminopropionitrile (BAPN) on skin and bone collagen. *Clin. Orthop. & Rel. Res.*, **83**: 245.

Henrichsen, E. (1958). Alkaline phosphatase and calcification. *Acta Orthop. Scand.*, Suppl. 34, 1.

High, W. B. (1988). Effects of orally administered prostaglandin E-2 on cortical bone turnover in adult dogs: a histomorphometric study. *Bone*, **8**: 363.

Hill, D. J., Crawqce, C. J., Fowler, L., Holder, A. T., and Miller, R. D. G. (1984). Cultured fetal rat myoblasts release peptide growth factor which are immunologically and biologically similar to somatomedin. *J. Cell Physiol.*, **119**: 349.

Hirata, H., Dohi, T., Terada, H., Tanaka, S., Okamoto, H., and Trujimoto, A. (1983). Labelled-calcium release from rat mandibles exposed to prostaglandins *in vitro*. *Arch. Oral Biol.*, **28**: 963.

Hock, J. M., M. Centrella and E. Canalis. (1988). Transforming growth factor beta (TGF-beta-1) stimulates bone matrix apposition and bone cell replication in cultured rat calvaria. *Calcif. Tissue Int.* **42**: A32.

Holtrop, M. E., Raisz, L. G., and King, G. J. (1978). The response of osteoclasts to prostaglandin and osteoclast activating factor as measured by ultrastructural morphometry. In: Horton, J. E., Tarpley, T. M., and W. F. Davis (eds). *Proceedings, Mechanisms of Localized Bone Loss*. Information Retrieval Inc., Washington, D.C., 13.

Hooper, A. C. B. (1983). Skeletal dimensions in senescent laboratory mice. *Gerontology*, **29**: 221.

Horowitz, M. C., Ryaby, J. T., and Einhorn, T. A. (1988). Differentiation production of colony-stimulating factors by the murine osteoblastic cell line MCT3T. *Calcif. Tissue Int.*, **42 (Suppl.)**: A19 (Abstr. 74).

Horowitz, M. C., R. L. Jilka, R. Philbrick, J. T. Ryaby and T. A. Einhorn. (1989). Differential secretion of colony stimulating factors by osteoblasts. *Trans. Orthop. Res. Soc.* **14**: 88.

Horowitz, M. C., D. L. Coleman, P. M. Flood, T. S. Kupper and R. L. Jilka (1989a) Parathyroid hormone and lipopolysaccharide induce murine osteoblast-like cells to secrete a cytokine indistinguishable from granulocyte-macrophage colony stimulating factor. *J. Clin. Invest.* **83**: 149.

Howard, G. A., Bottemiller, B. L., Turner, R. T., Rader, J. I., and Baylink, D. J. (1981). Parathyroid hormone stimulates bone formation and resorption in organ culture: evidence for a coupling mechanism. *Proc. Natl. Acad. Sci., U.S.A.*, **78**: 3204.

Howes, R., Bowness, J. M., Grotendorst, G. R., Martin, G. R., and Reddi, A. H. (1988). Platelet-derived growth factor enhances demineralized bone matrix-induced cartilage and bone formation. *Calcif. Tissue Int.*, **42**: 34.

Hruza, Z. and Wachtlova, M. (1969). Diminution of bone blood flow and capillary network in rats during aging. *J. Gerontol.*, **24**: 315.

Hudson, T. G. F. (1964). Vanadium. Elsevier Publ. Co., Amsterdam.

Hughs, P. C. R., and Tanner, J. M. A (1970a). Longitudinal study of the growth of the black-hood rat. Method of measurement and rates of growth for skull limbs, pelvis, nose-rump and tail lengths. *J. Anat.*, **106**: 349.

Hughs, P. C. R., and Tanner, J. M. (1970b). The assessment of skeletal maturity in the growing rat. *J. Anat.*, **106**: 371.

Hughs, P. C. R., and Tanner, J. M. (1973). A radiographic study of the growth of the rat pelvis. *J. Anat.*, **114**: 439.

Hyldstrup, L., McNair, P., Jensen, G. F., and Transbol, I. (1986). Seasonal variations in indices of bone formation precede appropriate bone mineral changes in normal men. *Bone*, **7**: 167.

Hyldstrup, L., I. Clemmensen, B. A. Jensen, and I. Transbols. (1988) Non-invasive evaluation of bone formation: measurements of serum alkaline phosphatase, whole body retention of diphosphonate and serum osteocalcin in metabolic bone disorders and thyroid disease. *Scand. J. Clin. Lab. Invest.* **48**: 611.

Ibbotson, K. J., D'Souza, S. M., Smith, D. D., Carpenter, G., and Mundy, G. R. (1985). EGF receptor antiserum inhibits bone resorbing activity produced by a rat Leydig cell tumor associated with the humoral hypercalcemia of malignancy. *Endocrinol.*, **116**: 469.

Ibsen, K., and Urist, M. R. (1964). Relationship between pyrophosphate content and oxytetracycline labeling of bone salt. *Nature*, **203**: 761.

Ignotz, R. A., and Massague, J. (1987). Cell adhesion protein receptors as targets for transforming growth factor-β action. *Cell*, **51**: 189.

Irving, J. T., Le Bolt, S. A., and Schneider, E. L. (1981). Ectopic bone formation and aging. *Clin. Orthop. & Rel. Res.*, **154**: 249.

Ituarte, E. A., Ituarte, H. G., and Hahn, T. J. (1988). Insulin and glucose regulation of glycogen synthetase in rat calvarial osteoblastlike cells. *Calcif. Tissue Int.*, **42**: 351.

Jaffe, B. M., and Santoro, M. G. (1977). Prostaglandins and cancer. In: Ramwell, P. W. (ed). *The Prostaglandins*, Vol. 3, Plenum Publ. Co., N.Y., p. 329.

Jaffe, H. L. (1972). *Metabolic, Degenerative, and Inflammatory Diseases of Bones and Joints*. Lea and Febriger, Philadelphia.

Jeansonne, B. G., Feagin, F. F., McMinn, R. W., Shoemaker, R. L., and Rehm, W. S. (1979). Cell-to-cell communication of osteoblasts. *J. Dent. Res.*, **58**: 1415.

Jee, W. S. S., Park, H. Z., and Roberts, W. E. (1970). Corticosteroids and bone. *Am. J. Anat.*, **129**: 477.

Jee, W. S. S., Ueno, K., Deng, Y. P., and Woodbury, D. M. (1985). The effects of prostaglandin $E_2$ in growing rats: increased metaphyseal hard tissue and cortico-endosteal bone formation. *Calcif. Tissue Int.*, **37**: 148.

Jee, W. S. S., Ueno, K., Woodbury, D. M., Price, P., and Woodbury, L. A. (1987). The role of bone cells in increasing metaphyseal hard tissue in rapidly growing rats treated with prostaglandin R$_2$. *Bone*, **8**: 171.

Johnson, R. B., and Highison, G. J. (1983). A re-examination of the osteocytic network of interdental bone. *J. Submicrosc. Cytol.*, **15**: 619.

Jones, S. J. (1974). Secretory territories and the rate of matrix production of osteoblasts. *Calcif. Tissue Res.*, **14**: 309.

Jones, S. J., and Boyd, A. (1976a). Morphological changes in osteoblasts *in vitro*. *Cell Tissue Res.*, **166**: 101.

Jones, S. J., and Boyd, A. (1976b). Experimental study of changes in osteoblastic shape induced by calcitonin and parathyroid extract in an organ culture system. *Cell Tiss. Res.*, **169**: 449.

Jones, S. J., and Ness, A. R. (1977). A study of the arrangement of osteoblasts of rat calvarium cultured in medium with, or without, added parathyroid extract. *J. Cell Sci.*, **25**: 247.

Jones, S. J., Boyd, A., and Pawley, J. B. (1975). Osteoblasts and collagen orientation. *Cell. Tiss. Res.*, **159**: 73.

Jowsey, J. (1960). Age changes in human bone. *Clin. Orthop. & Rel. Res.*, **17**: 210.

Jowsey, J. (1964). Variations in bone mineralization with age and disease. In: Frost, H. M. (ed.). *Bone Biodynamics*, Little Brown and Co., Boston, 461.

Jowsey, J. (1966). Studies of haversian systems in man and some animals. *J. Anat.*, **100**: 857.

Jowsey, J. (1968). Age and species differences in bone. *Cornell Veterinarian* **58 (Suppl.)**: 74.

Jowsey, J., Kelly, P. J., Riggs, B. L., Bianco, A. J., Scholz, D. A., and Gershon-Cohen, J. (1969). Quantitative microradiographic studies of normal and osteoporotic bone. *J. Bone Joint Surg.*, **47A**: 785.

Jubiz, W., J. M. Canterbury, E. Reiss and F. H. Tyler. (1972). Circadian rhythm in serum parathyroid hormone concentration in human subjects. Correlation with serum calcium, phosphate, aluminum and growth hormone levels. *J. Clin. Invest.* **51**: 2040−2046.

Jundt, G., Berghauser, K.-H., Termine, J. D., and Schulz, A. (1987). Osteonectin − a differentiation marker of bone cells. *Cell Tissue Res.*, **248**: 409.

Kahn, A. J., and Simmons, D. J. (1977). Chondrocyte-to-osteocyte transformation in perichondrium-free epiphyseal cartilage. *Clin. Orthop. & Rel. Res.*, **129**: 299.

Kahn, A. J., Malone, J. D., and Teitelbaum, S. L. (1981). Osteoclast precursors, mononuclear phagocytes, and bone resorption. *Trans. Assoc. American Phys.*, **XCIV**: 267.

Kahn, S. E., and Arsenis, C. (1979). Identification, characterization and localization of a ($Ca^{2+}$ + $Mg^{2+}$) activated purine nucleoside triphosphate phosphohydrolase from calcifying cartilage. *Biochim. Biophys. Acta*, **569**: 52.

Kaplan, G. C., Eilon, G., Poser, J. W., and Jacobs, J. W. (1987). Constitutive biosynthesis of bone Gla protein in a human osteosarcoma cell line. *Endocrinol.*, **117**: 1235.

Kasperk, C. H., J. E. Wergedal, J. R. Farley, T. A. Linkhart, R. T. Turner, and D. J. Baylink (1989) Androgens directly stimulate proliferation of bone cells *in vitro*. *Endocrinol.* **124**: 1576.

Kay, L. L. Jr., Carnes, D. L. Jr., Weichselbaum, R., and Anast, C. S. (1983). Platelet-derived growth factor stimulates bone resorption by monocyte monolayers. *Endocrinology*, **112**: 761.

Keller, T. S., Spengler, D. M., and Carter, D. R. (1986). Geometric, elastic, and structural properties of maturing rat femora. *J. Biochem.*, **4**: 57.

Kelly, R. G., and Kanegis, L. A. (1967). Metabolism and tissue distribution of radioisotopically labeled minocycline. *Toxicol. Appl. Pharm.*, **11**: 171.

Kember, N. F. (1960). Cell division in endochondral ossification. A study of cell proliferation in rat bones by the method of tritiated thymidine autoradiography. *J. Bone Int. Surg.* **42-B**: 824−839.

Kerley, E. (1964). The microscopic determination of age in human bone. *Am. J. Phys. Anthrop.*, **23**: 149.

Key, L. L. Jr., Carnes, D. L. Jr., Weichselbaum, R., and Anast, C. (1983). Platelet-derived growth factor stimulates bone resorption by monocyte monolayers. *Endocrinol.*, **112**: 761.

Kiebzak, G. M., Smith, R., Gundberg, C. C., Howe, J. C., and Sacktor, B. (1988). Bone status of senescent male rats: chemical, morphometric, and mechanical analysis. *J. Bone Min. Res.*, **3**: 37.

Kimmel, D. B., and Jee, W. S. S. (1982). A quantitative histologic study of bone turnover in young adult beagles. *Anat. Rec.*, **203**: 31.

King, G. J., and Holtrop, M. E. (1975). Actin-like filaments in bone cells of cultured mouse calvaria as demonstrated by binding to heavy meromysin. *J. Cell Biol.*, **66**: 445.

Kita, K., Kawai, K., and Hirohata, K. (1987). Changes in bone marrow blood flow with aging. *J. Orthop. Res.*, **5**: 569.

Klagstrup, J., Melsen, F., and Moskilde, L. (1983). Thickness of bone formed at remodeling sites in normal human iliac trabecular bone: variations with age and sex. *Metab. Bone Dis. & Rel. Res.*, **5**: 17.

Klein, D. C., and Raisz, L. G. (1970). Prostaglandins — stimulation of bone resorption in tissue culture. *Endocrinol.*, **86**: 1436.

Klein, L. (1981). Steady-state relationship of calcium-45 between bone and blood: differences in growing dogs, chicks, and rats. *Science*, **214**: 190.

Klein-Nulend, J., Veldhuijzen, J. P., de Jong, M., and Burger, E. H. (1987a). Increased bone formation and decreased bone resorption in fetal mouse calvaria as a result of intermittent compressive force *in vitro*. *Bone and Mineral*, **2**: 441.

Klein-Nulend, J. (1987b). *Cellular responses of skeletal tissues to mechanical stimuli*. Free University Press, Amsterdam, p. 69.

Kodicek, E., and Thompson, G. A. (1964). Autoradiographic localization in bones of $[1\alpha-{}^3H]$ cholecalciferol. In: Fitton-Jackson, S., S. M. Partridge, R. D. Harkness and G. R. Tristam (eds), *Structure and Function of Connective Tissue*. Butteworths, London, p. 369.

Kohase, M., Henriksen-Destefano, D., Sehgal, P. B., and Vilcek, J. (1987). Dexamethasone inhibits feedback regulation of the mitogenic activity of tumor necrosis factor, interleukin-1, and epidermal growth factor in human fibroblasts. *J. Cellular Physiol.*, **132**: 271.

Kohler, P. (1986). Reimplantation of bone after autoclaving. Reconstruction of large diaphyseal defects in the rabbit. Doctoral Thesis. Karolinska Institute, Stockholm, Sweden.

Komoda, T., Nagata, A., Kiyoki, M., Miura, M., Koyama, I., Sakagishi, Y., and Kumegawa, M. (1988). Chloropromazine alters bone metabolism of rats *in vitro*. *Calcif. Tissue Int.*, **42**: 58.

Kream, B. E., Jose, M., Yamada, S., and DeLuca, H. F. (1977). Specific high affinity binding macromolecule for 1,25-dihydroxyvitamin $D_3$ in fetal bone. *Science*, **197**: 1086.

Kream, B. E., Rowe, D., Smith, M. D., Maher, V., and Majeska, R. (1986). Hormonal regulation of collagen synthesis in a clonal rat osteosarcoma cell line. *Endocrinol.*, **119**: 1922.

Krempien, B., and Ritz, E. (1978). Effects of parathyroid hormone on osteocytes. Ultrastructural evidence for anisotropic osteolysis and involvement of the cytoskeleton. *Metab. Bone. Dis. & Rel. Res.*, **1**: 55.

Kumegawa, M., Hiramatsu, M., Hatakeyama, K., Yajima, T., Kodama, H., Osaki, T., and Kurisu, K. (1983). Effects of epidermal growth factor on osteoblastic cells *in vitro*. *Calcif. Tissue Int.*, **35**: 542.

Kumegawa, M., Ikeda, E., Tanaka, S., Haneji, T., Yora, T., Sakagishi, Y., Minami, N., and Hiramatsu, M. (1984). The effects of prostaglandin $E_2$, parathyroid hormone, 1,25-dihydroxycholecalciferol, and cyclic nucleotide analogs on alkaline phosphatase activity in osteoblastic cells. *Calcif. Tissue Int.*, **36**: 72.

Kurihara, N., Ikeda, K., Hakeda, Y., Tsunoi, M., Maeda, M., and Kumegawa, M. (1984). Effect of 1,25-dihydroxyvitamin $D_3$ on alkaline phosphatase activity and collagen synthesis in osteoblastic cells, Clone MC3T3-E1. *Biochem. Biophys. Res. Commun.*, **119**: 767.

Kurihara, N., Ishizuka, S., Kiyoiki, M., Haketa, Y., Ikeda, K., and Kumegawa, M. (1986). Effects of 1,25-dihyroxyvitamin $D_3$ on osteoblastic MC3T3-E1 cells. *Endocrinol.*, **118**: 940.

Lafferty, F. W., Spencer, G. E., and Pearson, O. H. (1964). Effects of androgens, estrogens and high calcium intakes on bone formation and resorption in osteoporosis. *Am. J. Med.*, **36**: 514.

Lahtinen, T., Alhava, E. M., Karjalainen, P., and Romppanen, T. (1981). The effect of age on blood flow in the proximal femur in man. *J. Nucl. Med.*, **22**: 966.

Landis, W. J., and Glimcher, M. J. (1978). Electron diffraction and electron probe microanalysis of the mineral phase of bone tissue prepared by anhydrous techniques. *J. Ultrastr. Res.*, **63**: 188.

Lau, K.-H. W., J. C. Jennings and D. J. Baylink. (1988). Bovine skeletal growth factor stimulates protein phosphorylation of chicken bone cells *in vitro. Int. J. Biochem.* **20**: 1443.

Leaver, A. G. (1979). Noncollagenous proteins. In: Simmons, D. J. and Kunin, A. S. (eds). *Skeletal Research — An Experimental Approach.* Academic Press Inc., N. Y., p. 193.

Lee, W. R. (1964). Appositional bone formation in canine bone: a quantitative microscopic study using tetracycline markers. *J. Anat. (London)*, **98**: 665.

Lee, W. R., Marshall, J. H., and Sissons, H. A. (1965). Calcium accretion and bone formation in dogs. An experimental comparison of the results of $Ca^{45}$ kinetic analysis and tetracycline labelling. *J. Bone Joint Surg.*, **47B**: 157.

Leriche, R., and Policard, A. (1926). *Les Problems de la Physiologie Normale et Pathologique de l'Os.* Masson et Cie, Paris.

Lerner, U. H., M. Ransjo and A. Ljunggren. (1989). Bradykinin stimulates production of prostaglandin $E_2$ and prostacyclin in murine osteoblasts. *Bone and Mineral* **5**: 139.

Lian, J. B., Glimcher, M. J., Hauschka, P. V., Gallop, P. M., Cohen-Solal, L., and Reit, B. (1982). Alterations of the y-carboxyglutamic acid and osteocalcin concentrations in vitamin D-deficient chick bone. *J. Biol. Chem.*, **257**: 4999.

Lian, J. B., Tassinari, M., and Glowacki, J. (1984). Resorption of implanted bone prepared from normal and warfarin-treated rats. *J. Clin. Invest.*, **73**: 1223.

Liberman, U. A., Eil. C., Holst, P., Rosen, J. F., and Marx, S. J. (1983). Hereditary resistance to 1,25-dihydroxyvitamin D: defective function of receptors for 1,25-dihydroxyvitamin D in cells cultured from bone. *J. Clin. Endocrinol. Metab.*, **57**: 958.

Lindahl, A., Isgaard, J., Carlsson, L., and Isaksson, O. G. P. (1987). Differential effects of growth hormone and insulin-like growth factor I on colony formation of epiphyseal chondrocytes in suspension culture in rats of different ages. *Endocrinol.*, **121**: 1061.

Lindahl, O., and Lindgren, A. G. H. (1967). Cortical bone in man. I. Variation of the amount and density with age and sex. *Acta Orthop. Scand.*, **38**: 133.

Lindskog, S., Blomlof, L., and Hammarstrom, L. (1987). Comparative effects of parathyroid hormone on osteoblasts and cementoblasts. *J. Clin. Periodontol.*, **14**: 386.

Linkhart, S., Mohan, S., Linkhart, T. A., Kumegawa, M., and Baylink, D. J. (1986). Human skeletal growth factor stimulates collagen synthesis and inhibits proliferation in a clonal osteoblast cell line (MC3T3-E1). *J. Cellular Physiol.*, **128**: 307.

Lips, P., Courpron, P., and Meunier, P. J. (1978). Mean wall thickness of trabecular bone packets in the human iliac crest: changes with age. *Calcif. Tissue Res.*, **26**: 13.

Lohnes, D. and Jones, G. (1987). Side chain metabolism of vitamin $D_3$ in an osteosarcoma cell line UMR-106. *J. Biol. Chem.*, **262**: 14394.

Lomri, A., Marie, P. J., Escurat, M., and Portier, M.-M. (1987). Cytoskeletal protein synthesis and organization in cultured mouse osteoblastic cells. *FEBS Letters*, **222**: 311.

Lomri, A. and P. J. Marie (1988) Effect of parathyroid hormone and forskolin on cytoskeletal protein synthesis in cultured mouse osteoblastic cells. *Biochim. Biophys. Acta* **970**: 333.

Lorenz, M., and Plenk, H. Jr. (1977). A perfusion method of incubation to demonstrate horeseradish perodidase in bone. *Histochem.*, **53**: 257.

Lorenzo, J. A., and Raisz, L. G. (1982). Epidermal growth factor stimulates prostaglandin synthesis in fetal rat bone cultures when DNA synthesis is inhibited. *Clin. Res.*, **30 (2)**: 399A.

Lozupone, E. The rate of bony tissue deposition in the spongiosa of the extremities of long bones in the dog. *Anat. Anz. (Jena)* **166**: 175–185, 1988.

Luben, R. A., Wong, G. L., and Cohn, D. V. (1976). Biochemical characterization with parathormone and calcitonin of isolated bone cells: provisional identification of osteoclasts and osteoblasts. *Endocrinol.*, **99**: 526.

Lucas, P. A., P. A. Price and A. I. Caplan. (1988a). Chemotactic response of mesenchymal cells, fibroblasts, and osteoblast-like cells to bone Gla-protein. *Bone* **9**: 319–323.

Lucas, P. A. and A. I. Caplan. Chemotactic response of embryonic limb bud mesenchymal cells and muscle fibroblasts to transforming growth factor-β. Connect. *Tissue Res.* **18**: 1–7, 1988b.

Luk, S. C., Nopajaroonsri, C., and Simon, G. T. (1974). The ultrastructure of endosteum: a topographic study in young adult rabbits. *J. Ultrastr. Res.*, **46**: 165.

Lundy, M. W., Farley, J. R., and Baylink, D. J. (1986). Characterization of a rapidly responding animal model for fluoride stimulated bone formation. *Bone* **7**: 289.

MacPherson, J. N. and P. Tothill, P. (1978). Bone blood flow and age in the rat. *Clin. Sci. Mol. Med.*, **54**: 1411.

Macek, K., Deyl, Z., and Adam, M. (1980). The effect of age upon the content of γ-carboxyglutamic acid in rat mineralized tissue. *Exp. Geront.*, **15**: 1.

Mackie, E. J., Thesleff, I., and Chiquet-Ehrismann, R. (1987). Tenascin is associated with chondrogenic and osteogenic differentiation *in vivo* and promotes chondrogenesis *in vitro*. *J. Cell Biol.*, **105**: 2569.

Mahy, P. R. and M. R. Urist. (1988). Experimental heterotopic bone fomation induced by bone morphogenetic protein and recombinant human interleukin-1B. *Clin. Orthop. & Rel. Res.* **237**: 236–244.

Majeska, R. J., and Rodan, G. A. (1981). Hormonal regulation of alkaline phosphatase in an osteoblastic osteosarcoma cell line. *Calcif. Tissue Int.*, **33**: 297.

Majeska, R. J., and Rodan, G. A. (1982a). Alkaline phosphatase inhibition by parathyroid hormone and isoproterenol in a clonal rat osteosarcoma cell line. Possible mediation by cyclic AMP. *Calcif. Tissue Int.*, **34**: 59.

Majeska, R. J., and Rodan, G. A. (1982b). The effect of 1,25(OH)$_2$D$_3$ on alkaline phosphatase in osteoblastic osteosarcoma cells. *J. Biol. Chem.*, **257**: 3362.

Majeska, R. J., Rodan, S. B., and Rodan, G. A. (1980). Parathyroid hormone-responsive clonal cell lines from rat osteosarcoma. *Endocrinol.*, **107**: 1494.

Majeska, R. J., Nair, B. C., and Rodan, G. A. (1985). Glucocorticoid regulation of alkaline phosphatase in the osteoblastic osteosarcoma cell line ROS 17/2.8, *Endocrinol.*, **116**: 170.

Malluche, H. H., Faugere, M. C., Fanti, P., and Price, P. A. (1983). Bone GLA-protein — a biochemical index of bone formation and mineralization in uremic patients. *Calcif. Tissue Int.*, **35**: A38.

Malone, J. D., Teitelbaum, S. L., Griffin, G. L., Senior, R. M., and Kahn, A. J. (1982). Recruitment of osteoclast precursors by purified bone matrix constituents. *J. Cell Biol.*, **92**: 227.

Malone, J. D., M. Richards, and A. J. Kahn. (1986). Human peripheral monocytes express putative receptors for neuroexcitatory amino acids. *Proc. Natl. Acad. Sci. U.S.A.* **83**: 3307.

Manolagas, S. C., Anderson, D. C., and Lumb, G. A. (1979). Glucocorticoids regulate the concentration of 1,25-dihydroxycholecalciferol receptors in bone. *Nature*, **177**: 314.

Manolagas, S. C., Burton, D. W., and Deftos, L. J. (1981). 1,25-dihydroxyvitamin $D_3$ stimulates the alkaline phosphatase activity of osteoblast-like cells. *J. Biol. Chem.*, **256**: 7115.

Marcus, R., and Orner, F. B. (1977). Cyclic AMP production in rat calvaria *in vitro*: interaction of prostaglandins with parathyroid hormone. *Endocrinol.*, **101**: 1570.

Margulies, J. Y., Simkin, A., Leichter, I., Bivas, A., Steinberg, R., Giladi, M., Stein, M., Kashtan, H., and Milgrom, C. (1986). Effect of intense physical activity on the bone-mineral content in the lower limbs of young adults. *J. Bone Jnt. Surg.*, **68-A (7)**: 1090.

Mariano-Menez, M. R., Wakley, G. K., Farley, S. M., and Baylink, D. J. (1989). Fluoride metabolism and the osteoporotic patient. In: Simmons, D. J. (ed.). *Nutrition and Bone Development*. Oxford University Press, N.Y., (in press).

Marie, P. J., Garba, M. T., Hott, M., and Miravet, L. (1985). Effect of low doses of stable strontium on bone metabolism in rats. *Mineral Electrolyte Metab.*, **11**: 5.

Marie, P. J., Hott, M., and Perheentupa, J. (1988). Effects of epidermal growth factor on bone formation and resorption *in vivo*. *Calcif. Tissue Int.*, **42 (Suppl.)**: A22 (Abstr. 86).

Mark, M. P., Prince, C. W., Gay, S., Austin, R. L., Bhown, M., Finkelman, R. D., and Butler, W. T. (1987b). A comparative immunocytochemical study on the subcellular distributions of 44 kDa bone phosphoprotein and bone Y-carboxyglutamic acid (Gla)-containing protein in osteoblasts. *J. Bone Min. Res.*, **2 (4)**: 337.

Mark, M. P., Prince, C. W., Osawa, T., Gay. S., Bronckers, A. L. J. J., and Butler, W. T. (1987c). Immunohistochemical demonstration of a 44kDal phosphoprotein in developing rat bones. *J. Histochem. Cytochem.*, **35**: 707.

Mark, M. P., Prince, C. W., Gay, S., Austin, R. L., and Butler, W. T. (1988). 44-k Dal bone phosphoprotein (osteopontin) antigenicity at ectopic sites in newborn rats: kidney and nervous tissues. *Cell Tissue Res.*, **251**: 23.

Markowitz, M. E., Rosen, J. F., and Mizruchi, M. (1985). Effects of 1,25-dihydroxyvitamin $D_3$ on circadian mineral rhythms in humans. *Calcif. Tissue Int.*, **37**: 351.

Markowitz, J. E., C. M. Gundberg and J. F. Rosen. (1987). The circadian rhythm of serum osteocalcin concentrations: Effects of 1,25-Dihydroxyvitamin D administration. *Calcif. Tissue Int.* **40**: 179−183.

Marotti, G. (1976). Map of bone formation rate values recorded throughout the skeleton of the dog. In: Z. F. G. Jaworski (ed). *Bone Morphometry*. University of Ottawa Press, p. 202.

Marshall, W. A. (1975). Seasonal variation in growth rates of normal and blind children. *Human Biol.*, **43**: 502.

Martin, D. L., and Armelagos, G. J. (1979). Morphometrics of compact bone: an example from Sudanese Nubia. *Am. J. Phys. Anthrop.*, **51**: 571.

Martin, R. B. (1987). Osteonal remodeling in response to screw implantation in the canine femora. *J. Orthop. Res.*, **5**: 445.

Martin, R. K., Albright, J. P., Jee, W. S. S., Taylor, G. N., and Clarke, W. R. (1981). Bone loss in the beagle tibia: influence of age, weight, and sex. *Calcif. Tissue Int.*, **33**: 233.

Masoud, I., Shapiro, F., and Moses, A. (1986). Longitudinal roetgencephalometric study of the growth of the New Zealand white rabbit: Cumulative and biweekly incremental growth rates for skull and mandible. *J. Craniofac. Gen. Develop. Biol.*, **6**: 259.

Massler, M., and Schour, I. (1951). The growth pattern of the cranial vault in the albino rat as measured by vital staining with Alizarin red "S". *Anat. Rec.*, **110**: 83.

Matsushita, M., T. Tsuboyama, R. Kasai, H. Okumura, T. Yamamuro, K. Higuchi, K. Higushi, A. Kohno, T. Yonezu, A. Utani, M. Umezawa, and T. Takeda. (1986). Age related changes in bone mass in the senescence-accelerated mouse (SAM). SAM-R/3 and SAM-P/6 as new murine models for senile osteoporosis. *Am. J. Pathol.* **125**: 276.

Matthews, J. L., Davis, W. L., Margin, J. H., and Talmage, R. (1975). The endosteal cell response to exogenous stimuli, an electron microscope study. In: Slavkin, H. (ed). *Extracellular Matrix Influences on Gene Expression*. Academic Press Inc., N.Y., p. 735.

Matthews, J. L., Martin, J. H., and Carson, F. L. (1978). Ultrastructure of calcifylaxis in skin. *Metab. Bone Dis. & Rel. Res.*, **1**: 219.

Matthews, J. L. (1982). Bone structure and ultrastructure. In: Urist, M. R. (ed). *Fundamental and Clinical Bone Physiology*. J. B. Lippincott Co, Philadelphia, p. 4.

Matthews, J. L., and Talmage, R. V. (1981). Influence of parathyroid hormone on bone cell ultrastructure. *Clin. Orthop. & Rel. Res.*, **156**: 27.

Mazess, R. B., Barden, H., Towsley, M., and Engle, V. Bone mineral density of the spine and radius in normal young women. *Am. Soc. Bone Min. Res.*, June 1985, Abstr.

McCarthy, T. L., M. Centrella and E. Canalis. (1989) Parathyroid hormone enhances the transcript and polypeptide levels of insulin-like growth factor I in osteoblast-enriched cultures from fetal rat bone. *Endocrinol.* **124**: 1247.

McCulloch, C. A. G. and J. N. M. Heersche. (1988). Lifetime of the osteoblast in mouse periodontium. *Anat. Rec.* **222**: 128−135.

McDonald, B. R., Gallagher, J. A., Ahnfelt-Ronne, I., Beresford, J. N., Gowen, M., and Russell, R. G. G. (1984). Effects of bovine parathyroid hormone and 1,25-dihydroxyvitamin $D_3$ on the production of prostaglandins by cells derived from human bone. *FEBS Letters*, **169**: 49.

Melcher, A. H., McCulloch, C. A. G., Cheong, T., Nemeth, E., and Shiga, A. (1987). Cells from bone synthesize cementum-like and bone-like tissue *in vitro* and may migrate into the periodontal ligament *in vivo*. *J. Periodont. Res.*, **22**: 246.

Melick, R. A., Farrugia, W., and Quelch, K. J. (1985). Plasma osteocalcin in man. *Austr. N. Zeal. J. Med.*, **15**: 410.

Melsen, F., and Mosekilde, L. (1977). Morphometric and dynamic studies of bone changes in hyperthyroidism. *Acta Pathol. Microbiol. Scand.*, **[A]. 85**: 141.

Melsen, F., and Mosekilde, L. (1978). Tetracycline double-labeling of iliac trabecular bone in 41 normal individuals. *Calcif. Tissue Res.*, **26**: 99.

Melsen, F., Melsen, B., Mosekilde, L., and Bergmann, S. (1978). Histomorphometric analysis of normal bone from the iliac crest. *Acta Path. Microbiol. Scand.*, Sect. A, **86**: 70.

Melsen, F., Mosekilde, L., and Kragstrup, J. (1983). Metabolic bone diseases as evaluated by bone histomorphometry. In: Recker, R. R. (ed). *Bone Histomorphometry: Techniques and Interpretation*. CRC Press, Boca Raton, FL, p. 265.

Menton, D. N., Simmons, D. J., Orr, B. V., and Plurad, S. B. (1982). A cellular investment of bone marrow. *Anat. Rec.*, **203**: 157.

Menton, D. N., Simmons, D. J., Chang, S.-L., and Orr, B. Y. (1984). From bone lining cell to osteocyte — a S. E. M. study. *Anat. Rec.*, **209**: 29.

Merz, W., and Schenk, R. (1970). A quantitative histological study on bone formation in human cancellous bone. *Acta Anat.*, **76**: 1.

Miller, S. C., Bowman, B. M., Smith, J. M., and Jee, W. S. S. (1980). Characterization of endosteal bone-lining cells from fatty marrow bone sites in adult beagles. *Anat. Rec.* **198**: 163.

Mohan, S., and Radha, E. (1980). Hydroxyproline excretion and collagen catabolism in rats of different age groups. *Biochem. Med.*, **24**: 1.

Mohan, S., Jennings, J. C., Linkhart, T. A., and Baylink, D. J. (1986). Isolation and purification of a low-molecular weight skeletal growth factor from human bones. *Biochim. Biophys. Acta*, **884**: 234.

Mohan, S., Linkhart, T., Jennings, J., and Baylink, D. (1987b). Chemical and biological characterization of low-molecular-weight human skeletal growth factor. *Biochim. Biophys. Acta*, **884**: 243.

Mohan, S., J. C. Jennings, T. A. Linkhart and D. J. Baylink (1988) Primary structure of human skeletal growth factor: homology with human insulin-like growth factor-II. *Biochim. Biophys. Acta* **966**: 44.

Morel, G., Boivin, G., David, L., Dubois, P. M., and Meunier, P. J. (1985). Immunocytochemical evidence for endogenous calcitonin and parathyroid hormone in osteoblasts from the calvaria of neonatal mice. Absence of endogenous estradiol and estradiol receptors. *Cell Tissue Res.*, **240**: 89.

Moss, M. L. (1954). Differential growth analysis of bone morphology. *Am. J. Phys. Anthrop.*, n.s. **12**: 71.

Moss, M. L., and Baer, M. J. (1956). Differential growth of the rat skull. *Growth*, **20**: 107.

Muhlrad, A., Bab, I., and Sela, J. (1981). Dynamic changes in bone cells and extracellular matrix vesicles during healing of alveolar bone in rats. *Metab. Bone Dis. & Rel. Res.*, **2**: 347.

Mulkins, M. A., Manolagas, S. C., Deftos, L. J., and Sussman, H. H. (1983). 1,25-dihdyroxyvitamin $D_3$ increases bone alkaline phosphatase isoenzyme levels in human osteogenic sarcoma cells. *J. Biol. Chem.*, **258**: 6219.

Mundy, G. R., Varani, J., Orr, W., Gondek, M. D., and Ward, P. A. (1978). Resorbing bone is chemotactic for monocytes. *Science*, **276**: 132.

Murthy, G. P., Rajalkakshmi, R., and Ramakrishnan, C. V. (1986). Developmental pattern of alkaline phosphatase in soluble and particulate fractions of rat skull cap and femur. *Calcif. Tissue Int.*, **39**: 185.

Mustoe, T. A., Pierce, G. F., Thomason, A., Grimates, P., Sporn, M. B., and Deuel, T. F. (1987). Accelerated healing of incisional wounds in rats induced by transforming growth factor-β. *Science*, **237**: 1333.

Myubi-Muamba, J.-M., Gevers, G., and Dequeker, J. (1987). Studies on EDTA extracts and collagenase digests from osteoporotic cancellous bone of the femoral head. *Clin. Biochem.*, **20**: 221.

Nakamura, Y., Hirashita, A., and Kuwabara, Y. (1984). The localization of acid phosphatase activity in osteoblasts incident to experimental tooth movement. *Acta Histochemica Cytochemica*, **17**: 571.

Nakatani, Y., Tsunoi, M., Hakeda, Y., Kurihara, N., Fujita, K., and Kumegawa, M. (1984). Effect of parathyroid hormone on cAMP production and alkaline phosphatase activity in osteoblastic clone MC3T3−El. *Biochem. Biophys. Res. Commun.*, **123**: 894.

Neuman, M. W., and Neuman, W. F. (1958). *The Chemical Dynamics of Bone Mineral*. University of Chicago Press, Chicago, IL.

Neuman, W. F. (1964). Blood-bone exchange. In: Frost, H. M. (ed). *Bone Biodvnamics*, Little Brown and Co., Boston, p. 393.

Neuman, W. F., and Ramp, W. K. (1971). The concept of a bone membrane. In: Nichols, G. Jr. and Wasserman, R. H. (eds). *Cellular Mechanisms for Calcium Transfer and Homeostasis*. Academic Press Inc., N. Y., p. 197.

Neuman, W. F., Neuman, M. F., Sammon, P. J., and Casanett, G. W. (1975). The metabolism of labeled parathyroid hormone. *Calcif. Tissue Res.*, **18**: 263.

Ng, K. W., Partridge, N. C., Niall, M., and Martin, T. J. (1983a). Epidermal growth factor receptors in clonal lines of a rat osteogenic sarcoma and in osteoblast-rich rat bone cells. *Calcif. Tissue Int.*, **35**: 298.

Ng, K. W., Partridge, N. C., Niall, M., and Martin, T. J. (1983b). Stimulation of DNA synthesis by epidermal growth factor in osteoblast-like cells. *Calcif. Tissue Int.*, **35**: 624.

Ng, K. W., Gummer, P. R., Michelangeli, V. P., Bateman, J. F., Mascara, T., Cole, W. G., and Martin, T. J. (1988). Regulation of alkaline phosphatase expression in a neonatal rat clonal calvarial cell strain by retinoic acid. *J. Bone Min. Res.*, **3**: 53.

Nielsen, F. H. (1986). Other elements: Sb, Ba, B, Br, Cs, Ge, Rb, Ag, Sr., Sn, Ti, Zr, Be, Bi,

Ga, Au, In, Nb, Sc, Te, Ti, W. In: Merz, W. (ed). *Trace Elements in Human and Animal Nutrition.* Vol. 2, Academic Press Inc., N.Y., 415.

Nielsen, H. K., Thomsen, K., Eriksen, E. F., Charles, P., Storm, T., and Mosekilde, L. (1988). The effects of high-dose glucocorticoid administration on serum bone gamma carboxyglutamic acid-containing protein, serum alkaline phosphatase and vitamin D metabolites in normal subjects. *Bone and Mineral,* **4**: 105.

Nielsen, H. K., P. Charles and L. Moskilde (1988a). The effect of single oral doses of prednisone on the circadian rhythm of serum osteocalcin in normal subjects. *J. Clin. Endocrinol Metab.* **67**: 1025–1030.

Nishimoto, S. K., and Price, P. A. (1979). Proof that the y-carboxyglutamic acid-containing bone protein is synthesized in calf bone. *J. Biol. Chem.,* **254**: 437.

Nishimoto, S. K., and Price, P. A. (1980). Secretion of the vitamin K-dependent protein of bone by rat osteosarcoma cells. *J. Biol. Chem.,* **255**: 6579.

Nishimoto, S. K., and Price, P. A. (1985). The vitamin K-dependent bone protein is accumulated with cultured osteosarcoma cells in the presence of vitamin K antagonist warfarin. *J. Biol. Chem.,* **260**: 2832.

Nishimoto, S. K., Chang, C. H., Gendler, E., Stryker, W. F., and Nimni, M. E. (1985). The effect of aging on bone formation in rats: biochemical and histological evidence for decreased bone formation capacity. *Calcif. Tissue Int.,* **37**: 617.

Nishimoto, S. K., Stryker, W. F., and Nimni, M. E. (1987). Calcification of osteoblastlike rat osteosarcoma cells in agarose suspension cultures. *Calcif. Tissue Int.,* **41**: 274.

Noda, M., and Rodan, G. A. (1986). Type-β transforming growth factor inhibits proliferation and expression of alkaline phosphatase in murine osteoblast-like cells. *Biochem. Biophys. Res. Comm.,* **140**: 56.

Noda, M., and Rodan, G. A. (1987). Type β transforming growth factor (TGFβ) regulation of alkaline phosphatase expression and other phenotype-related mRNAs in osteoblastic rat osteosarcoma cells. *J. Cellular Physiol.,* **133**: 426.

Noda, M. (1989) Transcriptional regulation of osteocalcin production by transforming growth factor-b in rat osteoblast-like cells. *Endocrinology* **124**: 612.

Noda, M. and G. A. Rodan (1989) Transcriptional regulation of osteopontin production in rat osteoblast-like cells by parathyroid hormone. *J. Cell Biol.* **108**: 713.

Noda, M., K. Yoon, S. B. Rodan, C. W. Prince, W. T. Butler, and G. A. Rodan. (1988a). Transforming growth factor b1 stimulates and parathyroid hormone inhibits osteopontin gene expression in rat osteosarcoma (ROSD 17/2.8) cells. *J Bone Min. Res.* **3**: S218.

Noda, M., K. Yoon, C. W. Prince, W. T. Butler and G. A. Rodan. (1988b). Transcriptional regulation of osteopontin production in rat osteosarcoma cells by Type β transforming growth factor. *J. Biol. Chem.* **263**: 13916–13921.

Norimatsu, H. C., Vander Wiel, C. J., and Talmage, R. V. (1979). Morphological support of a role for cells lining bone surfaces in maintenance of plasma calcium concentrations. *Clin. Orthop. & Rel. Res.,* **138**: 254.

Norimatsu, H. (1980). The rapid effects of calcitonin on lining cell-osteocyte complex. *Bone Metab.,* (Jpn). **13**: 407.

Nuki, K., Soskolne, W. A., and Raisz, L. G. (1981). Bone resorbing activity of gingiva from beagle dogs following metronidazole and indomethacin therapy. *J. Periodont. Res.,* **16**: 205.

Nuti, R., Galli, M., Righi, G., Turchetti, V., Franci, B., and Martorelli, M. T. (1983). iCT and iPTH levels in Paget's disease of bone. Chronobiological aspects. *Calcif. Tissue Int.,* **35 (Suppl)**: A45.

Oberg, T., Frajers, C-M., Friberg, V., and Lohmander, S. (1969). Collagen formation and growth in the mandibular joint of the guinea pig as revealed by autoradiography with [³H]-proline. *Acta Odont. Scand.,* **27**: 425.

Ogata, K., and Simmons, D. J. (1976). Effect of intra-articular injections of methyprednisolone acetate on body weight in rats — a circadian rhythm. J. Interdisc. *Cycle Res.*, **7**: 223.

Ogata, K., and Simmons, D. J. (1981). Chronotherapeutic effects of intra-articular injections of methyprednisolone acetate. In: Walker, C. A., C. M. Winget and K. F. A. Soliman (eds). *Chronopharmacology and Chronotherapeutics.* Florida A & M University Foundation, Tallahassee, Fl, 295.

Ohmdahl, J. L., and DeLuca, H. F. (1971). Strontium induced rickets: metabolic basis. *Science,* **174**: 949.

Okimura, T., Ohmori, H., Kuborta, Y., and Yamamoto, I. (1979). Effects of anti-inflammatory and immunomodulating agents on the release of β-glucuronidase and collagenase from cultured macrophages of guinea pig. *Biochem. Pharmacol.*, **28**: 2729.

Olderg, A., A. Franzen and D. Heinegard. (1986). Cloning and sequence analysis of rat bone sialoprotein (osteopontin) cDNA reveals an argly-asp cell binding sequence. *Proc. Natl. Acad. Sci. U.S.A.* **83**: 8819.

Ophaug, R. H., Wong, K. M., and Singer, L. (1979). Lack of effect of fluoride on urinary cAMP excretion in rats. *J. Dental Res.*, **58**: 2036.

Ortner, D. J. (1975). Aging effects on osteon remodeling. *Calcif. Tissue Res.*, **18**: 27.

Osaki, Y., Tsunoi, M., Hakeda, Y., Kurisu, K., and Kumegawa, M. (1984). Immunocyto-chemical study of collagen in epidermal growth factor (EGF)-treated osteoblastic cells. *J. Histochem. Cytochem.*, **32**: 1231.

Otsuka, K., Sodek, J., and Limeback, H. (1984). Synthesis of collagenase and collagenase inhibitors by osteoblast-like cells in culture. *Eur. J. Biochem.*, **145**: 123.

Oudet, C. L., and Petrovic, A. G. (1982). Daytime and seasons are sources of variations for cartilage and bone growth rate. In: Dixon, A. D. and B. G. Sarnat (eds). *Factors and Mechanisms Influencing Bone Growth*, A. R. Liss Inc., N.Y., 481.

Oursler, M. J., and Osdoby, P. (1988). Osteoclast development in marrow cultured in calvaria-conditioned media. *Develop. Biol.*, **127**: 170.

Owen, M. (1963). Cell population kinetics of an osteogenic tissue. *J. Cell Biol.*, **19**: 19.

Owen, M. (1985). Lineage of osteogenic cells and their relationship to the stromal system. In: Peck, W. A. (ed). *Bone and Mineral Research*, Vol. 3, 1.

Owen, M. E., J. Cave and C. J. Joyner. (1987). Clonal analysis *in vitro* of osteogenic differen-tiation of marrow CFU-F *J. Cell Sci.* **87**: 731−738.

Pacifici, R., Civitelli, R., Rifas, L., Halstead, L., and Avioli, L. V. (1988). Does interleukin-1 affect intracellular calcium in osteoblast-like cells (UMR 106)? *J. Bone Min. Res.*, **3**: 107.

Paradis, G. R., and Kelly, P. J. (1975). Blood flow and mineral deposition in canine tibial fractures. *J. Bone Joint Surg.*, **220**.

Parfitt, A. M. (1983). The physiologic and clinical significance of bone histomorphometric data. In: Recker, R. R. (ed.): *Bone Histomorphometry: Techniques and Interpretation.* CRC Press, Boca Raton, FL, 143.

Partridge, N. C., Alcorn, D., Michelangeli, V. P., Kemp, B. E., Ryan, G. B., and Martin, T. J. (1981). Functional properties of hormonally responsive normal and malignant rat osteo-blast cells. *Endocrinol.*, **108**: 213.

Partridge, N. C., Alcorn, D., Michelangeli, V. P., Ryan, G., and Martin, T. J. (1983). Morphological and biochemical characterization of four clonal osteogenic sarcoma cell lines of rat origin. *Cancer Res.*, **43**: 4308.

Partridge, N. C., Jeffrey, J. J., Ehlich, L. S., Teitelbaum, S. L., Fliszar, C., Welgus, H. G., and Kahn, A. J. (1987). Hormonal regulation of the production of collagenase and a collagenase inhibitor activity by rat osteogenic sarcoma cells. *Endocrinol.*, **120**: 1956.

Patterson-Buckendahl, P. E., Grindeland, R. E., Martin, R. B., Cann, C. E., and Arnaud, S. B. (1985). Osteocalcin as an indicator of bone metabolism during spaceflight. *Physiologist,* **28**: S227.

Patterson-Buckendahl, P., Arnaud, S. B., Mechanic, G. L., Martin, R. B., Grindeland, R. E., and Cann, C. E. (1987). Fragility and composition of growing rat bone after one week in spaceflight. *Am. J. Physiol.*, **252**: R240.

Peck, W. A., and Messinger, K. (1970). Nucleoside and ribonucleic acid metabolism in isolated bone cells (effects of insulin and cortisol *in vitro*). *J. Biol. Chem.* **245**: 2722.

Peck, W. A., and Rifas, L. (1982). Regulation of osteoblast activity and the osteoblast-osteocyte transformation. In: Massry, S., J. Letteri, and E. R. Ritz (eds.). *Regulation of Phosphate and Mineral Metabolism.* Plenum, New York, 393.

Peck, W. A., Burks, J. K., and Kohler, G. (1979). Selective enhancement of bone cell proliferation by a factor derived from cultured bone cells. *Calcif. Tissue Int.*, **28**: 150.

Pedersen, U., Melsen, F., Kragstrup, J., and Charles, P. (1984). Histomorphometric analysis of iliac trabecular bone in otosclerosis. *Acta Otolaryngol. (Stockh)* **97**: 305.

Peress, H. S., Anderson, H. C., and Sajdera, S. W. (1974). The lipids of matrix vesicles. *Calcif. Tissue Res.*, **14**: 275,.

Petkovich, P. M., Wrana, J. L., Grigoriadis, A. E., Heersche, J. N. M., and Sodek, J. (1987). 1,25-dihydroxyvitamin $D_3$ increases epidermal growth factor receptors and transforming growth factor β-like activity in a bone-derived cell line. *J. Biol. Chem.*, **262**: 13424.

Petrovic, A., Stutzmann, J., and Oudet, C. (1981). Turn-over of human alveolar bone removed either in the day or in the night. *J. Interdisc. Cycle Res.*, **12**: 161.

Pfeilschifter, J., D'Souza, S., and Mundy, G. R. (1986). Transforming growth factor β (TGFβ) is released from resorbing bone and stimulates osteoblast activity. *J. Bone Min. Res.*, **1** (Suppl.): 246 (Abstract).

Pfeilschifter, J., D'Souza, S. M., and Mundy, G. R. (1987). Effects of transforming growth factor-β on osteoblastic osteosarcoma cells. *Endocrinol.*, **121**: 212.

Piez, K. A. (1968). Cross-linking of collagen and elastin. *Ann. Rev. Biochem.*, **37**: 547.

Pines, M., Santora, A., Gierschik, P., Menczel, J., and Spiegel, A. (1986). The inhibitory guanine nucleotide regulatory protein modulates agonist-stimulated c-AMP production in rat osteosarcoma cells. *Bone and Mineral*, **1**: 15.

Pirok, D. J., Ramser, J. R., Takahashi, H., Villanueva, A. R., and Frost, H. M. (1966). Normal histological, tetracycline, and dynamic parameters in human mineralized bone sections. *Henry Ford Hosp. Med. Bull.*, **14**: 195.

Pisano, M. M., and Greene, R. M. (1986). Hormone and growth factor involvement in craniofacial development. *IRCS Med. Sci.*, **14**: 635.

Plas, A. van der and Nijweide, P. J. (1988). Cell-cell interactions in the osteogenic compartment of bone. *Bone*, **9**: 107.

Plato, C. C., and Norris, A. H. (1980). Bone measurements of the second metacarpal and grip strength. *Human Biol.*, **52**: 131.

Polla, B. S., Healky, A. M., Bryne, M., and Krane, S. M. (1987). 1,25-dihydroxyvitamin $D_3$ induces collagen binding to the human monocyte line U937. *J. Clin. Invest.*, **80**: 962.

Pols, H. A. P., J. P. T. M. van Leeuwen, J. P. Schilte, T. J. Visser and J. C. Birkenhager. (1988). Heterogenous up-regulation of the 1,25-dihyroxyvitamin $D_3$ receptor by parathyroid hormone (PTH) and PTH-like peptid on osteoblast-like cells. *Biochem. Biophys. Res. Commun.* **156**: 588−594.

Ponseti, I. V., and Aleu, F. (1958). Fracture healing in rats treated with aminoacetonitrile. *J. Bone Joint Surg.*, **40**−**A**: 1093.

Posner, A. S., and Betts, F. (1975). Synthetic amorphous calcium phosphate and its relation to bone mineral structure. *Accounts of Chem. Res.*, **8**: 273.

Postlewaite, A. E., and Kang, A. H. (1976). Collagen and collagen peptide-induced chemotaxis of human blood monocytes. *J. Exp. Med.*, **143**: 1299.

Price, P. A. (1985). Vitamin K-dependent formation of bone Gla protein (osteocalcin) and its function. *Vitamins and Hormones*, **42**: 65.

Price, P. A., and Baukol, S. A. (1980). 1,25-dihydroxyvitamin $D_3$ increases synthesis of the vitamin D-dependent bone protein by osteosarcoma cells. *J. Biol. Chem.*, **255**: 11660.

Price, P. A., and Baukol, S. A. (1981). 1,25-dihydroxyvitamin $D_3$ increases serum levels of the vitamin D-dependent bone protein. *Biochem. Biophys. Res. Commun.*, **99**: 928.

Price, P. A., and Nishimoto, S. K. (1980). Radioimmunoassay for the vitamin D-dependent protein of bone and its discovery in plasma. *Proc. Nat. Acad. Sci., U.S.A.*, **77**: 2234.

Price, P. A., and Williamson, M. K. (1981). Effects of warfarin on bone. *J. Biol Chem.*, **256**: 12754.

Price, P. A., Lothringer, J. W., and Nishimoto, S. K. (1980). Absence of the Vitamin K dependent bone protein in fetal rat mineral. Evidence for another y-carboxyglutamic acid-containing component in bone. *J. Biol. Chem.*, **255**: 2938.

Price, P. A., Parthemore, J. G., and Deftos, L. J. (1980). New biochemical marker for bone metabolism: measurement by radioimmunoassay of bone Gla protein in the plasma of normal subjects and patients with bone diseases. *J. Clin. Invest.*, **66**: 878.

Price, P. A., Williamson, M. K., and Lothringer, J. W. (1981). Origin of the vitamin K dependent bone protein found in plasma and its clearance by kidney and bone. *J. Biol. Chem.*, **256**: 12760.

Price, P. A., Urist, M. R., and Otawara, Y. (1983). Matrix GLA protein, a new y-carboxyglutamic acid-containing protein which is associated with the organic matrix of bone. *Biochem. Biophys. Res. Commun.*, **117**: 765.

Prince, C. W., and Butler, W. T. (1987). 1,25-dihydroxyvitamin $D_3$ regulates the biosynthesis of osteopontin, a bone-derived cell attachment protein, in clonal osteoblast-like osteosarcoma cells. *Collagen Rel. Res.*, **7**: 305.

Pritchard, J. J. (1976). The osteoblast. In: Bourne, G. H. (ed.). *The Biochemistry and Physiology of Bone*. Vol. 1, Academic Press Inc., N.Y., 19.

Puche, R. C., Romano, M. C., Locatto, M. E., and Ferrettie, J. L. (1973). The effect of insulin on bone resorption. *Calcif. Tissue Res.*, **12**: 8.

Puzas, J. E., and Brand, J. S. (1979). Parathyroid hormone stimulation of collagenase secretion by isolated bone cells. *Endocrinol.*, **104**: 559.

Puzas, J. E., Drivdahl, R. H., Howard, G. A., and Baylink, D. J. (1981). Endogenous inhibitor of bone cell proliferation. *Proc. Soc. Exp. Biol. Med.*, **116**: 113.

Quarles, L. D., Gitelman, H. J., and Drezner, M. K. (1988). Induction of *de novo* bone formation in the beagle. A novel effect of aluminum. *J. Clin. Invest.*, **81**: 1056.

Radom, S., Zulawski, M., and Dahlig, E. (1972). Circadian rhythm of total urinary hydroxyproline excretion and 3-H hydroxyproline test. *Clin. Chim. Acta*, **39**: 277.

Rahn, B. A., and Perren, S. M. (1970). Calcein blue as a fluorescent label in bone. *Experientia*, **26**: 519.

Raisz, L. G., and Martin, T. J. (1983). Prostaglandins in bone and mineral metabolism. In: Peck, W. A. (ed.). *Bone and Mineral Research*, Elsevier, Amsterdam, p. 286.

Raisz, L. G., H. A. Simmons, A. L. Sandberg and E. Canalis. (1980). Direct stimulation of bone resorption by epidermal growth factor. *Endocrinol.* **107**: 270–273.

Raman, A. (1969). Appositional growth rate in rat bones using the tetracycline labeling method. *Acta Orthop. Scand.*, **40**: 193.

Ransjo, M., and Lerner, U. H. (1987). Effects of cholera toxin on cyclic AMP accumulation and bone resorption in cultured mouse calvaria. *Biochim. Biphys. Acta*, **930**: 378.

Rao, G. V. G., and Draper, H. H. (1969). Age-related changes in the bones of adult mice. *J. Gerontol.*, **24**: 149.

Rao, L. G., Heersche, J. N. M., Marchuk, L. L., and Sturtridge, W. (1981). Immunohistochemical demonstration of calcitonin binding to specific cell types in fixed rat bone tissue. *Endocrinol.*, **108**: 1972.

Redhead, C. R., and Baker, P. F. (1988). Control of intracellular pH in rat calvarial osteoblasts: coexistence of both chloride-bicarbonate and sodium-hydrogen exchange. *Calcif. Tissue Int.*, **42**: 237.

Reid, I. R., Civitelli, R., Avioli, L. V., and Hruska, K. A. (1987). PTH depresses cytosolic pH and DNA synthesis in osteoblast-like cells. *J. Bone Min. Res.*, 2 (Suppl.): Abstr. 127.

Reinholt, F. P., Hjerpe, A., Jansson, K., and Engfeldt, B. (1983). Stereological studies on matrix vesicle distribution in the epiphyseal growth plate during healing of low phosphate, vitamin D deficiency rickets. *Virchows Archiv. (Cell Pathology) B*, **44**: 357.

Reynolds, E. L., and Sontag, L. W. (1944). Seasonal variations in weight, height and appearance of ossification centers. *J. Pediatrics*, **24**: 524.

Rhinelander, F. W. (1968). The normal microcirculation of dipahyseal cortex and its response to fracture. *J. Bone Joint Surg.*, **50A**: 784.

Rhinelander, F. W., and Baragry, R. A. (1962). Microangiography in bone healing. I. Undisplaced closed fracture. *J. Bone Joint Surg.*, **44A**: 1273.

Rhinelander, F. W., Phillips, R. W., Steer, W.-M., and Beer, J. C. (1968). Microangiography in bone healing. II. Displaced closed fractures. *J. Bone Joint Surg.*, **50A**: 643.

Ribelin, W. E., Masri, M. S., and DeEds, F. (1960). Fluorescence of bone after quercetin ingestion. *Proc. Soc. Exp. Biol. Med.*, **103**: 271.

Riesenfeld, A. (1972). Functional and hormonal control of pelvic morphology in the rat. *Acta Anat.*, **82**: 231.

Riesenfeld, A. (1981). Age changes in bone size and mass in two strains of senescent rats. *Acta Anat.*, **109**: 64.

Rifas, L., Shen, V., Mitchell, K., and Peck, W. A. (1984). Macrophage-derived growth factor for osteoblast-like cells and chondrocytes. *Proc. Natl. Acad. Sci. U.S.A.*, **81**: 4558.

Rifkin, B. R., Baker, R. L., Somerman, M. J., Pointon, S. 'E., Coleman, S. J., and Yu, W. Y. A. (1980). Osteoid resorption by mononuclear cells *in vitro*. *Cell Tissue Res.*, **210**: 493.

Roberto, M. (1978). Quantitative evaluation of postnatal bone growth in the auditory ossicles of the dog. *Ann. Otol. Rhinol. Laryngol.*, **87**: 370.

Roberts, W. E., Mozsary, P. G., and Klingler, E. (1982). Nuclear size as a cell-kinetic marker for osteoblast differentiation. *Am. J. Anat.*, **165**: 373.

Robinson, R. A. (1960). Chemical analysis and electron microscopy of bone. In: Roadahl, K., Nicholson, J. T. and Brown, E. M. Jr. (eds.). *Bone as a Tissue*. McGraw Hill Book Co., Inc., 186.

Robison, R. (1923). Possible significance of the hexosophosphoric esters in ossification. *Biochem. J.*, **17**: 286.

Rodan, G. A., and Martin, T. J. (1981). Role of osteoblasts in hormonal control of bone resorption — a hypothesis. *Calcif. Tissues Int.*, **33**: 349.

Rodan, G. A., and Rodan, S. B. (1983). Further characterization of hormone adenylate cyclase coupling in desensitized ROS 17/2.8 cells. *Calcif. Tissue Int.*, **35**: 687.

Rodan, S. B., and Rodan, G. A. (1986). Dexamethasone effects on β-adrenergic receptors and adenylate cyclase regulatory proteins $G_s$ and $G_i$ in ROS 17/2.8 cells. *Endocrinol.*, **118**: 2510.

Rodan, S. B., Fisher, M. K., Egan, J. J., Epstein, P. M., and Rodan, G. A. (1984). Effect of dexamethasone on parathyroid hormone stimulation of adenylate cyclase in ROS 17/2.8 cells. *Endocrinol.*, **115**: 951.

Rodan, S. B., Imai, Y., Thiede, M. A., Weselows, G., Thompson, D., Bar-Shavit, Z., and Rodan, G. A. (1987). Characterization of a human osteosarcoma cell line (Saos-2) with osteoblastic properties. *Cancer Res.*, **47**: 4961.

Rodan, S. B., Heath, J. K., Chin, J., Schmidt, J. A., and Rodan, G. A. (1988). Interleukin-1 receptors on transformed human and rat osteoblastic cells. *Calc. Tissue Int. 42(Suppl.):* **A19** (Abstr.71).

Roodman, G. D., Ibbotson, K. J., MacDonald, B. R., Kuehl, T. J., and Mundy, G. R. (1985). 1,25-dihydroxyvitamin $D_3$ causes formation of multinucleated cells with several osteoclast characteristics in cultures of primate marrow. *Proc. Natl. Acad. Sci., U.S.A.*, **82**: 8213.

Rosen, O.M. (1987). After insulin binds. *Science*, **237**: 1452.

Rosenberg, G. D., Simmons, D. J., Halberg, H., Nelson, W., and Burstein, A. (1981). Skeletal effects of methylprednisolone sodium succinate administration on an everyday or alternate day chronopharmacologic dose schedule. In: Halberg, F., L. E. Scheving, E. W. Powell and D. K. Hayes (eds.). *Proc. XIII International Congress on Chronobiology.* Il Ponte Publ. House, Milan., p. 231.

Rouleau, M. F., Warshawsky, H., and Goltzman, D. (1986). Parathyroid hormone binding *in vivo* to renal, hepatic, and skeletal tissues of the rat using a radioautoradiographic approach. *Endocrinol.*, **118**: 919.

Rouleau, M. F., J. Mitchell and D. Goltzman. (1988). *In vivo* distribution of parathyroid hormone receptors in bone: Evidence that a predominant osseous target cell is not the mature osteoblast. *Endocrinol.* **123**: 187−191.

Royce, P. M., and Barnes, M. J. (1988). Interaction of embryonic chick calvarial bone cells with collagen substrata: attachment characteristics and growth behavior. *Conn. Tissue Res.*, **17**: 55.

Rubin, C. T., and Lanyon, L. E. (1984). Regulation of bone formation by applied dynamic loads. *J. Bone Joint Surg.*, **66-A**: 397.

Ruff, C. B., and Hayes, W. C. (1982). Subperiosteal expansion and cortical remodeling of the human femur and tibia with age. *Science*, **317**: 945.

Russell, J. E., Simmons, D. J., Huber, B., and Roos, B. (1983). Meal timing as a Zeitgeber for skeletal DNA and collagen synthesis rhythm. *Endocrinol.*, **113**: 2035.

Russell, J. E., Walker, W. V., and Simmons, D. J. (1984a). Adrenal/parathyroid regulation of DNA, collagen, and protein synthesis in rat epiphyseal cartilage and bone. *J. Endocrinol.*, **103**: 49.

Russell, J. E., Grazman, B., and Simmons, D. J. (1948b). Mineralization in rat metaphyseal bone exhibits a circadian stage dependency. *Proc. Soc. Exp. Biol. Med.*, **176**: 342.

Russell, J. E., Price, P. A., and Simmons, D. J. (1984c). Synchronous circadian rhythms for rat serum BGP protein and osteoblast collagen synthesis. *Clin. Res.*, **32**: 53A.

Sakamoto, M., and Sakamoto, S. (1984a). Immunocytochemical localization of collagenase in isolated mouse bone cells. *Biomed. Res.*, **5**: 29.

Sakamoto, S., and Sakamoto, M. (1984b). Isolation and characterization of collagenase synthesized by mouse bone cells in culture. *Biomed. Res.*, **5**: 39.

Saksena, S. K., Steele, R., and Harper, M. J. K. (1973). Effects of exogenous oestradiol and progesterone on serum levels of prostaglandin F and luteinizing hormone in chronically ovariectomized rats. *J. Reprod. Fert.*, **3**: 495.

Sandberg, A. L., Raisz, L. G., Wahl, L. M., and Simmons, H. A. (1982). Enhancement of complement-mediated prostaglandin synthesis and bone resorption by arachnidonic acid and inhibition by cortisol. *Prostagl. Leukotrienes and Medicine*, **8**: 419.

Sandberg, M., H. Autio-Harmainen and E. Vuorio. Localization of the expression of Type I, III, and IV collagen, TGF-β, and c-fos genes in developing human calvarial bones. *Develop. Biol.* **130**: 324−334, 1988.

Sandy, J. R., S. Meghji, A. M. Scutt, W. Harvey, M. Harris and M. C. Meikle. (1989). Murine osteoblasts release bone-resorbing factors of high and low molecular weights: stimulation by mechanical deformation. *Bone and Mineral* **5:** 155−1689.

Santoro, M. G., Jaffe, B. M., and Simmons, D. J. (1977). Bone resorption *in vitro* and *in vivo* in

PGE-treated mice. *Proc. Soc. Exp. Biol. Med.*, **156**: 373.

Sasaki, T., Tomingawa, H., and Higashi, S. (1984). Endocytotic activity of kitten odontoblasts in early dentinogenesis. 1. Thin section and freeze-fracture study. *J. Anat.*, **138**: 485.

Sasaki, T., Yamaguchi, A., Shohei, Y., and Yoshiki, S. (1985). Uptake of horseradish peroxidase by bone cells during endochondral bone development. *Cell Tissue Res.*, **239**: 547.

Sato, K., Kasono, K., Fujii, Y., Kawakami, M., Tsushima, T., and Shizume, K. (1987). Tumor necrosis factor type a (Cachectin) stimulates mouse osteoblast-like cells (MC3T3-El) to produce macrophage-colony stimulating activity and prostaglandin $E_2$. *Biochem. Biophys. Res. Commun.*, **145**: 323.

Saville, P. D., and Smith, P. M. (1966). Relation between axial and appendicular skeletal calcium and body weight in the rat. *Anat. Rec.*, **156**: 455.

Schaafsma, G., van Beresteyn, E. C. H., Raymakers, J. A., and Duursma, S. A. (1987). Nutritional aspects of osteoporosis. *Wld. Rev. Nutr. Diet.*, **49**: 121.

Schen, S., Villanueva, A. R., and Frost, H. M. (1965). Number of osteoblasts per unit area of osteoid seam in cortical human bone. *Canad. J. Physiol. Pharmacol.*, **43**: 319.

Schmid, Ch., Steiner, Th., and Froesch, E. R. (1983). Insulin-like growth factors stimulate synthesis of nucleic acids and glycogen in cultured calvarial cells. *Calcif. Tissue Int.*, **35**: 578.

Schmid, C., Ernst, M., Frankenfeldt, C., and Froesch, E. R. (1988). Collagen mRNA regulation in osteoblastic cells: glucocorticoid inhibition reversed by insulin-like growth factor (IGF) I. *Calcif. Tissue Int.*, **42** (Suppl.): A24 (Abstr. 95).

Schoenecker, P. L., Bitz, M., and Whiteside, L. A. (1978). The acute effect of position of immobilization on capital femoral epiphyseal blood flow. *J. Bone Joint Surg.*, **60A**: 899.

Schoenle, E., Zapi, J., Humbel, R. E., and Froesch, E. R. (1982). Insulin-like growth factor I stimulates growth in hypophysectomized rats. *Nature*, **296**: 252.

Schulz, A., and Delling, G. (1976). Age-related changes of new bone formation. Determination of histomorphometric parameters of the iliac crest trabecular bone. In: Jaworski, Z. F. G. ed). *Bone Mophometry*. University of Ottawa Press, Ottawa, p. 189.

Schwartz, P. L., Wettenhall, R. E. H., Truedel, M. A., and Burnstein, J. (1970). A long-term effect of insulin on collagen synthesis by newborn rat bone *in vitro*. *Diabetes*, **19**: 465.

Scott, D. M., Kent, G. N., and Cohn, D. V. (1980). Collagen synthesis in cultured osteoblast-like cells. *Arch. Biochem. Biophys.*, **201**: 384.

Sela, J., Amir, D., Schwartz, Z., and Weinberg, H. (1987). Changes in the distribution of extracellular matrix vesicles during healing of rat tibial bone (computerized morphometry and electron microscopy) *Bone*, **8**: 245.

Senior, R. M., Griffin, G. L., Huang, J. S., Walz, D. A., and Deuel, T. F. (1983). Chemotactic activity of platelet alpha granule proteins for fibroblasts. *J. Cell Biol.*, **96**: 383.

Seppa, H., Grotendorst, G., Seppa, S., Schiffmann, E., and Martin, G. R. (1982). Platelet-derived growth factor is chemotactic for fibroblasts. *J. Cell Biol.*, **92**: 584.

Seyedin, S. M., A. Y. Thompson, H. Bentz, D. M. Rosen, J. M. McPherson, A. Conti, N. R. Siegel, G. R. Gallupi and K. A. Piez. Cartilage-inducing factor-A; Apparent identity to transforming growth factor-β. *J. Biol. Chem.* **261**: 5693−5695, 1986.

Shapiro, F. (1988). Cortical bone repair. The relationship of the lacunar-canalicular system and intercellular gap junctions to the repair process. *J. Bone Int. Surg.* **70-A**: 1067.

Shen, V., G. Kohler, J. J. Jeffrey and W. A. Peck. (1989). Bone resorbing asgents promote and interferon-Y inhibits bone cell collagenase production. *J. Bone Min. Res.* **3**: 657.

Shipley, P. G., Park, E. A., McCollum, E. V., Simmonds, N., and Kinney, E. M. (1922). Studies on experimental rickets. XX. The effects of strontium administration on the histological structure of the growing bones. *Bull. Johns Hopkins. Hosp.*, **33**: 216.

Shteyer, A., Gazit, D., Passi-Even, L., Bab, I., Majeska, R. J., Gronowicz, G., Lurie, A., and Rodan, G. (1986). Formation of calcifying matrix by osteosarcoma cells in diffusion chambers *in vivo. Calcif. Tissue Int.*, **39**: 49.

Shulman, L. B., Greenspan, R., and Bauer, R. (1972). Pretransplant periodontal ligament enzymolysis to prolong tooth allograft survival. In: Mandl, I. (ed). *Collagenase.* Gordon and Breach Science Publ. N.Y., p. 93.

Shupnik, M. A., Yip, N. Y.-Y., and Tashjian, A. H. (1980). Characterization and regulation of receptors for epidermal growth factor in mouse calvaria. *Endocrinol.*, **107**: 1738.

Sibonga, J., S. Mohan, S. Nishimoto., E. Holton, T. Linkhart, G. Wakley and D. Baylink. (1989). Impairment of bone formation (BF) in response to skeletal unloading is associated with a bone derived growth factor deficit. *Clin. Res.* **37**: 135A.

Siegel, R. C. (1976). Collagen cross-linking, synthesis of collagen cross links *in vitro* which highly purified lysyl oxidase. *J. Biol. Chem.*, **251**: 5786.

Silve, C. M., Hradek, G. T., Jones, A. L., and Arnaud, C. D. (1982). Parathyroid hormone receptor in intact embryonic chicken bone: characterization and cellular localization. *J. Cell Biol.*, **94**: 379.

Silve, C., Grosse, B., Tau, C., Garabedian, M., Fritsch, J., Delmas, P. D., Cournot-Witmer, G., and Balsan, S. (1986). Response to parathyroid hormone and 1,25-dihydroxyvitamin $D_3$ of bone-derived cells isolated from normal children and children with abnormalities in skeletal development. *J. Clin. Endocrinol. Metab.*, **62**: 583.

Simkin, A., Leichter, I., and Ayalon, J. (1986). The effect of limb loading exercizes on the bone density in postmenopausal osteoporotic women. *Bone*, **7 (5)**: 418.

Simmons, D. J. (1963). Cellular changes in the bones of mice as studied with tritiated thymidine and the effects of estrogen. *Clin. Orthop. & Rel. Res.* **26**: 176−189.

Simmons, D. J. (1966). Collagen formation and endosteal ossification in estrogen-treated mice. *Proc. Soc. Exp. Biol. Med.*, **121**: 1165.

Simmons, D. J. (1976). Comparative physiology of bone. In: Bourne, G. H. (ed.). *The Biochemistry and Physiology of Bone*, Vol. 4, Academic Press, N.Y., p. 445.

Simmons, D. J. (1979). Experimental design and the implications of circadian skeletal rhythmicity. In: Simmons, D. J. and A. S. Kunin (eds.). *Skeletal Research-An Experimental Approach*, Academic Press Inc., N.Y., p. 567.

Simmons, D. J. (1985). Options for bone aging with the microscope. *Yearbook Physical Anthrop.*, **28**: 249.

Simmons, D. J., Pankovich A. M., and Budy, A. M. (1965). Osteolathyrism in mice and inhibition of the endosteal bone reaction in estrogen-treated mice by aminoacetonitrile. *Am. J. Anat.*, **116**:387.

Simmons, D. J., Bratberg, J. J., Lesker, P. A., and Aab, L. (1976). What is the best time of day to schedule a bone graft operation? *Clin. Orthop. & Rel. Res.*, **116**: 227.

Simmons, D. J., Lesker, P. A., Cohen, M., and McDonald, D. (1977). Chronobiology of fracture healing. In: Lassmann G. and F. Seitelberger (eds.). *Rhythmische Funktionen in Biologischen Systemen.* Facultas-Verlaq, Wein, p. 140.

Simmons, D. J., Teitelbaum, S. L., and Rosenberg, G. D. (1981). Tetracycline induced changes in calcification rate in rabbit bone. *Metab. Bone Dis. & Rel. Res.*, **3**: 51.

Simmons, D. J., Kent, G. N., Jilka, R. L., Scott, R., Fallon, M., and Cohn, D. V. (1982). The formation of bone by isolated cultured osteoblasts in millipore diffusion chambers. *Calcif. Tissue Int.*, **34**: 291.

Simmons, D. J., Parvin, C., Smith, K. C., France, P., and Kazarian, L. (1986). Effect of rotopositioning on the growth and maturation of mandibular bone in immobilized Rhesus monkeys. *Aviat. Space Environ. Med.*, **57**: 157.

Simmons, D. J., Russell, J. E., and Daughaday, W. H. (1986b). Lack of a correlation between the circadian rhythm of epiphyseal growth cartilage DNA synthesis and serum somatomedin-C in growing rats. *J. Bone Min. Res.*, **1**: 107.

Simmons, D. J., Menton, D. N., Russell, J. E., Smith, R., and Walker, W. V. (1988). Bone cell populations and histomorphometric correlates to function. *Anat. Rec.*

Slootweg, S. C., Van Buul-Offers, S. C., Heerman-Erlee, M. P. M., van Zoelen, E. J. J., and Duursma, S. A. (1988). Production of IGF-I and II and their binding proteins by fetal mouse osteoblasts. *Calcif. Tissue Int.*, **42** (Supp.): A36 (Abstr. 141).

Slovik, D. M., Rosenthal, D. I., Doppelt, S. H., Potts Jr., J. T., Daly, M. A., Campbell, J. A., and Neer, R. M. (1986). Restoration of spinal bone in osteoporotic men by treatment with human parathyroid hormone (1−34) and 1,25-dihydroxyvitamin D. *J. Bone Min. Res.*, **1(4)**: 377.

Smith, D. M., and Johnston, C. C. (1974). Hormonal responsiveness of adenylate cyclase activity from separated bone cells. *Endocrinol.*, **95**: 130.

Sodek, J., and Heersche, J. N. M. (1981). Uptake of collagenolytic enzymes by bone cells during isolation from embryonic rat calvaria. *Calcif. Tissue Int.*, **33**: 255.

Sodek, J., Bellows, C. G., Aubin, J. E., Limeback, H., Otsuka, K., and Yao, K.-L. (1985). Differences in collagen gene expression in subclones and long-term cultures of clonally derived rat bone cell populations. In: Butler, W. T. (ed). *The Chemistry and Biology of Mineralized Tissues.* Ebsco Media Inc., Birmingham, p. 303.

Somerman, M., Schiffman, E., Reddi, A. H., and Termine, J. (1982). Regulation of the attachment and migration of bone cells *in vitro*. *J. Periodont. Res.*, **17**: 527.

Somerman, M. J., Hotchkiss, R. N., Bowers, M. R., and Termine, J. (1983). Comparison of fetal and adult human bone: identification of a chemotactic factor in fetal bone. *Metab. Bone Dis. & Rel. Res.*, **5**: 75.

Somerman, M. J., Prince, C. W., Sauk, J. J., Foster, R. A., and Butler, W. T. (1987). Mechanism of fibroblast attachment to bone extracellular matrix: role of a 44 kilodalton bone phosphoprotein. *J. Bone Min. Res.*, **2(3)**: 259.

Soni, N. N. (1969). Microradiographic-topographic study of growth rates in mandibles and maxillas of guinea pig. *J. Dent. Res.*, **48**: 298.

Soni, N. N. (1970). Determination of growth rates by tetracycline labeling in young guinea pig mandibles. *J. Dent. Res.*, **49**: 1099.

Soni, N. N., and Messer, K. B. (1971). Determination of growth rate by tetracycline labelling in guinea pig maxillas. *Anat. Rec.*, **166**: 569.

Sontag, W. (1986). Quantitative measurements of periosteal and cortical-endosteal bone formation and resorption in the midshaft of female rat femur. *Bone*, **7**: 55.

Spies, Y. H., Price, P. A., Deftos, J. L., and Manolagas, S. C. (1986). Phenotype-associated changes in the effects of 1,25−dihydroxyvitamin $D_3$ on alkaline phosphatase and bone GLA protein of rat osteoblastic cells. *Endocrinology*, **118**: 1340.

Starcher, B. C., Hill, C. H., and Madras, I. G. (1980). Effect of zinc deficiency on bone collagenase and collagen turnover. *J. Nutr.*, **110**: 2095.

Stashenko, P., Dewhirst, R. D., Rooney, M. L., Desjardins, L. A., and Heeley, J. D. (1987). Interleukin-lb is a potentent inhibitor of bone formation *in vitro*. *J. Bone Min. Res.*, **2**: 559.

Stauffer, M., Baylink, D., Wergedal, J., and Rich, C. (1972). Bone repletion in calcium deficient rats fed a high calcium diet. *Calcif. Tissue Res.*, **9**: 163.

Stepan, J. J., Presl. J., Broulik, P., and Pacovsky, V. (1987). Serum osteocalcin levels and alkaline phosphatase isoenzyme after oophorectomy and in primary hyperparathyroidism. *J. Clin. Endocrinol. Metab.*, **64**: 1079.

Stern, P. H., and Raisz, L. G. (1979). Organ culture of bone. In: Simmons, D. J. and A. S. Kunin (eds). *Skeletal Research- An Experimental Approach.* Academic Press Inc., N.Y., pp. 21.

Stern, P. J., Bruno, L. P., and Hopson, C. N. (1985). Skeletal deformities after burn injuries. An animal model. *Trans. Orthop. Res. Soc.*, **10**: 175.

Storey, E. (1961). Strontium "rickets": Bone calcium and strontium changes. *Australasian Ann. Med.*, **10**: 213.

Stromqvist, B. (1985). Scintimetric evaluation of bone metabolism. *Acta Orthop. Scand.*, **56**: 174.

Stronski, S. A., Bettschen-Camin, L., Wetterwald, A., Felix, R., Trechsel, U., and Fleisch, H. (1988). Bisphosphonates inhibit 1,25−dihydroxyvitamin $D_3$−induced increase of osteocalcin in plasma of rats *in vivo* and in culture medium of rat calvaria *in vitro*. *Calcif. Tissue Int.*, **42**: 248.

Sudo, H., Kodama, H.-A., Amagai, Y., Yamamoto, S., and Kasai, S. (1983). *In vitro* differentiation and calcification in a new clonal osteogenic cell line derived from newborn mouse calvaria. *J. Cell Biol.*, **96**: 191.

Suttie, J. M., P. F. Fennessie, P. D. Gluckman and I. D. Corson. (1988). Elevated plasma IGF-1 levels in stage prevented from growing antlers. *Endocrinol.* **122**: 3005−3006.

Syftestad, G. T., and Urist, M. R. (1982). Bone aging. *Clin. Orthop. & Rel. Res.*, **162**: 288.

Tabuchi, C., Simmons, D. J., Fausto, A., Russell, J. E., Binderman, I., and Avioli, L. V. (1986). The bone deficit in ovariectomized rats: the functional contribution of the marrow stromal cell population and the effect of oral dihydrotachysterol treatment. *J. Clin. Invest.*, **78**: 637.

Takagi, M., Parmley, R. T., and Denys, F. R. (1981). Endocytic activity and ultrastructural cytochemistry of lysosome-related organelles in epiphyseal chondrocytes. *J. Ultrastr. Res.*, **74**: 69.

Takahashi, H., Epker, B., and Frost, H. M. (1965). Relation between age and size of osteons in man. *Henry Ford Hosp. Bull.*, **13**: 25.

Takahashi, T., Kurihara, N., Takahashi, K., and Kumegawa, M. (1986). An ultrastructural study of phagocytosis in bone by osteoblastic cells; from fetal mouse calvaria *in vitro*. *Arch. oral Biol.*, **31**: 703.

Talmage, R. V. (1969). Calcium homeostasis − calcium transport − parathyroid action. *Clin. Orthop. & Rel. Res.*, **67**: 210.

Talmage, R. V. (1970). Morphological and physiological considerations in a new concept of calcium transport in bone. *Am. J. Anat.*, **129**: 467.

Talmage, R. V., Cooper, C. W., and Toverud, S. U. (1983). The physiological significance of calcitonin. In: Peck, W. A. (ed). *Bone and Mineral Research*, Vol. 1, p. 74.

Talmage, R. V., Stinnett, S. S., Landwehr, J. T., Vincent, L. M., and McCartney, W. H. (1986). Age-related loss of bone mineral density in non-athletic and athletic women. *Bone and Mineral*, **1**: 115.

Tam, C. S., Harrison, J. E., and Cruikshank, B. (1978). Bone apposition rate as an index of bone metabolism. *Metabolism*, **27**: 143.

Tashjian A. H. Jr., Voelkel, E. F., McDonough, J., and Levine, L. (1975). Hydrocortisone inhibits prostaglandin production by mouse fibrosarcoma cells. *Nature*, **258**: 739.

Tashjian, A. H., and Levine, L. (1978). Epidermal growth factor stimulates prostaglandin production and bone resorption in cultured mouse calvaria. *Biochem Biophys. Res. Commun.*, **85**: 966.

Tashjian, A. H., E. F. Voelkel, M. Lazzars, F. R. Singer, A. B. Roberts, R. Derynck, M. E. Winkler, and L. Levine. (1985). Alpha and beta human transforming growth factors stimulate prostaglandin production and bone resorption in cultured mouse calvaria. *Proc. Natl. Acad. Sci. U.S.A.* **82**: 4535−4538.

Tatakis, D. N., Schneeberger, G., and Dziak, R. (1988). Recombinant interleukin-l stimulates prostaglandin $E_2$ production by osteoblastic cells: synergy with parathyroid hormone. *Calcif. Tissue Int.*, **42**: 358.

Ten Cate, A. R., and Deporter, D. A. (1974). The role of the fibroblast in collagen turnover in the functioning periodontal ligament of the mouse. *Arch. Oral Biol.*, **19**: 339.

Termine, J. D., and Posner, A. S. (1967). Amorphous/crystalline interrelationships in bone mineral. *Calcif. Tissue Res.*, **1**: 8.

Termine, J. D., Kleinman, H. K., Whitson, S. W., Conn, K. M., McGarvey, M. L., and Martin, G. R. (1981). Osteonectin, a bone-specific protein linking mineral to collagen. *Cell*, **26**: 99.

Thesleff, I, T. Kantomaa, E. Mackie and R. Chiquet-Ehrismann. (1988). Immunohisto-chemical localization of the matrix glycoprotein tenascin in the skull of the growing rat. *Arch. oral Biol.* **33**: 383–390.

Thomsen, K., Riis, B., and Christiansen, C. (1986). Effect of estrogen/gestagen and 24R,25– dihydroxyvitamin $D_3$ therapy on bone formation in postmenopausal women. *J. Bone Min. Res.*, **1**: 503.

Tomson, M. B., and Nancollas, G. H. (1978). Mineralization kinetics: a constant composition approach. *Science, 200*: 1059.

Tondevold, E., and Eliasen, P. (1982). Blood flow rates in canine cortical and cancellous bone measured with $^{99}Tc^m$-labelled human albumin microspheres. *Acta Orthop. Scand.*, **53**: 7.

Tonna, E. A. (1958). Histologic and histochemical studies on the periosteum of male and female rats at different ages. *J. Gerontol.*, **13**: 14.

Tonna, E. A. (1961). The cellular complement of the skeletal system studied autoradio-graphically during growth and aging. *J. Biophys. Biochem. Cytol.*, **9**: 813.

Tonna, E. A. (1975). Electron microscopy of aging skeletal cells. III. The periosteum. *Lab. Invest.*, **31**: 609.

Tonna, E.A. (1976). Topographic labelling method using [$^3$H]-proline autoradiography in assessing of ageing paradontal bone in the mouse. *Arch. Oral Biol.*, **21**: 729.

Tonna, E. A. (1979). Bone tracers: cell and tissue level techniques. In: Simmons, D. J. and A. S. Kunin (eds.). Skeletal Research-An Experimental Approach. *Academic Press Inc., N.Y.,* pp. 487.

Tonna, E. A. (1985). Aging of the skeletal system and supporting tissue. In: Cristofalo, V. J. (ed.). *Handbook of Cell Biology and Aging.* CRC Press, Boca Raton, FL, p. 195.

Tonna, E. A., and Cronkite, E. P. (1962). Changes in the skeletal cell proliferative response to trauma concomitant with aging. *J. Bone Joint Surg.*, **44A**: 1557.

Tonna, E. A., and Lampen, N. (1972). Electron microscopy of aging skeletal cells. I. Centrioles and solitary cilia. *J. Gerontol.*, **27**: 316.

Tonna, E. A., and Pillsbury, N. (1959). Mitochondrial changes associated with aging of periosteal osteoblasts. *Anat. Rec.*, **134**: 739.

Tonna, E. A., and Severson, A. R. (1971). Changes in localization and distribution of adenosine triphosphatase activity in skeletal tissues of the mouse concomitant with aging. *J. Gerontol.*, **26**: 186.

Tonna, E. A., Singh, I. J., and Sandhu, H. S. (1987). Autoradiographic investigation of circadian rhythms in alveolar bone periosteum and cementum in young mice. *Histol. Histopath.*, **2**: 129.

Tothill, P., Hooper, G., McCarthy, I. D., and Hughes, S. P. F. (1985). The variation with flow-rate of the extraction of bone-seeking tracers in recirculation experiments. *Calcif. Tissue Int.*, **37**: 312.

Triffitt, J. T. (1987). The special proteins of bone tissue. *Clin. Sci.*, **72**: 399.

Triffitt, J. T., Terepka, A. R., and Neuman, E. F. (1968). A comparative study of exchange *in vivo* of major constituents of bone mineral. *Calc. Tissue Res.*, **2**: 165.

Triffitt, J. T., Gebauer, U., Ashton, B. A., Owen, M., and Reynolds, J. J. (1976). Origin of plasma $a_2HS$- glycoprotein and its accumulation in bone. *Nature*, **262**: 226.

Triffitt, J. T., Owen, M. E., Ashton, B. A., and Wilson, J. M. (1978). Plasma disappearance of rabbit α₂HS-glycoprotein and its uptake by bone tissue. *Calcif. Tissue Res.*, **26**: 155.

Trueta, J., and Caladias, A. N. (1984). A study of the blood supply of long bones. *Surg. Gynecol. Obstet.*, **118**: 485.

Tsutsumi, C., Kakuta, K., Hosoya, N., Orimo, H., Hoshiba, K., and Moriuchi, S. (1987). Bone γ-carboxyglutamic acid-containing protein (BGP)-induced changes in chick embryonic calvaria *in vitro J. Nutr. Sci. Vitaminol.*, **33**: 157.

Turner, R. T., Vandersteenhoven, J. J., and Bell, N. H. (1987). The effects of ovariectomy and 17β-estradiol on cortical bone histomorphometry in growing rats. *J. Bone Min. Res.*, **2**: 115.

Uchida, A., T. Kikuchi, and Y. Shimomura. (1988). Osteogenic capacity of cultured human periosteal cells. *Acta Orthop. Scand.* **59**: 29−33.

Ueda, K., Saito, A., Nakano, H., Aoshima, M., Yakota, M., Muraoka, R., and Iwaya, T. (1980). Cortical hyperostosis following long-term administration of prostaglandin E in infants with cyanotic congenital heart disease. *J. Pediatrics*, **97**: 834.

Ueno, K., Haba, T., Woodbury, D., Price, R., Anderson, R., and Jee, W. S. S. (1985). The effects of prostaglandin E₂ in rapidly growing rats: depressed longitudinal and radial growth and increased metaphyseal hard tissue mass. *Bone*, **6**: 79.

Urist, M. R., DeLange, R. J., and Finerman, G. A. M. (1983). Bone cell differentiation and growth factors. *Science*, **220**: 680.

Vaes, G. M., and Nichols Jr., G. (1962). Metabolism of glycine-1-C¹⁴ by bone *in vitro*: Effects of hormones and other factors. *Endocrinology*, **70**: 890.

Vaes, G., Eeckhout, Y., and Druetz, J. E. (1976). A latent neutral protease released by bone in culture. *Arch. Int. Physiologie Biochimie*, **84**: 666.

Valk, I. M., Chabloz, A. M. E. L., and Van Gilst, W. (1983). Intradaily variation of the human lower leg length and short term growth − a longitudinal study in fourteen children. *Growth XLVII*: 397.

VanGerven, D. P., Armelagos, G. J., and Bartley, M. H. (1969). Roengenographic and direct measurement of femoral cortical involution in a prehistoric Mississippian population. *Am. J. Phys. Anthrop.*, **31**: 23.

VanGerven, D. P., and Armelagos, G. J. (1970). Cortical involution in prehistoric Mississippian femoral. *J. Gerontol.*, **25**: 20.

VanWinkle, B. A., and Neustein, J. (1987). Management of open fractures with sterilization of large, contaminated, extruded cortical fragments. *Clin. Orthop. & Rel. Res.*, **223**: 275.

Vanderhoeft, P. J., Kelly, P. J., Janes, J. M., and Peterson, L. F. A. (1963). Growth and structure of bone distal to an arteriovenous fistula: quantitative analysis of tetracycline-induced transverse growth patterns. *J. Bone Joint Surg.*, **45B**: 582.

Vassilopoulou-Sellin, R., Lock, R. L., II, Oyedeji, C. O., and Saman, N. A. (1987). Cartilage sulfation inhibitor from rat liver curtails growth of embryonic chicken cartilage. *Metabolism*, **36**: 89.

Vater, C. A., Harris Jr., E. D., and Siegel, R. C. (1979). Native cross-links in collagen fibrils induce resistance to human synovial collagenase. *Biochem J.*, **181**: 639.

Vedi, S., Compston, J. E., Webb, A., and Tighe, J. R. (1983). Histomorphometric analysis of dynamic parameters of trabecular bone formation in the iliac crest of normal British subjects. *Metab. Bone Dis. & Rel. Res.*, **5**: 69.

Venencie, P. Y., G. A. Boffa, P. D. Delmas, O. Verola, I. Benkaidali, J. Frija, B. Pillet and A Puissant. (1988). Pachydermoperiostosis with gastric hypertrophy, anemia, and increased serum bone Gla-protein levels. *Arch. Dermatol.* **124**: 1813−1834.

Vermeer, C. (1984). The binding of Gla-containing proteins to phospholipids. *FEBS Letters*, **173**: 169.

Vigorita, V. J., and Suda, M. K. (1983). The microscopic morphology of fluoride-induced bone. *Clin. Orthop. & Rel. Res.*, **177**: 274.

Vilmann, H. (1968). The growth of the parietal bone in the albino rat studied by roentgenoce-phalometry and vital staining. *Arch. Oral Biol.*, **13**: 887.

Vilmann, H. (1969). The *in vivo* staining of bone with alizarin red *S. J. Anat.*, **105**: 533.

Vilmann, H. (1972). The growth of the cranial vault in the albino rat. *Arch. oral Biol.*, **17**: 399.

Vilmann, H. (1976). Growth of the nasal bone in the rat. *Arch. Oral Biol.*, **21**: 623.

Voelkel, D. F., Tashjian Jr., A. H., and Levine, L. (1980). Cyclooxygenase products of arachnidonic acid metabolism by mouse bone in organ culture. *Biochim. Biophys. Acta*, **620**: 418.

Volpi, G., Palazzini, S., Cane, V., Remaggi, F., and Muglia, M. A. Morphometric analysis of osteoblast dynamics in the chick embryo tibia. *Anat. Embryol.*, **162**: 393.

Waite, L. C. (1972). Carbonic anhydrase inhibitors, parathyroid hormone and calcium meta-bolism. *Endocrinol.*, **91**: 1160.

Walker, D. G., Lapiere, C. M., and Gross, J. (1968). A collagenolytic factor in rat bone promoted by parathyroid extract. *Biochem. Biophys. Res. Commun.*, **15**: 397.

Walker, W. V., Russell, J. E., Simmons, D. J., Scheving, L. E., Cornelissen, G., and Halberg, F. (1985). Effect of a synthetic adrenocorticotrophin analogue, ACTH 1–17, on DNA synthesis in murine metaphyseal bone. *Biochem. Pharmacol.*, **34**: 1191.

Wallwork, J., and Sandstead, H. (1989). Zinc nutriture and bone metabolism. In: Simmons, D. J. (ed). *Nutrition and Bone Development*. Oxford University Press, N.Y., (in Press).

Wang, G.-J., Hubbard, S. L., Reger, S. I., Miller, E. D., and Stamp, W. G. (1983). Femoral blood flow in long term steroid therapy: Study of rabbit model. *Southern Med. J.*, **76**: 1530.

Weaks-Dybvig, M., Sanavi, F., Zander, H., and Rifkin, B. R. (1982). The effect of indomethacin on alveolar bone loss in experimental periodontitis. *J. Periodont. Res.*, **17**: 90.

Weatherell, J. A. (1960). Chlorozol fast pink as an *in vivo* stain for unmineralized bone and tooth matrix. *Stain Tech.*, **35**: 139.

Weiner, S., and Price, P. A. (1986). Disaggregation of bone into crystals. *Calcif. Tissue Int.*, **39**: 365.

Weinger, J. M., and Holtrop, M. E. (1974). An ultrastructural study of bone cells. The occurrence of microtubules, microfilaments and tight junctions. *Calcif. Tissue Res.*, **14**: 15.

Weinstein, R. S. and N. H. Bell. Diminished rates of bone formation of normal black adults. *New Engl. J. Med.* **319**: 1698–1701, 1988

Weintroub, S., and Reddi, A. H. (1988). Influence of irradiation on the osteoinductive potential of demineralized bone matrix. *Calcif. Tissue Int.*, **42**: 255.

Weir, E. C., M. Centrella, R. E. Matus, M. L. Brooks, T. Wu and K. L. Insogna. (1988). Adenylate cyclase stimulating, bone resorbing and B TGF-like activities in canine apocrine cell adenocarcinoma of the anal sac. *Calcif. Tissue Int.* **43**: 359–365.

Wellmitz, G., Petzold, E., Jentzch, K. D., Heder, G., and Buntrock, P. (1980). The effect of brain fraction with fibroblast growth factor activity on regeneration and differentiation of articular cartilage. *Exp. Pathol.*, **18**: 282.

Wergedal, J. E., and Baylink, D. J. (1984). Characterization of cells isolated and cultured from human bone. *Proc. Soc. Exp. Biol. Med.*, **176**: 60.

Wergedal, J. E., Farley, J. R., and Baylink, D. J. (1984). Proliferation and phosphatase activities in human bone cells treated with fluoride and skeletal growth factor *in vitro*. *Trans. Orthop. Res. Soc.*, **9**: 38.

Wettenhall, R. E. H., Schwartz, P. L., and Burnstein, J. (1969). Actions of insulin and growth hormone on collagen and chondroitin sulfate synthesis in bone organ cultures. *Diabetes*, **18**: 280.

Wezeman, F. H. (1976). 25–hydroxyvitamin $D_3$: autoradiographic evidence of sites of action in epiphyseal cartilage and bone. *Science*, **194**: 1069.

Whiteside, L. A., and Lesker, P. A. (1978). The effects of extraperiosteal and subperiosteal dissection. *J. Bone Joint Surg.*, **60A**: 26.

Whiteside, L. A., Ogata, K., Lesker, P., and Reynolds, F. C. (1978). Acute effects of periosteal stripping and medullary reaming on regional bone blood flow. *Clin. Orthop. & Rel. Res.*, **131**: 266.

Whitson, S. W. (1972). Tight junction formation in the osteon. *Clin. Orthop. & Rel. Res.*, **86**: 206.

Whitson, S. W., Harrison, W., Dunlap, M. K., Bowers Jr. D. E., Fisher, L. W., Robey, P. G., and Termine, J. D. (1984). Fetal bovine bone cells synthesize bone-specific matrix proteins. *J. Cell Biol.*, **99**: 607.

Wiestner, M., Fischer, S., Dessau, W., and Muller, P. K. (1981). Collagen types synthesized by isolated calvarium cells. *Exp. Cell Res.*, **133**: 115.

Wijngaert, F. P. van der, Tas, M. C., van der Meer, J. W. M., and Burger, E. H. (1987). Growth of osteoclast precursor-like cells from whole mouse bone marrow: Inhibitory effect of CSF-l. *Bone and Mineral*, **3**: 97, (1987).

Williams, D. C., Boder, G. B., Toomey, R. E., Paul, D. C., Hillman, C. C., King, K. L., Van Frank, R. M., and Johnston, C. C. (1980). Mineralization and metabolic response in serially passaged adult rat bone cells. *Calcif. Tissue Int.*, **30**: 233.

Williams, L. T., Antroniades, H. N., and Goetzl, E. J. (1983). Platelet-derived growth fractor stimulates 3T3 cell mitogenesis and leukocyte chemotaxis through different structural determinants. *J. Clin. Invest.*, **72**: 1759.

Wong, G. L. (1982). Characterization of subpopulations of OC and OB bone cells obtained by sedimentation at unit gravity. *Calcif. Tissues Int.*, **34**: 67.

Wong, G. L. (1986). Skeletal effects of parathyroid hormone. In: Peck, W. A.(ed). *Bone and Mineral Research*, Vol. 4, pp. 103.

Wong, G. L., Luben, R. A., and Cohn, D. V. (1977). 1,25-dihydroxycholecalciferol and parathyroid: effects on isolated osteoclast-like and osteoblast-like cells. *Science*, **197**: 663.

Wong, G. L., Roberts, R., and Miller, E. (1987). Production of and response to growth-stimulating activity in isolated bone cells. *J. Bone Min. Res.*, **2**: 23.

Worsfold, M., C. A. Sharp and M. W. J. Davie (1988). Serum osteocalcin and other indices of bone formation: an 8-decade population study in healthy men and women. *Clin. Chim. Acta* **178**: 225.

Wrana, J. L., Maeno, M., Hawrylyshyn, B., Yao, K-L., Domenicucci, C., and Sodek, J. (1988). Differential effects of transforming growth factor-b on the synthesis of extracellular matrix proteins by normal fetal rat calvarial bone cell populations. *J. Cell Biol.*, **106**: 915.

Wrobel, J. (1983). Diurnal variations of calcium transport in the small intestine of adrenalectomized, nephrectomized and vitamin D-treated rats. *Calcif Tissue Int.*, **35**: 352.

Wronski, T. J., Smith, J. M., and Jee, W. S. S. (1981). Variations in mineral apposition rate of trabecular bone within the beagle skeleton. *Calcif. Tissue Int.*, **33**: 583.

Wronski, T. J., Lowry, P. L., Walsh, C. C., and Ignaszewski, L. A. (1986). Skeletal alterations in ovariectomized rats. *Calcif. Tissue Int.*, **37**: 324.

Wronski, T. J., Walsh, C. C., and Ignaszewski, L. A. (1987a). Histologic evidence for osteopenia and increased bone turnover in ovariectomized rats. *Bone*, **7**: 119.

Wronski, T. J., Cintron, M., and Dann, L. M. (1987b). Temporal variations in bone turnover in ovariectomized rats. *J. Bone Min. Res.*, **2** (Suppl. 1): Abstract 472.

Wronski, T. J., Dann L. M. and Horner. S. L. (1989). Time course of vertebral osteopenia in ovariectomized rats. *Calcif. Tissues Int.* (In press).

Wu, K., Schubeck, K. E., Frost, H. M., and Villanueva, A. R. (1970). Haversian bone formation rates determined by a new method in a mastodon and in human diabetes mellitus and osteoporosis. *Calcif. Tissue Res.*, **6**: 204.

Wuthier, R. E., Linder, R. E., Warner, L. P., Gore, S. T., and Borg, T. K., (1978). Non-enzymatic isolation of matrix vesicles: characteristics and initial studies on $^{45}$Ca and $^{32}$P-orthophosphate metabolism. *Metab. Bone Dis. & Rel. Res.*, **1**: 125.

Yajima, M., Okano, K., Yamada, Y., Fujibayashi, S., Suzuki, S., Naito, S., Sasagawa, K., Ohira, K., Nawa, C., Kou, S., Sekita, N., and Someya, K. (1988). Effects of various cell growth factors and cyclosporin A on cloned osteoblastic cell line MC3T3—El cells. *Calcif. Tissue Int.*, **42** (Suppl.): A27 (Abstract 106).

Yamaguchi, M., Oishi, H., and Suketa, Y. (1987). Stimulatory effects of zinc on bone formation in tissue culture. *Biochem. Pharmacol.*, **36**: 4007.

Yamoaka, K., Marion, S. L., Gallegos, A., and Haussler, M. R. (1986). 1,25-dihydroxyvitamin $D_3$ enhances the growth of tumors in athymic mice inoculated with receptor rich osteosarcoma cells. *Biochem. Biophys. Res. Commun.*, **139**: 1292.

Yee, J. A. (1983). Properties of osteoblast-like cells isolated from the cortical endosteal surface of adult rabbits. *Calcif. Tissue Int.*, **35**: 571.

Yee, J. A. (1985). Stimulation of alkaline phosphatase activity in cultured neonatal mouse calvarial bone cells by parathyroid hormone. *Calcif. Tissue Int.*, **37**: 530.

Yeh, C. K., and Rodan, G. A. (1984). Tensile forces enhance prostaglandin-E synthesis in osteoblastic cells grown on collagen ribbons. *Calcif. Tissue Int.*, **36**: 567.

Yonaga, T., and Morimoto, S. (1979). A calcitonin-like action of prostaglandin $E_1$. *Prostaglandins*, **17**: 801.

Yoon, K., Buenaga, R., and Rodan, G. A. (1987). Tissue specificity and developmental expression of rat osteopontin. *Biochem. Biophys. Res. Commun.*, **148 (3)**: 1129.

Yoon, K., S. J. C. Rutledge, R. F. Buenaga and G. A. Rodan (1988) Characterization of the rat osteocalcin gene: stimulation of a promoter activity by 1,25-dihydroxyvitamin $D_3$. *Biochemistry* **27**: 8521.

Yoshikawa, K. (1971). Histochemical and autoradiographic study of osteolathyrism in skeletal and periodontal tissues. *Acta Histochem. Cytochem.*, **4**: 11.

Yoshioka, T., Sato, B., Matsumoto, K., and Ono, K. (1980). Steroid receptors in osteoblasts. *Clin. Orthop. & Rel. Res.*, **148**: 297.

Young. R. W., (1962). Cell proliferation and specialization during endochondral osteogenesis in young rats. *J. Cell Biol.* **14**: 357–370.

Yu, J.-H., Wells, H., Ryan Jr. W. J., and Lloyd, W. S. (1976). Effects of prostaglandns and other drugs on the cyclic AMP content of cultured bone cells. *Prostaglandins*, **12**: 501.

# 7

# Mechanisms of Bone Formation *In Vitro*

## P. J. NIJWEIDE
*Laboratory for Cell Biology and Histology,*
*University of Leiden, Medical Faculty,*
*Leiden, The Netherlands*


*AND*


## E. H. BURGER
*Department of Oral Cell Biology,*
*Academic Center of Dentistry ACTA,*
*Vrije Universiteit, HV Amsterdam,*
*The Netherlands*

General introduction
Organ and tissue culture of bone
    Introduction
    The long bone system
    The calvarium system
    Periosteal tissue
Culture of isolated bone cells
Culture conditions
    The medium
    The gasphase
Osteogenesis in vitro
    Introduction
    Bone matrix formation and calcification in tissue and organ culture

## General Introduction

Tissue culture in its most general sense, comprising cell, tissue and organ culture, is about 100 years old. In the early years roughly between 1880 and 1920 the circumstances under which cells could be kept alive outside the body were tested by investigators such as Roux, Harrison, Burrows, Carrel and others (Witkowski, 1986). After 1920 culture methods became more and more sophisticated, permitting cell proliferation and cell differentiation *in vitro*.

The field of bone research was, surprisingly, one of the first areas where culture systems were used to investigate developmental, metabolic, endo-crinological etc. processes. 60 years ago Fell (1928) introduced organ culture as a method to study embryonic development. To this day her methods for organ, tissue and even cell culture (Fell, 1932) are used to answer a wide variety of questions. The major additions to the culture methods of the '20's and '30's concern the use of better defined media, the development of various cell isolation procedures and the use of (tumor) cell lines. The foundation however was already firmly established.

Organ culture proved to be preeminently suitable to investigate the action of vitamins and hormones on bone. Gaillard was one of the first investigators to demonstrate the direct action of a diffusible product from cocultured parathyroid tissue (Gaillard, 1955) and later of parathyroid extract (Gaillard, 1960) on bone tissue in culture. These studies were followed by an increasing number of similar studies by Gaillard and by other investigators with numerous other hormones, vitamins and factors. Soon, however, even organ culture was found to be too complex a system to define the precise actions of culture additives such as hormones. This led to the development of bone cell cultures (Peck *et al.*, 1964). Complete osteo-genesis, i.e. bone matrix formation and calcification, however, proved more difficult in cell cultures in comparison with organ cultures. Nevertheless, in the last decade, several bone cell culture systems which allow bone formation have been described (see Chapter 5).

## Organ and Tissue Culture of Bone

### Introduction

Since the introduction of culture methods in bone research, two organ culture systems have mainly been used: the calvarium and the long bone system. To a lesser extent, but for *in vitro* osteogenesis studies perhaps as important, periosteal tissue dissected from long bones or calvaria has also been used. Calvaria, limb bones or periostea from, generally, fetal or neonatal chick, mouse or rat are dissected and explanted on/in a semisolid or fluid medium. All three systems have their advantages and disadvantages. The cellular composition of the calvarium, provided that the chondrocranium is not included, is less complicated than that of the long bone rudiment and is therefore more suitable for metabolic studies. Formation and activity of, and, especially, interrelation between the various tissues responsible for bone formation, modeling and remodeling, are better studied in long bones. In long bones growth plate cartilage, intramembranous and endochondral bone, periosteum and bone marrow are intricately related. Long bone cultures are therefore more suitable for developmental studies requiring, often sophisticated, histological, (immuno) histochemical or autoradiographical methods.

Periosteal tissue has been found to be very appropriate to study the initiation of osteoblast differentiation and osteogenesis *in vitro*. It provides the link between organ and cell culture.

### The Long Bone System

The long bone system was introduced by Fell and associates (Fell, 1928; Fell and Robison, 1929). They showed for the first time that very early mesenchymal limb bud anlagen, from the chick embryo, could be induced to develop and differentiate into cartilagenous long bones showing all the different stages of cartilage and bone cell differentiation and the formation of calcified bone (for a review see Fell, 1956). Since that time the embryonic and fetal development of chick long bone, *in vivo* and *in vitro*, has been extensively described (for a review see Caplan and Pechak, 1987). The development of the chick embryo has been subdivided by Hamburger and Hamilton (1951) into a number of more of less discrete stages describing the successive events in long bone development (Caplan and Pechak, 1987). This system makes it possible to study organogenesis, including osteogenesis, *in vitro* starting from defined developmental stages, and to monitor the influences of external circumstances on these processes.

However, if the results obtained with *in vitro* cultures are to be extrapolated to humans, the use of chick bone has a drawback. Avian long bone organogenesis is clearly different from that in mammals (Hall, 1987). In the chick embryo, initial mineralisation of the primitive bone collar occurs without concurrent mineralisation of cartilage and unlike mammalian osteoclasts, avian osteoclasts resorb uncalcified cartilage matrix during the formation of the primitive marrow cavity (Silvestrini, 1979; Caplan *et al.*, 1983). Furthermore, the actual formation of a marrow cavity in chick long bones is difficult to attain in culture (Gaillard *et al.*, 1979). These and other considerations prompted many investigators to turn to fetal long bones of mammalian origin, notably mouse and rat (Fig. 1) Fell and Mellanby, 1952; Gaillard, 1960; Raisz and Niemann, 1969). Since their introduction, mouse and rat long bones have been used in numerous studies. Most of these, however, concern bone resorption, not bone formation.

## The Calvarium System

In 1955 Gaillard showed that parathyroid tissue secreted product(s) *in vitro* which stimulated resorption in cocultured fragments of fetal mouse calvaria. After this publication many investigators used the calvarium system, either calvarium halves or fragments dissected from the parietal bones. Again mouse, rat and chick are the most commonly used experimental animals. Apart from the comparatively simple cellular composition, ease of dissection and handling are advantages in using calvaria. Furthermore, calvaria of near-term, fetal animals contain enough calcium to monitor resorption via the release of calcium ions into the culture medium (Heersche, 1969). Indeed the calvarium system has proved to be a very sensitive *in vitro* system for the study of resorption and its (hormonal) regulation (Stern and Krieger, 1983).

Only very few studies are available in which the intramembranous ossification of the calvarium has been investigated (Marvaso and Bernard, 1977; Klein Nulend *et al.*, 1987). Over the last 20 years calvaria from fetal or neonatal mice, rats and chicks have been used extensively as sources of enzymatically isolated bone cells (see Chapter 5).

## Periosteal Tissue

One of the methods of choice to study osteogenesis *in vitro* is the culture of periosteal tissue. The advantages are obvious. The process of *de novo* bone formation can be studied separate from interfering resorption. As a tissue, the periosteum offers the three dimensional structure needed for a regular bone formation pattern, which is often missing in cell cultures. The method

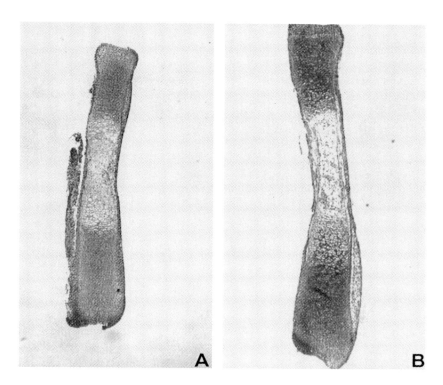

**Fig. 1** A. Non-cultured radius of 15-day-old fetal mouse.
B. Similar radius after two days of culture. Note the longitudinal growth and the formation of a marrow cavity surrounded by a bone collar. Staining azur-eosin, magnification 40 X.

was initiated by Fell (1932). She studied the osteogenic capacity of the periosteum dissected from limb bones of embryonic chicks at different stages of development. Periosteal tissue from 6–10 days old embryos formed bone in most explants. Readily recognizable osteoblasts were present in the cultures after 2–4 days. Well developed osteoid matrix was present around day 7, and calcifications could be shown around day 12. In some cases cartilage nodules were also formed. Periosteum from late embryos or young chicks was less osteogenic, probably as a result of damage to the osteogenic layer during its removal from the bone surface. The periosteum at that development stage is tough and rather firmly attached to the bone. Mechanical damage to the osteoblast and preosteoblast layers might easily result from stripping off the periosteum (Fell, 1932).

Many years later the culture of periosteal tissue was reintroduced. Periostea of 17–18 day-old fetal chick calvaria, folded double with the osteogenic layer inside, formed a layer of osteoid bordered by newly differentiated osteoblasts within 2–6 days (Fig 2; Nijweide, 1975). The osteoid calcified readily upon addition of 5–10 mM β-glycerophosphate to the culture medium (Tenenbaum and Heersche, 1982). The ultrastructure of the bone formed *in vitro* was virtually identical to bone formed *in vivo* (Tenenbaum *et al.*, 1986b). Generally, osteoid formation and calcification only occur in the center of the explant, i.e. in the fold. Tenenbaum and Heersche (1986) however, showed that osteogenesis also took place at the originally bone-facing side of an unfolded periosteum, cultured with that side facing upwards. They suggested that limiting the diffusion of locally produced factors creates a suitable microenvironment for osteo-differentiation (see Chapter 2). Although the culture of periosteal tissue shows promising results, until now not much use has been made of the method. The fact that it is fairly difficult to remove the periosteum more or less intact from fetal mammalian bone may be one of the more important reasons for this.

## Culture of Isolated Bone Cells

Peck and coworkers (1964) initiated the use of bone cell cultures. They isolated cells from frontal and parietal bones of fetal or neonatal rat calvaria by collagenase digestion of the surrounding uncalcified matrix. The isolated cells were viable and proliferated during culture. The authors immediately recognized, however, the problem of identification of the cells in culture. Although the cultured cells possessed alkaline phosphatase activity (an osteoblast marker) their nature could not be unambiguously defined. Several groups have tried to isolate more defined and homogeneous cell populations. Cohn and coworkers (Wong and Cohn, 1974; 1975; Luben *et al.*, 1976; Boonekamp *et al.*, 1984) isolated osteoblast enriched populations by sequential digestion of mouse calvaria (see Chapter 5). Their rationale was to remove the outer layers of the periosteum by successive collagenase treatments. The osteoblasts would then be liberated in the later digests. Although their efforts succeeded in increasing the osteoblastic nature of their osteoblast-like (PT) cell populations (Wong and Cohn, 1974; Luben *et al.*, 1976), the

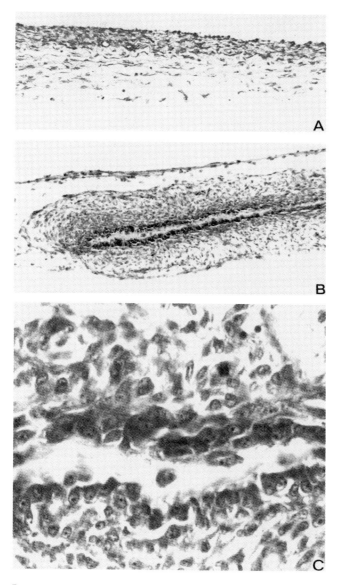

**Fig. 2**  A. Periosteum dissected from the calvarium of a 18-day-old fetal chick cultured
unfolded for 3 days. Magnification 90 ×. B. Similar periosteum cultured folded
double with the osteogenic layer inside. Note the formation of two rows of
basophilic osteoblasts, with osteoid in between, in the center of the culture.
Magnification 90 ×. C. Detail of the osteogenic center of a double folded, cultured
periosteum. Magnification 600 ×. Azur-eosin staining.

populations were clearly not free from other cell types such as osteoclast precursors (Burger *et al.*, 1986; Jilka, 1986). Wong (1982) and Wong & Kocour (1983) have devised a number of additional cell separation techniques to increase the homogeneity of the populations but they apparently had only limited success.

Other investigators have tried to improve the osteoblastic character of their bone cell populations by removing the fibroblastic outer periosteum before isolating the cells from the surface of the calvarium using enzymatic digestion (Yagiela and Woodbury, 1977; Nijweide *et al.*, 1981). This method proved valid in so far as two populations (Nijweide *et al.* 1981) were obtained one of which (OB) was still osteogenic after prolonged culture times, while the other (PF, isolated from the dissected outer periosteum) was not (Nijweide *et al.*, 1982a). An isolation technique which avoids the use of enzymes was proposed by Ecarot-Charrier *et al.* (1983). The method involved placing glass fragments on the endocranial surface of neonatal mouse calvaria after the removal of the outer periosteum. Osteoblasts migrated from the bone onto the glass fragments (Jones and Boyde, 1977) and subsequently, when the glass fragments were seeded in culture dishes, from the glass onto the bottom of the dishes. The isolated cells showed high levels of type I collagen synthesis. In the presence of 10 mM β-glycerophosphate, the collagen matrix calcified during culture. The pattern of mineralisation closely resembled that seen *in vivo*.

Recently, Beresford *et al.* (1983) have reported on the isolation of human bone cells. They dissected trabecular fragments from human bone obtained at surgery or biopsy. The fragments were cut into small particles, washed intensively to remove marrow cells, and seeded into culture dishes. The cell outgrowth was cultured until confluency was obtained, replated and used for various studies. The cell cultures possessed several osteoblastic characteristics such as responsiveness to calcium-regulating hormones, ability to synthesize type I collagen and osteocalcin (Beresford *et al.*, 1984), but were heterogeneous in several respects. An attempt to improve the homogeneity with a technique of aqueous two-phase partition was apparently not successful (Sharpe *et al.*, 1984). Furthermore, the osteogenic potential of the cells could not be established in an *in vivo* diffusion chamber assay (Ashton *et al.*, 1985).

Gehron Robey and Termine (1985) adapted the method described above. They treated the bone fragments with collagenase for two hours to remove more thoroughly all marrow and loosely adhering cells. After many weeks of culture in a low calcium medium (Binderman and Somjen, 1982) the outgrowing cells were able to produce and calcify matrix in the presence of 10 mM β-glycerophosphate. The idea of establishing cultures of endosteal osteoblasts by outgrowth of cells from bone fragments was introduced by

Fell (1932). She explanted fragments of late fetal or neonatal chick bones, thoroughly cleaned of superficially adherent cells, and observed outgrowth of cells from cavities within the bone which were capable of matrix formation and calcification.

The method of isolating and culturing endosteal osteoblast-like cells has a number of advantages compared to the fetal or neonatal calvarium cell systems, one of which is of course the possibility of using (adult) human cells. On the other hand the method is more time consuming, requiring a long culture time (weeks) to establish enough cultures for biochemical assays. Whether the use of adult cells instead of fetal cells is an important advantage has not been clearly established (Williams *et al.*, 1980). Of course, at first sight extrapolation of *in vitro* results to the *in vivo* situation seems more feasible when adult bone cells are used. However, a fully differentiated osteoblast in fetal tissue is not essentially different from an osteoblast in adult tissue. Indeed, many mechanisms involved in embryonic bone organogenesis are reiterated during fracture healing of adult bone (see Volume 7). This question deserves closer attention in future research. Several authors have stressed the importance of isolating bone cells without using enzymatic digestion procedures (Smith and Johnston, 1974; Ecarot-Charrier *et al.*, 1983; Gehron Robey and Termine, 1985). There is, however, no convincing evidence that collagenase treatment has a detrimental effect on the osteoblast phenotypic expression. Osteogenic potential has been shown in both collagenase- and non-collagenase-isolated bone cells (Nefusi *et al.*, 1985).

Yet another approach to the study of osteogenesis in cell cultures was used by Osdoby and Caplan (1976; 1979; 1980). They isolated limb bud mesenchymal cells from chick embryos at different stages of development (Hamburger and Hamilton, 1951). Cells isolated from early stages could differentiate, *in vitro*, into various cell types (chondrocytes, myocytes, osteoblasts) and could be manipulated in their differentiation direction by e.g. changes in seeding density. Between stages 24 and 28 cells became committed, some of them to the osteogenic cell lineage.

In addition to bone tissue or its mesenchymal anlage, potentially osteogenic cells are also present in adult bone marrow (Friedenstein, 1976; Owen, 1985). The isolation of these cells is relatively easy. Bone marrow cells dissociated after gentle mechanical disruption, can be seeded in low concentrations to ensure clonal growth of the fibroblastic cells (Friedenstein, 1976; 1980). Within two weeks the majority of the hemopoietic cells die and separate fibroblastic colonies are visible (Ashton *et al.*, 1980). Originally, the osteogenic character of the stromal fibroblasts was established by grafting clones of stromal fibroblasts under the renal capsule of syngeneic recipients (Friendenstein, 1980) or by implantation into diffusion chambers *in vivo*

(Ashton *et al.*, 1980). More recently, several reports have described bone formation and calcification *in vitro* (Tibone and Bernard, 1982; Howlett *et al.*, 1986; Luria *et al.*, 1987). In contrast to bone cells enzymatically isolated from fetal tissues, stromal cells have not been extensively used in biochemical and endocrinological studies. A serious drawback of the bone marrow culture system is its extreme heterogeneity.

One of the major advances in the study of the cell biology of bone in recent years, has been the development of osteoblastic cell lines by several research groups. These cell lines are either tumor derived, such as the rat osteosarcoma cell lines UMR (Partridge *et al.*, 1981) and ROS (Majeska *et al.*, 1983), or clonal lines derived from normal bone such as the mouse calvarial cell lines MC3T3-E1 (Sudo *et al.*, 1983), MMB-1 (Walters *et al.*, 1982) and rat calvarial cell lines (Williams *et al.*, 1980; Aubin *et al.*, 1982). The advantage of using clonal lines of normal or tumor origin as compared to freshly isolated, non-clonal cells, lies in the availability of large numbers of cells, the homogeneity of the cell cultures and the expected invariability of the phenotype. However, in the long run even these clonal cell lines appear unstable to some extent (Heersche *et al.*, 1985; Majeska and Rodan, 1985).

## Culture Conditions

### The Medium

Growth of bone *in vitro* started on the surface of a clot composed of plasma and embryonic extract (Fell, 1928). During the first decades of the development of bone culture, the plasma clot was the method of choice, either the hanging-drop method or the watch-glass method (Fell, 1956). Since then, minor changes have been made, but essentially the plasma clot or semi-solid medium is still being used. Sometimes the plasma is exchanged for agar. The embryonic extract in the clot was not only necessary for solidification of the plasma but also as a stimulator of growth and differentiation. Gaillard (1935) and others (Miszurski, 1939; Miyazaki *et al.*, 1957) observed that press-juice of chick embryos not only promoted growth and differentiation but also that, depending on the age of the chick embryos, one process was favoured above the other. Extracts of early embryos (7 day) primarily promoted proliferation, that of later embryos (13–18 day) promoted differentiation. Gaillard advised using extracts of embryos of increasing age during long-term culture. Considering the increased knowledge we now have on hormones and (growth) factors, it would be interesting to reinvestigate this issue (Mayne *et al.*, 1976).

Apart from plasma and embryonic extract semisolid media (and fluid media) generally contain serum. Freshly made homologous serum is generally to be prefered. For convenience sake, however, new born calf of fetal calf serum is most often used. These sera have the advantage of being commercially available in large batches of uniform quality.

Since the composition of semi-solid medium is undefined an increasing number of investigators have turned to fluid, more or less synthetic, media. Furthermore, the use of a fluid medium has the advantage that samples can be added or removed without disturbing the culture. In most cases fluid medium is composed of a balanced salt solution to which various amino acids, vitamins etc. are added (Biggers *et al.*, 1961; Reynolds, 1972; Burks and Peck, 1978). One of the most important vitamins to be added is ascorbic acid (vitamin C). This vitamin is involved in the production of collagen and is therefore of vital importance to bone matrix formation *in vitro* (Reynolds, 1972). Usually $50-200$ µg/ml are added to culture media, in organ as well as cell cultures. In general, growth, differentiation and especially bone formation are more difficult to attain in completely synthetic media than in media that contain 'natural' components. The synthetic media are therefore almost always enriched with $5-20\%$ serum and sometimes with embryonic extract (Nijweide *et al.*, 1981; 1982a; Osdoby and Caplan, 1979).

## The Gasphase

In the early years of the development of bone tissue culture techniques, the gasphase used was air. At present, most of the available culture media are based on 5% $CO_2$ in air. The higher $CO_2$ tension appears to stimulate both cell proliferation in cell cultures and bone formation and calcification in organ cultures (Nijweide *et al.*, 1982b). The $O_2$ tension is also of importance. However, the various tissues in, for example, long bones have different requirements. Low $O_2$ tension promotes differentiation of cartilage, high tension inhibits chondrocyte maturation but stimulates bone matrix formation and calcification (Basset, 1962; Hall, 1970; Reynolds, 1972; Nijweide *et al.*, 1982b). The importance of sufficient gas exchange is illustrated by the type of cultures that have been and are successfully used for bone and bone cell cultures. Tissue explants are either placed on top of a semi-solid medium, or on a stainless steel grid whose surface is at the same level as the medium, or on a lenspaper floating on top of the medium (Reynolds, 1972; Freshney, 1983). In all three methods the tissue is kept at the interphase between gasphase and fluid to ensure a good exchange. A non-stationary culture method is the rollertube culture in which the explant is alternately taken in and out of the (fluid) culture medium by the circling movement of the rollerdrum (Miyazaki *et al.*, 1957; Freshney, 1983).

If the tissues or isolated cells are cultured on the bottom of a culture dish

**Table I**
Effect of medium volume on calcification (C) and resorption (R) *in vitro.*

| fetal age at explanation | 15 | | 16 | | 17 | |
|---|---|---|---|---|---|---|
| volume | C | R | C | R | C | R |
| 100 µl | ± | − | ND | ND | ND | ND |
| 150 µl | ++ | ++ | ++ | ++ | ++ | ++ |
| 200 µl | ++ | ± | ++ | ++ | ++ | ++ |
| 250 µl | ± | − | ++ | + | ++ | ++ |

Metatarsal bones (n=4) of various fetal ages were cultured in a fluid medium (α MEM, 10% FCS, 10 mM β-glycerophosphate) in wells of a 24 well plate. At explantation 15/16 day-old bones were not calcified and 17 day-old bones had a small calcified area; none of the bones showed any resorption. Calcification and resorption during culture were scored by determination of the length of the calcified area resp. marrow cavity.

++ good, + moderate, ± little, − no calcification/resorption
ND: not done

in stationary culture, the level of the fluid above must be carefully adapted to the cells or tissues cultured. This is illustrated in an experiment in which we compared calcification and resorption in fetal metatarsal bones in a 24-well tissue culture plate (Table I). The amount of fluid and therefore the fluid level required for good calcification and resorption depended very much on the age and size of the explanted bone.

## Osteogenesis *In Vitro*

### Introduction

Osteogenesis is a multistep process. It can be divided into three parts, each of which is in itself of a complex character: 1. proliferation of progenitor and precursor cells, differentiation into active osteoblasts; 2. bone matrix production, i.e. production of collagenous and non-collagenous bone proteins; 3. calcification of bone matrix, i.e. cell regulated concentration and deposition of, primarily, calcium and phosphate at the site of calcification. In spite of extensive research over many years we still know surprisingly little about bone formation and its regulation. One of the reasons for this is that we don't have many, if any, reliable means to stimulate bone formation *in vitro* (or *in vivo*). One often learns a lot about a process by being able to manipulate it. Another obstruction to the understanding of bone formation is the complexity of the process. Bone formation is the result of a long sequence of related events. Interference with any of these events may stop the entire process. Despite these problems, *in vitro* culture studies have helped to increase our understanding and to acquire information about the (hormonal) regulation of specific parts of the process of bone formation. Most of these studies are concerned with the regulation of osteoblastic cell proliferation, alkaline phosphatase activity as a marker for osteoblast differentiation and collagen production as a measure of osteoblast function. (In 1983 Raisz and Kream published an excellent paper on the state of the art on these questions. Chapters 4−6 and 8 in this volume have updated the information).

In this chapter we will restrict ourselves to discussing the conditions, *in vitro*, that allow osteogenesis, including specifically calcification. Collagen production or proline incorporation is a convenient measure but not necessarily an absolute indicator of bone formation. Calcification of bone matrix is pre-eminently so.

## Bone Matrix Formation and Calcification in Tissue and Organ Culture

There is no definite evidence that the mechanisms of bone formation, i.e. matrix formation and calcification, in tissue and organ culture are essentially different from the mechanisms *in vivo*. Light microscopically and electron microscopically, bone formation in organ (e.g. Marvaso and Bernard, 1977; Schwartz *et. al.*, 1985) or tissue (Tenenbaum *et al.*, 1986b; Luria *et al.*, 1987) culture closely resembles bone formation *in vivo* (see Chapter 6). One of the few differences that have been reported is the appearance of a seam of dark staining material (the lamina limitans) around the calcified areas which were already present at the moment of explantation (Scherft, 1978). These laminae are probably formed as a response to the temporary arrest of the calcification process during the dissection and explantation procedures.

Although calcification, when it occurs *in vitro*, appears to be normal, it is often absent or severely slowed down (for review see Stern and Raisz, 1979). Recently, Tenenbaum and Heersche (1982) have shown that the additon of organic phosphate to the culture medium strongly stimulates calcification. Its presence is not needed under optimal culture conditions, but has a beneficial and useful effect in more or less synthetic media (see Chapter 2).

As the biochemical aspects of bone matrix formation *in vivo* are not yet fully understood, the biochemical comparison of *in vitro* with *in vivo* formed bone matrix is very difficult. Histochemical differences have been reported (Mazza *et al.*, 1979). However, in that particular study calcification of *in vitro* formed matrix did not occur. It is difficult therefore to surmise whether the matrix was not calcified because it was abnormal or stained differently because it had not been calcified.

Bone matrix collagen consists almost entirely of type I collagen. Typing of the collagen produced *in vitro* has therefore become one of the biochemical methods mostly used to determine whether bone matrix is produced *in vitro* and whether that matrix is similar to that produced *in vivo*. In addition to collagen, osteoblasts secrete a number of other matrix components, including osteocalcin (Hauschka *et al.*, 1975; Price *et al.*, 1976; Groot *et al.*, 1986), osteonectin (Termine *et al.*, 1981; Jundt *et al.*, 1987) and osteopontin (Prince *et al.*, 1987; Mark *et al.*, 1987a, b). Several of these non-collagenous proteins have now been demonstrated in bone tissue and cell cultures (e.g. Beresford *et al.*, 1984; Whitson *et al.*, 1984; Gehron Robey and Termine, 1985; Bellows *et al.*, 1986; Gerstenfeld *et al.*, 1987). It will be the challenge of future research to establish the precise function of these proteins in the process of bone formation. Biochemical determination of the levels of production *in vitro* will then help us to define the differentiation stage and activities of bone cells in tissue culture.

## Calcification in Cell Cultures

*In situ* and in organ cultures, mature osteoblasts can be recognized histologically, histochemically and recently, immunocytochemically. Osteoblasts have a typical, plumb morphology in the tissue, are basophilic, have high alkaline phosphatase activity on their cell surface and possess receptors for parathyroid hormone (PTH) and 1,25 dihydroxyvitamin $D_3$ (1,25 $(OH)_2D_3$) (for a review see Rodan and Rodan, 1984). Recently, polyclonal and monoclonal antibodies, specific for various osteogenic differentiation stages, have been developed for the mouse, rat and chick (Tsuru *et al.*, 1984; Nijweide and Mulder, 1986; Nijweide *et al.*, 1988). These antibodies may help us in the future to acquire a better understanding of the origin and differentiation of the osteoblast (Owen, 1985; Nijweide *et al.*, 1986). They may also help to define the differentiation status of each individual osteoblast-like cell in cell cultures. Osteoblasts tend to loose some of their specific characteristics *in vitro*, especially when cultured as a monolayer. In cell cultures in which multilayers are formed, osteoblasts often reassume their specific morphology. The osteogenic potential of isolated putative osteoblasts has been demonstrated in many ways. Primary bone marrow stromal cells, but also other types, have been shown to form calcified bone matrix in diffusion chambers implanted *in vivo* (Ashton *et al.*, 1980; Bab *et al.*, 1984; Ashton *et al.*, 1984; Shteyer *et al.*, 1986) or grafted under the renal capsule (Friedenstein, 1980). Osteoblasts isolated from fetal or 20-day-old rat calvaria (Boonekamp *et al.*, 1984) and injected into the posterior tibial muscle of syngeneic rats produced solid blocks of woven and laminar bone within 8 weeks (Moskalewski *et al.*, 1983; Groot *et al.*, 1983). The possibility, although remote, of induction of bone forming cells in the host can be avoided by transplantation on the chorioallantoic membrane of quail eggs (Hamburger, 1942). Host and quail cells are readily recognized in histological sections (Le Douarin, 1973). Osteoblast-like cells isolated from fetal chick calvaria and cultured for 6 days formed trabecular calcified bone on the chorioallantoic membrane within 6 days (Nijweide *et al.*, 1982a).

Binderman *et al.* (1974) were among the first to show calcification in cultures of isolated calvarial cells (rat) in the culture dish. Mineral appeared in the preformed matrix after 8 weeks of culture. Electronmicroscopically, the calcification process resembled calcification *in vivo*. From this publication onwards many investigators have tried to show calcification in cultures of cells of various origin and species. Success was limited however. Many failures were probably attributable to the long culture time needed for calcification and the fact that calcification occurs, perhaps exclusively, in areas surrounded by cells, i.e. in multilayer cultures or multilayer areas of cultures (Osdody and Caplan, 1976; Williams *et al.*, 1980). The need for three dimensional structure for calcification can be demonstrated by scraping together the cells of a non-calcifying monolayer of chicken osteoblasts (Nijweide *et al.*, 1981) and culturing the obtained cell aggregate on a semi-solid coagulum rich in plasma, serum and embryonic extract. Within a few days the preformed matrix in the aggregate calcifies (Fig. 3; Nijweide, unpublished results).

A break through in the study of *in vitro* mineralisation of cell cultures was the introduction of β-glycerophosphate to the culture medium (Tenenbaum and Heersche, 1982). The rationale for the use of β-glycerophosphate is the availability of organic phosphate around cells with a high alkaline phosphatase activity. The addition of β-glycerophosphate to culture media proved very advantagous. Calcification in the presence of organic phosphate has been demonstrated in cultures of osteoblast-like cells isolated from calvaria of fetal chicks (Gerstenfeld *et al.*, 1987), rats (Nefussi *et al.*, 1985; Bellows *et al.*, 1986; Bellows *et al.*, 1987), mice (Ecarot-Charrier *et al.*, 1983) and calf (Whitson *et al.*, 1986). Calcification was also found in cultures of human bone cells (Gehron Robey and Termine, 1985) and cultures of osteoblastic cell line (e.g. Sudo *et. al.*, 1983; Koshihara *et al.*, 1987).

## Regulation of Bone Formation

As already mentioned, bone formation is a complicated multistep process. Each of these steps can be affected or regulated by various hormones or factors. Often the same hormone or factor acts on more than one step,

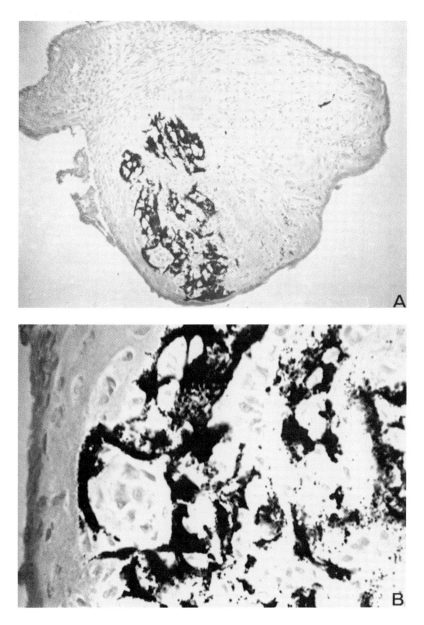

**Fig. 3** A. Osteoblasts isolated from a 18-day-old chick calvarium cultured for 6 days as
monolayer, then scraped together and cultured for an additional three days as a
cell aggregate on a semi-solid medium in the presence of 2 mM glycerophosphate.
Magnification 75 ×. B. Detail, magnification 300 ×. Von Kossa staining.

sometimes with opposite effects or profound differences in time scale (Raisz and Kream, 1983; Heersche, this volume). Besides hormones or (local) growth factors, stretching and pressure forces are perhaps as important for bone formation. There are many examples *in vivo* of the importance of gravitational and muscular stresses for bone formation (e.g. Proc. Kroc Foundation Conference, Calcif. Tissue Int. 36, S1–116, 1984). Development of valid *in vitro* culture systems to address this question has proven difficult. However, a number of methods have now been devised to apply stretching and pressure forces on organ and bone cell cultures. Mechanical stress has been shown to stimulate proliferation (Rodan *et al.*, 1975; Hasegawa *et al.*, 1985) and protein synthesis (Meikle *et al.*, 1979; Hasegawa *et al.*, 1985) in organ and cell cultures of bone. Intermittend pressure especially has profound effects on cell differentiation in bone (Hall, 1968; Copray *et al.*, 1985). In organ cultures of long bone rudiments as well as fetal calvaria, intermittent hydrostatic force stimulated matrix mineralisation (Klein Nulend *et al.*, 1986; 1987). The study of the effects of mechanical stress on bone development and bone formation *in vitro* is still in its infancy but promises to be a fruitful area of research, since mechanical stress is one of the few adjustable factors that appears to stimulate bone formation and calcification. Most hormonal and other regulatory mechanisms are inhibitory.

The benificial effect of organic phosphates is one of the few examples where calcification as a separate process is affected as the effect cannot be traced back to changes in e.g. matrix formation/composition or differentiation status of the bone forming cells. It offers the possibility of reproducible *in vitro* calcification, something that was often absent before its introduction (Tenenbaum and Heersche, 1982). The use of β-glycerophosphate in mineralising culture systems is now widespread. Electronmicroscopical studies of cell and organ culture calcification in the presence of β-glycerophosphate did not find differences with *in vivo* calcification. Still, we have to be careful. β-Glycerophosphate is not physiologically available for calcification. Other organic phosphates may be present in blood or tissue fluid (Tenenbaum *et al.*, 1986a) but their concentration is probably much less that 5–10 mM. High concentrations such as 10 mM β-glycerophosphate have been shown to cause precipitation of calcium phosphate in the medium (Kodama *et al.*, 1986), and to be inhibitory for cell growth (Ashton *et al.*, 1986). In our own experience the concentration of β-glycerophosphate has to be carefully adjusted to the type of culture. Metatarsal bones of 15- or 16-day-old mice, which are not yet calcified at the time of explantation need 10 mM to induce *in vitro* calcification in fluid media. As soon as calcification has started in these bones or when freshly explanted 17-day-old fetal bones are used in which calcification *in vivo* has already started, the concentration of β-glycerophosphate should be decreased to 2 mM and later even to 0,2 mM to avoid abnormal calcification (Nijweide, unpublished results).

## Summary and Conclusions

The study of bone formation using *in vitro* methods started in the early days of tissue culture. In the course of time a large number of *in vitro* systems have been put forward as model systems for the study of bone metabolism. In some of these systems bone formation was described, in a smaller number calcification of the bone matrix. More recently, the isolation and culture of osteoblast-like cells was introduced. Culture of cells freshly isolated from fetal or adult bone or of cells from cell lines, either derived from osteogenic tumors or normal bone, is now common practice.

In most of these cell culture systems matrix formation and calcification have been demonstrated, although the addition of excessive amounts of organic phosphates to the culture medium is almost always required. The precise mode of action of organic phosphate, primarily β-glycerophosphate, has to be established in the near future. A careful and extensive biochemical and microscopical study of this organic phosphate-induced calcification is still lacking. Such a study is urgently needed and should demonstrate whether it represents physiological mineralisation or whether organic phosphate induced calcification merely demonstrates the presence of high alkaline phosphatase activity in the tissue. The study may also deepen our understanding of the process of biomineralisation.

Several new developments promise a sharp increase in interest in and knowledge of, osteogenesis in the coming years. The tissue and cell culture experience acquired over the years has set the stage. The rapidly increasing information about bone specific proteins will enable us to monitor bone formation much better than in the past, when one depended almost solely on collagen type I production. The intricate relation between bone matrix composition and calcification needs to be clarified.

Differentiation within the osteogenic cell line is one of the key processes that govern bone formation. Several groups have begun the production of (monoclonal) antibodies directed against differentiation stage-specific cellular or matrix-derived antigens. Such probes may contribute to our understanding of the diversity of osteogenic phenotype that has been found in cultures of freshly isolated cell populations as well as in cloned cell lines.

## References

Ashton, B. A., Allen, T. D., Howlett, C. R., Eaglesom, C. C.. Hattori, A., and Owen, M. (1980). Formation of bone and cartilage by marrow stromal cells in diffusion chambers *in vivo*. *Clin. Orthop. Rel. Res.*, **151**: 294–307.

Ashton, B. A., Eaglesom, C. C., Bab, I., and Owen, M. E. (1984). Distribution of fibroblastic colony forming cells in rabbit bone marrow and assay of their osteogenic potential by an in vivo diffusion chamber method. *Calcif. Tissue Int.*, **36**: 83−86.

Ashton, B. A., Abdullah, F., Cave, J., Williamson, M., Sykes, B. C., Couch, M., and Poser, J. W. (1985). Characterization of cells with high alkaline phosphatase activity derived from human bone and marrow: preliminary assessment of their osteogenicity. *Bone*, **6**: 313−319.

Ashton, B. A., Couch, M., and Owen, M. (1986). The influence of β-glycerophosphate on human bone derived cells. In: *Cell mediated calcification and matrix vesicles*. S. Y. Ali (ed.). Excerpta Medica, Amsterdam, New York, Oxford, pp. 349−352.

Aubin, J. E., Heersche, J. N. M., Merrilees, M. J., and Sodek, J. (1982). Isolation of bone cell clones with differences in growth, hormone responses, and extra cellular matrix production. *J. Cell Biol.*, **92**: 452−461.

Bab, I., Ashton, B. A., Syftestad, G. T., and Owen, M. E. (1984). Assessment of an *in vivo* diffusion chamber method as a quantitative assay for osteogenesis. *Calcif. Tissue Int.*, **36**: 77−82.

Basset, C. A. L. (1982). Current concepts of bone formation. *J. Bone Joint Surg.*, **44**A: 1217−1244.

Bellows, C. G., Aubin, J. E., Heersche, J. N. M., and Antosz, M. E. (1986). Mineralised bone nodules formed *in vitro* from enzymatically released rat calvaria cell populations. *Calcif. Tissue Int.*, **38**: 143−154.

Bellows, C. G., Aubin, J. E., and Heersche, J. N. M. (1987). Physiological concentrations of glucocorticoids stimulate formation of bone nodules from isolated rat calvaria cell *in vitro*. *Endocrinology*, **121**: 1985−1992.

Beresford, J. N., Gallagher, J. A., Gowen, M., McGuire, M. K. B., Poser, J., and Russell, R. G. G. (1983). Human bone cells in culture. A novel system for the investigation of bone cell metabolism. *Clin. Sci.* **64**: 38−39.

Beresford, J. N., Gallagher, J. A., Poser, J. W., and Russell, R. G. G. (1984). Production of osteocalcin by human bone cells *in vitro*. Effects of 1,25 $(OH)_2D_3$, 24, $25(OH)_2D_3$, parathyroid hormone, and glucocorticoids. *Metab. Bone Dis. Rel. Res.*, **5**: 229−234.

Biggers, J. D., Gwatkin, R. B. L., and Heyner, S. (1961). Growth of embryonic avian and mammalian tibiae on a relatively simple chemically defined medium. *Exptl. Cell Res.*, **25**: 41−58.

Binderman, I., Duksin, D., Harell, A., Katzir, E., and Sacks, L. (1974). Formation of bone tissue in culture from isolated bone cells. *J. Cell Biol.*, **61**: 427−439.

Binderman, I., and Somjen, D. (1982). Serum factors and calcium modulate growth of osteoblast-like cells in culture. In: *Current advances in skeletogenesis*: M. Silberman, H. C. Slavkin (eds.). Elsevier Science Publishers BV, Amsterdam, pp. 338−342.

Boonekamp, P. M., Hekkelman, J. W., Hamilton, J. W., Cohn, D. V., and Jilka, R. L. (1984). Effect of culture on the hormone responsiveness of bone cells isolated by an improved sequential digestion procedure. *Proc. K. Ned. Acad. Wet.*, B **87**: 371−381.

Burger, E. H., Boonekamp, P. M., and Nijweide, P. J. (1986). Osteoblast and osteoclast precursors in primary cultures of calvarial bone cells. *Anat. Rec.*, **214**: 32−40.

Burks, J. K., and Peck, W. A. (1978). Bone cells: a serum-free medium supports proliferation in primary culture. *Science*, **199**: 542−544.

Caplan, A. I., Syftestad, G. and Osdoby Ph. (1983). The development of embryonic bone and cartilage in tissue culture. *Clin. Orthop. Rel. Res.*, **174**: 243−263.

Caplan, A. I., and Pechak, D. G. (1987). The cellular and molecular embryology of bone formation. In: *Bone and Mineral Research* **5**: W. A. Peck (ed.) Elsevier Science Publishers BV, Amsterdam, pp. 117−183.

Copray, J. C. V. M., Jansen, H. W. B., and Duterloo, H. S. (1985). Effect of compressive forces on phosphatase activity in mandibular condylar cartilage of the rat. *J. Anat.*, **140**: 479–489.

Ecarot-Charrier, B., Glorieux, F. H., van der Rest, M., and Pereira, G. (1983). Osteoblasts isolated from mouse calvaria initiate matrix mineralization, *J. Cell Biol.*, **96**: 639–643.

Fell, H. B. (1928). Experiments on the differentiation *in vitro* of cartilage and bone. Part I. *Arch. Exptl. Zellforsch.*, **7**: 390–410.

Fell, H. B., and Robison, R. (1929). The growth, development and phosphatase activity of embryonic avian femora and limb-buds cultivated *in vitro*. *Biochem. J.*, **23**: 767–784.

Fell, H. B. (1932). The osteogenic capacity *in vitro* of periosteum and endosteum isolated from the limb skeleton of fowl embryos and young chicks. *J. Anat.*, **66**: 157–180.

Fell, H. B., and Mellanby, E. (1952). The effect of hypervitaminosis A on embryonic limb-bones cultivated in vitro. *J. Phys.*, **116**: 320–349.

Fell, H. B. (1956). Skeletal development in tissue culture. In: *The biochemistry and physiology of bone*, G. H. Bourne (ed.). Acad. Press, New York, pp. 401–441.

Freshney, R. I. (1983). *Culture of animal cells*. Alan R. Liss, Inc., New York.

Friedenstein, A. J. (1976). Precursor cells of mechanocytes. *Int. Rev. Cytol.*, **47**: 327–359.

Friedenstein, A. J. (1980). Stromal mechanisms of bone marrow: cloning *in vitro* and retransplantation in vivo. In: *Immunobiology of bone marrow transplantation*. S. Thienfelder (ed.). Springer-Verlag, Berlin, pp. 19–29.

Gaillard, P. J. (1935). Development changes in the composition of the body fluids in relation to growth and differentiation of tissue cultures. *Protoplasma*, **23**: 145–174.

Gaillard, P. J. (1955). Parathyroid gland tissue and bone in vitro. *Exp. Cell Res.*, (Suppl.) **3**: 154–169.

Gaillard, P. J. (1960). The influence of parathormone on the explanted radius of albino mouse embryos. *Proc. K. Ned. Akad. Wet.*, C **63**: 25–37.

Gaillard, P. J. (1961). The influence of parathyroid extract on the explanted radius of albino mouse embryos II. *Proc. K. Ned. Akad. Wet.*, C **64**: 119–128.

Gaillard, P. J., Herrmann-Erlee, M. P. M., Hekkelman, J. W., Burger, E. H., and Nijweide, P. J. (1979). Skeletal tissue in culture. *Clin. Orthop. Rel. Res.*, **142**: 196–214.

Gehron Robey, P., and Termine, J. D. (1985). Human bone cells in vitro. *Calcif. Tissue Int.*, **37**: 453–460.

Gehron Robey, P., Kirshner, J. A., Conn, K. M., and Termine, J. D. (1985). Biosynthesis of non-collagenous proteins by bone cells in vitro. In: *Current advances in skeletogenesis*. A. Ornoy, R. Harell, J. Sela (eds.). Elsevier Science Publishers BV, Amsterdam, pp. 461–466.

Gerstenfeld, L. C., Chipman, S. D., Glowacki, J., and Lian, J. B. (1987). Expression of differentiated function by mineralizing cultures of chicken osteoblasts. *Develop. Biol.*, **122**: 49–60.

Groot, C. G., Moskalewski, S., Scherft, J. P., and Boonekamp, P. M. (1983). Electron microscopy of bone formed by syngeneic transplanted calvarial osteoblasts. *Cell. Biol. Int. Rep.*, **7**: 322.

Groot, C. G., Danes, J. K., Blok, J., Hoogendijk, A., and Hauschka, P. V. (1986). Light and electron microscopic demonstration of osteocalcin antigenicity in embryonic and adult rat bone. *Bone*, **7**: 379–385.

Hall, B. K. (1968). In vitro studies on the mechanical evocation of adventitious cartilage in the chick. *J. Exp. Zool.*, **168**: 283–306.

Hall, B. K. (1970). Cellular differentiation in skeletal tissues. *Biol. Rev.*, **45**: 455–484.

Hall B. K. (1987). Earliest evidence of cartilage and bone development in embryonic life. *Clin. Orthop. Rel. Res.*, **225**: 255–272

Hamburger, V. (1942). In: *A manual of experimental embryology*. University of Chicago Press. pp. 158–163.

Hamburger, V., and Hamilton, H. L. (1951). A series of normal stages in the development of the chick embryo. *J. of Morphology*, **88**: 48−92.

Hasegawa, S., Sato, S., Saito, S., Suzuki, Y., and Brunette, D. M. (1985). Mechanical stretching increases the number of cultured bone cells synthesizing DNA and alters their pattern of protein synthesis. *Calcif. Tissue Int.*, **37**: 431−436.

Hauschka, P. V., Lian, J. B., and Gallop, P. M. (1975). Direct identification of the calcium-binding amino acid carboxy-glutamate in mineral tissue. *Proc. Natl. Acad. Sci. USA*, **72**: 3925−3929.

Heersche, J. N. M. (1969). The effect of thyrocalcitonin and parathyroid hormone on bone metabolism in tissue culture. *Proc. K. Ned. Akad. Wet.*, C **72**: 286−298.

Heersche, J. N. M., Aubin, J. E., Grigoriadis, A. E., and Moriya, Y. (1985). Hormone responsiveness of bone cell populations. In: *The chemistry and biology of mineralized tissues*. W. T. Butler (ed.), pp. 286−295.

Howlett, C. R., Cavé, J., Williamson, M., Farmer, J., Ali, S. Y., Bab, I., and Owen, M. E. (1986). Mineralization in *in vitro* cultures of rabbit marrow stromal cells. *Clin. Orthop. Rel. Res.*, **213**: 251−263.

Jilka, R. L. (1986). Parathyroid hormone − stimulated development of osteoclasts in cultures of cells from neonatal murine calvaria. *Bone*, **7**: 29−40.

Jones, S. J., and Boyde, A. (1977). The migration of osteoblasts. *Cell. Tissue Res.*, **184**: 179−193.

Jundt, G., Berghäuser, K. H., Termine, J. D., and Schulz, A. (1987). Osteonectin − a differentiation marker of bone cells. *Cell Tissue Res.*, **248**: 409−415.

Kodama, H., Amagai, Y., Sudo, H., Ohno, T., and Iijima, K. (1986). Culture conditions affecting differentiation and calcification in the MC3T3-E1 osteogenic cell line. In: *Cell mediated calcification and matrix vesicles*. S. Y. Ali (ed.) Excerpta Medica, Amsterdam, New York, Oxford, pp. 297−302.

Koshihara, Y., Kawamura, M., Oda, H., and Higaki, S. (1987). In vitro calcification in human osteoblastic cell line derived form periosteum. *Biochem. Biophys. Res. Commun.*, **145**: 651−657.

Klein Nulend, J., Veldhuijzen, J. P., and Burger, E. H. (1986). Increased calcification of growth plate cartilage as a result of compressive force *in vitro*. *Arthr. Rheum.*, **29**: 1002−1009.

Klein Nulend, J., Veldhuijzen, J. P., de Jong, M., and Burger, E. H. (1987). Increased bone formation and decreased bone resorption in fetal mouse calvaria as a result of intermittent compressive force *in vitro*. *Bone & Mineral*, **2**: 441−448.

Le Douarin, N. (1973). A biological cell labeling technique and its use in experimental embryology, *Dev. Biol.*, **30**: 217−222.

Luben, R. A., Wong, G. L., and Cohn, D. V. (1976). Biochemical characterization with parathormone and calcitonin of isolated bone cells: provisional identification of osteoclasts and osteoblasts. *Endocrinology*, **99**: 526−534.

Luria, E. A., Owen, M. E., Friedenstein, A. J., Morris, J. F., and Kuznetsow, S. A. (1987). Bone formation in organ cultures of bone marrow. *Cell Tissue Res.*, **248**: 449−454.

Majeska, R. J., and Rodan, G. A. (1985). Culture and activity of osteoblasts and osteoblast-like cells. In: *The chemistry and biology of mineralized tissues*. W. T. Butler (ed.), pp. 279−285.

Mark, M. P., Prince, C. W., Gay, S., Austin, R. L., Bhown, M., Finkelman, R. D., and Butler, W. T. (1987a). A comparative immunocytochemical study on the subcellular distributions of 44 kDa bone phosphoprotein and bone Y-carboxyglutamic acid (Gla)-containing protein in osteoblasts. *J. Bone Min. Res.*, **2**: 337−345.

Mark, M. P., Prince, C. W., Oosawa, T., Gay, S., Bronckers, A. L. J. J., and Butler, W. T. (1987b). Immunohistochemical demonstration of a 44-kD phosphoprotein in developing rat bones. *J. Histochem. Cytochem.*, **35**: 707−715.

Marvaso, V., and Bernard, G. W. (1977). Initial intramembraneous osteogenesis *in vitro*. Am. J. Anat., **149**: 453–468.

Mayne, R., Vail, M. S., and Miller, E. J. (1976). The effect of embryo extract on the types of collagen synthesized by cultured chick chondrocytes. *Develop. Biol.*, **54**: 230–240.

Mazza, A., Felluga, B., and Curci, G. (1979). A histochemical study of the matrix of long bones of the mouse embryo grown *in vitro*. *Metab. Bone. Dis. Rel. Res.*, **2**: 65–72.

Meikle, M. C., Reynolds, J. J., Sellers, A., and Diryle, J. T. (1979). Rabbit cranial sutures *in vitro*: a new experimental model for studying the response of fibrous joints to mechanical stress. *Calcif. Tissue Int.*, **28**: 137–144.

Miszurski, B. (1939). Further contribution to the influence of extracts from embryos of different age on the growth of cartilage and ossification *in vitro*. *Arch. exptl. Zellforsch.*, **23**: 80–83.

Miyazaki, Y., Katsuta, H., Aoyama, Y., Endo, H., Takaoka, T., and Oishi, Y. (1957). Studies on the mechanism of ossification in tissue culture. *Japan J. Exp. Med.*, **27**: 331–342.

Moskalewski, S., Boonekamp, P. M., and Scherft, J. P. (1983). Bone formation by isolated calvarial osteoblasts in syngeneic and allogeneic transplants: light microcopic observations. *Am. J. Anat.*, **167**: 249–263.

Nefussi, J. R., Boy-Lefevre, M. L., Boulekbache, A., and Forest, N. (1985). Mineralization in vitro of matrix formed by osteoblasts isolated by collagenase digestion. *Differentiation*, **29**: 160–168.

Nijweide, P. J. (1975). Embryonic chicken periosteum in tissue culture, osteoid formation and calcium uptake. *Proc. K. Ned. Akad. Wet.*, C **78**: 410–417.

Nijweide, P. J., van der Plas, A., and Scherft, J. P. (1981). Biochemical and histological studies on various bone cell preparations. *Calcif. Tissue Int.*, **33**: 529–540.

Nijweide, P. J., van Iperen-van Gent, A. S., Kawilarang-de Haas, E. W. M., van der Plas, A., and Wassenaar, A. M. (1982a). Bone formation and calcification by isolated osteoblast-like cells. *J. Cell Biol.*, **93**: 318–323.

Nijweide, P. J., Burger, E. H., Hekkelman, J. W., Herrmann-Erlee, M. P. M., and Gaillard, P. J. (1982b). Regulatory mechanisms in the development of bone and cartilage: the use of tissue culture techniques in the study of the development of embryonic bone and cartilage: a perspective. In: *Factors and mechanisms influencing bone growth*. Alan R. Liss Inc. New York, pp. 457–480.

Nijweide, P. J., and Mulder. R. J. P. (1986). Identification of osteocytes in osteoblast-like cell cultures using a monoclonal antibody specifically directed against osteocytes. *Histochemistry*, **84**: 342–347.

Nijweide, P. J., Burger, E. H., and Feyen, J. H. M. (1986). Cells of bone: proliferation, differentiation and hormonal regulation. *Physiol. Rev.*, **66**: 855–885.

Nijweide, P. J., van der Plas, A., and Olthof, A. A. (1988). Osteoblastic differentiation. In: Cell and molecular biology of hard tissues. Wiley, Chichester (Ciba Found. Symp. 136), 61–77.

Osbody, P., and Caplan, A. I. (1976). The possible differentiation of osteogenic elements in vitro from chick limb mesodermal cells. *Develop. Biol.*, **52**: 283–299.

Osdoby, P., and Caplan, A. I. (1979). Osteogenesis in cultures of limb mesenchymal cells. *Develop. Biol.*, **73**: 84–102.

Osdoby, P., and Caplan, A. I. (1980). A scanning electron microscopic investigation of *in vitro* osteogenesis. *Calcif. Tissue Int.*, **30**: 43–50.

Owen, M. (1985). Lineage of osteogenic cells and their relationship to the stromal system. In: *Bone and Mineral Research* **3**: W. A. Peck (ed.). Elsevier Science Publishers BV, Amsterdam, pp. 1–23.

Partridge, N. C., Alcorn, D., Michelangeli, V. P., Kemp, B. E., Ryan, G. B., and Martin, T. J.

(1981). Functional properties of hormonally responsive cultured normal and malignant rat osteoblastic cells. *Endocrinology*, **108**: 213−219.

Peck, W. A., Birge, S. J., and Fedak, S. A. (1964). Bone cells: biochemical and biological studies after enzymatic isolation. *Science*, **146**: 1476−1477.

Price, P. A., Otsuka, A. S., Poser, J. W., Krislaponis, J., and Raman, N. (1976). Characterization of a γ-carboxyglutamic acid-containing protein from bone. *Proc. Nat. Acad. Sci. USA*, **73**: 1447−1451.

Prince, C. W., Oosawa, T., Butler, W. T., Tomana, M., Bhown, A. S., Bhown, M., and Schohenloher, R. E. (1987). Isolation, characterization, and biosynthesis of a phosphorylated glycoprotein from rat bone. *J. Biol. Chem.*, **262**: 2900−2906.

Raisz, L. G., and Niemann, I. (1969). Effect of phosphate, calcium and magnesium on bone resorption and hormonal responses in tissue culture. *Endocrinology*, **85**: 446−452.

Raisz, L. G., and Kream, B. E. (1983). Regulation of bone formation. *New Eng. J. Med.*, **309**: 29−35 and 83−89.

Reynolds, J. J. (1972). Skeletal tissue in culture. In: *The biochemistry and physiology of bone*, G. H. Bourne (ed.). Acad. Press, New York and London, vol. 1, second edition, pp. 69−126.

Robison, R. (1923). The possible significance of hexosephosphoric esters in ossification. *Biochem. J.*, **17**: 286−293.

Rodan, G. A., Mensi, T., and Harvey, A. (1975). A quantitative method for the application of compressive forces to bone in tissue culture. *Calcif. Tissue Res.*, **18**: 125−131.

Rodan, G. A., and Rodan, S. B. (1984). Expression of the osteoblastic phenotype. In: *Bone and Mineral Research* **2**: W. A. Peck (ed.), Elsevier, pp. 244−285.

Sherft, J. P. (1978). The lamina limitans of the organic bone matrix: formation in vitro. *J. Ultrastruct. Res.*, **64**: 173−184.

Schwartz, Z., Ornoy, A., and Soskolne, W. A. (1985). An in vitro assay of bone development using fetal long bones of mice: morphological studies. *Acta Anat.*, **124**: 197−205.

Sharpe, P. T., MacDonald, B. R., Gallagher, J. A., Treffry, T. E., and Russell, R. G. G. (1984). Studies on the growth of human bone-derived cells in culture using aqueous two-phase partition. *Bioscience Reports*, **4**: 415−419.

Sheyter, A., Gazit, D., Passi-Even, L., Bab, I., Majeska, R., Gronowicz, G., Lurie, A., and Rodan, G. (1986). Formation of calcifying matrix by osteosarcoma cells in diffusion chambers *in vivo*. *Calcif. Tissue Int.*, **39**: 49−54.

Silvestrini, G., Ricordi, M. E., and Bonucci, E. (1979). Resorption of uncalcified cartilage in the diaphysis of the chick embryo. *Cell Tissue Res.*, **196**: 221−224.

Smith, D. M., and Johnston, C. C. (1974). Hormonal responsiveness of adenylate cyclase activity form separated bone cells. *Endocrinology*, **95**: 130−139.

Stern, P. H., and Raisz, L. G. (1979). Organ culture of bone. In: *Skeletal Research*, D. J. Simmons and A. S. Kunin (eds.). Acad. Press, New York, San Francisco, London, pp. 21−59.

Stern, P. H., and Krieger, N. S. (1983). Comparison of fetal rat limb bones and neonatal mouse calvaria: effects of parathyroid hormone and 1,25 dihydroxy vitamin $D_3$. *Calcif. Tissue Int.*, **35**: 172−176.

Sudo, H., Kodama, H., Amagai, Y., Yamamoto, S., and Kasai, S. (1983). *In vitro* differentiation and calcification in a new clonal osteogenic cell line derived form newborn calvaria. *J. Cell Biol.*, **96**: 191−198.

Tenenbaum, H. C., and Heersche, J. N. M. (1982). Differentiation of osteoblasts and formation of mineralized bone *in vitro*. *Calcif. Tissue Int.*, **34**: 76−79.

Tenenbaum, H. C., and Heersche, J. N. M. (1986). Differentiation of osteoid-producing cells *in vitro*: possible evidence for the requirement of a micro environment. *Calcif. Tissue Int.*, **38**: 262−267.

Tenenbaum, H. C., Heersche, J. N. H., and Palangio, K. G. (1986a). Control of mineralization of bone *in vitro*. In: *Cell mediated calcification and matrix vesicles*. S. Y. Ali (ed.), Excerpta Medica, Amsterdam, New York, Oxford, pp. 315−319.

Tenenbaum, H. C., Palangio, K. G., Holmyard, D. P., and Pritzker, K. P. H. (1986b). An ultrastructural study of osteogenesis in chick periosteum in vitro. *Bone* **7**: 295−302.

Termine, J. D., Kleinman, H. K., Whitson, S. W., Conn, K. M., McGarvey, M. L., and Martin, G. R. (1981). Osteonectin, a bone-specific protein linking mineral to collagen. *Cell* **26**: 99−105.

Tibone, K. W., and Bernard, G. W. (1982). A new in vitro model of intramembranous osteogenesis from adult bone marrow stem cells. In: *Factors and mechanisms influencing bone growth*. A. D. Dixon, B. G. Sarnat (eds.). Alan. A. Liss, Inc. New York, pp. 107−123.

Tsuru, S., Kitani, H., Oguchi, M., Mashiko, M., Zinnaka, Y., and Shimomura, Y. (1984). Separation of osteoblast-like cells from bone marrow by fluorescence-activated cell sorting. *J. Histochem. Cytochem.*, **32**: 43−48.

Walters, M. R., Rosen, D. M., Norman, A. W., and Luben, R. A. (1982). 1,25-Dihydroxy-vitamin D receptors in an established bone cell line. *J. Biol. Chem.*, **257**: 7481−7484.

Whitson, S. W., Harrison, W., Dunlap, M. K., Bowers, D. E., Fisher, L. W., Gehron Robey, P., and Termine, J. D. (1984). Fetal bovine bone cells synthesize bone-specific proteins. *J. Cell Biol.*, **99**: 607−614.

Williams, D. C., Boder, G. B., Toomey, R. E., Paul, D. C., Hillman, C. C., King, K. L., van Frank, R. M., and Johnston, C. C. (1980). Mineralization and metabolism response in serially passaged adult rat bone cells. *Calcif. Tissue Int.*, **30**: 233−246.

Witkowski, J. A. (1986). Honor Fell. *TIBS* **11**: 486−488.

Wong, G. L., and Cohn, D. V. (1974). Separation of parathyroid hormone and calcitonin-sensitive cells from non-responsive cells. *Nature*, **252**: 713−715.

Wong, G. L., and Cohn, D. V. (1975). Target cells in bone for parathormone and calcitonin are different: enrichment for each cell type by sequential digestion of mouse calvaria and selective adhesion to polymeric surfaces. *Proc. Natl. Acad. Sci. USA*, **72**: 3167−3171.

Wong, G. L. (1982). Characterization of subpopulations of OC and OB bone cells obtained by sedimentation at unit gravity. *Calcif. Tissue Int.*, **34**: 67−75.

Wong, G. L., and Kocour, B. A. (1983). Differential serum dependence of cultured osteoclastic and osteoblastic bone cells. *Calcif. Tissue Int.*, **35**: 778−782.

Yagiela, J. A., and Woodbury, D. M. (1977). Enzymatic isolation of osteoblasts from fetal rat calvaria. *Anat. Rec.*, **188**: 287−306.

# 8

# Regulation of Cellular Activity of Bone-Forming Cells

## JOHAN N. M. HEERSCHE AND JANE E. AUBIN

*Medical Research Council Group in Periodontal Physiology,*
*Faculty of Dentistry,*
*University of Toronto,*
*Toronto, Ontario*
*Canada*

## Introduction

Cells from the osteoblast lineage, i.e. osteoblasts, osteocytes and lining
cells, have two major functions; namely, deposition and subsequent mineralization of the organic bone matrix and regulation of osteoclastic bone
resorption. Regulation of the cellular activity of osteoblasts therefore has to
be considered in the light of both these processes: regulation of formation
and mineralization of bone matrix and regulation of certain aspects of
osteoclastic resorption, such as the regulation of access of osteoclasts to the
bone matrix, regulation of osteoclast activity and regulation of osteoclast
numbers.

In this chapter we will first give a brief overview of the different classes of
regulatory molecules and the mechanisms through which they are thought
to operate, then discuss the regulation of osteoblastic activity as it pertains
to matrix deposition and then review the role of cells from the osteoblast
lineage in the regulation of osteoclastic bone resorption.

## Classes of Regulatory Molecules and their Mechanism of Action

Signals from the extracellular environment are received by specialized
receptor molecules, located either in the nucleus or on the external surface
of the cell membrane. A brief discussion of the general principles involved is
given here to facilitate an understanding of the mechanisms involved in
regulating osteoblast numbers and osteoblast activities.

One major category of regulatory molecules are hormones and growth
factors that do not cross cell membranes and interact with receptors
located on the external surface of their target cells. In many cases, the cell
surface receptors are associated with a cyclic AMP (cAMP) generating
system. Parathyroid hormone (PTH), prostaglandins (PG's), glucagon,
epinephrine and norepinephrine are examples of hormones that have effects
on osteoblasts and that act through this mechanism.

Some hormones with this mechanism of action also operate through a
class of cell surface receptors where hormone-receptor interaction results in
the intracellular release of messenger molecules derived from phosphoin-
ositides, increases in intracellular calcium concentration and subsequent
activation of protein kinase C. The hormone concentrations required for
activation of these receptors may be several orders of magnitude lower than
those at which the cAMP-mediated events occur (Wakelam *et al.*, 1986).
The action of at least some of the calcium-regulating hormones could be
mediated via this pathway as well, but no detailed information is available
at the present time.

Many growth factors with effects on bone cells, for example Epidermal Growth Factor (EGF), Fibroblast Growth Factor (FGF), Platelet Derived Growth Factor (PDGF), Transforming Growth Factor (TGF) α and β, and also insulin and Insulin-like Growth Factors (IGF) act via a third category of receptors on the external surface of target cells (see chapter 4). Here the signal appears to be transmitted across the cell membrane by the receptor molecule itself, resulting in most cases in rapid phosphorylation of a tyrosine-kinase that is part of the receptor molecule. Many of these factors also induce receptor-mediated inositol lipid turnover, $Ca^{2+}$ efflux and protein kinase C activation.

Hormones and other agonists that do cross cell membranes (e.g. steroid hormones, thyroid hormones) generally act via intracellular receptors that are located in the nucleus or the cytoplasm and are, or become associated with, specific sites on the genome. Hormone-receptor interaction leads to gene activation, mRNA synthesis and synthesis of specific hormone-induced proteins. Estrogens, retinoids, vitamin D metabolites and thyroid hormones are examples of hormones that have direct effects on bone cells and act through this mechanism.

The response of cells to extracellular signals is frequently modulated by regulation of the number of receptors for these signals. Numerous examples have been found where the number of receptors for certain agonists are either increased (up-regulation) or decreased (down-regulation) in response to other agonists. Examples for osteoblast-like cell populations are that the number of receptors for PTH in ROS 17/2 cells is up-regulated by hydrocortisone (Yamamoto, 1985), that the number of receptors for $1,25(OH)_2D_3$ is up-regulated by glucocorticoids (Chen *et al.*, 1982), retinoic acid (Petkovich *et al.*, 1984) and $1,25(OH)_2D_3$ (Costa *et al.*, 1985), and that the number of receptors for PTH is down-regulated by PTH itself and by $1,25(OH)_2D_3$ (Yamamoto, 1985).

Differentiation of some cell populations can also lead to changes in receptor levels. For example, Nerve Growth Factor (NGF)-induced differentiation of the rat PC12 pheochromocytoma cell line was accompanied by a dramatic drop in EGF receptors (Boonstra *et al.*, 1987) and proliferating myoblast cells, committed to terminal differentiation by removal of FGF, lose both their EGF receptors (Lim and Hauschka, 1984) and FGF receptors (Olwin and Hauschka, 1988). Similar phenomena may occur in bone cells: In a recent study of the binding of $^{125}I$-EGF in the distal end of the femur and the mandibular alveolar bone *in vivo*, specific binding sites were observed on cells with abundant endocytic components, on RER rich cells, and on cells histologically resembling undifferentiated precursor cells, but not on osteoblasts (Martineau-Doize *et al.*, 1988).

## Regulation of Bone Formation, Osteoblastic Activity and Osteoblast Proliferation

The question to be discussed in this section is how modulation of matrix deposition by osteoblasts contributes to the increase or decrease in bone mass that has been found to be associated with changes in the concentrations of PTH, vitamin D metabolites, corticosteroids, estrogens, insulin, cytokines and other growth factors.

In cultured fetal bone tissue in organ culture, collagen synthesis is stimulated by insulin (Kream et al., 1985) and IGF-I (Canalis, 1980) and inhibited by PTH (Kream et al., 1980), $1,25(OH)_2D_3$ (Raisz et al., 1978) and EGF (Canalis, 1983). Factors such as prostaglandins (Chyum and Raisz, 1984) and corticosteroids (Hahn et al., 1984) have been found to either stimulate or inhibit collagen synthesis in this system, depending on hormone concentrations and culture conditions. In another system, the clonal osteoblast-like rat osteosarcoma cell line ROS 17/2.8, PTH and $1,25(OH)_2D_3$ also inhibited collagen synthesis (Kream et al., 1986). However, collagen synthesis in this cell line was not affected by prostaglandin or EGF. Since ROS 17/2 cells do not respond to $PGE_2$ and have no receptors for EGF (Rodan and Rodan, 1984), this latter finding was not surprising. In another clonal osteoblast-like cell line, MC 3T3E1, EGF decreased collagen synthesis (Hata et al., 1983) while $1,25(OH)_2D_3$ stimulated collagen synthesis (Kuniharu et al., 1984). These data indicate that results obtained using clonal cell lines with osteoblast-like characteristics are not always comparable to results obtained using cultured calvariae and, moreover, that results obtained with different osteoblast-like cell lines can also differ considerably. This raises the question of whether the differences between various clonal osteoblast-like cell lines represent differences between osteoblast populations in vivo, or whether the properties of different clonal cell lines correlate with the properties of osteogenic cells at specific stages of differentiation.

There is some evidence to suggest that differences exist between different parts of the skeleton in terms of their responses to regulatory factors. Both in vivo (Ueda et al., 1980) and in vitro (Nefussi and Baron, 1985) prostaglandins appear to selectively stimulate periosteal bone formation. The observation that in sarcoidosis (a granulomatous disease associated with uncontrolled, increased production of $1,25(OH)_2D_3$), the small bones of the hands and feet are predominantly affected (Longcope ad Freiman, 1952) also indicates that populations of bone cells in different parts of the skeleton respond differently to systemic regulators of bone metabolism. A similar conclusion can be drawn from the observation that fluoride appears to increase selectively the amount of trabecular bone while having no effect on, or possibly even decreasing, the amount of cortical bone (Gutteridge *et al.*, 1984) and from the observation that excess glucocorticoid in patients results in a significant loss of trabecular bone (vertebrae, ribs) with much less change in cortical bone mass (Hahn *et al.*, 1974; Dykman *et al.*, 1985). This latter pattern of bone loss is also observed in patients with primary hyperparathyroidism (Dykman *et al.*, 1985), and it seems likely that the increased bone resorption observed with glucocorticoid excess is a result of secondary hyperparathyroidism associated with reduced intestinal calcium absorption.

Parathyroid hormone and vitamin D metabolites have long been recognized as primary regulators of bone metabolism. Similarly, abnormalities in bone metabolism in response to excess glucocorticoids and associated with estrogen deficiency or diabetes were recognized quite early. However, the direct effects of these factors on osteoblast metabolism are still largely unknown, although it is becoming increasingly clear that many of these hormones may act on bone via regulation of synthesis and release of growth factors by specific cell populations in bone.

## Parathyroid Hormone (PTH)

*In vivo* parathyroid hormone (PTH) increases both osteoblastic and osteoclastic activity, resulting in accelerated bone turnover, decreased bone mass and replacement of the cell population adjacent to the bone surface by fibrous connective tissue. *In vitro*, however, Gaillard (1955) observed a clear stimulation of osteoclastic bone resorption and an inhibition of osteoblastic function when chick or mouse parathyroid tissue was co-cultured with parietal bone fragments of mouse embryos. Later experiments by Gaillard and several other investigators using purified PTH and cultures of embryonic long bones or calvariae from either mouse or rat (Gaillard 1961; Kroon, 1959; Raisz *et al.*, 1968) have confirmed these observations. Thus, an obvious problem regarding the effects of PTH on bone metabolism becomes apparent. Whereas PTH *in vivo* stimulates osteoblastic activity (see, for example, Gennant *et al.*, 1975), PTH *in vitro* inhibits osteoblastic activity. At least a partial explanation of the disparity between the *in vivo* and *in vitro* effects of PTH may have been found when we (Tam *et al.*, 1982) observed that intermittent injections of PTH in parathyroidectomized rats stimulated bone formation without affecting resorption, while continuous infusion (in a sense comparable to the continuous presence of the hormone under tissue culture conditions) stimulated both resorption and formation.

The *in vitro* effects of PTH on the synthesis of matrix molecules by isolated osteoblast-like cells are generally inhibitory (Kream *et al.*, 1980; 1986), as are the effects on expression of alkaline phosphatase in cell populations derived from mouse calvariae (Wong *et al.*, 1977) and rat osteosarcoma-derived osteoblast-like cells (ROS 17/2; Majeska and Rodan, 1982). These inhibitory effects on characteristics usually associated with expression of the differentiated phenotype in osteoblast-like cells are in contrast to the effects of PTH on proliferation: Low concentrations of the hormone stimulate proliferation of UMR 106 rat osteosarcoma cells (Partridge et al., 1984) and of rat calvaria cells and ROS 17/2 cells (Majeska and Rodan, 1981). Thus, effects on proliferation seem to be associated with decreased expression of osteoblast-like characteristics and may represent the in vitro equivalent of the proliferation of cells with fibroblast-like phenotype observed in vivo in hyperparathyroidism.

In discussing the activity and modulation of activity of PTH, it has become important to consider the PTH-related protein (PTHrP; PTH-like protein-PLP; humoral hypercalcemia factor-HCF), not only in conditions such as the humoral hypercalcemia of malignancy, but also in normal tissues. A growing body of data suggests that PTHrP, although immunologically weakly related to PTH and sharing very limited sequence homology with PTH (8 of the first 13 amino acids shared, with sequence divergence thereafter), can elicit many of the biological activities of PTH on bone and kidney (Martin and Mundy, 1982; for recent discussions, see Burtis et al., 1987; Strewler et al., 1987; Moseley et al., 1987; Margin et al., 1987; Suva et al., 1987). Besides its ability to elicit a hypercalcemic response, these include stimulation of renal and osteoblastic adenylate cyclase (enhanced by dexamethasone just as is the PTH response itself) (Rodan et al., 1988), stimulation of renal 25-hydroxyvitamin D-hydroxylase, and reduction in alkaline phosphatase activity. Detailed assays of receptor binding (Nissenson et al., 1988), the many similar biological activities, and the fact that the PTH-antagonist [Tyr-34]bPTH-(7−34)$NH_2$ also inhibits PTHrP activities, have all pointed to the strong possibility that PTH and PTHrP share the same receptor, albeit with somewhat different binding characteristics. However, that a second category of receptors may exist, recognizing only one or the other hormone, or that not all the biological activities of PTH are shared by PTHrP, remains a possibility, especially in light of the recent observation that PTHrP (1−34) did not mimic the anabolic effect of hPTH (1−34) on rat bones in vivo (Hock et al., 1988).

## Vitamin $D_3$

The other factor long recognized to play a major role in bone metabolism is vitamin $D_3$. $1\alpha,25$-Dihydroxyvitamin $D_3$ (1,25-$(OH)_2D_3$) is the most biologically active metabolite of vitamin $D_3$ and is regarded primarily as an important regulator of calcium homeostasis (for a review, see Norman et al., 1982 and chapter 6 in volume 4). However, the widespread tissue distribution of intracellular $1,25\text{-}(OH)_2D_3$ receptors indicates that this metabolite has effects which extend beyond its role in calcium homeostasis (Henry and Norman, 1984) as its effects on, for example, monocyte and macrophage differentiation would support (Abe *et al.*, 1987). The primary effect of $1,25(OH)_2D_3$ excess on bone *in vivo* is an increase in bone resorption, reflected in increased numbers of osteoclasts and increased resorptive activity, and a clear deficiency in mineralization of newly formed bone matrix, resulting in increased osteoid surfaces and increased osteoid seam thickness (Parfitt, 1983). Interestingly, in vitamin D deficiency *in vivo*, circulating levels of $1,25(OH)_2D_3$ appear to be elevated or normal, while levels of $24,25(OH)_2D_3$ and $25(OH)D_3$ are decreased (Tam *et al.*, 1986). Whether the mineralization defect reflects an abnormality of osteoblastic function or is a result of lower than normal Ca and/or phosphate concentration in the extracellular fluids is not clear (Brommage and De Luca, 1985). Of interest in this regard is the observation that excess $1,25(OH)_2D_3$ also results in hyperosteoidosis (Hock *et al.* 1986).

The direct effects of $1,25(OH)_2D_3$ on isolated osteoblast-like cell populations are confusing: It inhibited collagen synthesis and stimulated osteocalcin synthesis in rat osteosarcoma cells (Kream *et al.*, 1986; Price and Baukol 1980) but stimulated collagen synthesis and fibronectin synthesis in human osteosarcoma cells (MG-63) (Franceschi *et al.*, 1985, 1988). The effects of $1,25(OH)_2D_3$ on cell proliferation of osteoblast-like cells are varied. $1,25(OH)_2D_3$ inhibited proliferation of osteoblast-like cells derived from mouse and rat calvariae (Chen *et al.*, 1983), whereas in ROS 17/2.8 cells, $1,25(OH)_2D_3$ inhibited cell growth at low cell density but increased cell growth at higher cell density (Majeska and Rodan, 1982). In contrast, in human bone cells $1,25(OH)_2D_3$ at a dose of $5 \times 10^{-12}$ mol/l stimulated cell proliferation, but inhibited cell proliferation at higher doses ($5 \times 10^{-9}$ – $5 \times 10^{-6}$ mol/l) (Skjodt *et al.*, 1985). To complicate things further, the effects of $1,25(OH)_2D_3$ on cell proliferation have also been shown to be dependent on the concentrations of serum used to supplement growth media (Rodan and Rodan, 1984), suggesting that growth factors originating from either cells or serum could be involved in mediating the effects of $1,25\text{-}(OH)_2D_3$. Indeed, in a series of experiments in which we studied the effects of $1,25(OH)_2D_3$ on a bone-derived cloned cell line (RCJ 1.20), we found that $1,25\text{-}(OH)_2D_3$ induced an increase in the number of receptors for EGF and potentiated the effect of EGF on anchorage-dependent growth and anchorage-independent growth of these cells (Petkovich *et al.*, 1987). $1,25\text{-}(OH)_2D_3$ also stimulated the secretion of a TGF-$\beta$-like compound. In view of the likely importance of TCF-$\beta$ and EGF in the regulation of osteoblastic and osteoclastic activity (discussed below), these results imply that at least some of the effects of $1,25(OH)_2D_3$ might be mediated through regulation of the secretion of and the responsiveness to growth factors of cells from the osteoblast lineage.

## Estrogen

Although it has been known that estrogen deficiency is associated with bone loss, and that estrogen replacement therapy prevents postmenopausal or post-ovariectomy osteoporosis, the mechanism whereby estrogen exerts its effects have been unclear until recently (Mazess, 1982; Riggs et al., 1972). Most data suggested that the effects of estrogens on bone were indirect: estrogen has no effect on collagen synthesis or bone resorption in cultured fetal rat calvariae (Canalis, 1978; Caputo et al., 1976) and no estrogen receptors could be found in bone tissue (van Paassen et al., 1978). With regard to osteoblastic activity, the major effect of estrogen deficiency appears to be a reduction in the formation surface, but not in the bone apposition rate (Arlot et al., 1984). This could result from an effect of estrogen on the differentiation of new osteoblasts. Recently, Gray et al. (1987) reported that estrogen decreased proliferation and increased alkaline phosphatase activity in UMR 106 cells, but had no effects on ROS 17/2.8 cells, thus suggesting that some osteoblast-like cell populations might be directly affected by estrogens. The even more recent detection of specific estrogen receptors in rat (ROS 17/2.8) and human (HOS-TE85) osteoblast-like osteosarcoma cells and in cultured normal human osteoblast-like cells (Komm et al., 1988; Eriksen et al., 1988) and the observation of increased mRNA levels for TGFβ and type I procollagen in estrogen treated HOS-TE85 cells (Komm et al., 1988) indicates even more strongly that estrogen has direct effects on osteoblast-like cells. It is of major interest to identify the precise cell type in bone that responds to estrogens.

## Glucocorticoids

Glucocorticoids also have clear effects on bone. In mammals, glucocorticoid excess is generally associated with net bone loss, due to a decrease in bone formation and an increase in bone resorption (for a review, see Baylink, 1983). In vitro, the direct effects of glucocorticoids on parameters of bone cell metabolism associated with formation appear to be stimulatory. First, it was found that dexamethasone stimulated osteogenesis and mineralization in cultured folded embryonic chick periostea (Tenenbaum and Heersche, 1985). By simultaneous quantitation of cell proliferation and the number of alkaline phosphatase positive cells in such cultures, evidence was obtained that dexamethasone stimulated proliferation of a population of cells that subsequently differentiated into osteoblasts, but inhibited further proliferation of possibly less differentiated progenitor cells (McCulloch and Tenenbaum, 1986). A stimulatory effect of dexamethasone on bone formation *in vitro* was also observed by Bellows *et al.* (1987), who observed that glucocorticoids increased the number of bone nodules appearing in cultures of fetal rat calvarial cell populations cultured in the presence of ascorbic acid and β-glycerophosphate. In addition, it was concluded from these data that two "classes" of osteoprogenitors might be present in such cultures: one capable of expressing bone formation without exogenous dexamethasone stimulation, and one expressing bone formation only in its presence. The possibility that these two populations of progenitor cells represent different stages of differentiation of cells in the osteoblast lineage is of particular interest, and the challenge is to identify these populations in intact bone tissue.

The well documented stimulatory effects of glucocorticoids on bone *in vitro* appear to be in conflict with the equally well documented observation that glucocorticoids *in vivo* stimulate bone resorption and inhibit bone formation. It seems likely that the stimulatory effects of corticosteroids on osteoblastic activity are masked in the *in vivo* situation by the development of secondary hyperparathyroidism as a result of the glucocorticoid-induced decrease in intestinal calcium absorption. The observation that the pattern of bone loss in hypercortisonism and hyperparathyroidism is similar (Dykman *et al.*, 1985) would support this possibility.

### Insulin

The only hormone clearly associated with stimulation of osteoblastic activity both *in vivo* and *in vitro* is insulin. *In vitro*, insulin stimulated collagen synthesis in cultured fetal rat bone (Canalis *et al.*, 1977; Kream *et al.*, 1985) while insulin deficiency *in vivo* is associated with a decreased bone mass and decreased osteoblastic activity (Hui *et al.*, 1985). It is not clear, however, how the observation that insulin decreased alkaline phosphatase activity of osteoblast-like osteosarcoma cells (Levy *et al.*, 1987) fits in with the generally stimulatory effects of insulin on osteoblasts. IGF has been shown to have effects similar to insulin (Canalis *et al.*, 1980)

### Growth factors

The effects of locally produced growth factors on collagen and DNA synthesis in bone tissue are being studied intensively (for a review see Canalis, 1985, and Chapter 4). Bone derived growth factor (BDGF) I, recently shown to be identical to TGF-β, and BDGF II, (or BDGF) now identified as beta 2 microglobulin ($\beta_2$M) (Centrella and Canalis, 1987; Canalis et al., 1987) are two growth factors extracted from and produced by fetal rat calvariae in vitro which can increase DNA and collagen synthesis in organ cultures of this same tissue. Fetal rat calvaria cultures also secrete and respond similarly to IGF-I (Canalis et al., 1988) and skeletal growth factor (SGF, Wergedal et al., 1986), now identified as IGF-II (La Tour et al., 1988). Adult bone matrix also contains these factors and others (see below). Whether these growth factors are released from bone matrix during bone resorption is not clear, but seems a distinct possibility, as sugggested, for example, for TGF-$\beta$ (Pfeilschifter and Mundy, 1987). If the assumption is correct that matrix TGF-$\beta$ is not degraded during the resorptive process, then TGF-$\beta$ (or other local growth factors) might function as the putative coupling factor between the resorptive and the formative phase of the remodelling process (see also, Jennings and Baylink, 1985). However, as pointed out by Baron et al., (1983) any factor released during the resorptive phase would have to act with a considerable time delay because of the time lag between the resorptive and formative phase in individual BMU's.

## TGF-$\beta$

The role of TGF-$\beta$ in the regulation of bone (and cartilage) differentiation and regulation of matrix deposition in bone (and cartilage) is not clear; opposite effects have been observed in different systems. Moreover, effects are clearly dependent on the presence or absence of other growth factors in the test system. In serum-containing medium under conditions in which colonies of bone forming osteoblasts normally develop, TGF-$\beta$ over a broad dose range (0.01−10 mg/ml) inhibited differentiation to functional osteoblasts of osteoprogenitor cells in populations derived from fetal rat calvariae (Antosz et al., 1988). This was true whether TGF-$\beta$ was present continuously or pulsed in for very short periods of time (15 min − 24 hrs). Using a different culture system, and using production of cAMP in response to PTH as the principal parameter for expression of an osteoblastic phenotype, TGF-$\beta$ stimulated the proliferation of progenitor cells giving rise to colonies, some of which comprised osteoblast-like cells (Guenther et al., 1988). Addition of anti-TGF-$\beta$ to cultures of rat calvaria osteoblast-like cells also resulted in a marked inhibition of osteoblast proliferation (Ernst et al., 1988). In keeping with the latter observation, TGF-$\beta$ stimulated osteoblast differentiation and cell replication in the osteoprogenitor zone of cultured rat calvariae (Hock et al., 1988) and also stimulated bone matrix apposition in this culture system. Opposite effects with regard to matrix apposition were found in human bone cell populations in which TGF-$\beta$ reduced matrix protein synthesis by 30%. Interestingly, however, comparison of fetal versus adult human bone cells showed that with increasing doses of TGF-β, growth of adult cells was slightly stimulated whereas growth of fetal cells was slightly inhibited (Gehron Robey *et al.*, 1988), suggesting that the nature of the osteoblastic cells or accessory cells recovered during the isolation is different in the adult versus the fetal cultures. Noda and Rodan (1987) found increased expression of osteoblastic characteristics (alkaline phosphatase activity) in response to TGF-β in ROS 17/2.8 *in vitro* and this effect was independent of the inhibition of cell proliferation. In contrast, TGF-β inhibited alkaline phosphatase activity in MC3T3-E1 cells in a manner also independent of its effects on proliferation (Noda and Rodan, 1986). Part of the problem in comparing the disparate activities of TGF-β is the wide variety of culture conditions under which effects of the growth factor have been assayed. For example, in some cases the full serum supplement (10−15% FCS) was present, in other cases reduced serum (0.2−2%) was used, and in other cases no serum was present. This alone, however, cannot account for all the different findings. Of interest is the possibility that the different model systems used comprise mixtures of osteoblastic cells at different stages of differentiation. For example, as has already been suggested (Centrella *et al.*, 1987; Pfeilschifter *et al.*, 1987; Noda and Rodan, 1986), the effects of TGF-β in inhibiting proliferation would be expected to be greater on less differentiated, more rapidly cycling cells so that effects on a population enriched in less differentiated cells would be more marked than in a more differentiated population. Finally, whether establishment to immortal growth (MC3T3-E1) or transformation (ROS 17/2.8) alters the nature of TGF-β effects remains to be elucidated. All these points need to be addressed more definitively in the models we use and in some cases this awaits new methods for identifying the cell types present (see below).

*FGF*

Not only whether a growth factor is present, but the form it is in is obviously crucial. This is true not only for TGF-β (active versus latent), but also for FGF and IGFs. For example, both acidic and basic FGFs (a and bFGF) are found in bone and bFGF in cartilage (bFGF = CDGF). The source of the FGFs found in bone is not yet clear, however, a variety of osteoblastic cells does respond to them: bFGF inhibited alkaline phosphatase activity, but stimulated osteopontin synthesis in ROS 17/2.8 cells (Rodan *et al.*, 1988); both a and bFGF regulated collagen synthesis and alkaline phosphatase activity in rat calvaria cells (Canalis *et al.*, 1988) and a and bFGF stimulated cell proliferation and osteocalcin synthesis in bovine bone cells (Globus *et al.*, 1988). FGF is very widely distributed and synthesized by many cells, ie. more widely distributed than PDGF, EGF, and TGF-α or β. However, its very tight association with heparin has been hypothesized to regulate its availability. Thus, FGF could be sequestered at high concentration in the extracellular matrix where it remains in association with heparin, and inactive, until it is released by, for example, enzymatic digestion with heparinase or other proteases released by macrophages or tumour cells or during interaction with heparin released by mast cells (Hauschka et al., 1986; Globus et al., 1988).

## IL-1

While the products of macrophages and other immune cells have long been studied in relation to resorption, dissecting out their activities on formation may help to clarify the intricacy of their roles as coupling agents. Moreover, osteoprogenitors or their more differentiated progeny may themselves secrete molecules formerly thought to be characteristic of stromal or hemopoietic populations. In this regard, bone cells cultured from newborn mouse calvariae have been reported to produce IL-1-like activity (Hanazawa et al., 1987) in addition to being able to respond to it. Both interleukin 1α (IL-1α) and interleukin 1β(IL-1β), have been shown to be potent bone resorbing agents in organ cultures in vitro with maximal activities in the range of $10^{-11}$ to $10^{-10}$ M (Gowen et al., 1983; Heath et al., 1985; Gowen and Mundy, 1986; Dewhirst et al., 1987; Stashenko et al., 1987).

There are now many reports that IL-1 can also stimulate parameters correlating with bone formation, including osteoblast proliferation (Gowen et al., 1985; Canalis, 1986; Smith et al., 1987), collagen synthesis (Smith et al., 1987), and alkaline phosphatase activity (Hanazawa et al., 1986). However, other studies showing inhibition of cell proliferation (Hanazawa et al., 1986; Stashenko et al., 1987), collagen synthesis (Canalis, 1986; Smith et al., 1987; Stashenko et al., 1987), and alkaline phosphatase activity (Stashenko et al., 1987) by osteoblasts in response to IL-1 lend further support to the concept that the osteoblastic model systems available represent heterogeneous populations and that the conditions under which agents are tested may alter the responses measured. In keeping with this, we recently found that IL-1α has complex biphasic effects on bone formation as measured by the formation of bone nodules in rat calvarial cell cultures: Both stimulation and inhibition of bone formation were observed depending on the concentration, time of addition and duration of treatment with IL-1α (Ellies et al., 1989). The concentrations which affected bone formation were similar to those which have been shown to stimulate osteoclastic bone resorption in organ cultures, suggesting that IL-1 could also play a role in the coupling of bone formation with bone resorption in vivo.

*EGF*

Not only Il-1, but many of the other agents tested for effects on osteoblast activity and bone formation have been found to have biphasic effects on the parameters measured, suggesting that their ability to regulate osteoblastic properties and differentiation are complex and implying that the effects they elicit may be dependent on both temporal aspects and local concentration, in addition to being influenced by whether other agents are present. An interesting example of this is EGF. When EGF was tested in the rat calvaria nodule system, continuous administration over 21 days caused a dose-related inhibition of nodule formation, even though cell proliferation was stimulated (Antosz *et al.*, 1988). In addition, no effects on protein or collagen synthesis were detectable at EGF concentrations that totally inhibited nodule formation. Interestingly, while short pulses of EGF (from 4h up to 48h over the first 3 days) caused a stimulation of nodule numbers, pulses of longer duration (>4 d) decreased the nodule number, even though all conditions were mitogenic for the population (Antosz *et al.*, 1987). However, even pulses of the same duration (i.e. 48 hours) could either stimulate (in early proliferating cultures) or inhibit (in later stationary phase, differentiating cultures) bone formation, emphasizing that the responsiveness of target cells may differ over their differentiation pathway.

## Heterogeneity of Osteoblast Populations.

The apparent inconsistencies in effects of many agents in different osteoblastic systems, or in the same model at different stages of culture could be sorted out, at least in part, by being able to define more precisely the subpopulation make-up of the cells or tissues we use. However, a major problem in analyzing the different steps leading from an uncommitted progenitor to a determined osteoprogenitor cell via the fully differentiated secretory osteoblast to either osteocyte or lining cell is the lack of appropriate markers for each stage of differentiation. Osteoblasts, pre-osteoblasts and osteocytes *in situ* have been characterized predominantly by morphological and histochemical criteria. To identify unambiguously cells earlier than the pre-osteoblast in the osteoblast lineage has not been possible, nor is it possible to determine whether any of the cells differing in morphological criteria also differ in other parameters (eg. responsiveness to hormones; synthesis of bone-related macromolecules) or whether the marked heterogeneity observed in cloned osteoblastic cell lines is physiologically significant.

Several possible avenues exist to investigate the reasons for the heterogeneity. One promising direction is the development of novel assays *functionally* identifying osteoprogenitor cells, eg. to identify a particular kind of osteoprogenitor by measuring its bone forming capacity without requiring either its isolation or even knowing any of its precise biochemical features (Bellows *et al.*, 1986; Nefussi *et al.*, 1985; Bellows and Aubin, 1989), analogous to the colony assays in use for many years for hemopoietic cells which have proven so useful in investigations of differentiation. A second approach is to identify new markers for cells of the osteoblast lineage, such as osteocalcin (Price, 1983) or osteopontin (44K phosphoprotein) (Mark *et al.*, 1987; Oldberg *et al.*, 1986). Other specific markers for osteoblastic cells may be found using the hybridoma technique, which is ideal for searching for unique cellular antigens representing cell populations at distinct stages of differentiation and maturation. Since osteoblast populations express hetero-geneous morphological and biochemical properties, there is every reason to believe that a range of stage specific, and unique, molecules are present. In support of this concept is the recent isolation of a monoclonal antibody directed against chicken osteocytes which does not stain other bone cells or a variety of other tissues (Nijweide and Mulder, 1986). The antibody recognizes a cell surface antigen present on osteocytes in bone and a proportion of cells isolated enzymatically from chicken calvaria and cultured for up to 6 days. It will be of interest to determine the biochemical and endocrinological properties of cells isolated on the basis of expressing this antigen. A panel of such antibodies, recognizing cells at other stages of osteoblast differentiation, would help to delineate different osteoblast sub-populations and to dissect the functional significance of the heterogeniety observed to date. Combined with other tools for identifying particular sub-populations, eg. those expressing osteoblast-related genes as determined by *in situ* hybridization, this route promises to become a powerful way to analyse the osteoblast lineage.

## The Role of Cells from the Osteoblast Lineage as Mediators of Resorptive Processes.

In support of a function for osteoblast-like cells in the physiological regu-lation of bone resorption are the following observations:
1) Osteoblasts have receptors for, and directly respond to, the bone-resorbing hormones PTH and $1,25(OH)_2D_3$ whereas osteoclasts do not (Chambers *et al.*, 1985); 2) osteoblasts, but not osteoclasts, produce pro-collagenase (Sakamoto *et al.*, 1978); 3) pro-collagenase secretion by, and/or content in, bone tissue is increased after stimulation with PTH (Sakamoto *et al.*, 1975; Eeckhout *et al.*, 1986); 4) calcitonin, which directly decreases the activity of osteoclasts but not of osteoblasts, has no effect on the degradation of non-mineralized bone collagen (Heersche, 1969) and no effect on procollagenase production by bone *in vitro* (Eeckhout *et al.*, 1986).

That cells from the osteogenic lineage may play an important role in regulating access of osteoclasts to the bone surface, and thus in regulating where resorption will occur, was suggested by Jones and Boyde (1976) and Rodan and Martin (1981), who stated that the main role of the osteoblast in regulating osteoclastic resorptive activity might be to regulate access of osteoclasts to the bone surface. In this view, all osteoclasts are potentially active resorbers, but are prevented from actually resorbing bone by cells from the osteoblast lineage that form a continuous protective layer over the bone surface.

In the adult (human) about 80% of the trabecular bone surface and about 95% of the intracortical surface is covered by inactive osteoblasts or lining cells (Parfitt, 1983) with no discernable osteoid remaining between the lining cells and the mineralized bone (Parfitt, 1984). Only a small percentage of the bone surface is covered by actively secreting osteoblasts in various stages of maturation. At these formation surfaces, a layer of osteoid is present between the osteoblasts and mineralized bone. Osteoclasts do not seem to be attracted to, or likely to resorb, areas of bone that are covered by either osteoid or non-mineralized collagen fibres. Thus, lining cell retraction alone might not be sufficient to initiate osteoclastic bone resorption. Chambers and Fuller (1985) have found that osteoblast-like cells cultured on bone covered by osteoid can degrade the osteoid layer, presumably through the release of collagenolytic enzymes. This observation is in agreement with previous observations demonstrating that degradation of nonmineralized osteoid is regulated differently from resorption of mineralized bone, and probably involves cells other than osteoclasts (Heersche, 1969; Brand and Raisz, 1972; Jilka and Cohn, 1983).

That degradation of nonmineralized collagen plays an important role in the initiation of bone resorption is strongly supported by the observations of Delaisse et al., (1985) who found that a synthetic inhibitor of mammalian tissue collagenase, CL1, almost completely inhibited the formation of resorption lacunae and degradation of matrix collagen in PTH-treated cultured fetal mouse calvariae. Thus, lining cells probably play a major role in determining when and where resorption by osteoclasts is initiated.

A further role for the osteoblast in regulating osteoclastic activity, i.e. direct stimulation of osteoclastic activity by hormone-induced secretion of resorptive molecules by osteoblasts, was also suggested by Rodan and Martin (1981). This was proven to exist by McSheehy and Chambers (1986) and Thomson et al. (1986), who showed that PTH, $1,25(OH)_2D_3$, and IL-1 stimulated osteoclastic activity indirectly by inducing osteoblast-like cells to release a soluble factor with osteoclast stimulating activity. The nature of the resorption stimulating activity is not yet clear. The first study describing such factors reported a single factor with a molecular weight of between 500–1,000 (McSheehy and Chambers, 1986). However, in a subsequent report, a factor with similar activities having a molecular weight of over 25,000 (Perry *et al.*, 1987) was described.

Since the cell populations derived from rat calvaria are highly heterogeneous (Aubin *et al.*, 1982), it is possible that different cell types produce different forms and varying amounts of osteoclast activating factors, and that these factors may have differing potencies. In part, this may reflect the different responses of the osteoblastic cells to the primary effector molecule. In this regard, it is important to note that differences have been observed in the effectiveness of UMR cells compared to ROS cells to promote osteoclast activity (McSheehy and Chambers, 1986). The aforementioned diversity of the cells from the osteogenic lineage that form the covering layer of cells on the bone surface (Parfitt, 1984), together with the observation that hyperparathyroidism results in the loss of predominantly cortical bone with apparent preservation of trabecular bone (Dykman *et al.*, 1985), only emphasizes the importance of osteoblast heterogeneity and diversity as a possible major factor in the local regulation of both formation and resorption processes.

## References

Abe, E., Ishimi, Y., Tanaka, H., Miyaura, C., Nagasawa, H., Hayashi, T. and Suda, T. (1987). The relationship between fusion and proliferation in mouse alveolar macrophages. *Endocrinology*, **121**: 271.

Antosz, M. and Aubin, J. E. (1988). Difference in the temporal characteristics of EGF and TGF-β effects on expression of the osteoblast phenotype in isolated rat calvaria cells *in vitro*. *J. Bone Mineral Res.*, **3**: (Suppl. 1), S 177.

Antusz, M. E., Bellows, C. G. and Aubin, J. E. (1987). Biphasic effects of epidermal growth factor on bone formation by isolated rat calvaria cells *in vitro*. *J. Bone Min. Res.*, **2**: 385

Arlot, M., Edouard, C., Meunier, P. J., Neer, R. M. and Reeve, J. (1984). Impaired osteoblast function in osteoporosis: Comparison between calcium balance and dynamic histomorphometry. *Brit. Med. J.*, **289**: 517.

Aubin, J. E., Heersche, J. N. M., Merrilees, M. J. and Sodek, J. (1982). Isolation of bone cell clones with differences in growth, hormone responses and extracellular matrix production. *J. Cell Biol.*, **92**: 427.

Baron, R., Vignery, A. and Horowitz, M. (1983). Lymphocytes, macrophages and the regulation of bone remodelling. In: *Bone and Mineral Research*, Annual 2 (ed. Peck, W. A.) Elsevier Science, Amsterdam, p. 175.

Baylink, D. J. (1983). Glucocorticoid-induced osteoporosis. *New Engl. J. Med.*, **309**: 306.

Bellows, C. G. and Aubin, J. E. (1989). Determination of numbers of osteoprogenitors present in isolated fetal rat calvaria cells *in vitro*. *Developmental Biol.*, **133**: 8.

Bellows, C. G., Aubin , J. E., and Heersche, J. N. M. (1987). Physiological concentrations of glucocorticoids stimulate formation of bone nodules from isolated rat calvaria cells *in vitro*. *Endocrinology*, **121**: 1985.

Bellows, C. G., Aubin, J. E., Heersche, J. N. M. and Antosz, M. E. (1986). Mineralized bone nodules formed *in vitro* from enzymatically released rat calvaria cell populations. *Calcif. Tiss. Int.*, **38**: 143.

Boonstra, J., Mummery, C. L., Feyen, A., de Hoog, W. J., van der Saag, P. T. and de Laat, S. W. (1987). Epidermal Growth Factor expression during morphological differentiation of pheochromocytoma cells, induced by nerve growth factor or dibutyrl cyclic AMP. *J. Cell. Physiol.*, **131**: 409.

Brand, J. S. and Raisz, L. G. (1972). Effects of thyrocalcitonin and phosphate ion on the parathyroid hormone stimulated resorption of bone. *Endocrinology*, **90**: 479.

Brommage, R. and DeLuca, H. (1985). Evidence that 1,25-Dihydroxyvitamin $D_3$ is the physiologically active metabolite of vitamin $D_3$. *Endocrine Reviews*, **6**: 491.

Burtis, W. J., Wu, T., Bunch, C., Wysolmerski, J. J., Insogna, K. L., Weir, E. C., Broadus, A. E. and Stewart, A. F. (1987). Identification of a novel 17,000 dalton PTH-like adenylate cyclase-stimulating protein from a tumor associated with humoral hypercalcemia of malignancy. *J. Biol. Chem.*, **262**: 7151.

Canalis, E. (1978). Effects of sex steroids on bone collagen synthesis *in vitro*. *Calcif. Tiss. Res.*, **25**: 105.

Canalis, E. (1980). Effect of insulin-like growth factor 1 on DNA and protein synthesis in cultured rat calvaria. *J. Clin. Invest.*, **66**, 70.

Canalis, E. (1983). Effect of hormones and growth factors on alkaline phosphatase activity and collagen synthesis in cultured rat calvariae. *Metabolism*, **31**, 14.

Canalis, E. (1985). Effect of growth factors on bone cell replication and differentiation. *Clin. Orthop.*, **183**: 246.

Canalis, E. (1986). Interleukin-1 has independent effects on deoxyribonucleic acid and collagen synthesis in cultures of rat calvariae. *Endocrinology*, **118**: 74.

Canalis, E. and Raisz, L. (1980). Effect of fibroblast growth factor on cultured fetal calvaria. *Metabolism*, **29**: 108.

Canalis, E., Centrella, M. and McCarthy, T. (1988). Effects of basic fibrobalst growth factor on cell replication and collagen synthesis in calvarial cultures. *Calcif. Tiss. Int.*, **42**: (Suppl.), A28.

Canalis, E., McCarthy, T. and Centrella, M. (1988). Isolation and characterization of insulin-like growth factor I (somatomedin C) from cultures of fetal rat calvariae. *Endocrinology*, **122**: 22.

Canalis, E., McCarthy, T., and Centrella, M. (1987). A bone-derived growth factor isolated from rat calvariae is $B_2$ microglobulin. *Endocrinology*, **121**: 1198.

Canalis, E. M., Dietrich, J. W., Masima, D. M., Raisz, L. G. (1977). Hormone control of bone collagen synthesis *in vitro*. *Endocrinology*, **100**: 668.

Caputo, C. B., Meadors, D., Raisz, L. G. (1976). Failure of estrogens and androgens to inhibit bone resorption in tissue culture. *Endocrinology*, **98**: 1065.

Centrella, M. and Canalis, E. (1985). Transforming and non-transforming growth factors are present in medium conditioned by fetal rat calvariae. *Proc. Natl. Acad. Sci. USA*, **82**: 7335.

Centrella, M. and Canalis, E. (1987). Isolation of EGF-dependent transforming growth factor (TGF-β-like) activity from culture medium conditioned by fetal rat calvariae. *J. Bone Min. Res.*, **2**: 29.

Centrella, M., Massague, J. and Canalis, E. (1986). Human platelet-derived transforming growth factor β stimulates parameters of bone growth in fetal rat calvariae. *Endocrinology*, **119**: 2306.

Centrella, M. McCarthy, T. L. and Canalis, E. (1987). Transforming growth factor B is a bifunctional regulator of replication and collagen synthesis in osteoblast-enriched cell cultures from fetal rat bone. *J. Biol. Chem.*, **262**: 2869.

Chambers, T. J. and Fuller, K. (1985). Bone cells predispose bone surfaces to resorption by exposure of mineral to osteoclastic contact. *J. Cell Sci.*, **76**: 155.

Chambers, T. J., McSheehy, P. M. J., Thomson, B. M. and Fuller, K. (1985). The effect of calcium regulating hormones and prostaglandins on bone resorption by osteoclasts disaggregated from neonatal rabbit bones. *Endocrinology*, **116**: 234.

Chen, T. L., Cone, C. M., and Feldman, D. (1983). Effects of 1,25-dihydroxyvitamin $D_3$ and glucocorticoids on the growth of rat and mouse osteoblast-like bone cells. *Calcif. Tiss. Int.*, **35**: 806.

Chen, T. L., Cone, C. M., Morey-Holton, E., and Feldman, D. (1982). Glucocorticoid regulation of 1,25($OH)_2$ vitamin $D_3$ receptors in cultured mouse bone cells. *J. Biol. Chem.*, **257**: 13563.

Chyun, Y. S., and Raisz, L. G. (1984). Stimulation of bone formation by Prostaglandin $E_2$. *Prostaglandins*, **27**: 97, (1984).

Costa, E. M., Hirst, M. A., and Feldman, D. (1985). Regulation of 1,25-dihydroxyvitamin $D_3$ receptors by vitamin D analogs in cultured mammalian cells. *Endocrinology*, **117**: 2204.

Delaisse, J. M., Eeckhout, Y., Sear, C., Galloway, A., McCullagh, K., and Vaes, G. (1985). A new synthetic inhibitor of mammalian tissue collagenase inhibits bone resorption in culture. *Biochem. Biophys. Res. Comm.*, **133**: 483.

Dewhirst, F. E., Ago, J. M., Peros, W. J., and Stashenko, P. (1987). Synergism between parathyroid hormone and interleukin 1 in stimulating bone resorption in organ culture. *J. Bone Min. Res.*, **2**: 127.

Dykman, T. R., Bluck, O. S., Murphy, W. A., Hahn, T. J., and Hahn, B. H. (1985). Evaluation of factors associated with glucocorticoid-induced osteopenia in patients with rheumatic diseases. *Arth. Rheum.*, **28**: 361.

Eeckhout, Y., Delaisse, J. M., and Vaes, G. (1986). Direct extraction and assay of bone tissue collagenase and its relation to parathyroid-hormone-induced bone resorption. *Biochem. J.*, **239**: 793.

Ellies, L. G., and Aubin, J. E. (1989). Time and concentration dependent stimulation and inhibition of bone formation *in vitro* by interleukin 1. *Bone and Mineral*, Submitted.

Eriksen, E. F., Colvard, D. S., Berg, N. J., Graham, M. L., Mann, K. G., Spelsberg, T. C., and Riggs, B. L. (1988). Evidence of estrogen receptors in normal human osteoblast-like cells. *Science*, **241**: 84.

Ernst, M., Schmid, C., Frankenfeldt, C., and Froesch, E. R. (1988). Estradiol stimulation of osteoblast proliferation *in vitro*: Mediator roles for TGF-β, $PGE_2$, insulin-like growth factor (IGF)I? *Calcif. Tiss. Int.*, **42**: (Suppl.), A30.

Franceschi, R. T., Linson, C. J., Peter, T. C., and Romano, P. R. (1985). Regulation of cellular adhesion and fibronectin synthesis by 1,25-dihydroxyvitamin $D_3$. *J. Biol. Chem.*, **262**: 4165.

Franceschi, R. T., Romano, P. R., and Park, K. Y. (1988). Regulation of collagen synthesis by 1,25-dihydroxyvitamin $D_3$. *J. Bone Min. Res.*, **3**: (Suppl. 1), Abstract 57, p. 583.

Gaillard, P. J. (1985). Parathyroid gland tissue and bone in vitro I. *Exp. Cell Res.*, (Suppl.) **38**: 154.

Gaillard, P. J. (1961). The influence of parathormone on the explanted radius of albino mouse embryos. *Proc. K. Ned. Akad. Wet.*, **C64**: 119.

Gehron Robey, P., Dominguez, P., Findlay, D. A., and Kopp, J. B. (1988). The effect of transforming growth factor β on human bone cells in vitro. *Calcif. Tiss. Int.*, **42**: (Suppl.) A34.

Gennant, H. K., Baron, J. M., Paloyan E., and Jowsey J. (1975). Osteosclerosis in primary hyperparathyroidism. *Am. J. Med.*, **59**: 104.

Globus, R. K., Patterson-Buckendahl, P., and Gospodarowicz, D. (1988). Regulation of bovine bone cell proliferation by fibroblast growth factor and transforming growth factor β.

*Endocrinology*, **123**: 98.

Gowen, M. and Mundy, G. R. (1986). Actions of recombinant interleukin 1, interleukin 2, and interferon-γ on bone resorption *in vitro. J. Immunol.*, **136**: 2478.

Gowen, M., Wood, D. D., Ihrie, E. J., McGuire, M. K. B., and Russell, R. G. G. (1983). An interleukin 1-like factor stimulates bone resorption *in vitro. Nature*, **306**: 378.

Gowen, M., Wood, D. D. and Russell, R. G. R. (1985). Stimulation of the proliferation of human bone cells *in vitro* by human monocyte products with interleukin-1 activity. *J. Clin Invest.*, **75**: 1223.

Gray, T. K., Flynn, T. C., Gray, K. M. and Nabell, L. M. (1987). 17B-estradiol acts directly on the clonal osteoblastic cell line UMR 106. *Proc. Natl. Acad. Sci. USA*, **84**: 6267.

Guenther, H. L., Cecchini, M. G., Elford, P. R. and Fleisch, H. (1988). Effects of transforming growth factor β upon bone cell populations grown either in monolayer or semisolid medium. *J. Bone·Mineral Res.*, **3**: 269.

Gutteridge, D. H., Price, R. I., *et al.* (1984). Fluoride in osteoporosis vertebral but not femoral fracture protection. *Am. Soc. Bone Min. Res.*, Proceedings, 6th Annual Meeting, A42.

Hahn, T. J., Boisseau, V. C., and Avioli, L. V. (1974). Effect of chronic corticosteroid administration on diaphyseal and metaphyseal bone mass. *J. Clin. Endocrinol. Metab.*, **39**: 274.

Hahn, T. J., Westbrook, S. L. and Halstead, L. R. (1984). Cortisol modulation of osteoblast metabolic activity in cultured neonatal rat bone. *Endocrinology*, **114**, 1864.

Hanazawa, S., Ohmori, Y., Amano, S., Hirose, K., Miyoshi, T., Kumegawa M., and Kitano, S. (1986). Human purified interleukin-1 inhibits DNA synthesis and cell growth of osteoblastic cell line (MC3T3-E1), but enhances alkaline phosphatase activity in the cells. *FEBS Lett.*, **203**: 279.

Hanazawa, S., Amano, S., Nakada, K., Ohmori, Y., Mujoshi, T., Hirose, K., and Kitano, S., (1987). Biological characterization of interleukin-1-like cytokine produced by cultured bone cells from newborn mouse calvaria. *Calcif. Tiss. Int.*, **41**: 31.

Hata, R., Hori, H., Nagai, Y., Tanaka, S., Kondo, M., Hiramatsu, M., Utsumi, N., and Kumegawa, M. (1983). Selective inhibition of type I collagen synthesis in osteoblastic cells by epidermal growth factor. *Endocrinology*, **115**: 867.

Hauschka, P. V., Mavrakos, M. D., Iafrati, M. D., Doleman, S. E., and Klagsbrun, M., (1986). Growth factors in bone matrix. *J. Biol. Chem.*, **261**: 12665.

Heath, J. K., Saklatvala, J., Meikle, M. C. Atkinson, S. J., Reynolds, J. J. (1985). Pig interleukin 1 (catabolin) is a potent stimulator of bone resorption *in vitro. Calcif. Tissue Int.*, **37**: 95.

Heersche, J. N. M. (1969). The effect of thyrocalcitonin and parathyroid hormone on bone metabolism in tissue culture: the effects of parathyroid hormone and thyrocalcitonin on the process of bone demineralization. *Proc. Kon. Ned. Akad. Wet.*, **C72**: 594.

Henry, H. L., and Norman, A. W. (1984). Vitamin D: Metabolism and Biological Actions. *Annu. Rev. Nutr.*, **4**: 493.

Hock, J. M., Centrella, M., and Canalis, E. (1988). Transforming growth factor beta (TGF-β-1) stimulates bone matrix apposition and bone cell replication in cultured rat calvaria. *Calcif. Tiss. Int.*, **42**: (Suppl.), A32.

Hock, J. M., Fonseca, J., Kemp, B. E., and Martin, T. J. (1988). Intermittent synthetic PTH-related peptide (PTHr Pl-34) does not mimic the anabolic effect of rat bones to parathyroid hormone (hPTHI-34) *in vivo. J. Bone Min. Res.*, **3**: (Suppl. 1), S105.

Hock, J. M., Gunnes-Hey, M., Poser, J., Olson, H., Bell, N. H., and Raisz, L. G. (1986). Stimulation of undermineralized matrix formation by 1,25-dihydroxyvitamin $D_3$ in long bones of rats. *Calc. Tiss. Int.*, **38**: 79.

Hui, S. L., Epstein, S., Johnston, C. C., Jr. (1985). A prospective study of bone mass in patients with type I diabetes. *J. Clin. Endocrinol. Metab.*, **60**: 74.

Jennings, J. C., and Baylink, D. J. (1985). Bovine skeletal growth factor: skeletal growth factor exists in small and large molecular weight forms. In: *The Chemistry and Biology of Mineralized Tissues*, (ed. Butler, W. T.) Ebsco Media, Birmingham, Alabama, p. 48.

Jilka, R. L., and Cohn, D. V. (1983). A collagenolytic response to parthormone, 1,25 dihydroxycholecalciferol $D_3$ and prostaglandin $E_2$ in bone of osteopetrotic (mi/mi) mice. *Endocrinology*, **112**: 945.

Jones, S. J., and Boyde, A. (1976). Experimental study of changes in osteoblastic shape induced by calcitonin and parathyroid extract in an organ culture system. *Cell Tiss. Res.*, **169**: 449.

Komm, B. S., Terpening, C. M., Benz, D. J., Graeme, K. A., Gallegos, A., Korc, M., Greene, G. L., O'Malley, B., and Haussler, M. R. (1988). Estrogen binding, receptor mRNA and biologic response in osteoblast-like osteosarcoma cells. *Science*, **241**: 81.

Kream, B. E., Rowe, D., Smith, M. D., Maher, V., and Majeska, R. (1986). Hormonal regulation of collagen synthesis in a clonal rat osteosarcoma cell line. *Endocrinology*, **119**: 1922.

Kream, B. E., Rowe, D. W., Gworek, S., and Raisz, L. G. (1980). Parathyroid hormone alters collagen synthesis and procollagen mRNA levels in fetal rat calvaria. *Proc. Natl. Acad. Sci. USA*, **77**: 5654.

Kream, B. E., Smith, M. D., Canalis, E., and Raisz, L. G. (1985). Characterization of the effect of insulin on collagen synthesis in fetal rat bone. *Endocrinology*, **116**: 296.

Kroon K. B. (1959). Effect of parathyroid extract on osteogenic tissue. *Acta Morphol. Neerl. Scand.*, **II-I**: 38.

Kunihara, N., Ikeda, K., Hakeda, Y., Tsunoi, M., Maeda, N., and Kumegawa, H. (1984). Effect of 1,25-dihydroxyvitamin $D_3$ on alkaline phosphatase activity and collagen synthesis in osteoblastic cells, clone MC3T3-E1. *Biochem. Biophys. Res. Commun.*, **119**: 767.

LaTour, D. A., Merriman, H. L., Kasperk, C. H., Linkhart, T. A., Mohan, S., Strong, D. D., and Baylink, D. J. (1988). The proto-oncogene c-fos—a potential regulator of bone cell proliferation—is induced by bone growth factors. *J. Bone Mineral Res.*, **3**: (Suppl. 1), S207.

Levy, J. R., Murray, E., Manolagas, S., Olefsky, J. M. (1987). Demonstration of insulin receptors and modulation of alkaline phosphatase activity by insulin in rat osteoblastic cells. *Endocrinology*, **119**: 1786.

Lim, R. W., and Hauschka, S. D. (1985). A rapid decrease in epidermal growth factor-binding capacity accompanies the terminal differentiation of mouse myoblasts *in vitro*. *J. Cell Biol.*, **98**: 739.

Longcope, W. T., and Freiman, D. G. (1952). A study of sarcoidosis, based on a combined investigation of 130 cases including 30 autopsies from the Johns Hopkins Hospital and Massachusetts General Hospital. *Medicine*, **31**: 1.

Majeska, R. J., and Rodan, G. A. (1982). Alkaline phosphatase inhibition by parathyroid hormone and isoproterenol in a clonal rat osteosarcoma cell line. Possible mediation by cyclic AMP. *Calcif. Tissue Int.*, **34**: 59.

Majeska, R. J., and Rodan, G. A. (1981). Low concentrations of parathyroid hormone enhance growth of clonal osteoblast-like cells in vitro. *Calcif. Tissue Int.*, **33**: 36A.

Majeska, R. J., and Rodan, G. A. (1982). The effect of $1,25(OH)_2D_3$ on alkaline phosphatase in osteoblastic osteosarcoma cells. *Journal of Biological Chemistry*, **257**: 3361.

Mangin, M., Webb, A. C., Dreyer, B., Posillico, J. T., Ikeda, K., Weir, E. C., Stewart, A. F., Bander, N. H., Milstone, L., Barton, D. E., Francke, U., and Broadus, A. E. (1988). Identification of a complementary DNA encoding a parathyroid hormone-like peptide from a human tumor associated with humoral hypercalcemia of malignancy. *Proc. Natl. Acad. Sci. U.S.A.*, **85**: 597.

Mark, M. P., Prince, C. W., Gay, S., Austin, R. L., Bhown, M., Finkelman, R. D., and Butler, W. T. (1987). A comparative immunocytochemical study on the subcellular distributions of 44KDa bone phosphoprotein and bone −carboxyglutamic acid (Gla)−containing protein in osteoblasts. *J. Bone Mineral Res.*, **2**: 337.

Martineau-Doize, B., Lai, W. H., Warshawsky, H., and Bergeron, J. J. M. (1988). *In vivo* demonstration of cell types in bone that harbor epidermal growth factor receptors. *Endocrinology*, **123**: 841.

Mazess, R. B. (1982). On aging bone loss. *Clin. Orthoped. Rel. Res.*, **165**: 239.

McCulloch, C. A. G., and Tenenbaum, H. C. (1986). Dexamethasone induces proliferation and terminal differentiation of osteogenic cells in tissue culture. *Anat. Rec.*, **215**: 397.

McSheehy, P. J., and Chambers, T. J. (1986). Osteoblast-like cells in the presence of parathyroid hormone release a soluble factor that stimulates osteoclastic bone resorption. *Endocrinology*, **119**: 1654.

Moseley, J. M., Kubota, M., Diefenbach-Jagger, H., Wettenhall, R. E. H., Kemp, B. E., Suva, L. J., Rodda, C. P., Ebeling, P. R., Hudson, P. J., Zajac, J. D., and Martin T. J., (1987). Parathyroid hormone-related protein purified from a human lung cancer line. *Proc. Natl. Acad. Sci. USA*, **84**: 5048−5052.

Mundy, G. R., and Martin, T. J. (1982). The hypercalcemia of malignancy: pathogenesis and treatment. *Metabolism*, **31**: 1247.

Nefussi, J. R., and Baron, R. (1985). $PGE_2$ stimulates both resorption and formation of bone *in vitro*: Differential responses of the periosteum and the endosteum in fetal rat long bone cultures. *Anat. Rec.*, **211**: 9.

Nefussi, J. -R., Boy-Lefebre, M. L., Boulebacke, H., and Forest, N. (1985). Mineralization *in vitro* of matrix formed by osteoblasts isolated by collagenase digestion. *Differentiation*, **29**: 160.

Nijweide, P. J., and Mulder, R. J. P. (1986). Identification of osteocytes in osteoblast-like cultures using a monoclonal antibody specifically directed against osteocytes. *Histochemistry*, **84**: 342.

Nissenson, R. A., Karpf, D., Bambino, T. (1987). Covalent labeling of a high-affinity, guanyl nucleotide-sensitive parathyroid hormone receptor in canine renal cortex. *Biochemistry*, **26**: 1874−1878.

Noda, M., and Rodan, R. A. (1987). Type B transforming growth factor (TGF-B) regulation of alkaline phosphatase expression and other phenotype-related mRNAs in osteoblastic rat osteosarcoma cells. *J. Cellular Physiol.*, **133**: 426.

Noda, M., and Rodan, G. A. (1986). Type B transforming growth factor inhibits proliferation and expression of alkaline phosphatase in murine osteoblast-like cells. *Biochem. Biophys. Res. Commun.*, **140**: 56.

Norman, A. W., Roth, J., and Orei, L. (1984). The vitamin D endocrine system: steroid metabolism, hormone receptors, biological response, calcium binding proteins. *Endocr. Rev.*, **3**: 331.

Oldberg, A., Franzen, A., and Heinegard, D. (1986). Cloning and sequence analysis of rat bone sialoprotein (osteopontin) cDNA reveals an Arg-Gly-Asp cell-binding sequence. *Proc. Natl. Acad. Sci.*, **83**: 8819.

Olwin, B. B., and Hauschka, S. D. (1988). Cell surface fibroblast growth factor and epidermal growth factor receptors are permanently lost during skeletal muscle terminal differentiation in culture. *J. Cell Biol.*, **107**: 761.

Parfitt, A. M. (1983). The physiologic and clinical significance of bone histomorphometric data. In: *Bone Histomorphometry* (ed. Recker, R.) CRC Press, Boca Raton, Fla., 143:

Parfitt, A. M. (1984). The cellular basis of bone remodelling: The quantum concept re-examined in light of recent advances in the cell biology of bone. *Calcif. Tiss. Int.*, **36**: 537.

Partridge, N. C., and Martin, T. J. (1984). Studies on the effects of parathyroid hormone on growth of UMR 106 osteogenic sarcoma cells. *Am. Soc. Bone Min. Res.*, Annual Meeting, Abstract p. A19.

Perry, H. M. (1986). Parathyroid hormone-lymphocyte interactions modulate bone resorption. *Endocrinology*, **119**: 2333.

Petkovich, P. M., Heersche, J. N. M., Tinker, D. O., and Jones, G. (1984). Retinoc acid stimutales 1,25-dihydroxyvitamin $D_3$ binding in rat osteosarcoma cells. *J. Biol. Chem.*, **259**: 8274.

Petkovich, P. M., Wrana, J. L., Grigoriadis, A. E., Heersche, J. N. M. and Sodek, J. (1987). 1,25-dihydroxyvitamin $D_3$ increases epidermal growth factor receptors and transforming growth factor β-like activity in a bone-derived cell line. *J. Biol. Chem.*, **262**: 13424.

Pfeilschifter, J., and Mundy, G. R. (1987). Modulation of type B transforming growth factor activity in bone cultures by osteotropic hormones. *Proc. Natl. Acad. Sci.*, **84**: 2024.

Pfeilschifter, J., D'Souza, S. M., and Mundy, G. R. (1987). Effects of transforming growth factor β on osteoblastic osteosarcoma cells. *Endocrinology*, **121**: 212.

Price, P. A. (1983). Non-collagen proteins of hard tissue. In: *Bone and Mineral Res.* (ed. Peck, W. A.) Excerpta Medica, Amsterdam, Vol. 1: pp. 157−191.

Price, P. A., and Baukol, S. A. (1980). 1,25-dihydroxyvitamin $D_3$ increases synthesis of the vitamin K-dependent bone protein by osteosarcoma cells. *J. Biol. Chem.*, **255**: 11660.

Raisz, L. G., Brand, J. S., Au, W. Y. W., Niemann, I., (1968). Interactions of parathyroid hormone and thyrocalcitonin on bone resorption in tissue culture. In: *Parathyroid Hormone and Thyrocalcitonin* (eds. Talmage R. V. and Belanger, L. F.), *Excerpta Medica*, I. C. S., **159**: 370.

Raisz, L. G., Maina, D. M., Gworek, S. C., Dietrich, J. W., and Canalis, E. M., (1978). Hormonal control of bone synthesis *in vitro*. Inhibitory effects of 1-hydroxylated vitamin D metabolites. *Endocrinology*, **102**, 731.

Riggs, L. R., Jowsey, J., Goldsmith, R. S., Kelly, P. J., Hoffman, D. L., and Arnaud, C. D., (1972). Short and long term effects of estrogen and synthetic anabolic hormone in post-menopausal osteoporosis. *J. Clin. Invest.*, **51**: 1659.

Rodan, G. A., and Martin, T. J., (1981). Role of osteoblasts in hormonal control of bone resorption. A hypothesis. *Calcif. Tissue Int.*, **33**: 349.

Rodan, G. A., and Rodan, S. B., (1984). Expression of the osteoblastic phenotype. In: Bone and Mineral Research, II. Ed. W. A. Peck. Elsevier, Amsterdam, p. 244.

Rodan, G. A., Rodan, S. B., and Majeska, R. J., (1982). In: *Current Advances in Skeletogenesis* (Silbermann, M., and Slavkin, M. C., eds.), Excerpta Medica, Amsterdam, p. 315.

Rodan, S. B., Noda, M., Wesolowski, G., Rosenblatt, M., and Rodan, G. A., (1988). Comparison of postreceptor effects of 1−34 human hypercalcemia factor and 1−34 human parathyroid hormone in rat osteosarcoma cells. *J. Clinical Invest.*, **81**: 924.

Rodan, S. B., Yoon, K., Wesolowski, G., and Rodan, G. A., (1988). Fibroblast growth factor enhances osteopontin and inhibits alkaline phosphatase expression independent of effects on cell proliferation in ROS 17/2.8 cells. *J. Bone Mineral Res.*, **3** (Suppl. 1), S144.

Sakamoto, S., Sakamoto, M., Goldhaber, P., and Glimcher, M., (1975). Collagenase and bone resorption: isolation of collagenase from culture medium containing serum after stimulation of bone resorption by addition of parathyroid hormone extract. *Biochim. Biophys. Res. Commun.*, **63**: 172.

Sakamoto, S., Sakamoto, M., Goldhaber, P., and Glimcher, M. J., (1978). Localization of tissue collagenase in bone by indirect immunofluorescent antibody technique. In: *Endocrinology of Calcium Metabolism* (eds. Copp, D. H. and Talmage, R. V.) p. 378, Excerpta Medica, Amsterdam-Oxford.

Skjodt, H., Gallagher, J. A., Beresford, J. N., Couch, M., Poser, J. W., and Russell, R. G. G.,

(1985). Vitamin D metabolites regulate osteocalcin synthesis and proliferation of human bone cells *in vitro. J. Endocr.*, **105**: 391.

Smith, D. D., Gowen, M., and Mundy, G. (1987). Effects of interferon-γ and other cytokines on collagen synthesis in fetal rat bone cultures. *Endocrinology*, **120**: 2494.

Stashenko, P., Dewhirst, F. R., Peros, W. J., Kent, R. L., and Ago, J. M., (1987). Synergistic interactions between interleukin 1, tumor necrosis factor, and lymphotixin in bone resorption. *J. Immunol.*, **138**, 1464.

Stashenko, P., Dewhirst, F. E., Rooney, M. L., DesJardins, L. A., and Heeley, J. D., (1987). IL-1B is a potent inhibitor of bone formation *in vitro. J. Bone Mineral Res.*, **6**: 559.

Strewler, G. J., Stern, P. H., Jacobs, J. W., Eveloff, J., Klein, R. F., Laung, S. C., Rosenblatt, M., and Nissenson, R. A., (1987). Parathyroid hormone-like protein from human renal carcinoma cells: structural and functional homology with parathyroid hormone. *J. Clin. Invest.*, **80**: 1803.

Suva, L. J., Winslow, G. A., Wettenhall, R., Hammonds, R. G., Moseley, J. M., Diefenbach-Jagger, H., Rodda, C. P., Kemp, B. E., Rodriguez, H., Chen, E. Y., Hudson, P. J., Martin, T. J., and Wood, W. I., (1987). A parathyroid hormone-related protein implicated in malignant hypercalcemia: cloning and expression. *Science*, **237**: 893.

Tam, C. S., Heersche, J. N. M., Jones, G., Murray, T. M., and Rasmussen, H., (1986). The effect of vitamin D on bone *in vivo. Endocrinology*, **118**: 2217.

Tam, C. S., Heersche, J. N. M., Murray, T. M., and Parsons, J. A., (1982). Parathyroid hormone stimulates the bone apposition rate independently of its resorptive action: differential effects of intermittent and continuous administration. *Endocrinology*, **110**: 506.

Tenenbaum, H. C., and Heersche, J. N. M., (1985). Dexamethasone stimulates osteogenesis in chick periosteum *in vitro. Endocrinology*, **117**, 2211.

Thomson, B. M., Saklatvala, J., and Chambers, T. J., (1986). Osteoblasts mediate interleukin 1 stimulation of bone resorption by rat osteoclasts. *J. Exp. Med.*, **164**: 104.

Ueda, K., Saito, A., Kanaro, H., Aoshima, M., Yokota, M., Muraoka, R., and Iwaya, T., (1980). Cortical hyperostosis following long-term administration of $PGE_2$ in infants with cyanotic congenital heart disease. *J. Pediatr.*, **97**: 834.

Van Paassen, H. C., Poortman, J., Borgart-Creutzburg, I. H. C., Thyssen, J. H. H., and Duursma, S. A., (1978). Oestrogen binding proteins in bone cell cyrosol. *Calcif. Tiss. Res.*, **25**: 249.

Wakelam *et al.* (1986). Activation of two signal transduction systems in hepatocytes by glucagon. *Nature*, **323**: 68.

Wergedal, J. E., Mohan, S., Taylor, A. K., and Baylink, D. J., (1986). Skeletal growth factor is produced by human osteoblast-like cells in culture. *Biochim. Biophys. Acta*, **889**: 163.

Wong, G. L., Luben, R. A., and Cohn, D. V., (1977). 1,25-Dihydroxycholecalciferol and parathormone: Effects on isolated osteoclast-like and osteoblast-like cells. *Science*, **197**: 663.

Yamamoto, I., (1985). Regulation of receptors for Parathyroid Hormone in rat osteosarcoma cells. *Japanese Journal Bone and Mineral Research*, **3**: 38.

# 9

# Bone-Forming Cells in Clinical Conditions

**A. Michael Parfitt**
*Henry Ford Hospital*
*Bone and Mineral Research Laboratory*
*Detroit, Michigan*

## Introduction and Scope:

The role of osteoblasts in the growth and development of the bones has been known for more than 100 years (Pritchard, 1972), but the importance of these cells in the conservation and maintenance of bone and in the pathogenesis of metabolic bone disease has been clearly established only in the last decade (Parfitt *et al.*, 1981a). With his usual prescience Albright had suspected that bone formation was defective in osteoporosis (Albright and Reifenstein, 1984), but confirmation of this suspicion became possible only when Frost introduced tetracycline labeling as a tool of clinical investigation (Frost, 1968). In this chapter I will summarize current knowledge of osteoblast function in the living adult human skeleton. Most of the knowledge has been gained from white women, since white men and blacks of either sex are less susceptible to metabolic bone disease, but qualifications based on sex or race will be indicated whenever possible. Information derived from other species and from *in vitro* studies at various levels of organization will be included to the extent that it makes *in vivo* observations in man more intelligible. A central aim is to define as exactly as possible what must be explained by studies at the cellular and molecular level, as described elsewhere in this volume and in this series, and to set some biologically plausible limits to the extrapolation from such studies to the level of the whole organism.

Osteoblasts normally assemble only at locations where osteoclasts have recently been active, and the spatial and temporal coupling between resorption and formation require examination in the broader context of the quantum concept of remodelling (Parfitt, 1984b) and the intermediary organization of the skeleton (Frost, 1985a). Because so much of our knowledge of the behavior of osteoblasts *in vivo* rests on double tetracycline labelling, what can legitimately be inferred from this method, and its assumptions and limitations, will be outlined (Parfitt, 1988a). Although dynamic histomorphometry is unable to identify the primary target of any skeletally active agent, for determining the cumulative summation of all effects, whether primary or secondary, direct or indirect, immediate or remote, it is not merely a good way; it is, in the present state of knowledge, the only way. Osteoblasts behave differently on different surfaces and in different architectural types of bone (Frost, 1985a), and the relative contributions of geometric and biologic factors to these differences will be explored.

The non-growing, remodelling skeleton is the main focus of this text, but contrasting osteoblasts from this system with the different activity of osteoblasts during growth and modelling places some aspects in clearer perspective. The structural differences between woven and lamellar bone reflect differences in their method of construction; whether an osteoblast is committed to produce one type of bone or another at the time of its birth, or whether it is pushed in a particular direction by systemic and local humoral agents is an unanswered question, important not only in itself, but to the relevance of different kinds of *in vitro* study to human physiology and pathology. Bone lining cells are often referred to as resting osteoblasts (Pritchard, 1972) and in young growing animals osteocytes may continue to form bone for some time after they become embedded beneath the surface (Baylink and Wergedal, 1971), but it is unlikely that either cell type is bone-forming in the adult human. Nevertheless, since they represent possible fates of an osteoblast, the nature and function of both lining cells and osteocytes and their role in disease must be examined.

The text is organized in two main sections. In the first, concepts of optimal osteoblast function and activity are developed, and in the second, these concepts are applied to the interpretation of findings in various nonoptimal circumstances including the effects of aging, disease and exposure to drugs. The distinction between optimal and non-optimal is made biologically rather than clinically. Although corresponding broadly to the clinical distinctions between health and disease, fit and unfit, and normal and abnormal, some of the semantic and logical problems introduced by these terms are avoided (Murphy, 1976).

## Bone Forming Cells in Optimal Conditions

A wide variety of *in vitro* studies indicate that osteoblasts are derived from the stromal cells of the bone marrow and from other resident connective tissue cells, and possess a characteristic repertoire of macromolecular synthetic mechanisms and hormonal receptors (Rodan and Rodan, 1983, Chapters 2, 3 and 8 herein).

## Osteoblasts in the Context of Quantal Remodelling

One quantum of bone remodelling consists of the erosion of one cavity on a bone surface by a team of osteoclasts and its refilling by a team of osteoblasts (Parfitt, 1984b). Usually more than 80% of any bone surface is in a state of quiescence with respect to remodelling, covered by a single layer of thin and flat lining cells that form the most obvious component of the cellular and connective tissue barrier that separates the mineralized bone from the soft tissue of the bone marrow (Parfitt, 1984b). All bone remodelling begins on a quiescent surface, and the conversion of a small region of surface from quiescence to remodeling activity is referred to as activation (Fig. 1). The initiation of resorption is the first observable evidence that activation has occurred (Baron et al., 1983a), but it is important to maintain the distinction between the event of activation and the process of resorption. Activation involves preparation of the bone surface (Parfitt, 1984b; Baron et al., 1983a) and proliferation of new blood vessels (Marotti and Zallone, 1980; Burkhardt et al., 1984) as well as recruitment of resorbing cells. Activation dictates where and when resorption will begin, and the frequency with which the event occurs is the major determinant of the whole-body rates of resorption and formation (Parfitt, 1988a). In conjunction with the mean life span of the remodelling cycle, the frequency of activation also determines the number of remodelling sites present at one time.

This simple definition of activation applies readily to the cancellous, endocortical and periosteal bone surfaces, but the situation for intracortical or haversian remodelling is more complex. When a cutting cone advances along an existing haversian canal, a succession of adjacent cross-sectional cavities are created, each representing the same sequence of quiescence, activation, resorption, formation, and back to quiescence (Parfitt, 1976a). But if, as is more usual (Tappen, 1977), the cutting cone originates in a Volkmann canal or on the endocortical surface, and advances without relation to an existing haversian canal (Fig. 2), the conversion of a quiescent surface to activity occurs only at the point of origin. The remodelling process creates a new haversian system, of which the canal's lining will be a new extension of the intracortical surface. But the two types of cortical remodelling have similar effects on bone turnover and for consistency in the calculation of activation frequency from tetracycline based measurements (Parfitt, 1983) it is convenient to disregard the difference between them.

Activation determines where and when osteoblasts will be needed, and resorption defines the nature and magnitude of the task they have been set (Jaworski, 1981). The size and shape of a resorption cavity reflects the collective work of a team of osteoclasts, which must depend not only on the number of cells recruited, the rate at which each cell resorbs bone and the active lifespan of each cell, but also on how the work of each resorbing cell

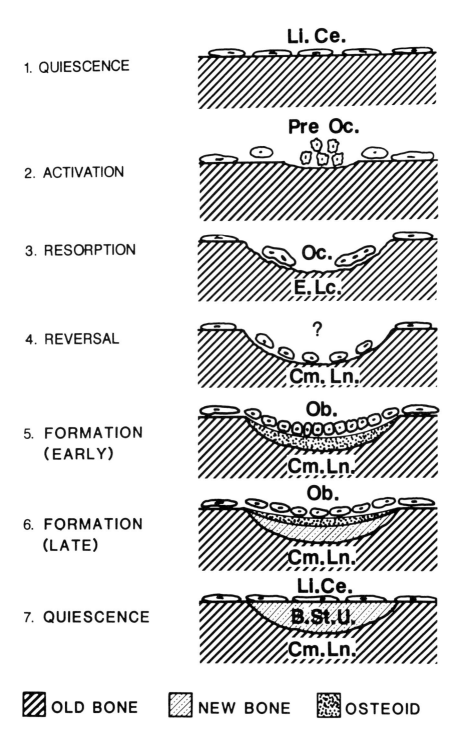

**Fig. 1** Normal remodeling sequence in adult human cancellous bone. Diagram illustrating erosion and repair of a single cavity. Li.Ce = Lining cell; Pre Oc = Preosteoclast (mononuclear); Oc = Osteoclast (multinucleated); E.Lc = Eroded lacuna; Cm Ln = Cement line (reversal line); Ob = Osteoblast; B.St.U = Bone structural unit. For definitions of stages see text. Modified from Parfitt, 1984b, with permission.

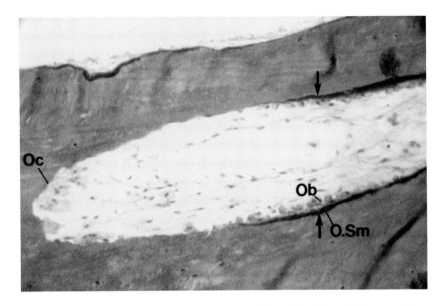

**Fig. 2** Cortical bone remodeling unit in human iliac bone. Osteoclasts (Oc) are eroding a longitudinal cavity from right to left into old bone without relation to an existing vascular channel. The cavity is being refilled centripetally by osteoblasts (Ob) lining an osteoid seam (O.Sm); it currently contains loose fibrous and vascular connective tissue, most of which will eventually be replaced by osteonal bone, leaving only a haversian canal. Arrows show approximate location of cross-section corresponding to Figure 3. Modified from Parfitt, 1988a, with permission.

is coordinated with that of its neighbor. By the time resorption is finished, the floor of the cavity has become smoother, and there follows a period of reversal during which, probably by mononuclear phagocytes (Baron *et al.*, 1983a), a thin layer of cement substance is deposited. This specialized form of bone matrix contains less collagen and mineral but more glycosaminoglycans and glycoproteins than regular bone matrix (Schaffler *et al.*, 1987), and initially is rich in acid phosphatase (Baron *et al.*, 1983a). Not much is known about the coupling mechanisms that ensure the arrival of osteoblasts in the right place, at the right time and in sufficient number, but both the release from resorbed bone of a substance that is mitogenic to osteoblast precursors (Farley *et al.*, 1987), and chemotaxis by constituents of cement substance are likely involved (Baron *et al.*, 1983a, Parfitt, 1984b).

For a few years between the completion of skeletal growth and consolidation and the onset of age-related bone loss, the refilling of cavities is complete; the bone surface is restored exactly to its previous location and the total volume of bone matrix remains constant (Parfitt, 1988a). But with increasing age refilling becomes less complete and the volume of bone matrix progressively declines. The loss of bone that results from incomplete refilling is irreversible, in the sense that each cycle of bone remodelling represents a transaction that, when completed, is irrevocable. The amount of bone deposited within a resorption cavity, like the amount of bone removed, reflects the collective work of a team of cells, and depends on the number of osteoblasts recruited, the rate at which each cell makes bone matrix, the active lifespan of each cell, and on how the work of each forming cell is coordinated with that of its neighbors. Consequently, the process of bone formation must be examined at three levels — the function of an individual osteoblast, the function of an osteoblast team (which depends also on the number of osteoblasts recruited for the team and how they work together) and the frequency with which new teams are assembled (which depends on the frequency of the initiating event of activation).

## Methods of Studying Human Osteoblasts

The examination of tissue sections by light or electron microscopy can provide information on the size, shape and structure of osteoblasts, the nature, location and amount of bone matrix recently made by osteoblasts, the extent of bone surface where formation is currently occurring, and the rate of appositional bone growth. Various substances made by osteoblasts can be measured in body fluids, but the levels are influenced mainly by the whole-body rate of bone formation and hence the rate of remodelling activation, and not by the activity of osteoblasts at the level of the team or the individual cell (Parfitt and Kleerekoper, 1984; Parfitt *et al.*, 1987a; Parfitt 1988a). Whole-body bone formation rate is measured most accurately and directly by radio-calcium kinetics (Charles *et al.*, 1987), but this is not as widely available as the biochemical methods. Cells cultured from explants of human bone are of similar phenotype to osteoblasts from other species (Beresford *et al.*, 1984; Gasser *et al.*, 1986) but it is not known from which *in vivo* cell type they are derived, and no consistent differences have yet been found between cells from normal subjects and cells from patients with metabolic bone disease (Gasser *et al.*, 1986; Wong *et al.*, 1987). Consequently, histologic methods remain pre-eminent in the clinical setting.

Human osteoblasts closely resemble in appearance those of other species (Villanueva *et al.*, 1983a). They have a maximum dimension of 15–20 μm that is often perpendicular to the bone surface, a nuclear profile (10 μm × 7 μm) usually at the pole furthest from the surface, and adjacent to the nucleus, a round, pale-staining or clear area — the juxta-nuclear vacuole or negative Golgi image (Pritchard, 1972). The cytoplasm stains deeply with basic aniline dyes and contains many granules that stain with methyl green pyronine (Dunstan and Evans 1980; Villanueva *et al.*, 1983a). Basophilia and pyroninophilia are cytochemical indices of RNA content and so reflect the intensity of protein synthesis, indicated also by its characteristic ultra-structural concomitants (Kahn *et al.*, 1983). The osteoblasts are arrayed in close proximity in a palisade and usually form only a single layer. Adjacent cells make contact by gap junctions (Doty, 1981), but there is no basement membrane and they do not provide the continuous barrier of a true epithelium (Kahn *et al.*, 1983).

Cells of this description are always separated from the mineralized bone surface by a layer or seam of, as yet unmineralized, bone matrix known as osteoid. Because of the local geometry, the profile of an osteoid seam appears in cortical bone as an annulus of circumference between 75 and 750 μm, and in cancellous bone as a crescent of length between 100 and 1500 μm, tapering at each end (Figs 3a and 4a). The seam merges into the thin layer of permanently unmineralized connective tissue (endosteal membrane) that separates lining cells from mineralized bone at quiescent surfaces (Parfitt, 1984); consequently, some criterion of minimum width must be adopted for defining the end of a seam. Based on resolution at magnifications convenient for quantitative microscopy, and on the tinctorial characteristics of the Villanueva bone stain, 2 μm is used in the author's laboratory. The thickness, surface extent and volume of osteoid are important quantitative indices of bone formation (Tables 1 and 2) and their mechanisms of control and functional and diagnostic significance (Parfitt, 1984a; Parfitt, 1988a; Parfitt, in press) are examined later. Described elsewhere are the relationships between these three-dimensional quantities and the primary two-dimensional, histologic measurements of width, perimeter length and area (Parfitt *et al.*, 1987b).

The interface between the cells and the osteoid is the site of matrix deposition, and the interface between the osteoid and the mineralized bone is the site of mineral deposition, so the existence of an osteoid seam is a

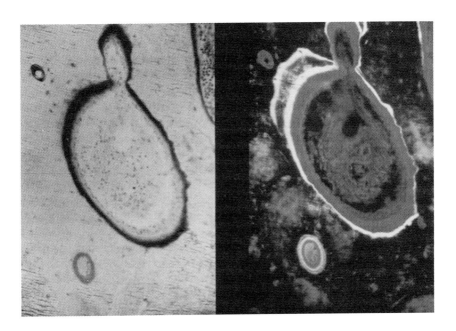

**Fig. 3** Cross-section through a cortical remodeling unit soon after onset of bone formation. The section is near a branching point, but the major branch would be located approximately as indicated in Figure 2. Left (a): bright field illumination to show osteoblasts and osteoid. Right (b): ultraviolet illumination to show bright bands of tetracycline fluorescence. The bone between the two labels in the left upper pole is of low mineral density because it has been recently made, and has large osteocytes because it was the bone made closest to the cement line. In the lower left-hand corner is a section through an almost completed unit where the seam is thin, the osteoblasts flat and the labels closer together. (x70)

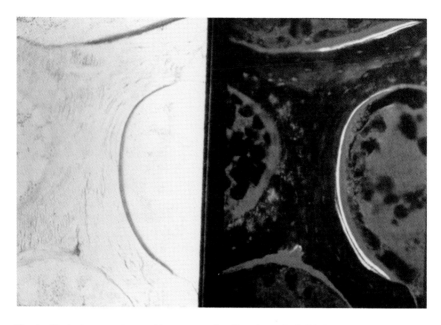

**Fig. 4** Typical crescentic osteoid seams in cancellous bone. Left (a): bright field illumination to show osteoid; the osteoblasts are not well stained. Right (b): ultraviolet illumination to show bright bands of tetracyline fluorescence. The seam profiles are crescents, in contrast to the annuli in Figure 3. (×75)

consequence of the spatial separation between these two aspects of bone formation (Parfitt, 1983). This in turn is a consequence of the temporal separation imposed by the need for matrix to mature before it can mineralize (Baylink *et al.*, 1980). Apparently homogeneous by light microscopy, osteoid contains several different zones by electron microscopy, the nascent collagen fibrils adjacent to the osteoblast showing increasing aggregation and alignment because of cross-linking before incorporation into mineralized bone (Fornasier, 1977; Kahn *et al.*, 1983). Other changes in preparation for mineralization (Parfitt, 1983) give rise to the histochemical features found at different distances from the osteoblast (Loe, 1959; Juster *et al.*, 1967).

**Table 1**
Tetracycline-based indices of bone formation and mineralization.

| | |
|---|---|
| Bone Surface (BS) | Total surface, whether mineralized or not |
| Osteoid Surface (OS) | Extent of surface currently *unmineralized* |
| Mineralizing Surface (MS) | Extent of surface currently *mineralizing* |
| Mineral apposition rate (MAR) | Mean interlabel distance/label interval |
| Adjusted apposition rate (Aj.AR) = | MAR * MS/OS |
| Mineralization lag time (Mlt) = | Mean osteoid thickness/Aj.AR |
| Formation Period (FP) = | Mean wall thickness (W.Th)/Aj.AR |
| Osteoblast vigor (% total/d) = | 1/FP * 100 |
| Bone formation rate (BFR)/BS = | MAR * MS/BS |
| Activation frequency (Ac.f) = | (BFR/BS)/W.Th. |

Definitions and abbreviations (Parfitt *et al.*, 1987b); for further details see text.

**Table 2**
Indices of bone formation and mineralization in the ilium.

| | *Cancellous* | *Endocortical* | *Intracortical* |
|---|---|---|---|
| Osteoid surface (%BS) | 10.1 ± 6.5 | 13.6 ± 8.7 | 11.9 ± 6.4 |
| Osteoid volume (%BV) | 1.50 ± 1.1 | —[a] | 0.32 ± 0.22 |
| Mineralizing surface (%BS) | 6.8 ± 3.3 | 7.3 ± 5.6 | 8.9 ± 6.2 |
| Osteoblast[b] surface (%BS) | 2.9 ± 1.7 | 3.3 ± 3.2 | 3.5 ± 3.3 |
| Osteoblast[b] surface (%OS) | 30.7 ± 16.3 | 26.0 ± 19.7 | 27.3 ± 22.0 |
| Mineralizing surface (%OS) | 70.8 ± 18.6 | 57.2 ± 28.5 | 67.7 ± 26.9 |
| Mineral apposition rate (μm/d) | 0.65 ± 0.11 | 0.63 ± 0.19 | 0.67 ± 0.19 |
| Osteoid apposition rate (μm/d) | 0.47 ± 0.16 | 0.40 ± 0.22 | 0.49 ± 0.23 |
| Osteoid thickness (μm) | 10.8 ± 2.2 | 9.7 ± 3.0 | 10.4 ± 2.6 |
| Mineralization lag time (d) | 25.8 ± 12.4 | 38.0 ± 29.6 | 34.2 ± 31.2 |
| Wall thickness (μm) | 41.8 ± 3.6 | 49.1 ± 5.1 | 54.3 ± 9.3 |
| Formation period[c] (d) | 95.2 ×/÷ 1.5 | 148 ×/÷ 2.1 | 130 ×/÷ 2.1 |
| Osteoblast vigor[c] (% total work/d) | 1.05 ×/÷ 1.5 | 0.68 ×/÷ 2.1 | 0.77 ×/÷ 2.1 |
| Bone formation rate (μm³/μm²BS/y) | 14.8 ± 6.2 | 16.6 ± 13.1 | 22.3 ± 17.9 |
| Activation frequency (/y) | 0.30 ± 0.13 | 0.29 ± 0.23 | 0.34 ± 0.27 |

Data obtained in 24 healthy, pre-menopausal women, aged less than 50 years, with measurements made separately on the cancellous, endocortical and intracortical subdivisions of the endosteal envelope. Data shown as means ± SD, with correction for three-dimensional expression (Parfitt *et al.*, 1987b). a. No volume is assigned to the endocortical surface. b. Includes types II and III combined. c. Geometric mean ×/÷ SD.

They likely include binding of phospholipids to collagen and of calcium to non-collagenous matrix proteins, accumulation of silicon (Landis *et al.*, 1986) and zinc (Vincent, 1963), and an initial increase in glycosaminoglycan content with a precipitous decline just before the onset of mineralization

(Baylink *et al.*, 1972). The time period required for these structural and bio-chemical changes — the osteoid maturation time — determines the earliest time point, after the onset of matrix synthesis at the birth of a new osteoid seam, that mineralization can begin.

An osteoid seam is generally an expression of the current activity of a team of osteoblasts, but histologic sections also contain information about the work of previous osteoblasts. The profile of the layer of cement substance deposited during the reversal phase is a cement line, and the region between a cement line and the closest quiescent bone surface is the profile of a new structural unit of bone made at some time in the past by one osteoblast team. In cortical bone the structural unit is the familiar haversian system or secondary osteon, a cylinder about 150−250 μm in diameter with a central canal. In cancellous bone the structural units are flattened and have a complex three-dimensional shape with interlocking prolongations (Kragstrup and Melsen, 1983a). The profile of a structural unit in a two-dimensional section is wider than but similar in shape to an osteoid seam — an annulus in cortical bone and a crescent in cancellous bone (Figs 5a and b). The perpendicular distance from the quiescent surface to the cement line at any location is known as wall thickness (Parfitt, 1983), and its mean value is an index of the depth of new bone deposited within resorption cavities by past osteoblast teams, averaged over the previous 1−20 years, the time depending on the local rate of bone turnover.

Within one structural unit the lamellae all run in a similar direction, but there is frequently a change in lamellar orientation at the boundary with older bone, and identification of this boundary using polarized light is the most commonly used basis for measurement of wall thickness (Lips *et al.*, 1978; Kragstrup *et al.*, 1982). What is likely the same boundary can be located by the color change from dark to light green (probably reflecting a change in mineral density) in Villanueva stained sections examined under ultraviolet light (Villanueva *et al.*, 1985). But if wall thickness measurement is based on positive identification of the cement line by staining, either with gallocyanine (Villanueva *et al.*, 1986) or toluidine blue (Recker *et al.*, 1988), significantly lower values are found (Villanueva *et al.*, 1985; Recker *et al.*, 1988). One explanation for this difference is that during the most recent remodeling episodes resorption remained wholly within a previous structural unit, and that osteoblasts present at different times at the same location respond to similar signals induced by mechanical strain, and so deposit collagen with similar orientation (Fig. 6), as an expression of what Frost has termed micromodelling (Frost, 1985a). Be that as it may, wall thickness measurements in different laboratories and in different groups of subjects cannot be compared unless the same method was used.

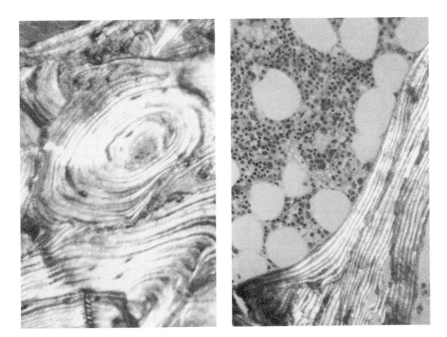

**Fig. 5** Profiles of a structural unit in cortical bone (left), forming a wide annulus, and in cancellous bone (right) forming a wide crescent. Note demarcation between new and old bone based on direction of lamellae. (×145)

## The Kinetics of Bone Formation

*In vivo* double-tetracycline labeling (Frost, 1968; Parfitt, 1983) introduces the critical dimension of time into bone histology. Tetracycline chelates calcium, and when its blood concentration is raised it binds reversibly to every bone surface accessible to the circulation, but with preference for the most recently formed mineral, which is of small crystal size and large surface area (Parfitt, 1983). During the few days after the end of a labeling period, tetracycline is permanently fixed at sites of currently active mineralization, where it is recognizable by its characteristic fluorescence under

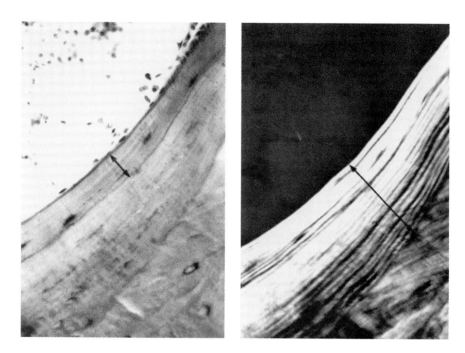

**Fig. 6** Comparison of two methods of measuring wall thickness. Gallocyanine stained section examined under regular light on left, and polarized light on right. The demarcation between newer and older bone based on cement line staining differs in location from the demarcation based on lamellar orientation. The cement line location is descernible under polarized light with this stain but usually not with other stains. If the cement line is an arrest line, the wall thickness based on lamellar orientation would be correct, but the fineness of the line and its wavy contour are more consistent with a reversal line. Note lining cells on the surface with flat and widely separated nuclei. (×175)

ultraviolet illumination. For convenience a band of fluorescence is also referred to as a label. Unlike radiocalcium, tetracycline accumulates in dead bone at sites that were forming *in vivo*, so there must be an additional, purely physicochemical mechanism of fixation (Parfitt, 1983; Aaron *et al.*, 1984). Sites of current mineralization are also identifiable by a band of granular structure and somewhat blurred outline that stains deeply with toluidine blue (Villanueva *et al.*, 1983b), and by a variety of other histo-chemical methods (Leblond and Weinstock, 1972; Parfitt, 1983). The min-eralization front so defined is invariably located at, but is not synonymous with, the osteoid-mineralized bone interface which persists until the osteoid seam disappears, whether or not mineralization is occurring.

A double band of fluorescence (Figs 3b and 4b) establishes unequivocally that bone formation occurred during the relevant time period, and permits measurement of the mineral apposition rate (Tables 1 and 2), but only a single label can be deposited if mineralization begins or ends between the periods of label administration. The best estimate of the extent of bone surface currently undergoing mineralization (Tables 1 and 2) is the mean length of the two labels, or the length of the second label, which is closer in time to the biopsy (Parfitt *et al.*, 1987b). If mineralization was continuous, all osteoid would be labeled except that which was most recently formed and which had not yet begun to mineralize, and the proportion of labeled osteoid would usually be greater than 85%. But in normal, young women the currently mineralizing surface averages only about 70% of the osteoid surface (Table 2), and in about half the subjects more than 30% of the osteoid is without any label. The proportion of osteoid undergoing mineral-ization is reported to be higher with histochemical methods of identification (Bordier and Tun Chot, 1972; Vedi *et al.*, 1982), but this reflects lower values for osteoid surface due to exclusion of thin seams.

One explanation proposed for the occurrence of unlabelled osteoid is that mineralization temporarily ceases and subsequently resumes (Frost, 1981). As will be discussed later, prolonged arrest of formation, giving rise to a so-called resting seam, is an important aspect of disordered osteoblast function in disease, but its occurrence in normal physiology is uncertain. Interruption of mineralization has been inferred in normal dogs because of the occasional absence of a second label despite the presence of osteoid (Hori *et al.*, 1985), but the oxy-tetracycline that was used can escape detection, because of all the standard labelling agents it has the least bright fluorescence. Further-more, in normal dogs (Schwartz and Recker, 1982) the relative proportions of single and double labelled surfaces agree closely with predictions from a theoretical algorithm (Frost, 1983), but if there were significant pauses in mineralization more single label would be found.

Excess single label consistent with interrupted mineralization has been found in one set of normal subjects (Keshawarz and Recker, 1986) but not in another (author's unpublished data). This difference could have been the result of making fluorescence measurements on thicker sections (Birkenhager-Frenkel and Birkenhager, 1987); these were 10 µm in the former study and 5 µm in the latter. Unlabelled osteoid occurs preferentially at the end of the osteoid seam life span when mineralization is much slower (Eriksen *et al.*, 1984). An alternative explanation is that too few tetracycline molecules are retained to exceed the threshold for visible fluorescence (Parfitt, 1984b; Parfitt, 1988a). When oxytetracycline is used as one of the labelling agents the total length of its label is consistently shorter than that of the other label (Villanueva and Parfitt, unpublished data), and the ease of detection of a label varies with the dose of tetracycline (Hattner *et al.*, 1977). The same mechanism could also account for an apparent excess of single label. Consequently, the occurrence of long term cessation of mineralization as a normal phenomenon remains unproven. In rapidly growing animals mineralization displays short term periodicity (Tam *et al.*, 1981; Simmons, 1981); whether the same occurs in mature, large animals is unknown.

The mineral apposition rate is widely but erroneously believed to reflect the process of mineralization independent of matrix synthesis, but mineralization cannot occur unless matrix is available. In experimental animals the rate of matrix apposition can be measured directly *in vivo* by radioautography of bone after administration of a labelled collagen precursor such as proline (Leblond and Weinstock, 1972; Marie *et al.*, 1985a). In human subjects only indirect measurement is possible, but in a completed structural unit the volumes of matrix and of mineralized bone are the same, and the distances travelled away from the cement line by the osteoblast-osteoid interface and by the osteoid-mineralized bone interface are the same. Consequently the mean rates of matrix apposition and mineral apposition averaged throughout the lifespan of an osteoid seam must be identical, even though, as described later, their instantaneous rates are systematically out of step.

Pending clarification of the significance of unlabelled osteoid, the best estimate of matrix apposition rate is the mineral apposition rate multiplied by the fraction of osteoid surface currently undergoing mineralization, as previously defined (Parfitt, 1983; Parfitt, 1988a), recognizing that this may be an underestimate. This quantity — the *adjusted apposition* rate (Tables 1 and 2) — can be referred to as the osteoid apposition rate in the absence of osteomalacia (Parfitt *et al.*, 1987). By contrast, the unadjusted mineral apposition rate is an estimate of the average velocity of mineral apposition during the first half or so of the osteoblasts lifespan when they are most active, although the peak instantaneous rates that occur soon after the onset of mineralization are substantially higher. Implicit in all these calculations is that the subject was in an approximate steady state at the time of the biopsy, and that measurements were made at an adequate number of locations, i.e. that sampling is unbiased with respect to both time and space.

Wall thickness is an estimate of the amount of bone matrix synthesized by a team of osteoblasts, and osteoid apposition rate is an estimate of how quickly the work of matrix synthesis can be performed. Wall thickness divided by osteoid apposition rate is an estimate of the time taken to complete the work, referred to as the formation period (Tables 1 and 2; Parfitt *et al.*, 1987b) or sigma (Frost, 1985a). This constitutes a natural time unit for the skeleton that affects the interpretation of all experiments that relate to bone remodelling *in vivo*, whether the planned experiments of the laboratory or the natural experiments of disease, since it is the shortest period needed to attain a new steady state after any intervention (Frost, 1973a). Amount of work, rate and time are interrelated, but under most circumstances time is the dependent variable. A team of osteoblasts strives to complete the task defined for it by the size of the resorption cavity, however long it should take, rather than to work only for a particular time, however little has been accomplished (Parfitt, 1976a).

Osteoid thickness is the amount of bone matrix remaining to be mineralized at any point on an osteoid seam, and osteoid thickness divided by osteoid apposition rate is an estimate of the average time interval between the deposition and mineralization of any infinitesimal volume of bone matrix (Fig. 7), referred to as the mineralization lag time (Tables 1 and 2; Parfitt, 1983; Parfitt, in press). At the birth of a particular osteoid seam, the lag time is synonymous with the osteoid maturation time as previously defined, but the lag time averaged throughout the life span of a seam is appreciably longer than the initial maturation time. The increase could result from a decline in the supply of mineral, since the net inward flux of calcium characteristic of osteoblasts must at some point change to the outward calcium gradient without net flux characteristic of lining cells (Parfitt, 1976a). To the extent that lag time exceeds maturation time the former is not an independent quantity but is an automatic consequence of the separately regulated rates of matrix and mineral apposition. Fortunately, this does not detract from its usefulness in the understanding of histomorphometric data.

The mineralizing surface expressed per unit of bone surface, rather than per unit of osteoid surface, multiplied by the mean mineral apposition rate gives the bone formation rate per unit of bone surface (Tables 1 and 2):

$$\text{BFR/BS}(\mu m^3/\mu m^2/y] = \text{MAR}(\mu m/d)*\text{MS/BS}*365 \dots\dots\dots\dots\dots (1)$$

Wall thickness is an estimate of the amount of bone made per activation event, so that bone formation rate divided by wall thickness is an estimate of the frequency of remodelling activation (Tables 1 and 2).

$$\text{Ac.f}(/y) = \text{BFR/BS}(\mu m^3/\mu m^2/y)/\text{W.Th}(\mu m) \dots\dots\dots\dots\dots\dots (2)$$

Since wall thickness varies only moderately, changes in formation rate are

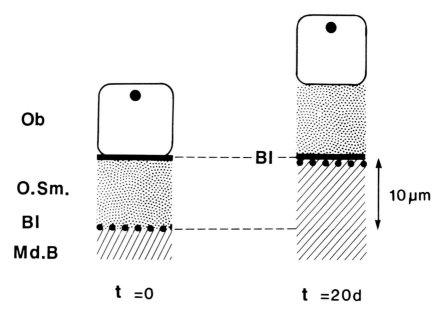

**Ob**

**O.Sm.**

**BI**

**Md.B**

t =0                                            t =20d

**Fig. 7** Calculation of mineralization lag time (Mlt). Ob = osteoblast; O.Sm = osteoid seam; BI = bone interface; Md.B = mineralized bone. At t = 0, the moiety of matrix immediately adjacent to the osteoblast (heavy solid line) has just been deposited. At t = 20 days, this moiety has just been reached by the advancing BI, which has traveled 10 μm (the thickness of the osteoid seam at t = 0) in 20 days for a mineral apposition rate of 0.5 μm/d. The thickness of the seam at t = 20 (the time of measurement) = 20 * matrix apposition rate (μm/d). In a steady state, mean thickness at t = 0 and at t = 20 are equal, and mean matrix and mineral apposition rates are equal. Modified from Parfitt (in press), with permission.

mainly the result of changes in the rate of remodelling activation (which determines the number of osteoblast teams created in unit time) rather than changes in the amount of bone made by the average team.

The volume, thickness and surface of osteoid are related as follows:
$$OV/BV(\%) = O.Th(\mu m) * OS/BS(\%) * BS/BV(\mu m^2/\mu m^3) \dots \dots \dots (3)$$

Each of these osteoid indices are separately related to the kinetic quantities defined earlier. As already mentioned, osteoid thickness is the product of osteoid apposition rate and mineralization lag time. Osteoid surface is determined by the average frequency with which new osteoid appears at any point on the bone surface (which in the steady state is the same as the rate of remodelling activation) and by the mean osteoid seam life span, or formation period. Osteoid volume is determined by the fractional rate of bone turnover (or volume-based bone formation rate) and the mean life span of an individual moiety of osteoid, which is the mineralization lag time. These relationships may be expressed:

$$O.Th(\mu m) = OAR(\mu m/d)*Mlt(d) \dots\dots\dots\dots\dots\dots\dots\dots\dots (4)$$

$$OS/BS(\%) = Ac.f(/d)*FP(d)*100 \dots\dots\dots\dots\dots\dots\dots\dots (5)$$

$$OV/BV(\%) = BFR/BS(\mu m^3/\mu m^2/d*Mlt(d)*BS/BV(\mu m^2/\mu m^3)*100 \dots (6)$$

Since wall thickness and bone surface/volume ratio vary little, the relationships between the static indices of osteoid accumulation and the kinetic indices of bone formation can be summarized as in Figure 8, and are depicted graphically in Figure 9. Note that each osteoid index is determined by different aspects of bone cell function, and in particular, that osteoid volume is independent of apposition rate, which in the steady state affects surface and thickness in opposite directions.

## The Life History of an Osteoblast and of an Osteoid Seam

Many of the cells found in close proximity to an osteoid seam, and therefore presumably associated with the process of bone formation, differ from the typical description of an osteoblast given earlier. Osteoid-related cells may be classified on morphologic grounds into four types (Villanueva et al., 1983a) that are believed to represent successive stages in the differentiation of a single cell line undergoing sequential changes in activity as well as in appearance (Parfitt et al., 1977; Parfitt, 1984b). Type I cells (Figure 10) have a large nucleus of elliptical profile with major and minor axes of approximately 15 and 9 μm containing 1−3 nucleoli and numerous chromatin granules that impart a speckled appearance; the cytoplasm is poorly stained and frequently invisible. Such cells are found in clusters close to a recently formed seam or in the deepest regions of a resorption cavity (Eriksen, 1986). These cells are believed to be preosteoblasts for two reasons. First, they are virtually identical in appearance with the cells found close to cancellous bone surfaces in the beagle that have the highest labelling index after tritiated thymidine administration (Kimmel, 1981a). Second, enlargement of the nucleus is a good indication that a cell is preparing to divide (Yen and Pardee, 1979), a morphometric criterion that has been validated specifically for osteoblasts and their precursors (Polig et al., 1984; Roberts and Morey, 1985).

Cells classified as type II (Fig. 11a and 11b) are the typical (cuboidal) osteoblasts described in a previous section, with the long axis usually perpendicular to the surface. Type III cells (intermediate osteoblasts) have profiles that are smaller and flatter in shape, with a long axis of 15−20 μm

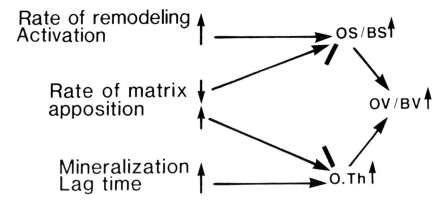

**Fig. 8**  Relationship between indices of osteoid accumulation and kinetic indices. A change in matrix apposition rate affects osteoid surface and thickness in opposite directions, because of reciprocal changes in formation period; in the steady state such changes have no influence on osteoid volume (indicated by heavy lines in front of arrows), which is determined only by the frequency of activation of remodeling and the mineralization lag time. Reprinted from Parfitt (in press), with permission.

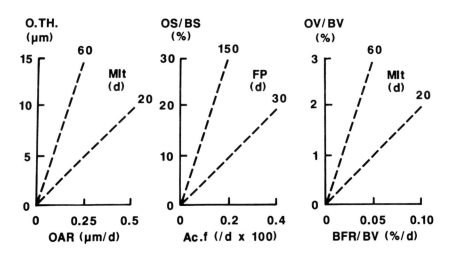

**Fig. 9**  Relationships between osteoid indices and kinetic aspects of osteoblast function. Abbreviations as in table 1. In each panel one kinetic quantity is plotted on the abscissa and the other is the slope of the corresponding line through the origin. Scales chosen to correspond appropriately to ranges expected in normal subjects. Units chosen to conform to equations in text.

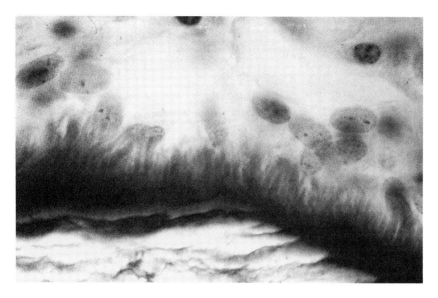

**Fig. 10** Type-I Cells (Pre-osteoblasts). Note large oval speckled nuclei with prominent nucleoli, pale-staining and barely visible cytoplasm and variable orientation and location. The fimbriated appearance of the osteoid is typical when a nascent seam is sectioned obliquely. (×280)

invariably parallel to the surface (Fig. 11c). The nucleus is also smaller and flatter than in Type II cells, with profile dimensions of approximately 10 × 4 μm. There is no juxtanuclear vacuole and the cytoplasm is less basophilic and contains fewer pyroninophilic granules. The profiles of Type IV cells (flat osteoblasts) and their nuclei are even thinner, flatter and more elongated and the cytoplasm is only weakly staining and contains few or, more usually, no pyroninophilic granules (Fig. 11d). The thinnest Type IV cells are indistinguishable from the lining cells that cover quiescent bone surfaces. It seems likely that Types II–IV represent a continuum of change in cell and nuclear shape and in intensity of basophilia and pyroninophilia, and the same morphologic sequence is found in diaphyseal bone growth (Volpi *et al.*, 1981) as well as in adult bone remodelling. Types II and III together correspond approximately to so-called "active" osteoblasts and Type IV to so-called "inactive" osteoblasts (Merz and Schenk, 1970; Bordier and tun Chot, 1972; Table 2).

The nuclear labeling studies necessary to prove developmental continuity between morphologically dissimilar cells cannot be performed in human subjects, but the interpretation proposed is supported by much indirect evidence. First, the different cell types are distributed, not at random, but such that most cells adjacent to the same osteoid seam are of similar morphology (Zallone, 1977). Consequently, the stage of evolution implied by the cell classification applies to the entire seam profile (Fig. 11). Second, the different cell types are consistently found at progressively greater distances from the cement line (Table 3), which serves as a marker for the passage of time (Parfitt *et al.*, 1981b). This inference is even stronger in cortical bone, where osteoblast morphology can be related also to the degree of radial closure (Marotti, 1977). Third, the nuclear height measured perpendicular to the bone surface, which provides a continuous measure rather than a discontinuous (and partly subjective) category of cell maturation, decreases progressively with increasing distance from the cement line (Eriksen *et al.*, 1984; Eriksen, 1986), as well as differing significantly between cell types (Polig *et al.*, 1984). Fourth, the sequential changes in morphology are accompanied by parallel changes in functional activity (Table 3), with a progressive decline in mineral apposition rate, fraction of osteoid labeled and osteoid thickness (Marotti, 1977, Parfitt *et al.*, 1981b; Eriksen, 1986).

These arguments imply that all members of the team of osteoblasts that will be responsible for rebuilding at a particular location must be assembled at about the same time, without the subsequent arrival of additional osteoblasts during construction, as some investigators have believed to be necessary (Johnson, 1964; Bordier *et al.*, 1977). During haversian remodelling in the beagle, the spatial distribution of labelled nuclei after administration of [3]H labelled thymidine indicates that new osteoblasts are formed only in the reversal region between the cutting and closing cones (Jaworski and Hooper, 1980) and do not continue to appear during centripetal closure of the osteon (Fig. 12). In human cortical bone, mitosis is observed only in the central connective tissue zone of the reversal region (Frost, 1965), from which pre-osteoblasts must presumably migrate towards the cement surface at the periphery (Fig. 12). Similar studies have not been performed in cancellous bone, but the location of pre-osteoblasts is inconsistent with continued osteoblast recruitment at the same site. Whatever the mechanisms of coupling, they have only a brief window of time in which to operate.

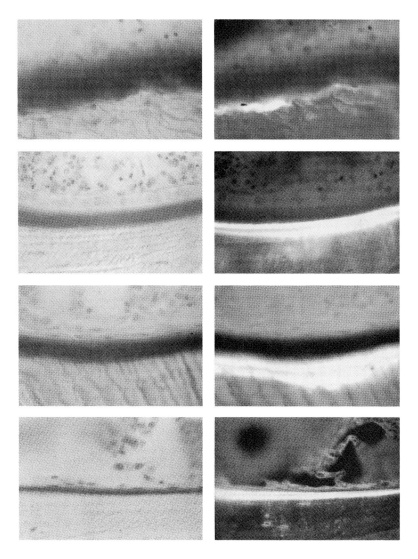

**Fig. 11** Sequential morphologic changes during the life span of osteoblasts. Bright field illumination on left to show osteoblasts and osteoid, ultraviolet illumination on right to show bright bands due to tetracycline fluorescence. a. Transition between Type I and Type II cells, with more regular orientation and location than in Figure 10; the cytoplasm is more basophilic and the nuclei are smaller, but pseudo-epithelial arrangement is not yet evident. b. Type II cells (cuboidal osteoblasts). c. Type III cells, with flatter and longer profiles. d. Type IV cells, showing further flattening of cells and more separation between nuclei. The distance between labels and the thickness of osteoid are not representative of the mean values in Table 3. (×385)

**Table 3**
Osteoblast differentiation.[a]

| | Osteoblast Type | | | |
| | II | III | IV | Combined |
|---|---|---|---|---|
| Extent (%OS) | 15 | 20 | 65 | 100 |
| Osteoid thickness (μm) | 17 | 12 | 7 | 9.5 |
| Mineralized thickness (μm) | 5 | 15 | 30 | 23.5 |
| Distance from Cm.Ln (μm) | 22 | 27 | 37 | 33 |
| Pyroninophilia | ++ | + | +− | + |
| Mineral apposition rate (μm/d) | 1.2 | 0.8 | 0.5 | 0.65 |
| Mineralizing surface (%OS) | 90 | 80 | 60 | 70 |
| Osteoid apposition rate | 1.5 | 0.6 | 0.2 | 0.45 |
| Mineralization lag time (d) | 11 | 20 | 35 | 28 |

a Structural and functional characteristics during morphologic transformation of osteoblasts through three stages of the life history of an osteoid seam. Representative composite values based on measurements in normal subjects and patients with osteoporosis (Villanueva et al., 1983a; Parfitt, 1983). The last column gives weighted averages over the entire osteoid surface. OS = Osteoid Surface; Cm.Ln = Cement line. Type I cells (pre-osteoblasts) are found apparently adjacent to about 1.5% of the osteoid surface, because of section obliquity, but are omitted for simplicity.

Multiple measurements at individual locations of osteoid thickness, mineralized bone thickness (distance between cement line and osteoid — bone interface) and total matrix thickness (distance from cement line to osteoid — marrow interface, or osteoid thickness plus mineralized bone thickness) can be used to construct growth curves which display movement away from the cement line as a function of time (Fig. 13), and represent the average kinetic history of individual bone-forming sites. In the first application of this idea the measurements were sorted according to osteoblast type (Parfitt et al., 1981b) but it is more efficient to sort them according to mineralized bone thickness (Eriksen, 1986), which allows the application of more sophisticated stereologic reconstruction methods (Eriksen et al., 1984). On such a plot the vertical distance between the growth lines for total matrix and for mineralized bone represents the osteoid thickness at a particular time, and the horizontal distance between the lines represents the time interval between deposition and mineralization of bone matrix (the mineralization lag time) at a particular distance from the cement line. The slope of the lines at any point is the instantaneous rate of matrix or mineral apposition.

Analysis of these curves indicates how the various aspects of osteoblast function change during the life history of an individual osteoid seam (Figure 14). The instantaneous values of the various quantities must be distinguished

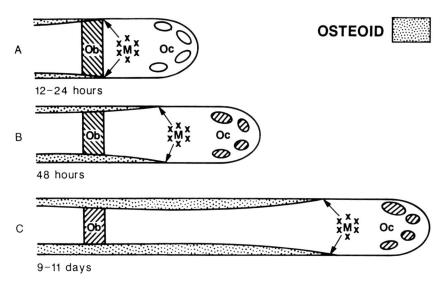

**Fig. 12**  Schematic representation of migration of labelled cells within cortical remodeling units. The zone of labelled osteoblasts (Ob) is initially located where bone formation has just begun. As the cutting cone advances to the right, the zone of labelled Ob remains in the same location relative to the bone, but becomes progressively further distant from the labelled osteoclasts (Oc). M = Zone of mitoses; the arrows indicate the presumed path of migration of pre-osteoblasts. Redrawn from Jaworski and Hooper (1980) with permission.

from the mean values obtained by histomorphometry as usually performed, which represent averages over the entire osteoid seam life span. Although more detailed measurements are available for cancellous bone, the overall sequence of events (Marotti, 1977), and the shape of the growth curves (Kelin and Frost, 1964) are very similar to those for cortical bone. The instantaneous rate of matrix apposition is most rapid (1.8−2.7 μm/d) at the onset, but falls quickly to about half the initial value. The osteoid seam increases rapidly in thickness to a maximum of about 15−20 μm, just before or shortly after the onset of mineralization 5−10 days later. The instantaneous rate of mineral apposition is also most rapid at the onset, but the peak rate is about half that of matrix apposition (0.9−1.3 μm/d). Thereafter, both rates progressively decline for the remaining life of the osteoid seam, but mineral apposition remains faster than matrix apposition. Consequently, the seam becomes progressively thinner and eventually disappears when formation is completed, leaving only the endosteal membrane, which is the last structure to be deposited by the osteoblast at the end of its active life span.

The cells of an osteoblast team, brought into existence at the same time

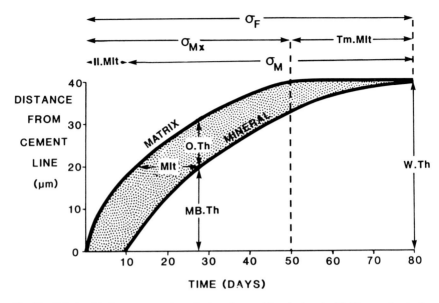

**Fig. 13** Relationship between matrix and mineral apposition during the life history of a single osteoid seam. The curved lines depict the distances of the edges of the matrix (osteoid) and of the mineral (bone interface) from the cement line as functions of time from the onset of matrix synthesis: the slopes of the lines at any point correspond to the instantaneous rates of matrix and mineral apposition. When the two curves meet, tne new structural unit is completed; at this point the vertical distance from the baseline is the wall thickness (W.Th) of the new unit (40 μm in this example) and the horizontal distance from the origin indicates the total duration of formation, or formation period ($\sigma_F$ — 80 days in this example). $\sigma_{Mx}$ — total duration of matrix synthesis (50 days), Tm.Mlt — terminal mineralization lag time (30 days), In.Mlt — initial mineralization lag time (10 days) (= osteoid maturation time), $\sigma_M$ — total duration of mineralization (70 days), MB.Th. = Mineralized bone thickness. The vertical distance between the two curved lines at any time represents the instantaneous osteoid seam thickness (O.Th) at that time. The horizontal distance between the curved lines at any distance from the cement line represents the instantaneous mineralization lag time (Mlt) at that distance. It follows that Mean O.Th.*$\sigma_F$ = Mean Mlt* W.Th. In the example shown, mean Mlt is 16 days, mean O.Th. = 8 μm, and mean adjusted apposition rate = 0.5 μm/d. Reprinted from Parfitt (in press), with permission.

and in the same place to undertake a common task, simultaneously undergo the same sequence of morphologic and functional changes. Virtually nothing is known about how this coordination is achieved, although it is likely to involve both local paracrine regulation (Kahn et al., 1983; Canalis, 1985) and some form of intercellular communication (Jeansonne et al., 1979; Khan et al., 1983). Even more remarkable than synchronization of function is the ability of osteoblasts to impose a structural order on their collective product that extends well beyond the immediate vicinity of a single cell. Osteoblasts must be able to control and systematically vary the orientation

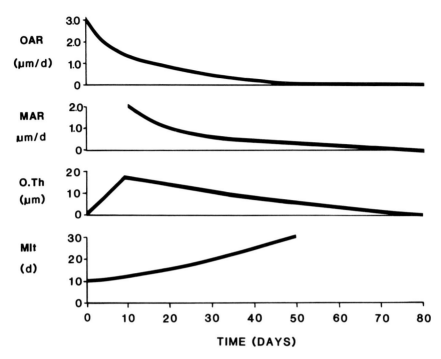

**Fig. 14** Changes in various indices of bone formation during the life history of an individual osteoid seam. Values correspond to the time course depicted in Figure 13. OAR — osteoid apposition rate; MAR — mineral apposition rate; O.Th. — osteoid thickness; Mlt — mineralization lag time. Reprinted from Parfitt (in press), with permission.

of the collagen fibers they produce in order to achieve the lamellated structure of mature bone, in which fiber direction remains more or less uniform within domains extending across the territories of many osteoblasts (Boyde, 1972). The alignment of the most superficial fibers closely matches the alignment of the osteoblasts in contact with them (Jones and Boyde, 1976), and there is suggestive evidence that control of alignment depends on the ability of osteoblasts to engage in limited movement over the surface (Boyde, 1972; Jones and Boyde, 1976). But how the collagen molecules made by adjacent cells are joined together to produce fibrils lying in the same direction remains a mystery.

The Osteoblast Team: Cell Number and Individual Cell Activity.

Differences in apposition rate are usually assumed to reflect differences in the activity of individual osteoblasts but must also depend on differences in cell density. The relevant index of activity is the volume of matrix synthesized per cell in unit time (production rate), and the relevant index of density is the number of cells per unit area of osteoid surface, which together define the following relationship:

Matrix apposition rate = Matrix production rate/cell*Cell density....(7)
$\quad$ ($\mu$m/d) $\qquad\qquad\qquad$ ($\mu$m$^3$/d) $\qquad\qquad\qquad$ (/$\mu$m$^2$)

This relationship is true whether expressed in terms of instantaneous values (Fig. 14) or mean values averaged throughout the seam lifespan. In the latter case the mean matrix apposition rate is the osteoid apposition rate as defined earlier. Unfortunately, there is no simple relationship between the number of osteoblast profiles in two-dimensional histologic sections and the number of osteoblasts in three-dimensional tissue (Gundersen, 1986). The few available direct measurements of osteoblast density are based on viewing the cell layer from above, either by light microscopy of thick longitudinal sections parallel to the closing cone of an osteon (Schen et al., 1965) or by scanning electron microscopy of intact bone surfaces (Jones, 1974). An alternative, less direct, method is to combine profile counts with determination of the average extension of osteoblasts in the third dimension from multiple serial sections (Marotti, 1977). The reciprocal of cell density is the contact area or secretory territory (Jones, 1974).

Wall thickness, like apposition rate, is also an expression of the integrated activity of the osteoblast team and must likewise depend both on cell activity and on cell density. The relevant index of activity is the average total volume of matrix synthesized by one osteoblast during its lifespan, referred to as matrix capacity, and the relevant index of density is the initial number of cells per unit area of cement surface. Because of the varying geometry of bone structural units, wall thickness depends also on the difference between initial cement surface area and final bone surface area (Jaworski and Wieczorek, 1985). This difference defines a dimensionless shape factor that is greater in cortical than in cancellous bone, as will be discussed later in more detail. With this proviso the following relationship will hold:

Wall thickness = Matrix capacity * Initial density * Shape factor ...(8)
$\quad$ ($\mu$m) $\qquad\qquad\qquad$ ($\mu$m$^3$) $\qquad\qquad\qquad$ ($\mu$m$^2$)

The relative constancy of wall thickness, which has a coefficient of variation of only 10−15% in any age group (Parfitt, 1988a) and no more than 20−25% throughout life (Landeros and Frost, 1964) probably reflects a relative constancy of both initial osteoblast density and matrix capacity (Jaworski and Wieczorek, 1985), since there is no evident reason why these two quantities should vary inversely.

Osteoid seam lifespan (formation period or sigma) is given by wall thickness divided by osteoid apposition rate, which defines the following relationship:

$$\frac{\text{Formation}}{\text{period (d)}} = \frac{\text{Mean matrix capacity } (\mu m^3)}{\text{Mean production rate } (\mu m^3/d)}$$

$$* \frac{\text{Initial density } (\mu m^2)}{\text{Mean density } (\mu m^2)}$$

$$* \text{ Shape Factor} \dots\dots\dots\dots\dots\dots\dots\dots\dots\dots\dots \quad (9)$$

The increase in secretory territory and consequent fall in cell density that occurs during the osteoid seam lifespan is more pronounced in cancellous than in cortical bone for the same geometrical reason mentioned earlier (Jaworski and Wieczorek, 1985), and so varies inversely with the shape factor. Consequently, the formation period is largely independent of cell density and is determined mainly by the two indices of osteoblast activity in matrix synthesis, the mean capacity and the mean rate of production. The formation period is currently the best index derivable by bone histomorphometry of individual osteoblast vigor (Frost, 1968), but formation period is inversely related to the fraction of its total lifetime output that an osteoblast can complete in one day, averaged throughout the osteoid seam lifespan, so that the reciprocal of formation period is directly related to osteoblast vigor (Tables 1 and 2), and has the advantage that a quantity with a lower limit of zero is more convenient to scale than a quantity with an upper limit of infinity.

The relationship between work, rate and time for an osteoblast team described earlier, and the analysis of team performance in terms of cell activity and cell number both suggest that each osteoblast has the potential to make a pre-determined total volume of bone matrix. Although plausible, this conclusion is not yet supported by any direct evidence and is in need of confirmation by measurements of three-dimensional osteoblast density, in conjunction with tetracycline-based remodelling kinetics. Nevertheless, as a reasonable working hypothesis, it suggests that a reduction in the number of osteoblasts recruited for a team will retard matrix apposition and reduce wall thickness in similar proportion, with little effect on formation period, and that a reduction in osteoblast vigor will slow down matrix apposition and prolong formation period in similar proportion with little effect on wall thickness (Fig. 15). This makes possible a preliminary examination of the relative contribution of these two components of osteoblast team performance in different circumstances.

The sequential changes in osteoblast morphology described earlier are accompanied by a loss of cells from the surface, both by transformation to osteocytes and by death (Parfitt, 1983), as will be discussed later in more detail. In haversian remodelling in the dog the initial secretory territory of osteoblasts is 100 $\mu m^2$, corresponding to a cell density of about 7,500/mm$^2$, allowing for gaps between the cells. Towards the end of radial closure secretory territory has increased to 224 $\mu m^2$, which corresponds to a cell density of about 2,000/mm$^2$, allowing for increased spacing between the cells (Marotti, 1977). For comparison, mean osteoblast density is about 4,500/mm$^2$ in human cortical remodelling (Schen *et al.*, 1965) and about 6,500/mm$^2$ in rat parietal bone (Jones, 1974). Reduction in cell density is undoubtedly one reason for the fall in apposition rate, but there is also a decline in osteoblast vigor. This has been demonstrated most clearly in dog cortical bone, with a 30% fall in matrix production per cell from 180 μm$^3$/d to approximately 130 μm$^3$/d, a change accompanied by a 45% decline in mean cell volume (Marotti, 1977). These data suggest that approximately 70% of the reduction in apposition rate results from loss of cells and 30% from decline in cell activity. Comparable measurements are not available in human bone, but during the first few weeks the fall with time in both matrix and mineral apposition is more rapid than the fall in nuclear height (Eriksen *et al.*, 1984).

There are large differences in activation frequency and bone formation rate between regions and between bones, with a distribution of remodeling activity that is probably characteristic of a particular species (Kimmel and Jee, 1982; Jaworski, 1987). To a large extent this reflects differences in mechanical strain in response to different patterns of load bearing and activity (Jaworski, 1987). Such differences could also account for the generally higher formation rates in men than in women (Melsen and Mosekilde, 1978). Remodeling is also influenced by the composition of the bone marrow. On surfaces in contact with hematopoietic marrow, the formation rate is higher (Wronski *et al.*, 1980) and apposition more rapid (Wronski *et al.*, 1981) than on surfaces in contact with fatty marrow. Red marrow has a higher blood flow (Gross *et al.*, 1979), a more extensive capillary network

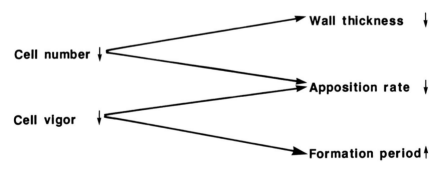

**Fig. 15** Relationships between osteoblast function and histologic indices. It is provisionally assumed that the average osteoblast makes the same total quantity of bone matrix during its lifetime; see text for further details.

(Burkhardt *et al.*, 1984), and greater abundance of precursor cells for both osteoclasts and osteoblasts (Vaughan, 1981; Baron *et al.*, 1983a; Kahn *et al.*, 1983) so it is not surprising that remodeling activation is more frequent. Apposition is presumably faster mainly because more cells are recruited for each team, but cell activity is probably also greater, because osteoblast size and vigor are correlated with vascular surface area (Marotti and Zallone, 1980).

Bone surfaces in continuity within the same bone can also manifest differences in remodeling. In the ilium, formation rates and wall-thickness both increase progressively from the cancellous to the endocortical to the intracortical or haversian surface, even though the rate of remodeling activation is not significantly different (Parfitt *et al.*, 1988; Table 2). Differences between the intracortical and cancellous surface are mainly the result of the geometric differences mentioned earlier. Assuming that cylindrical osteons have a cement line radius of 75 μm and a canal radius of 20 μm (Broulik *et al.*, 1982) the ratio of structural unit volume to initial cement surface area is 35 $\mu m^3/\mu m^2$. The shape factor required to convert this quantity to wall thickness (55 μm) is the ratio of initial surface area to mean surface area during closure, in this case 1.57. The calculations are more complex for cancellous bone, but if the structural units are segments through spheres of large radius, the ratio of volume to initial area is the same as in cortical bone but the shape factor is about 1.03 for a wall thickness (corrected for section obliquity) of 40 μm. However, these geometric factors do not adequately account for differences between the endocortical and cancellous surfaces, and an additional biologic difference is likely, such as in the number of osteoblasts recruited per activation event.

Pathologic conditions will be discussed more fully in the last section, but some general inferences can be made that shed light on the normal recruitment and activity of osteoblasts. An association between more frequent activation and more rapid apposition is found not only with local factors, such as erythoid hyperplasia (Weinstein and Lutcher, 1983) but also with systemic factors that influence bone remodeling, such as hyperthyroidism (Eriksen, 1986) and chronic renal failure with secondary hyperparathyroidism (Parfitt *et al.*, 1981b). But in normal menopause (Parfitt, in press) and in primary hyperparathyroidism (Eriksen, 1986) an increase in activation frequency is accompanied by a reduction in osteoid apposition rate, and there is no sex difference in osteoid apposition rate as there is in activation frequency (Melsen and Mosekilde, 1978). However, osteoid apposition rate cannot increase without an increase in activation frequency. It appears likely that the recruitment of osteoblast teams and the vigor of individual osteoblasts have some control factors in common and some that are specific to each function (Parfitt *et al.*, 1981b).

There are also instructive similarities and differences in the responses of osteoid apposition rate and wall-thickness to different conditions. Neither shows any difference between the sexes (Kragstrup et al., 1983b). Both are reduced in normal ageing and osteoporosis (Parfitt, 1988d) and in primary hyperparathyroidism (Eriksen, 1986), and both are increased in chronic renal failure (Parfitt et al., 1981). By contrast, in hypothyroidism (Eriksen, 1986), osteoid apposition rate and activation frequency are both markedly reduced, but wall-thickness is increased! This raises the possibility that a marked reduction in the number of osteoblast teams leads to an increase in the supply of precursor cells relative to demand, so that more osteoblasts can be recruited for each team. This would allow more bone matrix to be made despite the reduction in osteoblast vigor imposed by the general depression of cell metabolism.

## Osteoblasts in Growth and Repair

Most of the classic histologic studies of osteoblasts were carried out in embryonic or early neonatal bone, in which osteoblasts are much more numerous than in the adult skeleton (Pritchard, 1972). Osteoblast morphology is similar at all ages, but during growth the collective behavior of the cells is very different. Growth in the length of a bone occurs by enchondral ossification (Sissons, 1971; Kimmel, 1981b). The general scheme of growth in width is periosteal apposition of new bone without preceding resorption, and endocortical resorption of old bone without succeeding formation. This pattern is modified to maintain the shape of flared metaphyses, and to permit drift of the diaphysis relative to the body axis by eccentric rather than concentric growth (Smith, 1960; Frost, 1966). Slow growth occurs by simple apposition of circumferential lamellae, and rapid growth by lateral protrusion of perpendicular bars of bone which fuse to form longitudinal spaces that become filled by primary osteons, giving rise to so-called laminar or plexiform bone (Parfitt, 1976a). These processes, which change the size and shape of bones during growth, are referred to as modeling (Frost, 1966; Frost, 1985a), the term remodelling being restricted to the bone replacement mechanism in the adult skeleton described earlier.

The many differences between remodeling and modeling are summarized in Table 4. The most fundamental is that, in contrast to the cyclical erosion and repair of microscopic cavities with long periods of quiescence that is characteristic of remodeling, in modeling either resorption or formation occur continuously on the same surface for long periods of time without interruption (Parfitt, 1976a; Parfitt, 1984b). This has two related consequences: first, almost the entire periosteal and endocortical surface is engaged in either resorption or formation and there is little or no quiescent surface;

second, activation (in the sense of conversion of a quiescent to an active surface) is not required. Since the absolute change in cortical thickness is small in relation to the absolute change in external bone width, the velocity (distance travelled in unit time) of periosteal apposition and endocortical resorption can differ only slightly in a particular bone at one time, although both can vary widely between different bones and at different times. The mechanism of this close matching is unknown but it is presumably mediated by systemic rather than by local factors. Although the endocortical surface is predominantly resorptive during growth, if resorption is further stimulated by nutritional or hormonal manipulation, the additional deficit can be repaired by formation when the resorptive stimulus is removed (Baylink and Liu, 1979). Whether the mechanism of this local sequential coupling is similar to that in the adult remodeling skeleton is unknown.

The formation velocity or apposition rate is much faster during growth than after maturity. For example apposition rates of up to 70 μm/d occur at certain phases of growth in the young rabbit (Owen, 1971), and apposition rates of $3-10$ μm/d continue for long periods in the rat (Baylink *et al.*, 1970; Hammond and Storey, 1974). In human subjects the average rate of periosteal apposition is on the order of $2-3$ μm/d throughout the growth period, but during the most rapid growth the rate must be considerably higher. In the rat and rabbit the high rates of apposition are partly due to a high density of osteoblasts, which may be present in several overlapping layers, but the rate of matrix production is also higher than in the adult. For example, in rat parietal bone the apposition rate is 3 times higher than in human rib, reflecting a 50% increase in osteoblast density and a two-fold increase in matrix production per cell (Jones, 1974). Nevertheless, at the most rapidly growing surfaces the osteoblasts may only be active for a few days (Owen,

**Table 4**

Some differences between remodeling and modeling.

|  | Remodeling | Modeling |
|---|---|---|
| Timing | Cyclical | Continuous |
| Location of R and F | Same surface | Different surfaces |
| Extent | <20% of surface | >90% of surface |
| Activation[a] | Needed | Not needed |
| Apposition rate (μm/d) | 0.3 to 1.0 | 2 to 20 |
| Balance | Net loss | Net gain |
| Coupling | Local | Systemic |

R = resorption; F = formation
a. In sense of transformation of quiescent to active surface. Modified from Parfitt (1988a), with permission.

1971), so that the total matrix capacity as defined earlier could be similar at all ages.

Intracortical remodeling during growth is of lesser magnitude than the modeling changes just described, and is qualitatively different from that in the adult. About half of the currently active osteons manifest resorption on one side and formation on the other; because they appear to be moving laterally through the cortex they have been termed "waltzing" osteons (Epker and Frost, 1965), although "tangoing" osteons would be more accurate. However, the same appearance could be produced by an abrupt change in direction. If the former explanation is correct, the formation velocity on one side must be about the same as the resorption velocity on the other, a relationship that is characteristic of growth related processes but not of adult remodeling (Jaworski and Hooper, 1980; Jaworski, 1981). Another example of correspondence between resorption and formation velocities on different surfaces is the turnover of alveolar bone in relation to movement of a tooth under orthodontic manipulation (Baron et al., 1983a). Studies of cancellous bone remodeling during growth are sparse, but remodeling in the rat tail vertebrae appears to be both qualitatively and quantitatively similar to the human ilium (Baron et al., 1984).

Different types of bone are formed at different ages. Some are based on differences in the arrangement and quality of the collagen fibers (Smith, 1960; Pritchard, 1972; Parfitt, 1976a), but the two of greatest functional significance are woven or fibrous bone and lamellar bone (Collins 1966; Rasmussen and Bordier 1974; Table 5). As described earlier, lamellar bone is formed only in apposition to existing surfaces by coordinated osteoblasts making bone in a continuous layer on only one side. Woven bone is typically laid down directly in connective tissue, without the necessity for an adjacent free bone surface, by the rapid, uncoordinated, and non-polarised action of individual osteoblasts distributed at random. Each osteoblast surrounds itself on all sides with an island of new matrix without relation to its neighbors. Mineralization occurs rapidly and diffusely in the absence of clearly defined seams and without relation to collagen fibers, the process resembling the mineralization of cartilage rather than of mature bone (Boyde, 1972; Kahn et al., 1983).

The haphazard method of bone formation leads to a correspondingly haphazard structure, with collagen fibers running in all directions like carpet underfelt, in contrast to the regular grain of lamellar bone. Woven bone may resemble either cortical or cancellous lamellar bone in its three dimensional structure, but is usually intermediate between them in porosity and in the size of its soft tissue spaces (Hancox, 1972). The trabeculae are randomly arranged without relation to lines of stress, and are irregular in shape and variable in thickness. Osteocytes are more frequent and are scattered at random, with no relation to vascular channels. The lacunae are irregular in surface, and larger than in lamellar bone but more variable in size and shape (Frost, 1966; Boyde, 1972). Woven bone is invariably the first type of bone formed where no bone previously existed, and it is usually a temporary material whose normal fate is to be resorbed and replaced by lamellar bone.

Woven bone as described is characteristic of early embryonic development (Gardner, 1971), and consequently is sometimes referred to as fetal bone, but in the adult skeleton an intermediate type of bone formation is more common, in which bone that is lacking in lamellar structure, as determined by polarized microscopy, is laid down in apposition to an existing bone surface (Malluche and Faugere, 1986). Such bone can display all degrees of randomness of collagen fiber orientation, and is formed in fracture healing (Ham and Harris, 1971), in the periodontal ligament in response to orthodontic manipulation of a tooth (Storey, 1972) and in many pathologic situations described later. The osteoblasts are palisaded as in the formation of lamellar bone, and osteoid seams are well defined but woven in texture (Malluche and Faguere, 1986). Apposition rates are 50−100% greater than during the formation of lamellar bone, due to an increase both in cell density and in cell activity. Formation of ectopic bone, whether in the marrow cavity or outside the skeleton, begins in the manner described for embryonic bone but continues by apposition of adult-type, woven bone.

Recognition of the differences between growth and maturity in bone turnover and between woven and lamellar bone structure permits the description of five operationally distinct types of osteoblast activity (Parfitt, 1976a). 1, the noncoupled formation of woven bone *de novo* during early development, sometimes reactivated in later life; 2, the formation of woven bone coupled to previous chondroclastic resorption of calcified cartilage to form the primary spongiosa of enchondral ossification; 3, the formation of lamellar bone coupled to previous osteoclastic resorption of the primary

**Table 5**
Some differences between lamellar and woven bone.

| | Type of bone tissue | |
| | Lamellar | Woven |
| --- | --- | --- |
| Osteoblast organization | Monolayer | Isolated |
| Osteoblast activity | Polarized | Non-polarized |
| Fiber orientation | Regular | Irregular |
| Cell density | Low | High |
| Mineral density | High | Low |
| Production rate | Slow | Rapid |

spongiosa to form the secondary spongiosa; 4, the noncoupled formation of lamellar bone (both circumferential lamellae and primary osteons) on the periosteal surface of the diaphysis during postnatal growth; 5, the formation of lamellar bone coupled to previous osteoclastic resorption of lamellar bone during adult bone remodeling. In 2 and 3 the coupling is on a time scale of hours to days, but in 5 on a time scale of weeks and sometimes months. The first four all lead to a net gain of bone volume and mass, whereas the last leads for much of adult life to a net loss. Whether these activities are mediated by different cell types, or by the same cell types responding to different stimuli and different microenvironments, is not known.

## The Three Fates of an Osteoblast

As already stated, some osteoblasts become lining cells and some become osteocytes, but a significant proportion cannot be accounted for in either of these ways and must be presumed to have died during the life span of the seam. The relevant calculations, which assume an initial osteoblast density of $6,500/mm^2$ (Marotti, 1977), a lining cell density of $375/mm^2$ (Miller et al., 1980), an osteocyte density for cortical bone of $26,000/mm^3$ (Howard et al., 1985) and an 80% higher value for cancellous bone (Cane et al., 1982) are shown in Table 6 for both cortical and cancellous bone, assuming the geometrical shape factors previously calculated. In both types of bone the loss of osteoblasts is substantial (Johnson, 1964); but in cancellous bone a higher proportion finish up as either lining cells or osteocytes (Table 6). In every situation that has been appropriately studied, physiological or controlled cell death occurs by a process known as apoptosis (Wyllie et al., 1980), and the only study specifically addressing the issue suggested that osteoblasts die by the same mechanism (Kardos and Hubbard, 1982). Whether the three possible fates of an osteoblast are determined early in differentiation or occur randomly among equivalent cells is unknown, but would affect the significance of matrix capacity as defined earlier.

Lining cells represent the culmination of the morphologic transformation of osteoblasts described previously (Miller et al., 1980; Fig. 11). All the necessary transitional forms have been observed (Menton et al., 1984) and it is unnecessary to postulate a separate origin from the bone marrow unrelated to osteoblasts (Kahn et al., 1983). In the rat, lining cells are distinct from the marrow sac cells that enclose hematopoietic marrow (Menton et al., 1982; Menton et al., 1984) but in the dog only one cell layer can be found between the marrow and the bone (Deldar et al., 1985). Lining cell profiles are about 50 μm in length, with nuclei only 1−2 μm in thickness, often located near bone marrow capillaries (Miller and Jee, 1980). The cytoplasm does not exceed 0.5−1.0 μm in thickness and in

**Table 6**
Cell balance during remodeling.[a]

|                                          | Cortical  | Cancellous |
|------------------------------------------|-----------|------------|
| Initial osteoblast density $(/mm^2)$     | 6500      | 6500       |
| Corresponding final area $(mm^2)$        | 0.3       | 0.9        |
| Number of lining cells                   | 120(2%)   | 360(6%)    |
| Corresponding final volume $(mm^3)$      | 0.036     | 0.040      |
| Number of osteocytes                     | 940(14%)  | 1870(29%)  |
| Total cell number                        | 1060      | 2230       |
| Relative cell loss (%)                   | 84        | 65         |

a The measurements of osteoblast, lining cell and osteocyte density used in the calculations are cited in the text.

places must be so thin (less than 0.1 μm) as to be invisible by light microscopy, but by electronmicroscopy lining cells cover most of the quiescent bone surface (VanderWiel *et al.*, 1978), and gaps between the cells are not usually wider than 10 μm (Miller *et al.*, 1980). The thin edges of the cells may overlap and, like osteoblasts and osteocytes, they frequently make contact by gap junctions (Miller *et al.*, 1980). Lining cells have often been referred to as resting osteoblasts (Pritchard, 1972; Miller and Jee, 1987) and in birds they proliferate in response to estrogen and contribute to the formation of woven medullary bone (Bowman and Miller, 1986), but there is no evidence that they are able to regain the capacity to synthesize lamellar bone matrix in mammals. It seems reasonable to regard them as a distinct phenotype that, together with osteoblasts and osteoclasts, comprise the surface cells of bone (Miller and Jee, 1987).

Lining cells are in close proximity to the capillaries that run along the bone surface (Miller and Jee, 1980) and, via their cell processes running within canaliculi, they provide access to the circulation for osteocytes (Miller and Jee, 1980; Miller and Jee, 1987). Lining cells develop cytoplasmic contact with the marrow stromal cells from which they originated, and may participate in the regeneration of stromal cells and in their function of providing a suitable micro-environment for hematopoiesis (Deldar *et al.*, 1985). Quiescent surfaces are the primary site of mineral exchange between blood and bone, and regulation of this exchange by lining cells is an important component of calcium homeostasis (Parfitt, 1976a; Parfitt, 1987a), but detailed discussion will be deferred until the function of osteocytes has been examined. Finally, lining cells contribute in several ways to the activation of bone remodeling (Miller and Jee, 1987); by forming the primary target of several calciotropic hormones (Baron *et al.*, 1983a; Kahn *et al.*, 1983); by secreting collagenase to digest the endosteal membrane (Chambers *et al.*, 1985); by retraction to expose the mineralized bone surface (Parfitt, 1984b; Shen *et al.*, 1986); and probably by secretion of a variety of local regulatory substances (Parfitt, 1984b; Mundy and Roodman, 1987; Martin, 1987; Chambers, 1987). The fate of lining cells after activation is unknown, but it seems likely that they do not survive and that their average life span depends on the time interval between successive activation events at the same location, which is about three years in the ilium and up to 20 years on surfaces adjacent to fatty marrow.

Osteocytes are the most abundant cell type in bone. In cancellous bone with a surface/volume ratio of $15mm^2/mm^3$ there are approximately 10 times as many osteocytes as osteoblasts, and the preponderance is much greater in cortical bone. The transformation of osteoblasts to osteocytes, which is accompanied by a change in cell surface antigens (Nijweide and Mulder, 1986), has been described in detail (Boyde, 1972; Menton *et al.*, 1984). All osteocytes initially are enclosed by osteoid and may participate in its mineralization (Bordier *et al.*, 1977; Aaron, 1976). Around young osteocytes the synthesis of matrix and its mineralization continue for a short time (Baylink and Wergedal, 1971; Zallone *et al.*, 1983), but the composition of the intralacunar capsule and of the perilacunar bone made by osteocytes differs from that of interlacunar bone (Boyde, 1972; Parfitt, 1976a). Once this process is complete, the boundaries of lacunae do not change; there is no such phenomenon as osteocytic osteolysis (Parfitt, 1977; Boyde, 1981). The size of osteocytes and their lacunae depends on the size of the osteoblasts from which they arose, and so are larger in woven than in lamellar bone (Marotti *et al.*, 1985). Within each structural unit the lacunae are largest in the first-formed bone adjacent to the cement line, and smallest in the last-formed bone adjacent to the surface (Marotti, 1977). When new bone formation is stimulated by whatever means, the new lacunae may be made larger than usual and so remain, but lacunae made previously and already present are unaffected (Sissons *et al.*, 1985; Mercer and Crenshaw, 1985).

Osteocytes make contact by gap junctions, both with lining cells and with other osteocytes, via cell processes lying within canaliculae; contrary to earlier views, these extend across the cement line between adjacent structural units (Curtis *et al.*, 1985). The lacunar-canalicular network can maintain the viability of osteocytes provided they are not too far from a bone surface (Jaworski and Wieczorek, 1985), although the permissible distance may be greater than previously supposed (Curtis *et al.*, 1985). Osteocytes have a maximum life span of 20–25 years (Frost, 1960a; Hattner and Frost, 1963); many osteocytes are removed by remodeling before this span is reached, but even in cancellous bone in healthy subjects a significant proportion of osteocytes survive long enough for *in situ* death to be a plausible consequence, particularly in interstitial bone more than 75 μm from the surface (Parfitt *et al.*, 1987d). Osteocyte death is followed by hypermineralization of perilacunar and pericanalicular bone and eventually by plugging of lacunae and canaliculae by mineralized connective tissue, a phenomenon termed micropetrosis that is associated with increased brittleness (Frost, 1960b; Parfitt, 1987b). Osteocytes are probably able to detect mechanical strain via the generation of streaming potentials by deformation induced fluid flow (Eriksson, 1976; Frost, 1985b), but the signals that lead to adaptive bone remodeling on the surface are unknown. Osteocytes may also participate in the acquisition by bone of a strain memory that is dependent on the three-dimensional orientation of glycosaminoglycan molecules (Skerry *et al.*, 1987).

Lining cells and osteocytes together form a homeostatic system for regulation of the plasma calcium concentration that is partly independent of the remodeling system described earlier (Parfitt, 1976a; Parfitt, 1987a). Equilibration of calcium between blood and bone is inferred from the radioautographic demonstration of substantial uptake of labelled calcium at quiescent bone surfaces (Parfitt, 1981). Since there is little or no net flux, there has to be an equivalent outward movement of unlabelled calcium ions, a biologic equilibrium that must in some way be reconciled with the physico-chemical disequilibrium between bone mineral and systemic extra cellular fluid (ECF) (Parfitt, 1981; Parfitt, 1987a). Much evidence supports the existence of a separate bone ECF compartment that differs in composition from the systemic ECF, even though the lining cells provide only an incomplete and leaky barrier between them (Parfitt, 1981; Talmage *et al.*, 1983). The bone ECF extends throughout the canalicular and lacunar system, separating the mineral phase of bone from the bone cells, but also percolating through the submicroscopic channels between aggregates of crystals (Frost, 1973b).

Several theories concerning the blood-bone equilibrium postulate that lining cells maintain active outward transport of some ions-calcium, potassium or protons-but it seems more likely that the cells stabilize a less insoluble precursor such as brushite at the surface by secreting one or more inhibitors of transformation to hydroxyapatite (Parfitt, 1987a; Neuman *et al.*, 1987); whatever its nature, the same mechanism must also be provided by osteocytes, and must be susceptible to hormonal regulation (Norimatsu *et al.*, 1982; Parfitt, 1987a). The presence of non-apatite mineral of varying solubility on the surface could be related to the calcitonin-dependent, electron dense granules that appear beneath lining cells after feeding (Norimatsu *et al.*, 1982; Talmage *et al.*, 1983), and to the abundant particulate calcium in osteocytes (Nichols and Rogers, 1972). These particles, both extra and intracellular, probably represent a temporary storage form of bone mineral that participates in circadian changes in calcium balance

(Parfitt, 1981). The ability of the homeostatic system to regulate plasma calcium by determining the level of equilibration, and to stabilize plasma calcium by providing a short-term buffer mechanism, is enhanced by the large surface area for exchange provided by the canalicular-lacunar system, and by the percolation of bone ECF mentioned earlier (Frost, 1973b). Osteocytes are necessary for circulation through bone (Simmons et al., 1970) and for ion exchange with bone (Williams et al., 1987; Simonet et al., 1988), and could promote fluid movement by means of an osmotic pump, the efficiency of which is enhanced by counter-current flow inside and outside the cell processes with canaliculi (Frost, 1973b).

## Bone Forming Cells in Non-Optimal Conditions

A new osteoblast team is assembled at a time and place determined by an activation event, and the extent of its task is determined by the behavior of a preceding team of osteoclasts. The performance of the osteoblast team can be examined with respect to quantity of work (wall thickness), rate of work (osteoid apposition rate) and duration of work (formation period). These each relate in different ways to the number of osteoblasts initially recruited and the rate of their loss by death or further differentiation, and to the activity of individual osteoblasts. Ideally, all these aspects should be considered for each of the non-optimal conditions to be discussed, but there are extensive gaps in the available knowledge. In many clinical disorders, abnormal osteoblast recruitment or activity, either intraskeletal (Frame et al., 1987), or extraskeletal (Smith and Triffitt, 1986), can be inferred from radiographs or from standard histopathologic examination, but there has been too little study by the methods previously described to permit more than a brief qualitative description. The same applies to the important subject of benign and malignant tumors of bone-forming cells and their precursors. Such disorders may be mentioned briefly for the purpose of contrast or illustration, or else omitted altogether. Consequently the main emphasis will be on the role of osteoblasts in the pathogenesis of the three traditional forms of metabolic bone disease — osteoporosis, osteitis fibrosa and osteomalacia.

### The Effects of Age

The functions of all bodily systems reach a peak in young adulthood and thereafter decline progressively with increasing age (Hayflick, 1976), and the skeleton is no exception. For the scientific study of aging it is important to distinguish between effects on cells and on tissues due only to the passage of time, and effects secondary to age- or disease-related changes in other systems, but the information required to make these distinctions is frequently lacking; e.g. the difficulty in assigning relative importance to the effects of aging per se and of menopause or other endocrine changes. I have provisionally assumed that a decline in function is more likely to be a direct effect of age, and an enhancement of function more likely to be an indirect effect of age-related hormonal changes. It is also important to distinguish between the age of the body as a whole, and the age of individual cells (Hayflick, 1976; Baserga, 1985). Non-renewing cells such as neurons age in parallel with the body, but bone undergoes renewal. All neurons are necessarily older in an old than in a young person, but the ages of their osteoblasts may be very similar. The effects of aging are expressed mainly through the mechanisms of cell renewal, and the tissue, vascular and hormonal environment in which the osteoblasts must function.

## Changes in the amount and structure of bone

The most obvious effect of age on the skeleton is a decline in the amount of bone. The age at which this begins is uncertain, lying between 30 and 50 years, and is probably earlier in the axial than in the appendicular skeleton (Parfitt, 1988b). The trabeculae of cancellous bone become more widely separated (because some have been completely removed) and those remaining slowly become thinner. In the diaphyses, the boundary of cancellous bone tissue retreats towards the end of the bone so that in some locations cancellous bone disappears completely (Parfitt, 1988c), but some always remains in the vertebral bodies and ilium. In cortical bone the subendocortical regions become more porous and cancellous in structure, so that the marrow cavity gradually expands. Loss of bone from the endocortical surface is partly offset by very slow net apposition on the periosteal surface, but the usual net result is that the cortices become thinner. However, in extreme old age the rate of endocortical loss may fall below the rate of periosteal gain (Hui *et al.*, 1982).

It is both a necessary and a sufficient condition for net loss of bone to occur from a bone surface that the average quantity of bone made by a team of osteoblasts is less than the average quantity of bone removed by the preceding team of osteoclasts. Stated in another way, at any point on a surface bone will be lost if wall thickness at that point is less than the depth of the preceding resorption cavity at that point. The relative importance of these variables can be assessed in two ways. First, the performance of current osteoclast and osteoblast teams can be compared directly by complete remodeling sequence reconstruction (Eriksen, 1986), a method applicable to individual subjects, second the performance of previous osteoclast and osteoblast teams can be compared indirectly by measuring current activation frequency and mean wall thickness and estimating net bone loss from a particular surface (Parfitt *et al.*, 1987c), but this method is applicable only to groups of subjects. A limitation of both methods is that they cannot be used on the bone which has been lost, only on the bone that is still present for examination.

The most consistent age-related change in the function of osteoblast teams is a reduction in wall thickness on the cancellous bone surface (Parfitt, 1988a). This has been found with several different methods of measurement (Lips *et al.*, 1978; Kragstrup *et al.*, 1982; Villanueva *et al.*, 1985; Recker *et al.*, 1988) and in studies both of currently active (Eriksen, 1986) and previously active (Recker *et al.*, 1988) teams. Consideration of the mechanism and significance of this change must take account of the paradox that wall thickness does not fall with age on either the endocortical or the intracortical (or haversian) surfaces, at least in the ilium (Parfitt *et al.*, 1988; Table 7). The endocortical and cancellous bone surfaces are in continuity and in contact with the same bone marrow. The intracortical surface is in continuity with the endocortical surface, and is in contact with canalicular connective tissue and associated microcirculation, both derived from corresponding elements in the same bone marrow. All three surfaces are presumably perfused with blood and interstitial fluid of the same composition, ruling out any systemic contribution to the observed difference in osteoblast team performance with increasing age.

Could the fall in cancellous wall thickness with age be an artifact due to differential survival of trabeculae with different initial properties? Whenever there is focal remodeling balance, wall thickness is determined by resorption cavity depth. Trabeculae with deep cavities are more likely to be completely removed, and those with shallow cavities are more likely to survive (Parfitt *et al.*, 1987d). Consequently, wall thickness averaged over the entire surface would tend to fall with age even if wall thickness at any point on the surface remained constant. Since intracortical and endocortical bone loss is not accompanied by any net loss of surface, there is no differential survival of different regions, and no change in wall thickness with age would be expected. However, cancellous wall thickness probably begins to fall before there has been a significant reduction in total surface (Lips *et al.*, 1978; Recker *et al.*, 1988), and the frequency distribution of individual wall thickness measurements does not change in the manner expected from this mechanism (Eriksen *et al.*, 1984; Eriksen, 1986).

If the decline in wall thickness is genuine, then according to the model previously developed, the data suggest an age-related decline in the number of osteoblasts recruited for each team, in response to each activation event. The supply of osteoblast precursor cells could fall as a consequence of the

**Table 7**
Selected indices of osteoblast function in women.[a]

|  |  | Normal Subjects | | Osteoporosis |
| --- | --- | --- | --- | --- |
| Measurement | Surface | Age < 50y | Age > 50y | With Vert. Fx. |
| Wall thickness | Cancellous | 41.8 ± 3.6 | 38.7 ± 6.3 | 36.7 ± 6.1 |
| (μm) | Endocortical | 49.1 ± 5.1 | 49.2 ± 8.3 | 47.9 ± 6.1 |
|  | Intracortical | 54.3 ± 9.3 | 53.8 ± 7.2 | 53.9 ± 5.1 |
| Osteoid apposition | Cancellous | 0.47 ± 0.16 | 0.34 ± 0.15 | 0.24 ± 0.13 |
| Rate (μm/d) | Endocortical | 0.40 ± 0.22 | 0.35 ± 0.16 | 0.36 ± 0.19 |
|  | Intracortical | 0.49 ± 0.23 | 0.45 ± 0.23 | 0.42 ± 0.22 |
| Bone formation rate | Cancellous | 14.8 ± 6.2 | 20.7 ± 10.9 | 12.0 ± 11.8 |
| ($\mu m^3/\mu m^2 BS/y$) | Endocortical | 16.6 ± 13.1 | 24.8 ± 18.5 | 28.9 ± 25.2 |
|  | Intracortical | 22.3 ± 17.9 | 27.7 ± 16.2 | 27.4 ± 24.3 |

[a] Effect of age or menopause, and comparison with post-menopausal osteoporosis. Data expressed as means ± SD with correction for three-dimensional expression.

gradual replacement of hematopoietic by fatty marrow (Meunier *et al.*, 1971; Simmons 1981; Vaughan 1981). Alternatively, the intensity of the mitogenic signals generated by the coupling mechanism (Parfitt, 1984b; Canalis, 1985; Farley *et al.*, 1987) could decline with age. In either case there would need to be some circumstance unique to the cancellous bone surface. Changes in cell composition with age could occur at different rates in the central and peripheral zones of the marrow cavity (Deldar *et al.*, 1985). Alternatively, there could be regional differences in the response of the microcirculation to increasing age (Burkhardt *et al.*, 1984). Finally, declining physical activity could have a disproportionate effect on osteoblast recruitment in cancellous bone, which is more isolated from muscle tension than cortical bone, so that the minimum mechanical strain needed to sustain osteogenesis would be less easily achieved (Frost, 1987; Rubin and Lanyon, 1987).

## Changes in bone remodeling

In healthy women osteoblast teams not only make less bone with increasing age but they make it more slowly — osteoid apposition rate is about 25−30% less in healthy women older than 50 years than in younger women (Table 7). The fall in mineral apposition rate is modest, but the fall in the fraction of osteoid labelled is more substantial; possible interpretations of this were discussed under the Kinetics of Bone Formation. According to the model described earlier the fall in osteoid apposition rate is a consequence of an approximately 10% fall in the number of osteoblasts recruited for each team, and an approximately 20% fall in the average vigor of each osteoblast, with a corresponding prolongation of the formation period (Fig. 16). As for wall thickness, the changes are significant only on the cancellous surface; on the endocortical and intracortical surfaces the changes are in the same direction but are of smaller magnitude. Some explanations for focal decline in cell recruitment were given earlier. These explanations probably also contribute to a decline in cell vigor, but the release of various paracrine agents that stimulate individual cells could also undergo differential changes with age in different locations. Whether the same focal differences occur in men is unknown.

In normal subjects there is a significant, positive relationship between osteoid apposition rate and mean osteoid thickness (Fig. 17; Parfitt, 1984a). But the reduction in osteoid apposition after menopause is not accompanied by a fall in osteoid thickness, and the parameters of the regression equations are slightly different in the two groups (Parfitt 1984a). Consequently, there is an increase in mineralization lag time (O.Th/OAR) with age, most likely a reflection of delayed maturation of matrix rather than of a defect in mineralization (Parfitt, 1988a). This interpretation is supported by the absence of any change in lag time on the endocortical and intracortical surfaces; as will be mentioned in a later section, defects in mineralization are usually of similar severity on all surfaces. The association of delayed matrix maturation with impaired osteoblast vigor suggests that maturation is partly under osteoblast control, even though the changes are extracellular. Because of increases in both remodeling activation and formation period, osteoid surface also increases, with a corresponding increase in osteoid volume, but the values remain lower than in primary or secondary hyper-parathyroidism and much lower than in osteomalacia.

The falls in osteoblast recruitment and activity with age on the cancellous surface have several consequences. The effects of a fall in wall thickness depend on the corresponding changes in resorption cavity depth. Once the acute effects of menopause have subsided, resorption depth decreases, with a corresponding increase in interstitial bone thickness (Eriksen, 1986). A reduction in wall thickness of the same magnitude would be the expected response in order to maintain focal bone balance and preserve trabecular thickness. When the total cancellous space is examined, mean trabecular thickness does not change with age (Recker et al., 1988), because thinning in the central zone is balanced by the addition of new, thicker trabeculae at the periphery during the process of cancellization of the inner third of the cortex (Meema and Meema, 1988; Parfitt, 1988a). Trabecular thinning

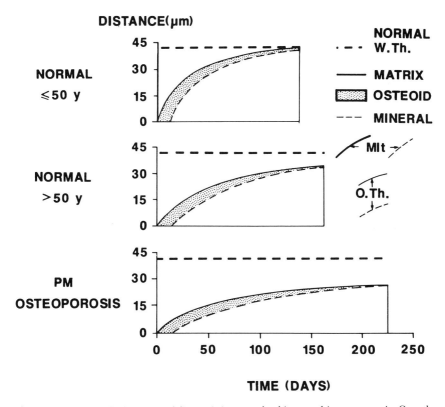

**Fig. 16** Evolution of a bone remodeling unit in normal subjects and in osteoporosis. Growth curves of matrix and mineral apposition constructed as in Figure 13. Note that the effect of age is to reduce wall-thickness and prolong formation period and that these age-related changes are more pronounced in patients with compression fracture. Modified from Parfitt, 1988a, with permission.

occurs when the osteoblast team fails to meet even the smaller task set by a less effective team of osteoclasts, with the result that trabeculae are more liable to perforation (Reeve, 1987) and more likely to undergo Euler buckling with load bearing (Kleerekoper *et al.*, 1987). The effects of a decline in osteoblast vigor and a corresponding prolongation of formation period will be discussed in the next section, in relation to the pathogenesis of fractures.

The lifelong net gain of bone on the periosteal surface is of potential clinical importance and some biologic interest, but its mechanism has received little attention. Some investigators have regarded it as a continuation of growth-related modeling at a very slow rate, but it seems more likely to be a form of remodeling in which the end result for each cycle is net gain

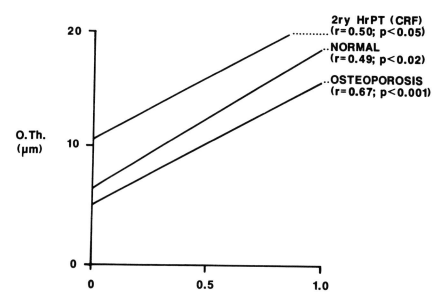

**Fig. 17** Relationship between osteoid thickness (O.Th) and osteoid apposition rate (OAR) in different conditions. Regression lines should be interpreted with caution, since each was estimated over a different range of OAR. There are significant differences between the intercepts, but not between the slopes. Data from Parfitt, 1984b.

rather than net loss as on the endosteal envelope (Parfitt, 1980). Fine detail radiography of the metacarpals indicates that a small proportion of the periosteal surface is normally undergoing shallow resorption (Meema, 1977), and the distribution of tetracycline labeling suggests that bone formation is discontinuous and cyclical rather than continuous (Epker and Frost, 1966). A remodelling based mechanism also accounts for the increase in the rate of periosteal gain after menopause, since the effect of an increase in remodelling activation is to amplify the magnitude of focal imbalance already present without changing its direction. Unfortunately, there are no data on resorption cavity depth or wall thickness on the periosteal envelope

## Sex Hormone Deficiency, Osteoporosis and Bone Fragility.

Age-related bone loss accelerates with menopause because of estrogen deficiency, but the remodeling mechanism is a combination of increased frequency of activation and consequent increase in the number of cell teams, and a qualitative abnormality in bone resorption such that teams of osteoclasts erode deeper than normal cavities, with little immediate change in the activity of osteoblast teams. More frequent activation and deeper resorption both increase the likelihood of trabecular plate perforation, which reduces three-dimensional connectivity and disproportionately impairs bone strength (Kleerekoper *et al.*, 1985). The recent discovery of estrogen receptors in osteoblast-like cells (Eriksen *et al.*, 1988) suggests that estrogen normally acts on lining cells in some manner to depress remodeling activation; the role of lining cells in the control of activation was discussed earlier. Estrogen may also act indirectly on bone by regulating the secretion of calcitonin, recently shown to be an effective substitute for estrogen in the prevention of early menopausal bone loss (Reginster *et al.*, 1987; MacIntyre *et al.*, 1988). Whether estrogen deficiency also contributes to the changes in osteoblast function described earlier (and attributed to age) is unknown, but available evidence suggests that these abnormalities are not reversed by estrogen replacement, the main effect of which is depression of remodeling activation and consequent reduction in the number of new osteoblast teams (Melsen *et al.*, 1989).

## Osteoblast dysfunction and bone fragility

A subnormal amount of bone, due to some combination of inadequate accumulation and excessive loss from untreated estrogen deficiency, or from other processes, is a necessary but not always a sufficient condition for the occurrence of fracture. The architectural effects on fragility were mentioned earlier. Among the population of women at risk, bone fragility is further increased by two abnormalities of osteoblast function that are confined to the cancellous surface in the ilium (Parfitt, 1988d), but present on all surfaces in the rib (Wu, 1973). A reduction in the rate of remodeling activation and consequent reduction in the frequency with which new teams of osteoblasts are assembled is a reversal of the age or menopause related trend, but a further fall in the rate of osteoid apposition and consequent prolongation of formation period is an exaggeration of the age or menopause related trend (Fig. 16; Table 7). In the ilium neither abnormality is found on either the endocortical or intracortical surface, on which formation rates tend to be as high or even higher than in healthy post-menopausal women (Brown *et al.*, 1987), and osteoid apposition rates very similar (Parfitt, 1988d; Table 7). Wall thickness is usually lower on the cancellous surface in patients with osteoporosis and vertebral fracture compared to healthy post-menopausal women (Darby and Meunier, 1981) especially at current remodeling sites in patients with low bone turnover

(Parfitt *et al.*, 1981b), but does not differ on the other subdivisions of the endosteal envelope.

As for the change with normal aging, the lower osteoid apposition rate is the result mainly of a fall in the fraction of osteoid labelled, but there is also a modest further reduction in mineral apposition rate (Meunier *et al.*, 1980a). In some patients the proportion of labelled osteoid is so small (sometimes absent altogether), that complete arrest of osteoblast activity seems a more likely explanation than retention of too little tetracycline to be detected. Such arrest may be prolonged but must be temporary, or else the entire surface would eventually be covered by osteoid. The concept of resting seams was originally developed from the study of cortical bone, in which the bone adjacent to osteoid seams is normally permeable to fuchsin when examined in fresh, unembedded, hand-ground sections, because recently deposited mineral is of relatively low density (Frost, 1966). The bone adjacent to a resting seam is impermeable to fuchsin, indicating a substantial increase in mineral density that would have taken several months, during which no further matrix synthesis could have occurred. This method cannot be applied to plastic embedded sections of cancellous bone, in which the existence of resting seams awaits confirmation by other methods such as microradiography. In cortical bone, resting seams were often found in states of tissue hypoxia (Frost, 1966), which may relate to the adverse effects of respiratory acidosis on the recruitment and function of osteoblasts (Malluche and Faugere, 1986).

According to the model developed previously, the lower osteoid apposition rate in osteoporosis is most evident at the beginning of the osteoid seam lifespan (Parfitt *et al.*, 1981), and reflects reductions both in the vigor of individual osteoblasts and in the number of osteoblasts recruited for each team. The most extreme example of osteoblast recruitment failure occurs when the cycle of remodeling is aborted, leaving a shallow resorption cavity covered by flat lining cells with no attempt at focal reconstruction. This phenomenon has been unequivocally demonstrated only in cortical bone (Jaworski *et al.*, 1972) but probably underlies the increase in the extent of eroded surface lacking osteoclasts (reversal surface) observed in some (Schenk *et al.*, 1969) but not in all (Recker *et al.*, 1988) studies of normal aging. In many patients with osteoporosis the extent of reversal surface is increased (Baron *et al.*, 1983b; Parfitt, 1988a), and there is an inverse relationship with the extent of osteoclast-covered surface, instead of the direct relationship found when the coupling of formation to resorption is normal (Baron *et al.*, 1981). Although often taken as evidence for increased bone resorption, this morphologic finding is an indication that osteoblast recruitment was delayed and possibly suppressed altogether.

Another consequence of osteoblast dysfunction in patients with compression fracture is a reduction in mean osteoid thickness, most readily detectable when measured directly rather than calculated indirectly from osteoid volume and surface (Parfitt *et al.*, 1981a). As in normal subjects there is a significant positive correlation between osteoid apposition rate and osteoid thickness, which partly accounts for the thinner seams in osteoporotic patients (Parfitt, 1984a). But in addition, the intercept in the regression equation is lower so that the seams are even thinner than would be predicted by the fall in osteoid apposition rate (Fig. 17). Because of the positive intercept there is a hyperbolic relationship between mineralization lag time and osteoid apposition rate, so that lag time is inevitably increased by a fall in osteoid apposition rate even in the absence of any defect in mineralization (Parfitt, in press). If the decrease in osteoblast vigor and consequent prolongation of formation period is relatively greater than the decrease in activation frequency, the osteoid surface will increase in extent. Consequently, mean osteoid volume is about the same as in normal subjects of similar age, although higher than in healthy pre-menopausal women.

Osteoid apposition rate in cancellous bone correlated with total skeletal blood flow in osteoporosis (Reeve *et al.*, 1988), but the significance of this is unclear. Since total skeletal blood flow is likely to reflect the whole-body rate of remodelling activation, this may be another example of the relationship between the rate of osteoblast team recruitment and the activity of osteoblast teams referred to earlier. Nevertheless, the fall in osteoid apposition rate is the best histomorphometric predictor of the whole-body rate of bone loss (Arlot *et al.*, 1984). The localization of two abnormalities of bone remodeling to one subdivision of the endocortical envelope implies the existence of factors that are not only *local* in the sense of being intrinsic to bone and not systemic, but also *focal*, in the sense of differing between different regions that are in continuity. The data also imply that, at least in some cases, osteoporosis is not just the low end of the normal frequency distribution for bone mass, but is a genuine disease that results from some disturbance in the local (or focal), regulation of bone remodeling (Raisz, 1988b).

*Possible contribution of fatigue microdamage to bone fragility*

Vertebral compression fractures result from biomechanical incompetence of cancellous rather than cortical bone, and the remodeling abnormalities just described are confined to cancellous bone, and so are likely to relate in some way to the increase in bone fragility. Bone, like other structural materials, is subject to fatigue damage, but unlike man-made structural materials it is able to repair itself (Frost, 1985b; Parfitt, 1987b). The repair mechanism must include a method of detecting fatigue microdamage, which probably involves the osteocytes and their cell processes, see earlier. This in some way initiates a focal remodeling process that removes the damaged bone and replaces it with new bone (Frost 1973b; Frost, 1985b), but the signalling mechanism is unknown. In order to prevent the accumulation of fatigue microdamage into macrodamage and overt fracture, repair must keep pace with production, but both of the remodeling abnormalities described have the potential for disturbing this balance unfavorably (Frost, 1986).

The age of a moiety of bone depends both on the probability that a remodeling process will be initiated on the nearest surface, and on the probability that the resorptive phase of a particular remodeling event will penetrate as far as the moiety, which in turn depends both on its distance from the surface and the mean and frequency distribution of resorption cavity depth (Parfitt et al., 1987d). Consequently, any fall in the rate of remodeling activation on a particular surface will increase the age of the bone beneath that surface, an effect which increases hyperbolically with increasing depth. An age-related reduction in mean resorption depth and consequent increase in interstitial bone thickness will amplify this trend, so that in patients with low cancellous bone turnover a substantially higher proportion than normal of the interstitial bone will be more than 20 years old (Parfitt et al., 1987d). Osteocytes have a finite life span, and in dogs total osteocyte volume falls significantly with age in both cortical and cancellous bone (Simonet et al., 1988). Osteocyte death would likely be accelerated by accumulation of very old bone, which would be expected to impair the detection of microdamage. The lining cells will also be older, and surface as well as deep bone more highly mineralized.

A reduction in osteoblast vigor and consequent prolongation of formation period would be expected to delay the repair of fatigue microdamage and so favor its accumulation (Frost, 1986). But fatigue fractures in cancellous bone heal by callus, and the formation of woven bone may be unimpaired despite profound retardation of lamellar bone formation (Frost, 1966). Consequently, the contribution of impaired osteoblast vigor to bone fragility is, at present, a reasonable inference rather than an established fact. Another challenge to the importance of qualitative factors in fracture pathogenesis is the discovery that in healthy American black subjects, a group with lower fracture rates than American whites, both the frequency of remodeling activation and the rate of mineral apposition are lower than in white subjects of similar age (Weinstein et al., 1988). Nevertheless, South African blacks have higher rates of bone turnover and an even lower rate of hip fracture than American blacks (C. Schnitzler; personal communication).

There are no data on the susceptibility of different ethnic groups to osteocyte death and fatigue microdamage of bone.

## Other forms of osteoporosis

Sex hormone deficiency also causes osteoporosis and vertebral fracture in men, but as in normal, post-menopausal women, the frequency of re-modeling activation and bone turnover are increased rather than decreased (Jackson *et al.*, 1987). Although the immediate effect of sex hormone de-ficiency on remodeling is similar in the two sexes, bone fragility in such patients is evidently not due to the remodeling defects so common in osteoporotic women. Trabecular thinning is a more characteristic mode of cancellous bone loss in men than in women (Aaron *et al.*, 1987), and thinner trabeculae are more liable to undergo perforation in response to an abnormal increase in remodeling activation (Reeve, 1987). The increased bone fragility is likely due to the combination of thin trabeculae that are less able to withstand buckling, and the architectural consequences of plate perforation and reduced connectivity (Kleerekoper *et al.*, 1987). By con-trast, men with idiopathic osteoporosis have the same remodeling defects as women with post-menopausal osteoporosis (Jackson *et al.*, 1987). Serum levels of calcitriol, the active metabolite of vitamin D, are reduced in both groups, but the contribution of this to the remodeling abnormalities is unknown.

Chronic exposure to excess glucocorticoid, whether endogenous (as in Cushings Syndrome) or exogenous (due to prescription of anti-inflammatory corticosteroids), also predisposes to osteoporosis. As after menopause, there is an initial period of rapid bone loss that is osteoclast-dependent and associated with high bone turnover, followed by slow bone loss that is osteoblast-dependent and associated with low bone turnover (Duncan *et al.*, 1973). As in post-menopausal osteoporosis, bone is lost preferentially from the axial rather than the appendicular skeleton, and there are the same remodeling defects — fewer osteoblast teams, each with fewer and less vigorous members (Bressot *et al.*, 1979). These defects are often more severe and present in a higher proportion of patients than in post-menopausal osteoporosis; whether they are similarly confined to the cancellous subdivision of the endosteal envelope is not known.

The same pattern of initial, rapid, osteoblast-mediated bone loss followed by later, slow, osteoblast-mediated bone loss is found also in osteoporosis occurring in various gastrointestinal and hepatobiliary diseases, in which, after the initial phase of high turnover due to secondary hyperpara-thyroidism, some unknown nutritional defect impairs osteoblast function

(Parfitt, *et al.*, 1985). The same sequence probably also occurs in traumatic osteodystrophy with transition to disuse osteoporosis (Parfitt, 1984c), but the osteoblast defects have been characterized in less detail (Minaire *et al.*, 1974). In the osteopenia of humoral hypercalcemia of malignancy, the course is compressed, and increased extent of resorption and decreased number and activity of osteoblasts are found simultaneously rather than successively (Stewart *et al.*, 1982). Occurrence of the same biphasic sequence in so many disorders that have little else in common probably reflects an intrinsic property of the skeleton, rather than any particular etiologic factor (Parfitt, 1988a).

### Therapeutic implications

To the extent that defects in bone forming cells contribute to bone loss and bone fragility, their identification and correction are obviously desirable. Furthermore, once sufficient bone has been lost for spontaneous fractures to occur, restoration of normal bone architecture and strength is impossible without the participation of osteoblasts, regardless of how the abnormal situation arose. Consequently, it is rational to attempt to treat established osteoporosis by manipulation of bone-forming cells. A frequently stated therapeutic aim is "stimulation of bone formation", but what is usually meant is finding some way to stimulate existing differentiated cells to work harder or for a longer time. Unfortunately, no certain method of accomplishing this is yet known. All modes of therapy with the potential for progressively increasing bone mass appear to work mainly, if not entirely, by increasing recruitment of new osteoblasts, either increasing the number of teams or the number of cells per team, or both. Furthermore, all such regimens currently under investigation may add bone to the axial skeleton at the expense of accelerating loss from the appendicular skeleton.

The oldest and most thoroughly studied method of increasing osteoblast recruitment is by administration of sodium fluoride (Riggs, 1983). It is unclear whether transformation of quiescent to forming surfaces occurs directly or following a brief episode of mini-resorption (Parfitt, 1988a). Fluoride directly stimulates osteoblast precursor proliferation (Farley *et al.*, 1983), and osteoblast number increases substantially, reaching a maximum at 3−6 months (Schenk *et al.*, 1970). The bone formed is initially partly woven in texture but eventually becomes remodeled to lamellar bone (Braincon and Meunier, 1981). But larger than normal osteocyte lacunae persist and there is usually a clear demarcation between the bone originally present and the new bone formed under the influence of fluoride (Vigorita and Suda, 1983). In patients who have been on treatment for several years many of the osteoid surfaces fail to take up tetracycline and many of the osteoblasts appear sick, with nuclei of aberrant shape and other signs of cell degeneration (Riggs, 1983; Vigorita and Suda, 1983). Despite this, spinal bone density increases continuously for at least the first four years (Riggs *et al.*, 1987), although prevention of further vertebral deformation has not yet been demonstrated.

According to the coherence concept (Frost, 1979), new osteoblast teams recruited in response to a pulsed stimulation of remodeling activation followed by depression of osteoclast activity will be able to overfill resorption cavities of smaller size, but the experimental validation of this concept is incomplete and published clinical trials are inconclusive (Anderson *et al.*, 1984; Pacifici *et al.*, 1988; Hodsman, 1988). Daily injections of human parathyroid hormone increase remodeling activation, as in endogenous hyperparathyroidism (Reeve *et al.*, 1980), but also increase wall thickness (Podbesek *et al.*, 1983), a response not found in endogenous hyperparathyroidism. This probably reflects a difference in the number of osteoblasts assembled for each team, due to the absence of any fall in plasma phosphate with the therapeutic regimen. In a variety of disorders there is a correlation between plasma phosphate and osteoid apposition rate (Parfitt and Villanueva, 1982), and supplemental phosphate appears to increase wall-thickness in patients with osteoporosis (Marie and Caulin, 1986), but whether the effect of phosphate is on osteoblast number or activity is unknown. Finally, aluminum administration to normal dogs causes a unique arborization of new bone into the marrow cavity (Quarles *et al.*, 1988), but the therapeutic implications of this observation have not yet been defined.

### Hyperparathyroidism and Osteitis Fibrosa.

Chronic hypersecretion of parathyroid hormone (PTH) is due to some combination of increased number and increased activity of secretary cells and can occur without regard to physiologic demand (primary), or in response to increased demand (secondary) (Parfitt and Kleerekoper, 1980). Primary hyperparathyroidism (HrPT) is usually of unknown etiology; is accompanied by hypercalcemia, and the glandular enlargement is due to a single adenoma or (less commonly) to hyperplasia of all glands. Secondary hyperparathyroidism is usually due to abnormal vitamin D metabolism due to intestinal or renal disease, and is accompanied (at least initially) by hypocalcemia,* the glands are enlarged because of hyperplasia (Parfitt, in press). The conditions of primary HrPT, secondary HrPT due to vitamin D deficiency and secondary HrPT due to chronic renal failure have differences as well as similarities that modify the effect of excess PTH on osteoblast number and activity (Table 8).

**Table 8**
Plasma composition in hyperparathyroidism.[a]

| Plasma | Primary | Secondary HrPT | |
| Constituent | HrPT | Vit. D- | CRF |
| --- | --- | --- | --- |
| PTH | ↑ | ↑ ↑ | ↑ ↑ ↑ |
| Calcium | ↑ | ↓ ↓ | ↓ |
| Phosphate | ↓ | ↓ | ↑ |
| Calcidiol | N | ↑ ↑ | N |
| Calcitriol | ↑ | N | ↓ |

[a] similarities and differences between different types that may modify effect of PTH excess on osteoblasts.

## Mild hyperparathyroidism and high turnover osteopenia

The most consistent long-term effect of HrPT on bone formation is an increase in the frequency of remodeling activation and consequent increase in the number of osteoblast teams. When PTH was infused continuously for several months in dogs, no alteration in the function of osteoblast teams was evident and, in particular, there was no defect corresponding to the depression of collagen synthesis found in acute *in vitro* experiments (Malluche *et al.*, 1982). In mild primary HrPT cancellous bone mass in the ilium is normal or increased (Delling *et al.*, 1979; Parfitt, 1986b; Melsen *et al.*, in press). On the cancellous surface current resorption depth is slightly reduced, and wall thickness is normal or somewhat less reduced (Ericksen, 1986; Melsen *et al.*, in press) so that the trabeculae tend to increase slowly in thickness. Both osteoid apposition rate and osteoblast nuclear height are significantly reduced, to a greater extent that any change in wall thickness, so that individual osteoblast vigor is impaired and formation period prolonged (Melsen *et al.*, in press). The absence of this abnormality in PTH infused dogs suggests that it is not a direct effect of PTH excess, but (as mentioned in the discussion of PTH as a treatment for osteoporosis) more likely an indirect effect due to hypophosphatemia (Parfitt and Villanueva, 1982).

As in normal subjects and patients with osteoporosis, in primary HrPT there is a significant positive correlation between osteoid thickness (Parfitt, 1984a). Mean osteoid thickness is normal and osteoid apposition rate is reduced, so that mineralization lag time is modestly increased. This is mainly a reflection of a further delay in osteoid maturation compared to the effect of normal ageing, rather than impairment of mineralization. But increased PTH secretion from any cause accelerates the catabolism of calciferol and calcidiol to biologically inactive metabolites (Clements *et al.*,

1987). Consequently, the vitamin D requirement is increased in HrPT, and in susceptible populations vitamin D depletion may result so that mineralization is impaired (Editorial, 1988). In vitamin D-replete patients with primary HrPT, osteoid surface and volume are increased 2–3 fold but this is mainly the result of increased remodeling activation and not of impaired mineralization. The number and activity of osteoblast teams are similar on the endocortical and intracortical surfaces, but resorption depth averaged over the duration of disease is increased on the endocortical surface with a consequent substantial reduction in cortical thickness (Parfitt *et al.*, 1987c).

An interesting feature of mild hyperparathyroidism, primary or secondary, is the increased external diameter of some appendicular bones, including the metacarpal (Parfitt, 1977b) and the mid-shaft of the radius (Parfitt, 1986). If, as previously postulated, each remodeling cycle on the periosteal surface adds rather than subtracts a small quantity of bone, then the increase in the rate of remodeling activation characteristic of hyperparathyroidism would be expected to amplify the rate of age-related periosteal gain, but, as with the effects of menopause, the gain is too small to offset the increased loss from the endocortical surface and prevent cortical thinning. Another disease in which increased remodeling activation is associated with periosteal expansion is acromegaly due to excess growth hormone (Dequeker, 1976), but the remodeling mechanisms have not been studied in detail. Increased periosteal gain is also produced by vigorous physical activity, such as the effects of tennis playing on the humerus (Martin *et al.*, 1987), but this is not offset by acceleration of endocortical loss and so leads to a corresponding increase in cortical thickness.

The mean size of osteocytic lacunae in undecalcified bone is normal in mild primary hyperparathyroidism, but in bone that has been partially demineralized with nitric acid, lacunar size is increased (Parfitt, 1976b). This is evidence, not for the mythical process of osteocytic osteolysis, but for an increase in the extent of metabolically hyperactive perilacunar bone, in which matrix solubility is increased as well as mineral density reduced. This phenomenon is not observed in hyperthyroidism, and so is not simply a non-specific consequence of reduced bone age, but an indication that the sphere of influence of the osteocyte is dependent in some way on PTH. The hypercalcemia of mild hyperparathyroidism is stable and non-progressive and results from an upward resetting of the level of equilibration between blood and bone at quiescent bone surfaces, not from an increase in net bone resorption (Parfitt, 1987a). Secondary mineralization would likely be accelerated, but the effect of this on surface bone density would be offset by the increase in activation frequency, which reduces the average time interval between successive remodeling events in the same location from about 3 years to about 18 months (Parfitt, 1987a).

In secondary HrPT due to vitamin D deficiency the histologic findings in iliac bone are very similar to primary HrPT, in direction, magnitude, relative deviation from normality of the different indices, and regression relationship between osteoid thickness and osteoid apposition rate (Parfitt, in press). There is a tendency for osteoid thickness to be slightly greater and osteoid apposition rate slightly lower, so that mineralization lag time is somewhat more prolonged. The mild mineralization defect may result from a lower plasma calcium and/or calcium x phosphate product, but the plasma levels are very similar to those in patients with secondary HrPT due to intestinal disease, who have normal plasma calcidiol levels but malabsorption of calcium as a direct result of the primary disease, rather than as an indirect result due to Vitamin D deficiency. In such patients the histologic findings more closely resemble those in primary HrPT, which suggests that the mild mineralization defect in patients with mild vitamin D deficiency is more likely a consequence of the low plasma calcidiol levels, possibly due to lack of substrate for synthesis of calcitriol in bone (Parfitt, in press).

## Severe hyperparathyroidism and osteitis fibrosa

Mild hyperparathyroid bone disease, whether primary or secondary, is characterized by increased surface remodeling and preferential loss of appendicular cortical bone, but severe hyperparathyroid bone disease is a qualitatively different disorder referred to as osteitis fibrosa (Collins, 1966; Woods, 1972; Parfitt, 1976b; Malluche and Faugere, 1986). This term is unsatisfactory since the lesions are not inflammatory, but no alternative method is available for identifying the two fundamentally different forms of hyperparathyroid bone disease. In osteitis fibrosa, osteoclast teams erode more deeply than normal, not just on the endocortical surface, but on the intracortical surface, leading to enlargement and coalescence of resorption cavities, on the cancellous surface, leading to dissecting intratrabecular resorption and on the periosteal surface, leading to a characteristic radiographic appearance (Meema, 1977). The large resorption cavities are partly refilled, not with normal lamellar bone, but with appositional woven bone and fibrous tissue. Fibrosis extends also along the cancellous surface, and in severe cases encroaches on the marrow, which undergoes osseous metaplasia with the production of non-appositional woven bone.

Osteitis fibrosa is neither a nonspecific response to unusually rapid bone resorption nor a reparative response to mechanical weakness of the skeleton, as have often been stated, but is a morphologically specific consequence of a substantial excess of PTH that exceeds some critical threshold. As a result, fibroblast and osteoblast proliferation are stimulated, and osteoblast differentiation is switched in the direction of woven rather than lamellar bone production. Osteitis fibrosa was first described in primary HrPT, in which it is the most specific but nowadays much the least common form of bone disease. Consequently, most of the knowledge about kinetic aspects of osteoblast function in osteitis fibrosa, based on tetracycline labeling, is the result of studying patients with chronic renal failure and severe secondary HrPT. It has proved much easier to prolong life than to control parathyroid hyperplasia, so that renal osteitis fibrosa has evolved from a rare curiosity to a common medical problem (Malluche and Faugere, 1986).

In early chronic renal failure, bone remodeling resembles that in mild primary HrPT with modestly increased activation frequency and its consequences on all surfaces; the same is found in mild experimental renal failure in dogs (Faugere et al., 1988). Appositional woven bone formation appears earlier in the course of disease and the threshold of PTH secretion needed for the production of osteitis fibrosa is eventually reached in the majority of patients in the absence of therapeutic intervention (Malluche and Faugere, 1986). In established renal osteitis fibrosa the frequency of remodeling activation is increased with consequent increases in the rate of recruitment of new osteoblast teams and in bone formation rates of about 5-fold (Parfitt, 1984a). Mean osteoid apposition rate is increased by about 20%, but the partition of this increase in activity between cell number and cell activity is uncertain because of the inaccuracy of wall thickness measurements in osteitis fibrosa.

There is a significant positive correlation between osteoid apposition rate and osteoid thickness, with a significantly higher intercept of the regression line (Fig. 17; Parfitt, 1984a), which probably results from unusually rapid matrix apposition in the early stages of the osteoblast lifespan (Parfitt et al., 1981b); osteoblast vigor is probably increased by the combination of severe hyperparathyroidism and hyperphosphatemia (Teitelbaum et al., 1980). As a result both of the higher osteoid apposition rate and of the higher regression intercept, mean osteoid thickness is increased by about 50%. The combination of increased thickness, surface and volume of osteoid would be impossible to differentiate from osteomalacia without tetracycline labeling, and according to the kinetic criteria described in the following section, osteomalacia is rare in chronic renal failure in the absence of other etiologic factors (Teitelbaum et al., 1980; Malluche and Faugere, 1986).

## Osteosclerosis

Cancellous bone mass is usually increased in chronic renal failure to a greater extent than in primary hyperparathyroidism. Although a higher than normal proportion of the bone is not mineralized, mineralized bone volume is often increased, sometimes to an extent that is radiographically apparent as osteosclerosis (Frame et al., 1987). This results from the combined effects of increased net appositional bone formation and osseous

metaplasia in the bone marrow, both consequences of the osteoblast proliferation and hyperactivity already mentioned. Metaplastic bone formation
leading to osteosclerosis is also a characteristic response to the presence in
the marrow of a metastatic tumor (Burkhardt *et al.*, 1982) and the connective tissue proliferation of myelofibrosis (Frame *et al.*, 1987). Before replacement of renal function by dialysis or transplantation became available,
metaphyseal osteosclerosis was especially common when chronic renal
failure began in childhood (Frame *et al.*, 1987), a clinical counterpart of the
response to PTH administration in growing rats (Kalu *et al.*, 1970; Parfitt,
1976b). In both situations the combination of PTH excess and hyperphosphatemia enhances the accumulation of cancellous bone during growth.

Vitamin D Deficiency and Osteomalacia.

Osteomalacia can occur in diverse clinical settings but in most types
there is either a primary disorder of vitamin D metabolism or a primary
(non-parathyroid hormone dependent) defect in the renal tubular reab-
sorption of phosphate (Parfitt, in press). In the former, hypocalcemia and
secondary hyperparathyroidism are usual and hypophosphatemia is mild,
whereas in the latter normocalcemia is the rule, secondary hyperparathyroidism is slight or absent and hypophosphatemia more severe. Although
alterations in vitamin D metabolism at many levels can cause osteomalacia,
vitamin D deficiency, either extrinsic (due to some combination of reduced
dietary intake and reduced production in skin) or intrinsic (due to intestinal
malabsorption and increased fecal loss) are most common. There are also
several less common etiologic categories. Some foreign substances (including
medications) can inhibit mineralization (Parfitt, submitted). In fibrogenesis
imperfecta ossium, the bone matrix consists of a tangled mass of very thin
and irregularly curved fibrils, with loss of normal birefringence, and is
essentially unmineralizable (Swan *et al.*, 1976). In axial osteomalacia the
osteoblasts in the axial skeleton are morphologically inactive but stain with
abnormal intensity for alkaline phophatase (Whyte *et al.*, 1981), and in
hypophosphatasia there is a genetic defect in the production of tissue non-
specific alkaline phosphatase, with accumulation and increased excretion of
inorganic pyrophosphate and phosphorylethanolamine (Fallon *et al.*, 1981).

*Role of Osteoblasts and other local factors in mineralization*

The complex and poorly understood process of mineralization will be
discussed in Volume 4 of this series. Mineralization occurs at the osteoid-
bone interface, so that all mineral ions deposited in bone must first pass
through or between the osteoblasts and through osteoid tissue, probably
along the canaliculae joining the osteocyte lacunae (Rasmussen and Bordier,

1974). The close morphologic relationship suggests that both osteoblasts and the osteoid osteocytes derived from them play a role in the packaging of minerals and their transport towards the site of deposition (Aaron, 1976; Bordier *et al.*, 1977). The importance of local factors is strengthened by the inconsistent relationship in clinical practice between plasma composition and the state of mineralization. For example, although there are significant correlations between plasma phosphate and osteoid apposition rate (positive) and between plasma calcium and osteoid seam thickness (negative), their magnitude is too small for useful prediction in individual patients (Parfitt and Villanueva, 1982). Furthermore, osteomalacia can be absent in some patients with a degree of persistent hypophosphatemia that in other patients would normally be regarded as sufficient explanation for their osteomalacia (de Vernejoul *et al.*, 1983).

In early Vitamin D-related osteomalacia some doubly labelled surfaces persist, at which the rate of mineral apposition is normal or only moderately reduced. This indicates that mineralization can proceed at the beginning of the osteoid seam lifespan although it terminates prematurely. Mineralizing and non-mineralizing osteoid seams are often close together, sometimes even in direct continuity, and are exposed to the same microcirculation, so that the difference between them cannot be explained in terms of serum chemical changes alone. Nevertheless, the mineralization defect is of similar severity on all subdivisions of the endosteal envelope, without the focal differences observed in osteoporosis. At doubly labelled seams a higher proportion of the surface is lined by osteoblasts (Meunier, 1983), suggesting that these cells, possibly in conjunction with the osteoid osteocytes (Bordier *et al.*, 1977), are able to promote mineralization in the face of a moderate reduction in plasma calcium phosphate ion product, but do so for a shorter period of time than normal in vitamin D depletion. When this function is lost, mineralization ceases even though matrix apposition continues slowly and the osteoid seam progressively gets thicker. There is an inverse correlation between osteoblast extent and osteoid thickness (Meunier, 1983), and in severe osteomalacia osteoblasts are few or absent altogether, mineralization never begins and double labels are not found.

The bone histologic data in patients with Vitamin D-related osteomalacia strongly suggest that deficiency of calcitriol or possibly of some other metabolite of vitamin D impairs some function of the osteoblast that favors mineralization. This proposal is consistent with the presence in osteoblasts of calcitriol receptors (Manolagas *et al*, 1980), the radiographic localization of labelled calcitriol in osteoblast nuclei (Stumpf *et al.*, 1981), the stimulation by calcitriol of the *in vitro* production by osteoblasts of alkaline phosphatase (Manolagas *et al.*, 1981) and osteocalcin (Lian *et al.*, 1985), the *in vivo* enhancement by calcitriol of mineral apposition rate in young mice (Marie *et al.*, 1985) and the morphologic changes induced by calcitriol in lining cells (Krempien and Klimpel, 1980). It seems likely that calcitriol could stimulate the inward transport of calcium and/or phosphate ions through or between cells at sites of mineralization, consistent with its known effect on the cells of the intestinal mucosa.

The concept that mineralization normally depends both on the availability of substrate ions via the circulation and on the activity of osteoblasts, although by no means rigorously established, enables many apparently conflicting data to be reconciled. How osteoblasts could influence mineralization is unknown. Concentration differences between mineralizing and non-mineralizing sites could be maintained by cells, or by structures derived from cells such as matrix vesicles, or by the ion-binding properties of macromolecules synthesized by cells. Furthermore, the exact chemical composition and three-dimensional structure of connective tissue matrixes, which depend on osteoblast function, are major determinants of where and when mineralization can occur, and abnormalities in collagen cross-linking and other changes in bone matrix maturation and composition have been found in vitamin D deficiency (Stern, 1980). The concept has the additional merit of unifying the pathogenesis of all major forms of osteomalacia, since hereditary or acquired defects in phosphate transport across the renal tubular epithelium could be accompanied by similar defects in transport across the quasi epithelium that covers bone surfaces (Marie and Glorieux, 1981).

## The evolution of osteomalacia — typical and variant forms

The abnormalities of osteoblast function in early vitamin D deficiency with secondary hyperparathyroidism were described in the preceding section. As the deficiency becomes more severe and/or more prolonged, osteoid surface extent, already increased because of hyperparathyroidism and more frequent remodeling activation, increases further because formation period is prolonged. When the osteoid surface exceeds about 70% of the bone surface, the normal positive relationship between adjusted apposition rate and osteoid thickness is reversed, so that as the former declines the latter increases instead of decreases (Fig. 18). This reversal is the cardinal kinetic characteristic of osteomalacia (Parfitt, 1981a; Parfitt, in press). Also, in contrast to the lack of correlation between osteoid thickness and surface in normal and osteoporotic subjects, in vitamin D deficiency there is a significant hyperbolic correlation (Fig. 18). Based on these relationships the mineralization defect of osteomalacia is conveniently defined as the concurrence of osteoid thickness (corrected for section obliquity) of greater than 12.5 μm and mineralization lag time longer than 100 days (Parfitt, in press).

The distinction between the presence or absence of some double tetra-

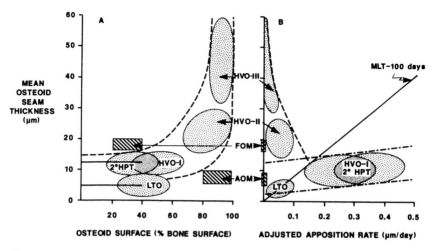

**Fig. 18**  Osteoid thickness relationships in osteomalacia. On left (a — static measurements) horizontal solid lines define mean and range for osteoid thickness and surface in normal subjects. The curved, interrupted lines denote the hyperbolic relationship found in patients with abnormal mineralization. On right (b — kinetic measurements) straight interrupted lines enclose the regression of osteoid thickness on adjusted apposition rate in normal and hyper-parathyroid subjects. Solid line represents a mineralization lag time (Mlt) of 100 days. HVO = hypovitaminosis D osteopathy) Stage i — secondary hyperparathyroidism, Stage ii — osteomalacia with some double-labels, Stage iii — osteomalacia with no double labels. LTO = low turnover osteopenia; FOM = focal osteomalacia, AOM — atypical osteomalacia. Reprinted from Rao (submitted), with permission.

cycline labels, which was mentioned earlier, provides a convenient further subdivision in the evolution and severity of the mineralization defect (Parfitt, in press). It also corresponds to the distinction between two types of osteoid seam in osteomalacia — those where some mineralized bone lies between the osteoid and the cement line, and those where the osteoid lies directly on the cement line. Since the total thickness of matrix that can be deposited by the osteoblast team is usually unaffected by osteomalacia, even though the rate of deposition is slowed, the maximum thickness of the osteoid seam is greater in the latter type. The two types of seam have in common that the loop normally formed by the growth curves of matrix apposition and mineralization (Fig. 13) never closes in the absence of treatment, which is the most fundamental characteristic of osteomalacia of all kinds (Fig. 19).

If defective mineralization is preceded by decreased rather than increased activation frequency, osteoid thickness will be disproportionately increased relative to osteoid surface, and osteoid volume will be normal or only slightly increased, a combination referred to as focal osteomalacia. With rare exceptions, focal osteomalacia is confined to defective mineralization induced by drugs, especially sodium etidronate, sodium fluoride and alumi-

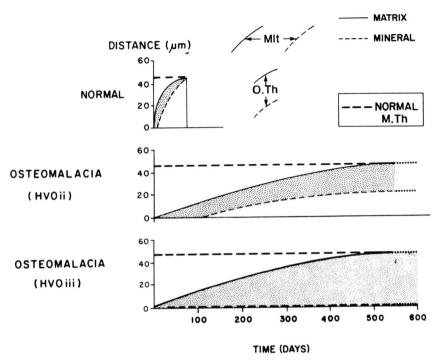

**Fig. 19** Evolution of a bone remodeling unit in osteomalacia. Growth curves of matrix and mineral apposition were constructed as in Figure 13. Note that in mild osteomalacia (HVO ii), mineralization is delayed in onset, retarded in rate and premature in termination, whereas in severe osteomalacia (HVO iii) no mineralization occurs at all. Modified from Parfitt, in press, with permission.

num in patients with chronic renal failure (Parfitt, submitted). If defective mineralization is accompanied by an equivalent retardation of matrix apposition, formation period will be markedly prolonged, osteoid surface and volume will be increased and lag time prolonged, and osteoid thickness may be normal, a combination referred to as atypical osteomalacia. This occurs in some patients with intestinal malabsorption in whom defective matrix synthesis is likely due to deficiency of some unidentified nutrient important for osteoblast health (Parfitt, in press), and in aluminum related bone disease, in which matrix synthesis is impaired by a direct toxic effect of aluminum on osteoblasts (Parfitt, 1988b). During the evolution of hypophosphatemic osteomalacia, matrix synthesis is presumably retarded by hypophosphatemia, but osteoid thickness eventually increases, and by the time bone biopsy is performed typical osteomalacia is present in most patients (Parfitt, in press).

The concept that defective mineralization and defective matrix synthesis are independent consequences of impaired osteoblast function provides a reasonable explanation for an otherwise confusing diversity of bone histomorphometric findings in the aforementioned three disorders — gastrointestinal and hepatobiliary bone disease, aluminum related bone disease, and chronic hypophosphatemia (Parfitt, 1988b; Parfitt, in press). In these disorders different patients may manifest varying combinations of low bone turnover and impaired osteoblast function indistinguishable from osteoporosis, high bone turnover, focal, atypical or generalized osteomalacia, and various intermediate and transitional states, with the exceptions that high turnover does not occur in uncomplicated primary hypophosphatemia, and focal osteomalacia is found only with aluminum. These different patterns can all be accounted for by independent defects of matrix synthesis and mineralization, in conjunction with secondary hyperparathyroidism and increased remodeling activation, each of the three functional abnormalities being of variable severity and time course in different patients (Parfitt, 1988b).

## Paget Disease: a qualitative disorder of bone formation.

The abnormalities of osteoblast function so far described can for the most part be regarded as quantitative deviations from normal in the amounts and rates of lamellar bone matrix formation and mineralization, in normal locations, by teams of osteoblasts that are normal except in their number and vigor of recruits. The single exception was osteitis fibrosa in severe hyperparathyroidism, together with the other causes of osteosclerosis that were briefly mentioned, in which there is formation of woven rather than lamellar bone. One other disease which shares this characteristic merits more detailed description. Referred to as osteitis deformans by those who disdain eponyms, Paget Disease is the most common example of a qualitative as well as a quantitative abnormality in bone formation (Collins, 1966; Woods, 1972 and see chapter 7 in Vol. 2). Although almost any bone can be affected, the disease is focal in distribution, usually beginning at one end of a long bone and gradually advancing toward the other. But the disease never appears in a new bone not already affected by the time the diagnosis is made, so that its localization was irrevocably determined many years earlier. There is suggestive but not conclusive evidence that the cause is a slow virus, but susceptibility to infection is probably influenced by genetic factors (Singer and Mills, 1983). Nothing is known about how the virus can induce characteristic changes in bone cell function in every new generation of cells in the affected region over many years. Conceivably, the abnormal nuclei transformed by the virus are immortal and the disease fundamentally neoplastic in nature (Rasmussen and Bordier, 1974).

The essential feature of Paget Disease is that normal bone is progressively replaced by bone of abnormal architecture. At the advancing edge are numerous foci of osteoclastic resorption that tend to enlarge and coalesce. Pagetic osteoclasts have many more nuclei than normal, and are generally larger and more irregular in size and shape (Rasmussen and Bordier, 1974; Meunier et al., 1980b). Within the space created are laid down irregular, randomly oriented trabeculae of primitive, coarse-fibered, woven-type bone without cartilage, lying within a highly vascular fibrous stroma that lacks either hematopoietic or fatty marrow (Collins, 1966; Singer et al., 1977). The new bone undergoes piecemeal resorption and replacement, in part by appositional woven bone and in part by small packets of lamellar bone, each composed of short lamellae whose grain varies randomly between adjacent packets, which are interspersed with remnants of the woven bone first formed (Woods, 1972; Singer et al., 1978). With time, as the advancing edge becomes more distant, activity in the older lesions may gradually subside, but the abnormal architecture persists. Bone surfaces become quiescent and fat cells reappear in the marrow (Milgram, 1977). Eventually almost all of the originally-formed, woven bone is replaced, and the irregularly shaped segments of lamellar bone with abrupt changes in orientation are joined together by prominent, extensively developed cement lines, conferring the characteristic mosaic pattern.

In patients with only one side of the pelvis affected, iliac biopsies from Pagetic lesions and from presumed normal bone can be compared. The possibility of bone biopsy usually arises only when the disease is well advanced, by which time new bone formation is almost entirely appositional. On the diseased side cancellous bone volume is increased approximately 2-fold (Meunier et al., 1980b), and about one-half of the total bone matrix is woven, with the proportion varying widely between different patients (Rasmussen and Bordier, 1974). All the surface indices of bone formation (Table 2) are increased about 5-fold. At sites of woven bone formation, the osteoblasts are more numerous and the cells and their nuclei are larger and more variable in size, shape and staining (Rasmussen and Bordier, 1974). The mineral and osteoid apposition rates are substantially increased (Meunier et al., 1980b; Parfitt and Villanueva, unpublished data), and total bone formation rates are about 10 times normal (Lee, 1957; Parfitt and Villanueva, unpublished data; Figure 20). A moderate increase in turnover in the apparently uninvolved ilium may be the result of secondary hyperparathyroidism (Meunier et al., 1980).

Whether the abnormal osteoblast function in Paget disease is the expected response to disordered bone resorption, or another manifestation of the disease is unclear. In favor of the former view are the well-established reparative role of woven bone formation, the close matching of whole body

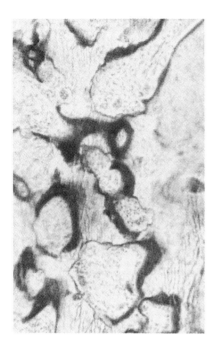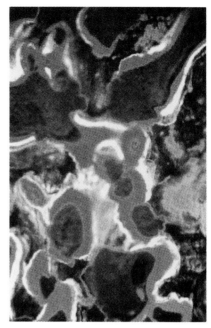

**Fig. 20** Disordered bone formation in Paget Disease. Left—bright field illumination to show osteoid; right—ultraviolet relation to show bright bands of tetracycline fluorescence. Note large excess of osteoid, extensive tetracycline uptake and abnormal bone structure. Although the fluorescent bands are wider than normal and somewhat blurred, double labels are evident in many places.

resorption and formation rates (Rasmussen and Bordier, 1974) and the sequential decline in biochemical markers of bone resorption and bone formation, consistent with the normal time scale of the remodeling cycle, when the recruitment and activity of osteoclasts are inhibited by the newer bisphosphonates (Frijlink *et al.*, 1979). In favor of the latter view are the abnormal morphology of Pagetic osteoblasts (Rasmussen and Bordier, 1974), the much earlier decline in some indices of bone formation when bone resorption is inhibited by calcitonin (Shai *et al.*, 1971; Simon *et al.*, 1984), the permanence of periosteal expansion and abnormal internal architecture (in contrast to the gradual restoration of normal bone shape and structure after fracture), the increase in total skeletal mass (Wallach *et al.*, 1975) and the absence of anything remotely resembling Paget disease, even with the largest increases in bone turnover due to hyperthyroidism. The increased risk of osteogenic sarcoma (Collins, 1966; Woods, 1972) does not necessarily imply that the osteoblasts are abnormal in Paget's disease, since the probability of mutation would be increased by more frequent mitosis in osteoblast precursor cells.

## Acknowledgement

The concepts presented in this chapter emerged gradually over 15 years of reflection and data analysis, to which many people have contributed. Particular thanks are due to Harold Frost for setting me on the right path, and to Tony Villanueva who made the most crucial observations.

## References

Aaron, J. E. (1976).Histology and microanatomy of bone. In: Nordin B. E. C. ed. *Calcium, Phosphate and Magnesium Metabolism.* Churchill-Livingstone, Edinburgh.

Aaron, J. E., Makins, N. B., Francis, R. M., Peacock M. (1987). Staining of the calcification front in human bone using contrasting fluorochromes in vitro. *J. Histochemistry and Cytochemistry*, **32**: 1251−1261.

Aaron, J. E., Makins, N. B., Sagreiya, K. (1987). The microanatomy of trabecular bone loss in normal ageing men and women. *Clin. Orthop.*, **215**: 260−271.

Albright, E., Reifenstein, E. G. (1948). *The parathyroid glands and metabolic bone disease.* Selected studies. Williams & Wilkins Co. Baltimore.

Anderson, C., Cape, R. D. T., Crilly, R. G., Hodsman, A. B., Wolfe, B. M. J. (1984). Preliminary observations of a form of coherence therapy for osteoporosis. *Calcif. Tissue. Int.*, **36**: 341−343.

Arlot, M., Edouard, C., Meunier, P. J., Neer, R. M., Reeve, J. (1984). Impaired osteoblast function in osteoporosis: comparison between calcium balance and dynamic histomorphometry. *Brit. Med. J.*, **289**: 517−520.

Baron, R., Vignery, A., Lang, R. (1981). Reversal phase and osteopenia: Defective coupling of resorption to formation in the pathogenesis of osteoporosis. In: DeLuca, H. F., Frost, H., Jee, W., Johnston, C., Parfitt, A. M., (1981). eds. *Osteoporosis: Recent Advances in Pathogenesis and Treatment.* Baltimore, University Park Press 311−320.

Baron, R., Vignery, A., Horowitz M. (1983a). Lymphocytes, macrophages and the regulation of bone remodeling. In: Peck, W. A., ed. *Bone & Mineral Research*, **2**, Elsevier, Amsterdam. 175−184.

Baron, R., Magee, S., Silverglate, A., Broadus, A., Lang, R. (1983b). Estimation of trabecular bone resorption by histomorphometry: Evidence for a prolonged reversal phase with normal resorption in post-menopausal osteoporosis and coupled increased resorption in primary hyperparathyroidism. In: Frame, B., Potts, J. T. Jr., eds. *Clinical Disorders of Bone and Mineral Metabolism.* Amsterdam, Excerpta Medica, 191−195.

Baron, R., Tross, R., Vignery, A. (1984). Evidence of sequential remodeling in rat trabecular bone: Morphology, dynamic histomorphometry, and changes during skeletal maturation. *Anat. Rec.*, **208**: 137−145.

Baserga, R. (1985). *The biology of cell reproduction.* Harvard University Press, Cambridge.

Baylink, D., Stauffer, M., Wergedal, J., Rich, C. (1970). Formation, mineralization and resorption of bone in vitamin D deficient rats. *J. Clin. Invest.*, **49**: 112−1134.

Baylink, D. J., Liu, C-C. (1979). The regulation of endosteal bone volume. *J. Periodontol.* **50**: 43−49.

Baylink, D. J., Wergedal, J. E. (1971). Bone formation by osteocytes. *Amer. J. Phys.*, **221**: 669−678.

Baylink, D., Wergedal, J., Thompson, E. (1972). Loss of protein polysaccharides at sites where bone mineralization is initiated. *J. Histochem. Cytochem.*, **20**: 279−292.

Baylink, D. J., Morey, E. R., Ivey, J. L., Stauffer, M. E. (1980). Vitamin D and bone, In: *Vitamin D: Molecular Biology and Clinical Nutrition*, Norman AW, ed. Marcel Dekker, New York, 387−453.

Beresford, J. N., Gallagher, J. A., Poser, J. W., Russell, R. G. G. (1984). Production of osteocalcin by human bone cells *in vitro*. Effects of $1,25(OH)_2D_3$, $24,25 (OH)_2D_3$, parathyroid hormone, and glucocorticoids. *Metab. Bone. Dis. Rel. Res.*, **5**: 229−234.

Birkenhager-Frenkel, D. H., Birkenhager, J. C. (1987). Bone appositional rate and percentage of doubly and singly labeled surfaces: Comparison of date from 5 and 20 μm sections. *Bone*, **8**: 7−12.

Bordier, P. H., Tun Chot, S. (1972). Quantitative histology of metabolic bone disease. *Clin. Endo. Metab.*, **1**: 197−215.

Bordier, P. H. Marie, P., Miravet, L., Ryckewaert, A., Rasmussen, H. (1977). Morphological and morphometrical characteristics of the mineralization front. A vitamin D regulated sequence of bone remodeling. In: Meunier, P. J. ed. *Bone Histomorphometry. Second International Workshop.*, Armour Montagu, Paris 335−354.

Bowman, B. M., Miller, S. C. (1986). The proliferation and differentiation of the bone-lining cell in estrogen-induced osteogenesis. *Bone*, **7**: 351−357.

Boyde, A. (1972). Scanning electron microscope studies of bone. In: Bourne, G. H., ed. *The Biochemistry and Physiology of Bone*, Vol I, 2nd Ed. New York, Academic Press, **1**: 259−310.

Boyde, A. (1981). Evidence against osteocytic osteolysis. In: Jee, W. S. S., Parfitt, A. M. eds. *Bone Histomorphometry*, Third International Workshop, Sun Valley, Armour Montagu, (Paris) pp. 239−255.

Bressot, C., Meunier, P. J., Chapuy, M. C., LeJeune, E., Edouard, C., Darby, A. J. (1979). Histomorphometric profile, pathophysiology and reversibility of corticosteroid-induced osteoporosis. *Metab. Bone Dis. Rel. Res.*, **1**: 303−311.

Briancon, D., Meunier, P. J. (1981). Treatment of osteoporosis with fluoride, calcium, and vitamin D. *Ortho. Clinics NA*, **12**: 629−648.

Broulik, P., Kragstrup, J., Mosekilde, L., Melsen, F. (1982). Osteon cross-section size in the iliac crest. *Acta Path. Microbiol. Immunol. Scand. Sect. A*, **90**: 339−344.

Brown, J. P., Delmas, P. D., Arlot, M., Meunier, P. J. (1987). Active bone turnover of the corticoendosteal envelope in postmenopausal osteoporosis. *J. Clin. Endocrin. Metab.*, **64**: 954−959.

Burkhardt, R., Frisch, B., Schlag, R., Sommerfield, W. (1982). Carcinomatous Osteodysplasia. *Skeletal Radiol.*, **8**: 169−178.

Burkhardt, R., Bartl, R., Frisch, B., Jager, K., Mahl, C., Hill, W., Kettner, G. (1984). The structural relationship of bone forming and endothelial cells of the bone marrow. In: Arlet, J., Ficat, R. D., Hungerford, D. S., eds. *Bone Circulation*, Williams and Wilkins, Baltimore, 2−14.

Canalis, E. (1985). Effect of growth factors on bone cell replication and differentiation. *Clin.*

*Orthop.*, **183**: 246−263.

Cane, V., Marotti, G., Volpi, G., Zaffe, D., Palazzini, S. (1982). Size and density of osteocyte lacunae in different regions of long bones. *Calcif. Tissue Int.*, **34**: 558−563.

Chambers, T. J. (1987). The regulation of osteoclastic function. In: Johansen, J. Riis, B., Christiansen, C., eds. *Osteoporosis*. Osteopress Aps, Copenhagen. 1987; pp. 756−761.

Chambers, T. J., Darby, J. A., Fuller, K. (1985). Mammalian collagenase predispose bone surfaces of osteoclastic resorption. *Cell Tissues Res.*, **241**: 671−675.

Charles, P., Eriksen, E. F., Mosekilde, L., Melsen, F., Jensen, F. T. (1987). Bone turnover and balanced evaluated by a combined calcium balance and calcium kinetic study and dynamic histomorphometry. *Metabolism*, **36**: 1118−1124.

Clements, M. R., Johnson, L., Fraser, D. R. (1987). A new mechanism for induced vitamin D deficiency in calcium deprivation. *Nature*, **325**: 62−65.

Collins, D. H. (1966). *Pathology of bone*. Butterworth, London.

Curtis, T. A., Ashrafi, S. H., Weber, D. F. (1985). Canalicular communication in the cortices of human long bones. *Anat. Rec.*, **212**: 336−344.

Darby, A. J., Meunier, P. J. (1981). Mean wall thickness and formation periods of trabecular bone packets in idiopathic osteoporosis. *Calcif. Tissue Int.*, **33**: 199−204.

Deldar, A. Lewis, H., Weiss, L. (1985). Bone lining cells and hematopoiesis: An electron microscopic study of canine bone marrow. *Anat. Rec.*, **213**: 187−201.

Delling, G., Schulz, A., Seifert, G. (1979). Histomorphometric analysis of bone changes in surgically proven primary hyperparathyroidism and nephrolithiasis − the importance of bone biopsy in diagnosis. *Path. Res. Pract.*, **166**: 90−100.

Dequeker, J. (1976). Quantitative radiology: Radiogrammetry of cortical bone. *Brit. J. Radiol.*, **49**: 912−920.

Doty, S. B. (1981). Morphological evidence of gap junctions between bone cells. *Calcif. Tissue. Int.*, **33**: 509−512.

Duncan, H. Hanson, C. A., Curtiss, A. (1973). The different effects of soluble and crystalline hydrocortisone on bone. *Calc. Tiss. Res.*, **12**: 159−168.

Dunstan, C. R. Evans, R. A. (1980). Quantitative bone histology: a new method. *Pathology*, **12**: 255−264.

Editorial. (1988). Acquired vitamin D deficiency and hyperparathyroidism. *Lancet*, 451−452.

Epker, B. N., Frost, H. M. (1965). The direction of transverse drifts of actively forming osteons in human rib cortex. J Bone Joint Surg. **47A**: 1211−1215.

Epker, B. N., Frost, H. M. (1966). Periosteal appositional bone growth from age two to age seventy in man − a tetracycline evaluation. *Anat. Rec.*, **154**: 573−578.

Eriksson, C. Electrical properties of bone. (1976). In: Bourne G.H., ed. *The Biochemistry and Physiology of Bone*. Vol IV, 2nd Ed, Academic Press, New York, 329−384.

Eriksen, E. F. (1986). Normal and pathological remodeling of human trabecular bone: Three dimensional reconstruction of the remodeling sequence in normals and in metabolic bone disease. *Endocrine Reviews*, **4**: 379−408.

Eriksen, E. F., Colvard, D. S., Berg, N. J., Graham, M. L., Mann, K. G., Spelsberg, T. C., Riggs, B. L. (1988). Evidence of estrogen receptors in normal human osteoblast-like cells. *Science*, **241**: 84−86.

Eriksen, E. F., Gundersen, H. J. G., Melsen, E., Mosekilde. L. (1984). Reconstruction of the formative site in iliac trabecular bone in 20 normal individuals employing a kinetic model for matrix and mineral apposition. *Metab. Bone Dis. & Rel. Res.*, **35**: 243−252.

Fallon, M. D., Teitelbaum, S. L., Weinstein, R. S., Goldfischer, S., Brown, D. M., Whyte, M. P. (1984). Hypophosphatasia: Clinicopathologic comparison of the infantile, childhood, and adult forms. *Medicine*, **63**: 12−24.

Farley, J. R., Wergedal, J. E., Baylink, D. J. (1983). Fluoride directly stimulates proliferation and alkaline phosphatase activity of bone-forming cells. *Science*, **222**: 330—332.

Farley, J. R., Tarbaux, N., Murphy, L. A., Masuda, T., Baylink, D. J. (1987). *In vitro* evidence that bone formation may be coupled to resorption by release of mitogen(s) from resorbing bone. *Metabolism*, **36**: 314—321.

Faugere, M-C., Friedler, R. M., Fanti, R., Malluche, H. H. (1988). Lack of histologic signs of Vit D deficiency in the early development of renal osteodystrophy. *J. Bone Min. Res.*, **3**: S95.

Fornasier, V. L. (1977). Osteoid: an ultrastructural study. *Human Pathology*, **8**: 243—254.

Frame, B., Honasoge, M., Kottamasu, S. R. (1987). *Osteosclerosis, hyperostosis and related disorders*. Elsevier, New York.

Frijlink, W. B., Bijvoet, O. L. M., teVelde, J., Heynen, G. (1979). Treatment of Paget's disease with (3-amino-1-hydroxypropylidene)-1, 1-bisphosphonate (A.P.D.). *Lancet*, **i**: 799—803.

Frost, H. M. 1960a *In vivo* osteocyte death. *J. Bone Joint Surg.*, **42A**: 138—143.

Frost, H. M. (1960b). Micropetrosis. *J. Bone Joint Surg.* **42A**: 144—150.

Frost, H. M. (1965). A synchronous group of mammalian cells whose *in vivo* behaviour can be studied. *Henry Ford Hosp. Med. Bull.*, **13**: 91—102.

Frost, H. M. (1966). *The Bone Dynamics in Osteoporosis and Osteomalacia*. Charles C. Thomas, Springfield, Il.

Frost, H. M. (1968). Tetracycline bone labeling in anatomy. *Am. J. Phys. Anthropology*, **29**: 183—196.

Frost, H. M. (1973a). The origin and nature of transients in human bone remodeling dynamics. In: Frame, B., Parfitt, A. M., Duncan, H., eds. *Clinical Aspects of Metabolic Bone Disease*, Amsterdam, Excerpta Medica ICS 270; 124—137.

Frost, H. M. (1973b). *Bone Modeling and Skeletal Modeling Errors*. Charles C. Thomas, Springfield, Il.

Frost, H. M. (1979). Treatment of osteoporosis by manipulation of coherent bone cell populations. *Clin. Orthop. Rel. Res.*, **143**: 227—244.

Frost, H. M. (1981). Resting seams: "On" and "Off" in lamellar bone-forming centers. In: Jee, W. S. S., Parfitt, A. M. (1981) eds. *Bone Histomorphometry: Third International Workshop*. Armour Montagu, Paris, 167—170.

Frost, H. M. (1983). Bone histomorphometry: Correction of the labeling "Escape Error" In: Recker, R. R., ed. *Bone Histomorphometry: Techniques and Interpretation*. CRC Press, Boca Raton, 133—142.

Frost, H. M. (1985a). The skeletal intermediary organization. A synthesis. In: Peck, W., Ed. *Bone & Min Res 3*, Elsevier, Amsterdam. 49—107.

Frost, H. M. (1985b). The pathomechanics of osteoporoses. *Clin. Orthop.* **200**: 198—228.

Frost, H. M. (1986). Bone microdamage: Factors that impair its repair. In: Uhthoff, H., Jaworski, Z. F. G., eds. *Current Concepts of Bone Fragility*. Berlin Heidelberg, Springer-Verlag, 123—146.

Frost, H. M. (1987). Bone "Mass" and the "Mechanostat": A proposal. *Anat. Rec.*, **219**: 1—9.

Gardner, E. (1971). Osteogenesis in the human embryo and fetus. In: Bourne G. H., ed. *The Biochemistry and Physiology of Bone*. Academic Press, New York, 77—118.

Gasser, K., Wilson, R., Rao, D., Hagler-Edwards, L., Riddle, J., Kleerekoper, M., Parfitt, A. M. (1986). Formation of mineralized connective tissue by human bone cells in vitro; studies in normal subjects and patients with osteoporosis. *J. Bone Min. Res.*, **1**: 122.

Gross, P. M., Heistad, D. D., Marcus, M. L. (1979). Neurohumoral regulation of blood flow to bones and marrow. *Amer. J. Physiol.*, 239 H440—H448.

Gundersen, H. J. G. (1986). Stereology of arbitrary particles. *J. Microsc.*, **143**: 3−45.

Ham, A. W., Harris, W. R. (1971). Repair and transplantation of bone. In: Bourne, G. H., ed. *The Biochemistry and Physiology of Bone*. Vol II, 2nd Ed. Academic Press, New York, 337−399.

Hammond, R. H., Storey, E. (1974). Measurement of growth and resorption of bone in the seventh caudal vertebra of the rat. *Calc. Tiss. Res.*, **15**: 11−20.

Hancox, N. M. (1972). *The Biology of Bone*. Cambridge, Cambridge University Press.

Hattner, R. S., Frost, H. M. (1963). Mean skeletal age: its calculation, and theoretical effects of skeletal tracer physiology and on the physical characteristics of bone. *Henry Ford Hosp. Med. Bull.*, **11**: 201−216.

Hattner, R. S., Ilnicki, L. P. Hodge, H. C. (1977). The dose-response relationship of tetracycline to the detectability of labeled osteons by fluorescence microscopy. In: Norman, A. W., Schaefer, K., Coburn, J. W., DeLuca, H. F., Fraser, D., Grigoleit, H. G., Herrath, D. V., eds. *Vitamin D, Biochemical, Chemical and Clinical Aspects Related to Calcium Metabolism*. de Gruyter, New York, 377−379.

Hayflick, L. (1976). The cell biology of human aging. *New Engl. J. Med.*, **295**: 1302−1308.

Hodsman, A. B. (1989). Effects of cyclical therapy for osteoporosis using an oral regimen of inorganic phosphate and sodium etidronate: A clinical and bone histomorphometric study. *Bone & Min.* **5**: 201−212.

Hori, M., Takahashi, H., Konno, T., Inoue, J., Haba, T. (1985). A classification of in vivo bone labels after double labeling in canine bones. *Bone*, **6**: 147−154.

Howard V., Reid S., Baddeley A., Boyde A. (1985). Unbiased estimation of particle density in the tandem scanning reflected light microscope. *J. Microscopy*, **138**: 203−212.

Hui, S. L. Wiske, P. S., Norton, J. A. Johnston, C. C. Jr. (1982). A prospective study of change in bone mass with age in postmenopausal women. *J. Chron. Dis.*, **35**: 715−725.

Jackson, J. A., Kleerekoper, M., Parfitt, A. M., Rao, D. S., Villanueva, A. R., Frame, B. (1987). Bone histomorphometry in hypogonadal and eugonadal men with spinal osteoporosis. *J. Clin. Endocrinol. Metab.*, **65**: 53−58.

Jaworski, Z. F. G., Hooper, C., (1980). Study of cell kinetics within evolving secondary haversian systems. *J. Anat.* **131**: 91−102.

Jaworski, Z. F. G. (1981). Physiology and pathology of bone remodeling. Cellular basis of bone structure in health and in osteoporosis. *Orthopedic Clinics of North America*, **12**: 485−512.

Jaworski, Z. F. G. (1987). Editorial: Does the mechanical usage (MU) inhibit bone "remodeling"? *Calcif. Tissue Int.* **41**: 2399−248.

Jaworski, Z. F. G., Meunier, P., Frost, H. M. (1972). Observations on 2 types of resorption cavities in human lamellar cortical bone. *Clin. Orthop*, **83**: 279.

Jaworski, Z. F. G, Wieczorek, E. (1985). Constants in lamellar bone formation determined by osteoblast kinetics. *Bone*, **6**: 361−363.

Jeansonne, B. G., Feagin, F. F., McMinn, R. W., Shoemaker, R. L., Rehm, W. S. (1979). Cell-to-cell communication of osteoblasts. *J. Dent. Res.*, **58**: 1415−1423.

Johnson, L. C. (1964). Morphologic analysis in pathology: the kinetics of disease and general biology of bone. In: Frost, H. M., ed. *Bone biodynamics*. Little, Brown and Co, Boston, 543−654.

Jones, S. J. (1974). Secretory territories and rate of matrix production of osteoblasts. *Calc. Tiss. Res.*, **14**: 309−315.

Jones, S. J., Boyde, A. (1976). Is there a relationship between osteoblasts and collagen orientation in bone? Israel *J. Med. Sci.*, **12**: 98−107.

Juster, M. Oligo, N., Laval-Jeantet, M. (1967). Lisere preosseux et tissu osteoide. In: Hioco, D. ed. *L'osteomalacie*, Masson, Paris.

Kahn, A. J., Fallon, M. D., Teitelbaum, S. L. (1983). Structure-function relationships in bone: An examination of events at the cellular level. In: Peck, W. A., ed. *Bone and Mineral Research*, 2. Elsevier, Amsterdam. pp. 125–174.

Kalu, D. N., Doyle, F. J., Pennock, J., Foster, G. V. (1970). Parathyroid hormone and experimental osteosclerosis. *Lancet*, 1: 1363–1366.

Kardos, T. B., Hubbard, M. J. (1982). Are matrix vesicles apoptotic bodies? In: Dixon, A. D., Sarnat, B. G., eds. *Factors and mechanisms influencing bone growth*. Alan R. Liss, New York. 45.

Kelin, M., Frost, H. M. (1964). Aging and the kinetics of human osteon formation. *J. Gerontology*, 19: 336–342.

Keshawarz, N. M., Recker, R. R. (1986). The label escape error: Comparison of measured and theoretical fraction of total bone–trabecular surface covered by single label in normals and patients with osteoporosis. *Bone*, 7: 83–87.

Kimmel, D. B. (1981a). A light microscopic description of osteoprogenitor cells of remodeling bone in the adult. In: Jee, W. S. S., Parfitt, A. M. eds. *Bone Histomorphometry; Third International Workshop*. Armour Montagu, Paris 181–188.

Kimmel, D. B. (1981b). Cellular basis of bone accumulation during growth: Implications for metabolic bone disease. In: DeLuca, H. F., Frost, H., Jee, W., Johnston, C., Parfitt, A. M. eds. *Osteoporosis: Recent Advances in Pathogenesis and Treatment*. Baltimore, University Park Press, 87–95.

Kimmel, D. B., Jee, W. S. S. (1982). A quantitative histologic study of bone turnover in young adults beagles. *Anat. Rec.*, 45: 203–231.

Kleerekoper, M., Villanueva, A. R., Stanciu, J., Rao, D. S., Parfitt, A. M. (1985). The role of three dimensional trabecular microstructure in the pathogenesis of vertebral compression fractures. *Calcif. Tissue Int.*, 37: 594–597.

Kleerekoper, M., Dickie, D., Feldkamp, L. A., Goldstein, S. A., Flynn, M. J., Parfitt, A. M. (1987). Cancellous bone architecture and bone strength. In: Christiansen, C., Johansen, C., Riis, B.J. eds *Osteoporosis 1987*. Osteopress Aps, Copenhagen, 294–300.

Kragstrup, J., Gundersen, H. J. G., Melsen, F., Mosekilde, L. (1982). Estimation of the three-dimensional wall thickness of completed remodeling sites in iliac trabecular bone. *Metab. Bone Dis. Rel. Res.*, 4: 113–119.

Kragstrup, J., Melsen, F. (1983a). Three-dimensional morphology of trabecular bone osteons reconstructed from serial sections. *Metab. Bone Dis. Relat. Res.*, 5: 127–130.

Kragstrup, J., Melsen, F., Mosekilde, L. (1983b). Thickness of bone formed at remodeling sites in normal human iliac trabecular bone: Variations with age and sex. *Metab. Bone. Dis. Rel. Res.*, 5: 17–21.

Krempien, B., Klimpel, F. (1980). Action of 1,25-dihydroxycholecalciferol on cartilage mineralization and on endosteal lining cells of bone. *Virchows Arch. A. Path. Anat. and Histol.* 388: 335–347.

Landeros, O., Frost, H. M. (1964). A cell system in which rate and amount of protein synthesis are separately controlled. *Science*, 145: 1323–1324.

Landis, W. J., Lee, D. D., Brenna, J. T., Chandra, S., Morrison, G. H. (1986). Detection and localization of silicon and associated elements in vertebrate bone tissue by imaging ion microscopy. *Calcif. Tissue Int*, 38: 52–59.

Leblond, C. P., Weinstock, M. (1972). Radioautographic studies of bone formation. In: Bourne, G. M., ed. *The Biochemistry and Physiology of Bone*. Vol. I, 2nd ed. Academic Press, New York.

Lee, W. R. (1967). Bone formation in Paget's disease. A quantitative microscopic study using tetracycline markers. *J. Bone Joint. Surg.*, 49B: 146–153.

Lian, J. B., Coutts, M., Canalis, E. (1985). Studies of hormonal regulation of osteocalcin synthesis in cultures fetal rat calvariae. *J. Biol. Chem.*, **260**: 8706−9710.

Lips, P., Courpron, P., Meunier, P. J. (1978). Mean wall thickness of trabecular bone packets in the human iliac crest: changes with age. *Calc. Tiss. Res.*, **26**: 13−17.

Loe, H. (1959). Bone tissue formation − a morphological and histochemical study. *Acta Odontol. Scand.*, (Suppl 27) **17**: 133−427.

Malluche, H. H., Faugere, M-C. (1986). *Atlas of Mineralized Bone Histology*, Karger, Basel.

Malluche, H. H., Sherman, D., Meyer, W., Tirz, E., Norman, A. W., Massry, S. G. (1982). Effects of long-term infusion of physiologic doses of 1−34 PTH on bone. *Am. J. Physiol.*, **242**: F197−201.

Manolagas, S. C., Burton, D. W., Deftos, L. J. (1981). 1,25-dihydroxyvitamin $D_3$ stimulates the alkaline phosphatase activity of osteoblast-like cells. *J. Biol. Chem.*, **256**: 7115−7117.

Manolagas, S. C., Haussler, M. R., Deftos, I. J. (1980). 1,25-dihydroxyvitamin $D_3$ receptor-like macromolecule in rat osteogenic sarcoma cell lines. *J. Biol. Chem.*, **255**: 4414−4417.

Marie, P. J., Caulin, F. (1986). Mechanisms underlying the effects of phosphate and calcitonin on bone histology in postmenopausal osteoporosis. *Bone*, **7**: 17−22.

Marie, P. J., Glorieux, F. H. (1981). Histomorphometric study of bone remodeling in hypo-phosphatemic vitamin D-resistant rickets. *Metab. Bone Dis. Rel. Res.*, **3**: 31−38.

Marie, P. J., Hott, M., Garba, M-T., (1985a). Inhibition of bone matrix apposition by (3-amino-1-hydroxypropylidene) -1,1-bisphosphonate (AHPrBP) in the mouse. *Bone*, **6**: 193−200.

Marie, P. J., Hott, M., Garba, M-T. (1985b). Contrasting effects of 1,25-dihydroxyvitamin $D_3$ on bone matrix and mineral appositional rates in the mouse. *Metabolism*, **34**: 777−783.

Marotti, G. (1977). Decrement in volume of osteoblasts during osteon formation and its effect on the size of the corresponding osteocytes. In: Meunier P.J. ed. *Bone Histomorphometry: Second International Workshop.* Paris, Armour Montagu, 299−310.

Marotti, G., Zallone, A. Z. (1980). Changes in the vascular network during the formation of haversian systems. *Acta Anat.*, **106**: 84−100.

Marotti, G., Remaggi, F., Zaffe, D. (1985). Quantitative investigation on osteocyte canaliculi in human compact and spongy bone. *Bone*, **6**: 335−337.

Martin, A. D., Bailey, D. A., Leicester, J. B., Gulka, I. (1987). Bone and muscle relationships in the foreams of lifetime tennis players. In: Christiansen, C., Johansen, J. S., Riis, B. J. *Osteoporosis 1987.* Osteopress Aps., Copenhagen, 599−600.

Martin, T. J. (1987). Cells of the osteoblast lineage in the regulation of bone turnover. In: Christiansen C., Johansen C., Riis B.J., eds. *Osteoporosis 1987.* Osteopress Aps, Copenhagen, 189−193.

MacIntyre, I., Whitehead, M. I., Banks, L. M., Stevenson, J. C., Wimalawansa, S. J., Healy, M. J. R. (1988). Calcitonin for prevention of postmenopausal bone loss. *Lancet*, **i**: 900−901.

Meema, H. E. (1977). Recognition of cortical bone resorption in metabolic disease *in vivo. Skel. Radiol.*, **2**: 11−19.

Meema, H. E., Meema, S. (1988). Longitudinal microradioscopic comparisons on endosteal and juxtaendosteal bone loss in premenopausal and postmenopausal women, and in those with end-stage renal disease. *Bone*, **8**: 343−350.

Melsen, F., Mosekilde, L., (1978) Tetracycline double-labeling of iliac trabecular bone in 41 normal adults. *Calcif. Tiss. Res.*, **26**: 99−102.

Melsen, F., Mosekilde, L., Eriksen, E. F., Charles, P., Steinicke, T. (1989). *In vivo* hormonal effects on trabecular bone remodeling, osteoid mineralization and skeletal turnover. In: Kleerekoper M., Krane S., eds. *Clinical Disorders of Bone and Mineral Metabolism.* Mary Ann Liebert Publishers, Inc. New York. p. 73−86.

Menton, D. N., Simmons, D. J., Orr, B. Y., Plurad, S. B. (1982). A cellular investment of bone marrow. *Anat. Rec.*, **203**: 157−164.

Menton, D. N., Simmons, D. J., Change S-L., Orr B. Y. (1984). From bone lining cell to osteocyte−An SEM study. *Anat. Rec.*, **209**: 29−39.

Mercer, R. R., Crenshaw, M. A. (1985). The role of osteocytes in bone resorption during lactation: Morphometric observations. *Bone*, **6**: 345−347.

Merz, W. A., Schenk, R. K. (1970). A quantitative histologic study of bone formation in human cancellous bone. *Acta Anat.*, **76**: 1−15.

Meunier, P. J. (1983). Histomorphometry of the skeleton. In: Peck, W. A., ed. *Bone and Mineral Research*, Annual 1, Excerpta Medica, Amsterdam. 191−222.

Meunier, P. J., Aaron, J., Edouard, G., Vignon, G. (1971). Osteoporosis and the replacement of cell populations of the marrow by adipose tissue. *Clin. Orthop. Rel. Res.*, **80**: 147−154.

Meunier, P. J., Courpron, C., Edouard, C., Alexandre, C., Bressot, C., Lips, P., Boyce, B. F. (1980a). Bone histomorphometry in osteoporotic states. In: Barzel U.S., ed. *Osteoporosis II*, Grune & Stratton, New York.

Meunier, P. J., Coindre, J. M., Edouard, C. M., Arlot, M. E. (1980b). Bone histomorphometry in Paget's disease. Quantitative and dynamic analysis of pagetic and nonpagetic bone tissue. *Arthritis and Rheumatism*, **23**: 1095−1103.

Milgram, J. W. (1977). Radiographical and pathological assessment of the activity of Paget's disease of bone. *Clin. Orth. Rel. Res.*, **127**: 43−54.

Miller, S. C., Bowman, B. M., Smith, J. M., Jee, W. S. S. (1980). Characterization of endosteal bone-lining cells from fatty marrow bone sites in adult beagles. *Anat. Rec.*, **198**: 163−173.

Miller, S. C., Jee, W. S. S. (1980). The microvascular bed of fatty bone marrow in the adult beagle. *Metab. Bone Dis. Rel. Res.*, **2**: 239−246.

Miller, S. C., Jee, W. S. S. (1987). The bone lining cell: A distinct phenotype? *Calcif. Tissue Int.*, **41**: 1−5.

Minaire, P., Meunier, P., Edouard, C., Bernard, J., Courpron, P., Bourret, J. (1974). Quantitative histological data on disuse osteoporosis: Comparison with biological data. *Calcif. Tissue Res.*, **17**: 57−73.

Mundy, G. R., Roodman, G. D. (1987). Osteoclast ontogeny and function. In: Peck, W. A., ed. *Bone and Mineral Research*, Elsevier, Amsterdam **5**: 209−279.

Murphy, E. A. (1986). *The logic of medicine*. Johns Hopkins University Press, Baltimore.

Neuman, M. W., Imai, K., Kawase, T., Saito, S. (1987). The calcium-buffering phase of bone mineral: Some clues to its form and formation. *J. Bones & Min. Res.* **3**: 171−181.

Nichols, G., Rogers, P. (1972). Bone cell calcium stores: Their size, location, and kinetics of exchange. *Calc. Tiss. Res.*, **9**: 80−94.

Nijweide, P. J. Mulder R. J. P. (1986). Identification of osteocytes in osteoblast-like cell cultures using a monoclonal antibody specifically directed against osteocytes. *Histochemistry*, **84**: 342−347.

Norimatsu, H., Yamamoto, T., Ozawa, H., Talmage, R. V. (1982). Changes in calcium phosphate on bone surfaces and in lining cells after the administration of parathyroid hormone or calcitonin. *Clin, Orthop. Rel. Res.*, **164**: 271−278.

Owen, M. (1971). Cellular dynamics of bone. In: Bourne, G. H., ed. The *Biochemistry and Physiology of Bone*, Vol. III, 2nd Ed., Academic Press. New York.

Pacifici, R., McMurtry, C., Vered, I., Rupich, R., Avioli, L. V. (1988). Coherence therapy does not prevent axial bone loss in osteoporotic women: A preliminary comparative study. *J. Clin. Endo. & Metab.*, **66**: 747−754.

Parfitt, A. M. (1976a). The actions of parathyroid hormone on bone. Relation to bone remodeling and turnover, calcium homeostasis and metabolic bone disease. I. Mechanisms of calcium transfer between blood and bone and their cellular basis. Morphologic and kinetic approaches to bone turnover. *Metabolism*, **25**: 809−844.

Parfitt, A. M. (1976b). The actions of parathyroid hormone on bone. Relation to bone remodelling and turnover, calcium homeostasis and metabolic bone disease. III. PTH and osteoblasts, the relationship between bone turnover and bone loss, and the state of the bones in primary hyperparathyroidism. *Metabolism*, **25**: 1033−1069.

Parfitt, A. M. (1977a). The cellular basis of bone turnover and bone loss. A rebuttal of the osteocytic resorption-bone flow theory. *Clin. Orthop.*, **127**: 236−247.

Parfitt, A. M. (1977b). Metacarpal cortical dimensions in hypoparathyroidism, primary hyperparathyroidism and chronic renal failure. *Calc. Tissue Res.*, **22 (Supplement)**: 329−331.

Parfitt, A. M. (1980). Richmond Smith as a clinical investigator: His work on adult periosteal bone expansion, and on nutritional and endocrine aspects of osteoporosis, in the light of current concepts. *HFH Med. J.*, **28**: 95−107.

Parfitt, A. M. (1981). Integration of skeletal and mineral homeostasis. In: DeLucca, H. F., Frost, H., Jee, W., Johnston, C., Parfitt, A. M. eds. *Osteoporosis: Recent Advances in Pathogenesis and Treatment*. Baltimore, University Park Press, 115−126.

Parfitt, A. M. (1983). The physiologic and clinical significant of bone histomorphometric data. In: Recker, R. ed. *Bone Histomorphometry. Techniques and Interpretations*. Boca Raton, CRC Press, 143−223.

Parfitt, A. M. (1984a). The cellular mechanisms of osteoid accumulation in metabolic bone disease. In: *Mineral Metabolism Research in Italy*, Vol. 4. Milano, Wichtig Editore, 3−9.

Parfitt, A. M. (1984b). The cellular basis of bone remodeling. The quantum concept re-examined in light of recent advances in cell biology of bone *Calc. Tissue Int.*, **36**: S37−S45.

Parfitt, A. M. (1984c). Bone as a source of urinary calcium-osseous hypercalciuria. In: Coe, F., ed. *Hypercalciuric States − Pathogenesis, Consequences and Treatment*. New York, Grune & Stratton, 313−378.

Parfitt, A. M. (1986). Accelerated cortical bone loss: primary and secondary hyperpara-thyroidism. In: Uhthoff, H., Jaworski, Z. F. G., eds. *Current Concepts of Bone Fragility*. Berlin Heidelberg, Springer-Verlag 279−285.

Parfitt, A. M. (1987a). Bone and plasma calcium homeostastis. *Bone,* **8**: 51−58.

Parfitt, A. M. (1987b). Pathogenesis of vertebral fracture: Qualitative abnormalities in bone architecture and bone age. In: Roche, A. F, ed. *Osteoporosis: Current Concepts*. Report of the Seventh Ross Conference on Medical Research. Ross Laboratories, Columbus, Ohio, 18−22.

Parfitt, A. M. (1988a). Bone remodeling: Relationship to the amount and structure of bone and the pathogenesis and prevention of fractures. In: Riggs, B. L., ed. *Osteoporosis − Etiology, Diagnosis and Management*. Raven Press, New York, 45−93.

Parfitt, A. M. (1988b). The localization of aluminum in bone: implications for the mechanism of fixation and for the pathogenesis of aluminum-related bone disease. Editorial, *Int. J. Artif. Organs* **11**: 79−90.

Parfitt, A. M. (1988c). The composition, structure and remodeling of bone: A basis for the interpretation of bone mineral measurements. In: Dequeker, J., Geusens, P., Wahner, H. W., eds. *Bone Mineral Measurements by Photon Absorptiometry: Methodological Problems*. Leuven University Press, Leuven 9−28.

Parfitt, A. M. (1989). Surface specific bone remodeling in health and disease. In: Kleerekoper, M., Krane, S., eds. Clinical Disorders of Bone and Mineral Metabolism. Mary Ann Liebert Publishers, Inc. New York. p. 7−14.

Parfitt, A. M. Osteomalacia and related disorders. In: Avioli, L. V., Krane, S. M. eds. *Metabolic Bone Disease*, 2nd ed. New York, Grune and Stratton.

Parfitt, A. M. Drug-Induced Osteomalacia. In: Posillico, J. T., Favus, M., eds. ASBMR Primer on Metabolic Bone Diseases (submitted for publication).

Parfitt, A. M., Kleerekoper, M. (1980). Clinical disorders of calcium, phosphorus and magnesium metabolism. In: Maxwell, M., Kleeman, C. R., eds. *Clinical Disorders of Fluid and Electrolyte Metabolism*, 3rd ed. New York, McGraw-Hill, 947−1152.

Parfitt, A. M., Kleerekoper, M. (1984). Diagnostic value of bone histomorphometry and comparison of histologic measurements and biochemical indices of bone remodeling. In: Christiansen, C., Arnaud, C. D., Nordin, B. E. C., Parfitt, A. M., Peck, W. A., Riggs, B. L. eds. *Osteoporosis*. Proc Copenhagen Intnl Symposium on Osteoporosis, June 3−8. Aalborg Stiftsbogtrykkeri, 103−109.

Parfitt, A. M., Villanueva, A. R., (1982). Hypophosphatemia and osteoblast function in human bone disease. In: Massry, S. G., Letteri, J. M., Ritz, E., eds. *Regulation of Phosphate and Mineral Metabolism, Adv. Exp. Med. Biol.*, **151**: 209−216.

Parfitt, A. M., Villanueva, A. R., Crouch, M. M., Mathews, C. H. E., Duncan, H. (1977). Classification of osteoid seams by combined use of cell morphology and tetracycline labelling. Evidence for intermittency of mineralization. In: Meunier, P. J., ed. *Bone Histomorphometry: Second International Workshop*. Paris, Armour Montagu, 299−310.

Parfitt, A. M., Mathews, C., Rao, D., Frame, B., Kleerekoper, M. Villanueva, A. R. (1981a). Impaired osteoblast function in metabolic bone disease. In: DeLuca, H. F., Frost, H., Jee, W., Johnston, C., Parfitt, A. M. eds. *Osteoporosis: Recent Advances in Pathogenesis and Treatment*. Baltimore, University Park Press, 321−330.

Parfitt, A. M., Villanueva, A. R., Mathews, C. H. E., Aswani, J. A. (1981b). Kinetics of matrix and mineral apposition in osteoporosis and renal osteodystrophy: Relationship to rate of turnover and to cell morphology. In: Jee, W. S. S., Parfitt, A. M., eds. *Bone Histomorphometry: Third International Workshop*. Paris, Armour-Montagu, 213−219.

Parfitt, A. M., Podenphant, J., Villanueva, A. R., Frame, B. (1985). Metabolic bone disease with and without osteomalacia after intestinal bypass surgery: A bone histomorphometric study. *Bone*, **6**: 211−220.

Parfitt, A. M., Simon, L. S., Villanueva, A. R., Krane, S. M. (1987a). Procollagen type I carboxy-terminal extension peptide in serum as a marker of collagen biosynthesis in bone. Correlation with iliac bone formation rates and comparison with total alkaline phosphatase. *J. Bone Mineral. Res.*, **2**: 427−436.

Parfitt, A. M., Drezner, M. K., Glorieux, F. H., Kanis, J. A., Malluche, H., Meunier, P. J., Ott, S. M., Recker, R. R. (1987b). Bone histomophometry nomenclature, symbols and units. Report of the ASBMR Histomorphometry Nomenclature Committee. *J. Bone Min. Res.*, **2**: 595−610.

Parfitt, A. M., Kleerekoper, M., Rao, D. S., Stanciu, J., Villanueva, A. R. (1987c). Cellular mechanisms of cortical thinning in primary hyperparathyroidism (PHPT). *J. Bone Min. Res.*, **2 (Suppl 1)**: 384.

Parfitt, A. M., Kleerekoper, M., Villanueva, A. R. (1987d). Increased bone age: Mechanisms and consequences. In: Christianses, C, Johansen, C, Riis, B. J., eds. *Osteoporosis 1987*. Osteopress Aps, Copenhagen. 301−308.

Parfitt, A. M., Villanueva, A. R., Rao, D. S. (1988). Surface differences in iliac bone re-modelling; contribution of geometric and biologic factors and effect of menopause. *J. Bone Min. Res.*, **3 (Suppl 1)**: S215.

Podbesek, R., Edouard, C., Meunier, P. J., Parsons, J. A., Reeve, J., Stevenson, R. W., Zanelli, J. M. (1983). Effects of two treatment regimens with synthetic human parathyroid hormone fragment on bone formation and the tissue balance of trabecular bone in greyhounds. *Endocrinol.*, **112**: 1000−1006.

Polig, E., Kimmel, D. B., Jee, W. S. S. (1984). Morphometry of bone cell nuclei and their location relative to bone surfaces. *Phys. Med. Biol.*, **29**: 939−952.

Pritchard, J. J. (1972). The osteoblast. In: Bourne, G. M. ed. *The biochemistry and Physiology of Bone.* Vol I, 2nd Ed, Academic Press, New York.

Quarles, L. D., Gitelman, H. J., Drezner, M. K. (1988). Induction of de novo bone formation in the beagle. A Novel Effect of Aluminum. *J. Clin. Invest.*, **81**: 1056−1066.

Raisz, L. G. (1988). Local and systemic factors in the pathogenesis of osteoporosis. *N. Engl. J. Med.*, **318**: 818−828.

Rao, D. S. Metabolic bone disease in gastrointestinal and biliary disorders. In: Posillico, J. T., Favus, M., eds. *ASBMR Primer on Metabolic Bone Diseases* (submitted for publication).

Rasmussen, H., Bordier, PhJ. (1974). *The physiological and cellular basis of metabolic bone disease.* Williams and Wilkins, Baltimore.

Recker, R. R., Kimmel, D. B., Parfitt, A. M., Davies, K. M., Keshwarz, N., Hinders, S. (1988). Static and tetracycline-based bone histomorphometric data from 34 normal postmenopausal females. *J. Bone Min. Res.*, **2**: 133−144.

Reeve, J. (1987). Bone turnover and trabecular plate survival after artificial menopause. *Br. Med. J.*, **295**: 757−760.

Reeve, J., Arlot, M., Wootton, R., Edouard, C., Tellez, M., Hest, R., Green, J. R., Meunier, P. J. (1988) Skeletal blood flow, iliac histomorphometry, and strontium kinetics in osteoporosis: A relationship between blood flow and corrected apposition rate. *J. Clin, Endo. Metab.*, **66**: 1124−1131.

Reeve, J., Meunier, P. J. Parsons, J. A., Bernat, M., Bijvoet, O. L. M., Courpron, P., Edouard, C., Klenerman, L., Neer, R. M., Renier, J. C., Slovik, D., Vismans, F. J. F. E. , Potts, J. T. Jr. (1980). Anabolic effect of human parathyroid hormone fragment on trabecular bone in involutional osteoporosis: a multicentre trial. *Br. Med. J.* **2**: 1340−1344.

Reginster, J. Y., Albert, A., Lecart, M. P., Lambelin, P., Denis, D., Deroisy, R., Fontaine, M. A., Franchimont, P. (1987). 1-Year controlled randomised trial of prevention of early postmenopausal bone loss by intranasal calcitonin. *Lancet*, **2**: 1481−1483.

Riggs, B. L. (1983). Treatment of osteoporosis with sodium fluoride: An appraisal. In: Peck, W. A., ed. *Bone & Min Res.*, Annual 2. Elsevier Science Publishers B.V., 366−393.

Riggs, B. L., Hodgson, S. F., Muhs, J., Wahner, H. W. (1987). Fluoride treatment of osteoporosis: Clinical and bone densitometric responses. In: Christiansen, C., Johansen, J. S., Riis, B. J. eds. *Osteoporosis* 1987. Osteopress Aps, Copenhagen, 817−823.

Roberts, W. E., Morey, E. R. (1985). Proliferation and differentiation sequence of osteoblast histogenesis under physiological conditions in rat periodontal ligament. *Am. J. Anat.*, **174**: 105−118.

Rodan, G. A., Rodan, S. E. (1983). Expression of the osteoblast phenotype. In: Peck, W. A., ed. *Bone & Mineral Research*, 2, Elsevier, Amsterdam.

Rubin, C. T., Lanyon, L. E. (1987). Osteoregulatory nature of mechanical stimuli: Function as a determinant for adaptive remodeling in bone. *J. Ortho. Res.*, **5**: 300−310.

Schaffler, M. B., Burr, D. B., Frederickson, R. G. (1987). Morphology of the osteonal cement line in human bone. *Anat. Record*, **217**: 223−228.

Schen, S., Villanueva, A. R., Frost, H. M. (1965). Number of osteoblasts per unit area of osteoid seam in cortical human bone. *Can. J. of Physiology and Pharmacology*, **43**: 319−325.

Schenk, R. K., Merz, W. A., Muller, J. (1969). A quantitative histological study on bone resorption in human cancellous bone. *Acta Anat.*, **74**: 44−53.

Schenk, R. K., Merz, W. A., Reutter, F. W. (1970). Fluoride in osteoporosis: Quantitative histological studies on bone structure and bone remodelling in serial biopsies of the iliac crest. In: Vischer, T. L., ed. *Fluoride in Medicine*, Hans Huber, Bern, Switzerland, 153−168.

Schwartz, M. P., Recker, R. R. (1982). The label escape error: Determination of the active bone-forming surface in histologic sections of bone measured by tetracycline double labels. *Metab. Bone Dis. Rel. Res.*, **4**: 237−241.

Shai, F., Baker, R. K., Wallach, S. (1971). The clinical and metabolic effects of porcine calcitonin on Paget's disease of bone. *J. Clin, Invest.*, **50**: 1927−1940.

Shen, V., Rifas, L., Kohler, G., Peck, W. A. (1986). Prostaglandins change cell shape and increase intercellular gap junctions in osteoblasts cultured from rat fetal calvaria. *J. Bone Min. Res.*, **1**: 243−249.

Simmons, D. J. (1981). Circadian Rhythms in bone. In: Jee, W. S. S., Parfitt, A. M., eds. *Bone Histomorphometry: Third International Workshop*. Armour Montagu, Paris, 137−149.

Simmons, D. J., Simmons, N. B., Marshall, J. H., (1970). The uptake of calcium-45 in the acellular-boned toadfish. *Calc. Tiss. Res.*, **5**: 206−221.

Simon, L. S., Krane, S. M., Wortman, P. D., Krane, I. M., Kovitz, K. L. (1984). Serum levels of Type I and III procollagen fragments in Paget's disease of bone. *J. Clin. Endocrinol. Metab.*, **58**: 110−120.

Simonet, W. T., Bronk, J. T., Pinto, M. R., Williams, E. A., Meadows, T. H., Kelly, P. J. (1988). Cortical and cancellous bone: Age-related changes in morphologic features, fluid spaces, and calcium homeostasis in dogs. *Mayo Clin. Proc.*, **63**: 154−160.

Singer, F. R., Mills, B. G. (1983). Paget's disease of bone: Etiologic and therapeutic aspects. In: Peck, W. A., ed. *Bone and Mineral Research*, Annual 2, Elsevier Science Publisher B.V., 394−421.

Singer, F. R., Schiller, A. L., Pyle, E.B., Krane, S.M. (1978). Paget's Disease of Bone. In: Avioli, L. V., Krane, S. M., eds. *Metabolic Bone Disease*, Volume II, Academic Press, Inc., New York, 489−575.

Sissons, H. A. (1971). The growth of bone. In: Bourne, G. H., ed. *The Biochemistry and Physiology of Bone*. Vol. 2, 2nd Ed. Academic Press, New York, 145−180.

Sissons, H. A., Kelman, G. J., Marotti, G., (1985). Bone resorption in calcium-deficient rats. *Bone* **6**: 345−347.

Skerry, T. M., Bitensky, L., Chayen, J., Lanyon, L. E., (1987). Strain memory in bone tissue? Is proteoglycan based persistence of strain history a cue for the control of adaptive bone remodelling? *Ortho. Trans.*, **11**: 277.

Smith, J. W. (1960). Collagen fibre patterns in mammalian bone. *J. Anat.* **94**: 329−344.

Smith, R., Triffitt, J. T. (1986). Bones in muscles: The problems of soft tissue ossification. *Quart. J. of Med.*, **235**: 985−990.

Stern, P. H. (1980). The D vitamins and bone. *Pharmacol. Rev.*, **32**: 47−80.

Stewart, A. F., Vignery, A., Silverglate, A., Ravin, N. D., LiVolsi, V., Broadus, A. E., Baron, R. (1982). Quantitative bone histomorphometry in humoral hypercalcemia of malignancy: Uncoupling of bone cell activity. *J. Clin. Endo. Metab.*, **55**: 219−227.

Storey, E. (1972). Growth and remodelling of bone and bones. *Am. J. Orthodont.*, **62**: 142−165.

Stumpf, W. E., Sar, M., DeLucca, H. F. (1981). Sites of action of 1,25 $(OH)_2$ Vitamin $D_3$ identified by thaw-mount autoradiography. In: Cohn, D. V., Talmage, R.V., Matthews J.L. *Hormonal control of calcium metabolism*. Amsterdam, Excerpta Medica, 222−229.

Swan, C. H. J., Shah, K., Brewer, D. B., Cooke, W. T. (1976). Fibrogenesis imperfecta ossium. *Quart. J. Med.*, **178**: 233−253.

Talmage, R. V., Cooper, C. W., Toverud, S. U. (1983). The physiological significance of calcitonin. In: Peck, W. A., ed. *Bone and Mineral Research*, Annual 1. Excerpta Medica, Amsterdam, 74−143.

Tam, C. S., Harrison, J. E., Heersche, J. N. M., Jones, G., Wilson, D. R., Parsons, J. A., Murray, T. M., (1981). Short term variation in the rate of apposition of mineralized bone matrix in small animals. In: Jee, W. S. S., Parfitt, A. M. eds. *Bone Histomorphometry: Third International Workshop*. Armour Montagu, Paris, 159−166.

Tappen, N. C. (1977). Three-dimensional studies of resorption spaces and developing osteons. *Am. J. Anat.*, **149**: 301−332.

Teitelbaum, S. L., Bergfeld, M. A., Freitag, J., Hruska, K. A., Slatopolsky E. (1980). Do parathyroid hormone and 1,25-Dihydroxyvitamin D modulate bone formation in uremia? *J. Clin. Endo. Metab.*, **51**: 247−251.

VanderWiel, C. J., Grubb, S. A., Talmage, R. V. (1978). The presence of lining cells on surfaces of human trabecular bone. *Clin. Ortho. Rel. Res.*, **134**: 350−355.

Vaughan, J. (1981). Osteogenesis and hematopoiesis. *Lancet* 133−136.

Vedi, S., Compston, J. E., Webb, A., Tighe, (1982). J. R. Histomorphometric analysis of bone biopsies from the iliac crest of normal British subjects. *Metab. Bone Dis. Rel. Res.*, **4**: 231−236.

de Vernejoul, M. C., Marie, P. J., Miravet, L., Ryckewaert, A. (1983). Chronic hypophosphatemia without osteomalacia. In: Frame, B., Potts, J. T. Jr., eds. *Clinical disorders of bone and mineral metabolism*. Amsterdam, Excerpta Medica, 232−236.

Vigorita, V. J., Suda, M. K. (1983). The microscopic morphology of fluoride-induced bone. *Clin. Orthop.* 177: 274−282.

Villanueva, A. R., Mathews, C. H. E., Parfitt, A. M. (1983a). Relationship between the size and shape of osteoblasts and the width of osteoid seams in bone. In: Takahashi, H., ed. *Handbook of Bone Morphometry*. Nishimara, 191−196.

Villanueva, A. R., Kujawa, M., Mathews, C. H. E., Parfitt, A. M., (1983b). Identification of the mineralization front: Comparison of a modified toluiding blue stain with tetracycline fluorescence. *Metab. Bone Dis. Rel. Res.*, **5**: 41−45.

Villanueva, A. R., Qui, M-C., Parfitt, A. M. (1985). Mean wall thickness in gallocyanine stained sections: Comparison with ultraviolet light (UVL) and polarized light (PL) microscopy. *Bone* **6**: 412.

Villanueva, A. R., Sypitkowski, C., Parfitt, A. M. (1986). A new method for identification of cement lines in undecalcified, plastic embedded sections of bone. *Stain Technol.* **61**: 83−88.

Vincent, J. (1963). Microscopic aspects of mineral metabolism in bone tissue with special reference to calcium, lead and zinc. *Clin. Orthoped.*, **20**: 161−174.

Volpi, G., Palazzini, S., Cane, V., Remaggi, F., Muglia, M. A. (1981). Morphometric analysis of osteoblast dynamics in the chick embryo tibia. *Anat. Embryol.*, **162**: 393−401.

Wallach, S., Avramides, A., Flores, A., Bellavia, J., Cohn, S. (1975). Skeletal turnover and total body elemental composition during extended calcitonin treatment of Paget's disease. *Metabolism*, **24**: 745−753.

Weinstein, R. S., Lutcher, C. L. (1983). Chronic erythroid hyperplasia and accelerated bone turnover. *Metab. Bone Dis. Rel. Res.*, **5**: 7−12.

Weinstein, R. S., Weinstein, D. L., Bell, N. H. (1988). Rates of bone formation and mineral apposition are diminished in normal black men and women. *J. Bone & Min. Res.*, **3 (Suppl 1)**: S89.

Whyte, M. P., Fallon, M. D., Murphy, W. A., Teitelbaum, S. L. (1981). Axial Osteomalacia. Clinical, laboratory and genetic investigation of affected mother and son. *Am. J. Med.*, **71**: 1041−1049.

Williams, E. A., Pinto, M. R. Kelly, P. J. (1987). Effects of age on cell size and ion uptake in canine cortical bone. *Mayo Clin. Proc.*, **62**: 15−21.

Wong, M. M., Ly, H., Rao, L. G., Hamilton, L., Ish-Shalom, S., Stockbridge, W., Tong, J., Transfeldt E., Murray, T. M. (1987). In vitro study of osteoblast-like (OBL) cells from patients with idiopathic osteoporosis (IOP): Preliminary observations on hormonal responsiveness and growth rates. In: Christiansen, C., Johansen, C., Riis, B. J., eds. *Osteoporosis 1987*. Osteopress Aps. Copenhagen, 234–236.

Woods, C. G. (1972). *Diagnostic orthopaedic pathology*. Blackwell Scientific Publications, Oxford.

Wronski, T. J., Smith, J. M., Jee, W. S. S. (1980). The microdistribution and retention of injected [239] Pu on trabecular bone surface of the beagle: Implications for the induction of osteosarcoma. *Radiation Res.*, **83**: 74–89.

Wronski, T. J., Smith, J. M., Jee, W. S. S. (1981). Variations in mineral apposition rate of trabecular bone within the beagle skeleton. *Calcif. Tissue. Int.* **33**: 583–586.

Wu, K. K. (1973). Haversian and endosteal bone formation rates in rib biopsies of 50 patients with senile and postmenopausal osteoporosis. *Henry Ford Hosp. Med. J.*, **21**: 143–153.

Wyllie, A. H., Kerr, J. F. R., Currie, A. R. (1980). Cell death: The significance of apoptosis. *Int. Rev. Cytol.*, **68**: 251–306.

Yen, A., Pardee, A. B. (1979). Role of nuclear size in cell growth initiation. *Science*, **204**: 1315–1317.

Zallone, A. Z. (1977). Relationships between shape and size of the osteoblasts and the accretion rate of trabecular bone surfaces. *Anat. Embryol.*, **152**: 65–72.

Zallone, A. Z., Teti, A., Primavera, M. V., Pace, G. (1983). Mature osteocytes behaviour in a repletion period: the occurence of osteoplastic activity. *Bas. Appl. Histochem.*, **27**: 191–204.

# 10

## Mutations Affecting Bone-Forming Cells

**David E. C. Cole and M. Michael Cohen, Jr.**
*Departments of Pediatrics and Oral Biology,*
*Dalhousie University,*
*Halifax, Nova Scotia*
*Canada*

Introduction
Fibrodysplasia ossificans progressiva
   Genetics
   Features and natural history
   Other similár conditions
   Pathogenesis
Hypophosphatasia
   The biology of alkaline phosphatase
   Hypophosphatasia
Osteosarcomas and the *c-fos* proto-oncogene
   Murine viral osteosarcomas
   The genetics of *c-fos*
   *c-fos* and bone development
Acknowledgments
References

## Introduction

Mutations are an essential part of evolution and contribute significantly to the expression of biological diversity. They are also a valuable source of new information on mechanisms of cellular metabolism. In vertebrate organisms, genomic or inherited mutations that affect only bone-forming

431

cells are apparently uncommon, presumably because they are incompatible with survival beyond the early stages of development. Moreover, there may be a relatively limited number of genes required to express the osteoblast phenotype.

This chapter focuses on three specific mutations that exemplify the progress that has been achieved in the understanding of human disorders. In the first instance, we review the clinical and biological features of a rare inherited condition of ectopic bone formation—*fibrodysplasia ossificans progressiva*. In the second, we summarize recent investigations that delineate the molecular basis of *hypophosphatasia*—an inherited disorder of bone characterized by a deficiency in alkaline phosphatase activity. With molecular cloning, it is now possible to identify the genetic antecedents of the disorder and to offer accurate genetic counselling for affected individuals and families at risk. Finally, we consider the rapid developments in our knowledge of the actions of the *c-fos protooncogene*, culminating in the demonstration that one of the roles for this gene in mammalian embryogenesis is in the development of bone. The *v-fos retroviral oncogene*, itself a mutated form of *c-fos*, was originally identified as a cause of mouse osteosarcoma and is clearly a mutation of direct relevance to an understanding of human neoplasia in calcified tissue.

## Fibrodysplasia Ossificans Progressiva

Fibrodysplasia ossificans progressiva (FOP) is a rare autosomal dominant condition with progressive ectopic ossification and distinctive skeletal malformations. Characteristic features include malformations of the large toe, reduction defects of all digits, deafness, baldness, and mental deficiency. Progressive disability due to ectopic calcification is saltatory, but severe restriction of movement eventually occurs and is especially evident in the shoulders and spine by the age of 10 years (Connor and Evans, 1982b; McKusick, 1972). A great many cases have been reported and by 1982, in excess of 550 instances had been noted (Connor and Evans, 1982a). Although many single cases appear in the literature, a number of large series have been followed (McKusick, 1972; Rogers and Geho, 1979; Tünte et al., 1967; Connor and Evans, 1982b). Caucasians are reported most commonly, but a number of Black patients have also been observed (Connor and Beighton, 1982; Shipton et al., 1985).

### Genetics

The overwhelming majority of cases are sporadic (McKusick, 1972; Tünte et al., 1967). Autosomal dominant inheritance is based on several instances of parent-to-child and male-to-male transmission (Burton-Fanning and Vaughan, 1901; Gaster, 1905) and on concordant monozygotic twins (Eaton *et al.*, 1957; Vastine *et al.*, 1948). Thus, most cases arise as new mutations. Genetic fitness appears to be close to zero, physical disability probably being the main reason, although infertility has been suggested (Tünte *et al.*, 1967).

Evidence from published reports to date indicates that in families in which the FOP gene is transmitted through two generations, penetrance is complete. However, variable expressivity is observed with respect to skeletal malformations and the extent of ectopic ossification. On occasion, a parent has exhibited only characteristic skeletal malformations, the child expressing the full FOP phenotype with ectopic ossification (Sympson, 1886). There is no evidence for genetic heterogeneity (Connor and Evans, 1982a).

With autosomal dominant inheritance, the expected 1:1 sex ratio has not been demonstrated. Some studies show that males are more frequently affected, ratios ranging from 4:1 to 3:2, although a female predilection as high as 67% of the patients was observed in one series (McKusick, 1972). The reasons for this are not entirely clear, but it seems obvious that problems of sample size in some studies and ascertainment bias in others play a major role.

A significant paternal age effect has been demonstrated for new mutations in three studies (Connor and Evans, 1982a; Rogers and Chase, 1979; Tünte *et al.*, 1967). A similar paternal age effect has also been found with other autosomal dominant mutations (eg. Apert syndrome, Marfan syndrome, achondroplasia) and indicates that, with increasing age, the chance of fertilization by a sperm which has a single gene replication error increases.

Connor and Evans (1982a), attempting complete ascertainment of FOP in the United Kingdom, indicated a point prevalence of $0.61 \times 10^{-6}$. They also calculated a direct estimate of the mutation rate of 1.8 (SE $\pm$ 1.04) $\times$ $10^{-6}$ mutations per gene per generation, a value comparable with other known human mutations.

## Features and Natural History

Clinical features include four possible types of malformation of the big toe, reduction defects of the digits, deafness, baldness, and mental deficiency. Findings in FOP, together with their frequencies, are presented in Table 1. All patients have skeletal abnormalities of the big toe which are present at birth (Fig. 1). Type I is the commonest; the big toes are short, lack a skin crease, and possess a single phalanx. In Type II, the big toes are of normal length but are stiff from early childhood and show progressive osseous fusion with age. In Type III, two phalanges are present which become rigid during the second decade due to osteophytic lipping. Variable

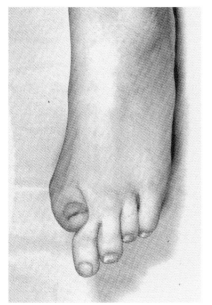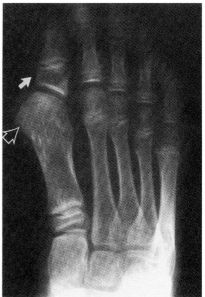

**Fig. 1**   Fibrodysplasia Ossificans Progressiva
A) Foreshortened large toe (Type I) in an affected patient.
B) Radiograph of Type I foreshortening in another patient. Note shortening in proximal phalanx (solid arrow) and widened, deviated first metatarsal (open arrow).

**Table 1**

Features of Fibrodysplasia Ossificans Progressiva

| Feature | Percentage |
|---|---|
| Abnormal hallux | 100 |
|    Type I (one phalanx) | 79 |
|    Type II (two phalanges with progressive bone fusion) | 9 |
|    Type III (two phalanges with osteophytic lipping) | 6 |
|    Type IV (variable reduction defects) | 6 |
| Short thumbs secondary to short first metacarpals | 59 |
| Clinodactyly, fifth finger | 44 |
| Short broad femoral necks | 55 |
| Ectopic calcification, site of onset | |
|    Neck | 38 |
|    Paraspinal region | 32 |
|    Head | 9 |
|    Limbs | 12 |
| Joint involvement | |
|    Spine | 100 |
|    Shoulder | 100 |
|    Elbow | 55 |
|    Wrist | 7 |
|    Hip | 59 |
|    Knee | 38 |
|    Ankle | 32 |
|    Temporomandibular | 71 |
| Deafness* | 24 |
| Diffuse thinning of hair** | 24 |
| Mental deficiency | 6 |

\* 63% of these were conductive
\*\* 75% of these were female
Adapted from data in Connor and Evans, 1982.

reduction defects are observed in Type IV. Other skeletal abnormalities include short thumbs due to short first metacarpals; clinodactyly of the fifth fingers; short broad femoral necks; abnormal cervical vertebrae with small bodies, large pedicles, and large spinous processes; progressive bony ankylosis of the cervical spine; and, occasionally, exostoses of the proximal tibiae (Connor and Evans, 1982b; McKusick, 1972; Rogers and Geho, 1979). The radiographic spectrum of abnormalities has been reviewed elsewhere (Cremin et al., 1982; Thickman et al., 1982).

Ectopic ossification is progressive and begins in early childhood. The site of onset is most commonly the neck or paraspinal region (Fig. 2A) and less commonly the head or limbs. When new lumps appear, reddening of the overlying skin may occur and may sometimes be associated with pain and tenderness. Certain areas within the connective tissues are especially prone to ossification, particularly the paraspinal muscles, limb girdle muscles, and the muscles of mastication. Involvement of joint capsules, ligaments, and plantar fasciae is common. In FOP patients, various factors are known to precipitate ectopic ossification such as muscle trauma, biopsy, surgical procedures to excise ectopic bone (Fig. 2B), intramuscular injections, careless venepuncture, and dental treatment (Connor and Evans, 1982b; McKusick, 1972; Rogers and Geho, 1979). All patients eventually develop restriction of movement and physical handicap. Episodes of ossification and subsequent disability are characteristically erratic and there are long periods of quiescence. Although ectopic ossification is most marked prior to puberty, new lumps may occur into the sixth and seventh decades. Ectopic calcification has the most severe effect on axial connective tissues, and limb involvement is most marked proximally (Fig. 3) (Connor and Evans, 1982b). Chest wall fixation may lead to diminished pulmonary reserve, and most patients eventually die from respiratory failure (Connor and Evans, 1981).

Other abnormalities such as deafness and baldness occur in approximately one quarter of all patients. Deafness may be conductive or sensorineural. The diffuse type of baldness, when present, becomes evident in middle age and the majority of affected individuals are female. It appears to be a primary feature of FOP, although it might conceivably represent a secondary effect of nutritional deficiency based on the inability to open the jaws. Mental deficiency is only found as a low frequency abnormality (Connor and Evans, 1982b; McKusick, 1972).

## Other Similar Conditions

A number of entities have similarities to FOP. Metaplastic bone formation in various organs and tissues may occur in association with inflammatory, neoplastic, and vascular disorders. It may be found in the deep soft tissues of paraplegic patients beneath the level of the spinal cord lesion. Metaplastic bone formation in the skin and subcutaneous tissue is known to occur with pilomatrixoma, a benign tumor (Kewalramani, 1977).

Myositis ossificans has histologic similarities to FOP. However, soft tissue lesions are solitary, grow rapidly, and are usually located in a limb. A previous history of trauma is often present (Ackerman, 1958).

Extraskeletally occurring osteosarcoma is rare [see below]. Although it resembles both FOP and myositis ossificans, most cases occur in adults and consist of large solitary masses in the extremities (Allan and Soule, 1971). FOP lesions are small and multinodular in character; extraskeletal osteo-

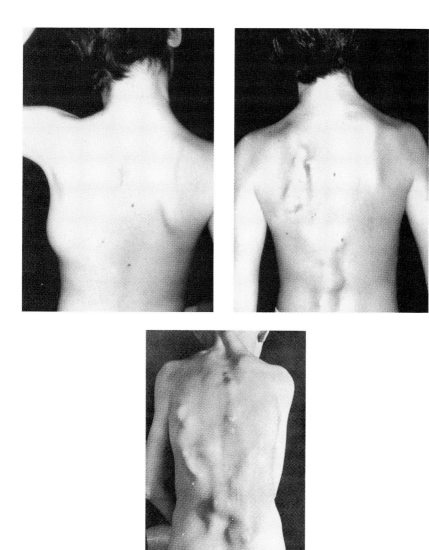

**Fig. 2**   Fibrodysplasia Ossificans Progressiva
A) Subscapular mass of ectopic bone in an 8 year old male.
B) Post-surgical recurrence in the same individual with abundant new bone formation. Note also the new lesions in the lumbar portion of the paraspinal muscles.
C) Advanced calcification in an older individual with muscle wasting and suggesting of posture due to fixation of joint angles. [Photo courtesy of Prof. P. E. Becker, Göttingen, Germany]

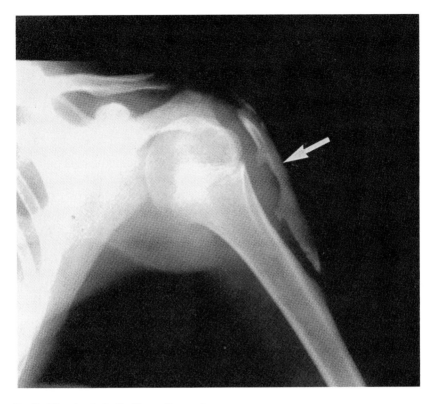

**Fig. 3**  Fibrodysplasia Ossificans Progressiva
Radiograph of shoulder showing calcification of the deltoid muscle and fascia (arrow) with normal skeletal modeling and mineral density.

sarcoma tends to occur as a large single tumor mass. Both myositis ossificans and extraosseous osteosarcoma resemble FOP in having the capacity to express fibrous, chondroid, and osseous tissue patterns. However, lesions of extraskeletal osteosarcoma are more cellular, have more atypia and more frequent mitoses, and produce malignant osteoid; these features are not present in FOP (Stout and Lattes, 1967; Allan and Soule, 1971).

Pathogenesis

FOP is a distinctive histopathologic entity which can be differentiated from other soft tissue ossifying lesions which ossify such as myositis ossificans, extraosseous osteosarcoma, and osseous metaplasia. Early FOP is characterized by multifocal, interconnecting nodules of spindle-shaped, fibroblastlike cells in a distinctive connective tissue matrix with bone spicules occupying the central area (Fig. 4). Foci of chondroid differentiation may sometimes be observed. Lesions evolve to become mature lamellar bone with adipose and hematopoietic tissue in the cancellous spaces; the rim of fibroblast-like cells is no longer evident. Such pathologic features suggest that the spindle-shaped cells, like periosteum, are precursors of the osseous tissue found in FOP lesions (Cramer et al., 1981).

Recent attempts to understand pathogenesis have viewed FOP lesions as a reaction to dystrophic calcification (Smith, 1975; Smith et al., 1966; Lutwak, 1964; Ruderman et al., 1979). Metaplastic bone formation has been observed with various lesions of the skin and subcutaneous tissue that are known to be associated with concurrent dystrophic calcifications (Roth, 1963). Studies of periosteal grafts also support the notion that aberrant periosteal differentiation may be the fundamental disturbance in FOP. Transplanted periosteum initially produces woven bone and later produces mature lamellar bone with adipose and hematopoietic marrow elements (Uddstromer and Ritsila, 1978; Skoog, 1967); poorly vascularized and non-immobilized periosteal grafts can make cartilage. Thus, ectopically placed periosteum can produce the full range of histologic patterns observed in FOP.

Evidence to date strongly suggests that the disturbance is not systemic, but multifocal. Clinical studies indicate that lesions tend to be located near flat bones, which are formed primarily by membranous ossification, and that the abdominal wall, perineum, and internal viscera are never involved. Biochemical studies have shown normal calcium and phosphate balance, normal levels of parathyroid hormone, normal tubular handling of phosphate, and normal responsiveness to parathyroid hormone stimulation (Connor and Beighton, 1982; Pitt and Hamilton, 1984). Bone scans typically show multiple foci of activity (Fig. 5). High levels of alkaline phosphatase have been demonstrated in surrounding connective tissue (Dixon et al., 1954). Conflicting results have been obtained by other investigators (Herrman et al., 1969; Beratis et al., 1976; Miller et al., 1977), but these studies considered only single patients using a spectrophotometric assay. Connor and Evans (1981) studied skin fibroblasts from 6 FOP patients and 27 normal controls in vitro using a more sensitive fluorometric assay system and found no abnormalities of alkaline phosphatase.

Associated hypoplasia of normally located osseous structures, such as the hallucal anomalies, is consistent with a reduction in a precursor cell pool derived from apparent migration; shape and location are maintained by the end-product, but size is reduced. Ultrastructural and histochemical studies also support the idea that fibroblast-like cells show evidence of osteogenic

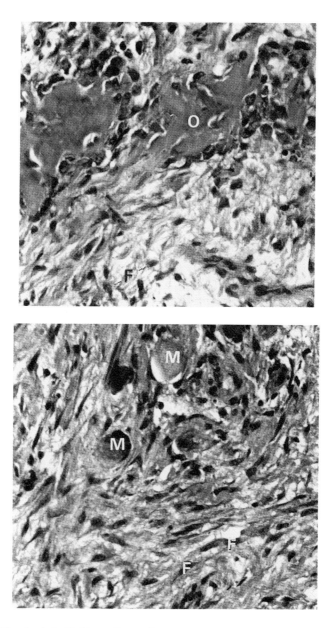

**Fig. 4**  Fibrodysplasia Ossificans Progressiva
A) Connective tissue with plump cellular fibroblasts (F), with area of osteoid (O) surrounded by osteoblasts.
B) Plump fibroblasts (F) infiltrating between muscle cells (M).

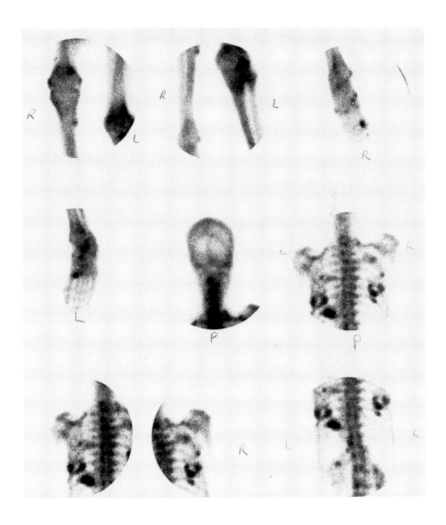

**Fig. 5** Fibrodysplasia Ossificans Progressiva
Series of radionuclide bone scans showing multiple foci of increased uptake (darker areas) over the knees (upper left and middle), spine (upper right), left foot (middle left), and the chest (middle right and lower 3 views). The patient's right (R) and left (L) are also indicated.

differentiation in FOP (Maxwell *et al.*, 1977). These mesenchymal cells are not all biologically the same and their differentiation is modified by perturbations in the cellular environment (Caplan and Pechak, 1987; see chapters 2 and 8 in this volume). The fact that fibroblast activity can be modulated pharmacologically (Reddi, 1985) may be exploited some day to develop rational therapy for FOP patients. The key to understanding the pathogenesis of FOP may lie in the elucidation of which genes control osteogenic transformation of mesenchymal cells in normal and diseased tissues.

## Hypophosphatasia

### The Biology of Alkaline Phosphatase

Alkaline phosphatase denotes a group of isoenzymes [orthophosphoric-monoester phosphohydrolases (alkaline optimum), EC 3.1.3.1.] characterized by optimal hydrolytic activity toward artificial phosphomonoesters at alkaline pH (Moss, 1982; McComb *et al.*, 1979, Whyte, 1989b). *In vitro* measurements of enzyme activity have been a part of clinical laboratory medicine for decades, but there is still considerable uncertainty about the precise composition of these proteins. Studies in different organisms and molecular sequencing of the structural genes has recently led to a better understanding of its structure and function.

### Bacteria and Yeast

Alkaline phosphatase is widely distributed among prokaryotic and eukaryotic organisms. The protein from *E. coli* has been sequenced (Bradshaw *et al.*, 1981) and the crystal structure has been mapped to sufficient resolution to establish the 3-dimensional structure (Fig. 6) (Wyckoff *et al.*, 1983; Sowadski *et al.*, 1985). Specified by a single gene called PhoA, (Chang *et al.*, 1986), a peptide of 47 kDa molecular weight is secreted into the periplasmic space of the bacterial envelope where it undergoes proteolytic cleavage and self-associates to form an enzymatically active dimer (Ishino *et al.*, 1987). In the process, the peptide acquires 2 zinc ions that are coordinately bound and participate in enzyme catalysis. In the third site, zinc or magnesium may be present (Coleman and Gettins, 1983)

In yeast (*Saccharomyces cerevisiae*), the PHO8 gene specifies an alkaline phosphatase containing considerable sequence identity with both the *E. coli* and human enzymes (Kaneko *et al.*, 1987). The most highly conserved regions are those surrounding the active sites for substrate and metal ligand binding. The N-terminus sequence is rich in basic and hydroxyl-containing

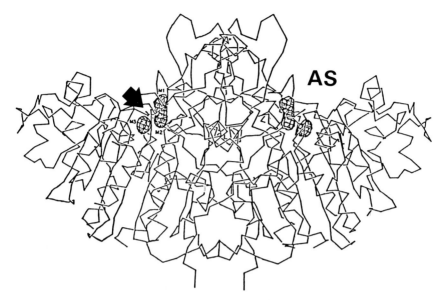

**Fig. 6** Alkaline phosphatase—preliminary 3 dimensional structure
Shown here is a trace of the carbon skeleton for the *E. coli* dimer with three metal-binding sites [M1, M2, M3 (arrow)] for each monomer. The active site (AS) of the enzyme can be distinguished as a pocket adjacent to the metal complex. [Reproduced with permission from Wyckoff 1983.]

amino acids and serves as a signal for translocation to intracellular vacuoles, where the active enzyme has been localized. The functional yeast enzyme is a dimer that undergoes N-glycosylation at specific asparagine residues (Kaneko *et al.*, 1987), a feature that appears to be common to all eukaryotic alkaline phosphatases. Yeast is a versatile tool for genetic analysis and it is likely to provide valuable insight into eukaryotic regulation of alkaline phosphatase gene expression.

*Human Isoenzymes and Isoforms*

In humans there are 3 major isoenzymes (Sargeant and Stinson, 1979; Moss, 1986; Stigbrand, 1984), (Table 2). One is associated with the intestine (IAP), another with the placenta (PLAP), and the third with different tissue-specific isoforms, including ones for bone, liver, and kidney (and now called the tissue non-specific alkaline phosphatase, TNSALP). Current biochemical evidence suggests that the IAP isoenzyme arose through duplication and divergence from an ancestral gene most closely related to TNSALP (Yora and Sakagishi, 1986; Komoda *et al.*, 1986). In primates,

**Table 2**

Alkaline Phosphatase:
Properties of Human Isoenzymes[1]

| Isozyme Type | Tissue Nonspecific (TNSALP) | Intestinal (IAP) | Placental (PLAP) |
|---|---|---|---|
| pH optimum | 10.1−10.2 | 10.1−10.2 | 10.7 |
| Heat Stability | | | |
| 56 C 15 min. | +/++ | ++ | +++ |
| 65 C 5 min. | − | − | +++ |
| Aminoacid Sensitivity | | | |
| L-phenylalanine (5−10mM) | ± | +++ | +++ |
| L-homoarginine (5−10mM) | +++ | ± | ± |
| Electrophoretic Migration | fast | slow | intermediate |
| Neuraminidase Sensitivity | + | − | + |
| Immunoreactive with antisera to: | | | |
| TNSALP | +++ | − | − |
| IAP | − | +++ | + |
| PLAP | − | + | +++ |
| Lectin binding | + | − | +++ |

[1] Adapted from Stigbrand (1984)

PLAP isoenzymes have arisen by a further duplication and divergence (Fig. 7), and there are likely other loci and multiple isoforms in this gene family (Henthorn *et al.*, 1987; Knoll, 1987).

The human placental isoenzyme [PLAP; MIM#17180][1] was the first eukaryotic form to be sequenced by analysis of proteolytic fragments. The amino acid sequence was subsequently confirmed by examining the nucleotide sequences for cloned cDNA (Kam, 1985; Millan, 1986; Henthorn *et al.*, 1986). The PLAP gene is also the only form with significant polymorphisms (Harris, 1983). Of the 3 common placental alleles, two (ALPp1 and ALPp3) differ at 13 sites and 7 of these result in an altered amino acid sequence. The origin of this diversity is not clear (Henthorn *et al.*, 1986), but study of

[1] Catalog numbers from *Mendelian Inheritance in Man* (MIM) by McKusick (1988).

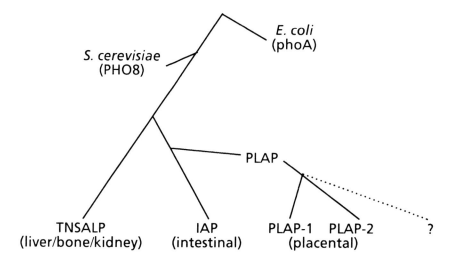

## HUMAN GENE FAMILY

**Fig. 7**  Alkaline phosphatase — phylogenetic tree
Postulated relationships between various alkaline phosphatase. Neither the length nor direction of the lines are quantitative, and there may be other related genes in the human family that are yet to be characterized.

similar allelism at the 21-hydroxylase locus (Higashi *et al.*, 1988) suggests that gene conversion is a likely mechanism. There is also recent evidence for a second placental gene (PLAP-2) that may not be expressed to any extent in term placenta, but is found in testis and thymus and occasionally in sera from patients with various neoplastic diseases (Knoll, 1987). This enzyme may be related to the so-called "PLAP-like" isoenzyme that has been the subject of several recent clinical reviews (Stigbrand, 1984; Moss, 1986). A similar isoenzyme has also been detected in human milk (Chuang, 1987).

The genes for human PLAP and IAP (MIM#17174) have been mapped to chromosome 2 using somatic cell hybridization techniques and chromosomal exclusion analysis. *In situ* hybridization with labelled probes generated from cloned cDNA show specific hybridization with the q34−q37 region of chromosome 2 (Griffin *et al.*, 1987). Since the divergence of placental and intestinal genes is likely a recent evolutionary event, it is not surprising that they should both be found close together in the human genome (Berger *et al.*, 1987; Millán, 1987; Henthorn *et al.*, 1986; Henthorn *et al.*, 1987).

Expression of different IAP proteins during development has been de-

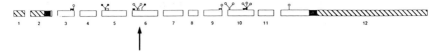

**Fig. 8**   Human alkaline phosphatase—gene structure
Schematic showing the 12 transcribed exons (rectangles) and untranslated regions (diagonal
stripes). The hydrophobic sequences for the signal peptide (exon 2) and the anchor-recognition
peptide (exon 12) are shown in black. Regions coding for the active site that are conserved
from *E. coli* are shown as small closed (β-sheets) or open (α-helices) rectangles above the
exons. Specifically conserved residues acting as metal ligands (white circles) and substrate
ligands (closed circles) are also shown. The site of the point mutation responsible for one form
of hypophosphatasia is indicated with an arrow. [Reproduced with permission from Weiss
*et al.* (1989b)]

scribed by several investigators (Mulivor, 1978; Miura, 1987; Besman and
Coleman, 1985) and the possibility of more than one locus for IAP has been
raised (Mueller *et al.*, 1985; Moss and Whitaker, 1987; Henthorn *et al.*,
1987).

The human TNSALP isoenzyme (MIM#17176) has been mapped to the
p36.1−p34 region of chromosome 1 by *in situ* studies (Smith *et al.*, 1988). It
is linked to the locus for the Rh blood group (Smith *et al.*, 1988; Greenberg
*et al.*, 1988) and is associated with several useful restriction fragment length
polymorphisms (RFLPs) (Ray *et al.*, 1988; Weiss *et al.*, 1987; Greenberg *et
al.*, 1988). Weiss and colleagues (1986) have cloned and sequenced the
cDNA for TNSALP alkaline phosphatase. When aligned, this sequence
shows significant positional identity with IAP and PLAP sequences but also
shares identity with *E. coli* and *S. cerevisiae* that it does not with the other
isoenzymes. Reports of the corresponding sequence in rats (Thiede *et al.*,
1988; Misumi *et al.*, 1988) indicate about 90% identity with the human
sequence, most of the differences being restricted to two small regions in the
carboxyterminal portion of the molecule. Subsequent analysis of genomic
DNA (Fig. 8) confirms that there is significant conservation of catalytically
important domains (Weiss *et al.*, 1988a). There appears to be only a single
copy of the TNSALP gene but the complexity of the non-translated regions
suggests considerable flexibility for regulating transcription.

*Properties of the Protein*

*Polypeptide Subunits*   In their native state, mammalian alkaline phosphatases probably exist as membrane-bound tetramers with subunits of 68
to 100 kD molecular weight (Coleman and Gettins, 1983; Sussman, 1984;

Hawrylak and Stinson, 1987). These values are greater than predicted from the primary sequence and more variable in size because of different post-translational modification.

The enzyme complex has an absolute requirement for zinc but displays optimal catalytic activity with addition of magnesium as well. Although several reports suggest a 2-to-1 ratio between metal site and peptide subunit, the stoichiometry for the assembled enzyme may vary from molecule to molecule (Coleman and Gettins, 1983).

In the amino terminal half of the polypeptide in humans, there are at least two asparagine residues available for N-glycosidic attachment of oligosaccharide side chains (Weiss et al., 1986). There is no agreement as yet on the precise composition of these side chains in the tissue-nonspecific form (TNSALP), but the structural studies of the placental isoenzyme indicate only a single, complex-type biantennary structure (Endo et al., 1988). The terminal sialic acid residues vary in number and contribute to the significant microheterogeneity of enzyme molecular weights and net charge under standard electrophoretic conditions (Moss, 1986; Gonchoroff and O'Brien, 1988). Removal of the terminal sialic acid residues does not result in complete homogeneity nor does removal of the remaining oligosaccharide side chain by endoglycosidases, and small differences in catalytic activity and sensitivity may remain. Other post-translational modifications may therefore be essential to the expression of the tissue-specific product (McComb et al., 1979).

*Membrane Association*  Isolation of membranes and other sub-cellular fractionation procedures suggest that most alkaline phosphatase activity is found in the plasma membrane and other studies indicate that it is an "ectoenzyme" expressed only on the outside surface of the cell (Whyte, 1989a). The release of alkaline phosphatase from the cell surface by phosphatidylinositol-specific phospholipase D (Davitz et al., 1987; Low and Prasad, 1988) is further evidence that this ectoenzyme is linked to the membrane by a novel covalent linkage between peptide and inositol phospholipid (Jemmerson and Low, 1987; Howard et al., 1987; Low, 1987; Low et al., 1986, Low and Saltiel, 1988) (Fig. 9). This configuration confers high lateral mobility on the membrane-bound enzyme (Noda et al., 1987) and probably contributes to stabilization of the tetrameric configuration (Hawrylak and Stinson, 1987; Takami et al., 1988). Because of the significant role of phosphatidylinositol in intracellular signalling pathways, this membrane attachment and release phenomenon may be associated with important regulatory functions of the cell in response to perturbations of cell homeostasis (Low et al., 1987; Sorimachi and Yasumura, 1988; Romero et al., 1988).

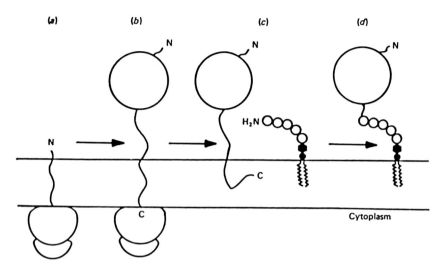

**Fig. 9** Alkaline phosphatase — membrane anchoring
Schematic of synthesis and attachment of alkaline phosphatase to the plasma membrane. Membrane bound ribosomes translocate nascent peptide to the lumen of the endoplasmic reticlum (a). After termination of synthesis (b), the C-termainal hydrophobic sequence is transiently anchored in the membrane (c). The transfer to a phosphoglycolipid precursor requires cleavage of a peptide bond [Asp-484 in human placental alkline phosphatase (Micanovic et al., 1988)] and formation of a new amide bond with the anchor (d). The mature protein is then translocated to the cell surface via conventional mechanisms. [Reproduced with permission from Low 1987].

*Catalytic Reaction*   Kinetically, alkaline phosphatase can be classified as a serine-dependent phosphohydrolase enzyme (McComb et al., 1979; Coleman and Gettins, 1983). This is a relatively common and probably very ancient enzymatic motif involving transfer of phosphate to a key serine hydroxyl group as an intermediate in the catalytic cascade. The serine phosphate then undergoes hydrolysis, releasing free phosphate after the parent alcohol has dissociated (Fig. 10). The reaction itself is markedly pH dependent as the name of the enzyme suggests. At artificially high pH (alkaline optimum), reaction is rapid and the rate limiting step is the release of phosphate from the enzyme; therefore, enzyme activity under these conditions is essentially independent of the nature of the substrate compound (Cocivera et al., 1980; Hall and Williams, 1986). The enzyme is readily assayed with synthetic substrates (e.g. p-nitrophenyl phosphate) at pH 10. At physiologically neutral pH, however, the rate limiting reaction step is the release of the

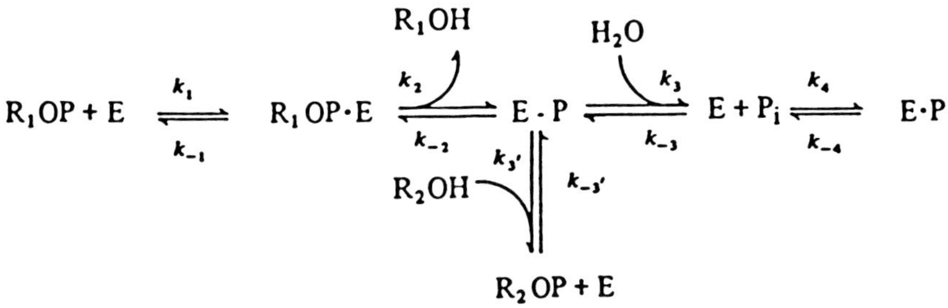

$$R_1OP + E \underset{k_{-1}}{\overset{k_1}{\rightleftharpoons}} R_1OP{\cdot}E \underset{k_{-2}}{\overset{k_2}{\rightleftharpoons}} E{\cdot}P \underset{k_{-3}}{\overset{k_3}{\rightleftharpoons}} E + P_i \underset{k_{-4}}{\overset{k_4}{\rightleftharpoons}} E{\cdot}P$$

with $R_1OH$ above the second equilibrium, $H_2O$ above the third, and the branch from $E{\cdot}P$ via $k_3'$ / $k_{-3}'$ and $R_2OH$ via $k_5'$ / $k_{-5'}$ leading to $R_2OP + E$.

**Fig. 10**   Alkaline phosphatase — reaction sequence
The usual reaction sequence involves: (i) adsorption of substrate ($R_1OP$) to the enzyme (E); (ii) transfer of the phosphate group to the enzyme to form a phosphoenzyme intermediate (E-P) and dissociation of the dephosphorylated product ($R_1OH$); and (iii) hydrolysis of the phosphoenzyme to release inorganic phosphate ($E + P_i$). The association of enzyme with free phosphate ($P_i$) and the phosphotransferase reaction involving a second substrate ($R_2OH$) are additional competing reactions, explaining the inhibition of the forward reaction by phosphate and other phosphate receptors [Reproduced with permission from Coleman and Gettins 1983]

dephosphorylated compound, which is consistent with the limited repertoire of natural substrates for this enzyme (Coleman and Gettins, 1983; Cocivera et al., 1980; Whyte, 1989b).

If an alcohol group is present in high concentration, alkaline phosphatases may catalyze a phosphate transfer from a phosphoester co-substrate. With human serum enzyme, this tranferase activity is apparently highly dependent on saturating concentrations of zinc ion (Stinson et al., 1987a) but the physiological significance of this alternate reaction is uncertain.

*Physiological Substrates*   At alkaline pH, alkaline phosphatase will hydrolyze most primary alcohol esters. Pyrophosphate, nucleotide di- and triphosphates, and phosphocreatine are also cleaved, although other enzymes with higher turnover and narrower specificity are thought to be more physiologically relevant (Whyte, 1989b; Caswell et al., 1986). Less is known about the action of alkaline phosphatase on phosphorylated macromolecules. Phosphotyrosine residues of nuclear histones are cleaved by the enzyme *in vitro* but a physiological role has not been defined. Intracellular phosphotyrosine residues generated by protein kinases appear to be hydrolyzed by a separate series of intracellular phosphatases, but alkaline phosphatase may also be active where it has access to substrate (Whyte, 1988; Whyte, 1989b; Sumikawa et al., 1987; Takahashi et al., 1987).

**Table 3**

---

Alkaline Phosphatase: Enzyme substrates

---

*Physiological*
  * phosphoethanolamine
  * pyridoxal-5'-phosphate
  * inorganic pyrophosphate
  * phosphatidic acid (Sumikawa *et al.*, 1987)[1]
  * phosphotyrosine, ?phosphoserine (Takahashi *et al.*, 1987)[1]
  * β-glycerophosphate[1]

*In vitro*
  * p-nitrophenyl phosphate (spectrophotometric)
  * 4-methylumbelliferyl phosphate (fluorometric)

---

[1] The precise role of alkaline phosphastase in the metabolism of these compound has not yet been clarified.

## Bone-derived Alkaline Phosphatase

The tissue non-specific alkaline phosphatase is readily distinguished from the other isoenzymes by its electrophoretic mobility, its sensitivity to inhibition by homoarginine but not phenylalanine or phenylalaninylglycyl-glycine, and its sensitivity to heat denaturation (Table 2). It has also been identified in leukocytes (Gainer *et al.*, 1982; Stinson *et al.*, 1985; Smith *et al.*, 1985). The liver and bone isoforms are distinguished electrophoretically and enzymatically. The bone isoform has an apparent isoelectric point (pI) of 4.21 (Griffiths and Black, 1987) which is higher than the liver isoform but lower than that for kidney, giving it intermediate mobility on electro-phoresis (Moss, 1982). Much of the residual charge heterogeneity of the bone isoform can be abolished by treatment with neuraminidase, suggesting a variable number of terminal sialic acid residues *in situ*. The bone isoform is also more sensitive to inhibition by denaturing agents, such as urea and guanidine hydrochloride (Shephard and Peake, 1986) and to inactivation by heat. It is also differentially bound by wheat germ lectin, presumably by virtue of the oligosaccharide composition. Characterization of these isoforms is reviewed elsewhere (Moss, 1986; Posen and Doherty, 1981; Griffiths and Black, 1987).

Bone alkaline phosphatase is constitutively expressed in the osteoblast and has been localized to the plasma membrane by a variety of histological techniques; see chapter 3. It is also present in matrix vesicles (Anderson, 1985), lending support to the concept that the vesicles are derived from the plasma membranes of mineralizing cell types (Rodan and Rodan, 1984).

**Table 4**

Alkaline Phosphatase: Postulated physiological functions[1]

1) Local Increase In Inorganic Phosphate Levels (Organophosphatase)
2) Destruction Of Inhibitors Of Hydroxyapatite Crystal Growth (Pyrophosphatase)
3) Phosphate Transport
4) $Ca^{++}$-Binding Protein
5) $Ca^{++}/Mg^{++}$ ATPase
6) Tyrosine-Specific Phosphoprotein Phosphatase

[1] Adapted from Whyte (1989b)

Synthesis and expression of the enzyme at the osteoblast cell surface is closely regulated and, if the phenomenon of autorelease (Sorimachi and Yasumura, 1988) also occurs in osteoblasts, would account for the predominance of the osseous fraction of TNSALP in the circulation.

Ever since alkaline phosphatase enzyme was first identified in calcifying mammalian cartilage, it has been considered to be important for bone mineralization (Bourne, 1973; Whyte, 1989a). However, the hypophosphatasia mutation remains the most compelling evidence for its essential role in skeletal metabolism (Whyte, 1989b; Ornoy et al., 1985). Histological evidence is supportive but biochemical studies, particularly those that examine the effects of enzyme inhibitors, have failed to identify unequivocally the mechanism by which the enzyme participates in mineralization. Among the proposed actions, pyrophosphatase activity appears to have the most physiological support, but its calcium-binding properties have received increasing attention lately (Register et al., 1986; de Bernard, 1986; McLean et al., 1987) (Table 4). [These hypotheses are discussed more fully in Chapter 3, this volume.] It has also been suggested that alkaline phosphatase may be essential for normal cell proliferation (Hösli and Vogt, 1979), but fibroblasts from individuals lacking the enzyme have normal morphology and growth characteristics (Whyte and Vrabel, 1987).

*Serum Isoenzymes and Isoforms*    Circulating alkaline phosphatase activity is almost entirely comprised of TNSALP isoforms, although PLAP isoenzyme is found in large amounts in pregnant women and some IAP may appear subsequent to a large meal. Fractionation by isoelectric focussing reveals at least 12 proteins of different isoelectric points and confirms that bone and liver isoforms account for most of the circulating activity (Griffiths and Black, 1987). During childhood and adolescence, total serum activity is a function of age, which is in large part reflective of the bone-derived isoform (Moss et al., 1982; Stepán et al., 1985; Schiele et al., 1983). Thus, total alkaline phosphatase is often used as a rough clinical index of skeletal activity, but direct measurement of the bone-derived isoform in serum is somewhat more sensitive (Farley *et al.*, 1986; Farley *et al.*, 1981). The clinical enzymology of serum alkaline phosphatases has been extensively reviewed elsewhere (Moss, 1986; Posen and Doherty, 1981).

**Hypophosphatasia**

Introduction

Hypophosphatasia is an inherited disorder of bone mineralization characterized by: (a) rachitic changes in childhood or osteomalacia in adult life; (b) absence of dental cementum and premature loss of teeth; and (c) decreased alkaline phosphatase enzyme activity. Hypophosphatasia was first identified as a separate entity by Rathbun in 1948, although there are earlier case reports (see Rasmussen, 1983). A wide range of presentations are described but all patients have some deficit in serum and tissue alkaline phosphatase activity. From a clinical perspective, most individuals can be classified as having either the neonatal, and infantile or childhood varieties (MIM #24150 and #24151), or the adult form (MIM #14630) of the disorder (Currarino, 1973; Fallon *et al.*, 1984; Kozlowski *et al.*, 1976; Rasmussen, 1983; Whyte, 1989b). Scriver and Cameron (1969) described a patient with clinical features of the childhood disorder but with normal serum alkaline phosphatase activity and designated this variant pseudohypophosphatasia.

Genetics

The birth prevalance of hypophosphatasia has been estimated to be 1/100,000 (Fraser, 1957) but this represents incomplete ascertainment because asymptomatic adults and milder forms of the disorder are excluded.

Both recessive and dominant modes of inheritance have been observed in different hypophosphatasia kindreds (Pimstone *et al.*, 1966; Rasmussen, 1983; Whyte *et al.*, 1982). The frequency of consanguinity and the recurrence rates for infantile hypophosphatasia are clearly indicative of a recessive mode (Pimstone *et al.*, 1966). The suggestion that hypophosphatasia is an autosomal dominant condition with homozygous lethality is in keeping with the data on the adult form of the disorder (Eastman and Bixler, 1983; Eastman and Bixler, 1982; Whyte *et al.*, 1982) but there is further heterogeneity (Fallon *et al.*, 1984) and there are examples of more than one presentation (e.g., infantile and adult or infantile and childhood) in the same sibship

(Weinstein and Whyte, 1981; Eastman and Bixler, 1982). Allelic diversity, compound heterozygosity, or the involvement of more than a single locus are possible explanations.

## Clinical Features

### Neonatal

In the neonatal form of hypophosphatasia, markedly impaired mineralization occurs *in utero*. The extremities are shortened, the long bones are deformed, and the cranial vault fails to mineralize. Polyhydramnios has been observed more frequently in hypophosphatasia pregnancies and premature stillbirths are not uncommon (Mulivor *et al.*, 1978; Rasmussen, 1983; Wolff *et al.*, 1982). Radiographs show small, sclerotic bones at the base of the skull and a membranous calvaria. The ribs are small, thin, and deformed. Sclerotic patches and spurs are also observed in the ribs and other tubular bones. In live births, the outcome depends on the extent of pulmonary and neurological compromise but demise often occurs within a few days (Currarino, 1973; Jelke, 1960; Kozlowski *et al.*, 1976; Mulivor *et al.*, 1978; Rasmussen, 1983; Teree *et al.*, 1968; Wolff *et al.*, 1982).

### Infantile

Such individuals commonly present some time after birth because of failure to thrive (Fallon, 1984; Pimstone *et al.*, 1966; Rasmussen, 1983). Apparently difficult to recognize in early radiographs, most affected newborns do well for a short period and then experience a wide variety of problems related to impaired bone growth. Hypercalcemia may be marked, explaining a history of irritability, poor feeding, anorexia, vomiting, hypotonia, polydipsia, polyuria, dehydration, and constipation. Changes in parathormone or vitamin D metabolism are apparently not contributing factors although increased immunoreactive PTH has been observed (Whyte and Seino, 1982; Maesaka *et al.*, 1988; Opshaug, *et al.*, 1982). Episodes of unexplained fever, tender bones, and respiratory distress are also described. Renal function may be impaired by hypercalciuria and traumatic fractures are frequently found (Fallon *et al.*, 1984; Jelke, 1960; Kozlowski *et al.*, 1976; Rasmussen, 1983; Teree and Klein 1968).

The anterior fontanel is often enlarged and may bulge. The membranous cranial sutures are also frequently widened and some degree of ocular prominence due to shallow orbits may be apparent within the first few months of life. The head circumference also increases more slowly than expected as premature sutural fusion sets in. Radiographs show widespread demineralization and rachitic changes in the metaphyses, but usually with less diaphyseal bowing than would be expected with severe metaphyseal disease (Fig. 11A) (Currarino, 1973; Kozlowski et al., 1976). In infants who survive, there is often spontaneous improvement in mineralization and remission of clinical problems (Pimstone et al., 1966; Whyte et al., 1986; Scriver and Cameron, 1969), except craniostenosis. While the sutures appear widened and membranous, intense osteoblastic activity may be detectable by nuclear scintigraphy (Sty et al., 1979). Moderate short stature in adulthood and premature loss of deciduous teeth (Figure 11B) are also common but the long-term outlook is otherwise good.

## Childhood

Childhood hypophosphatasia is a milder condition that often presents as "rickets" in the second and third year of life (Bruckner et al., 1969; Kozlowski et al., 1976). Signs of intracranial hypertension or failure to thrive are typical (Fallon et al., 1984; Kozlowski et al., 1976; Rasmussen, 1983). Some long bone deformity is not unusual but tends to improve with time. The most serious treatment complication in this group is also craniosynostosis. All sutures appear to be involved but ocular prominence due to shallow orbits can be quite characteristic. Other ocular signs include blue sclerae and keratopathy or conjunctival calcification due to hypercalcemia (Brenner et al., 1969; Fraser, 1957). Spontaneous remission of bone disease is not uncommon (Whyte et al., 1986). In at least one case, this has been accompanied by an increase in serum alkaline phosphatase activity (Wolff et al., 1982).

## Adult

The adult form is mild but osteomalacia may be associated with symptomatic pseudofractures, marked bone pain, and increased susceptibility to traumatic fracture (Bruckner et al., 1962; Coe et al., 1986; Pimstone et al., 1966; Rasmussen, 1983). The proximal femur is a frequent site of pseudofractures that extend to complete transverse fractures and loss of mobility (Fig. 12). In this group, a bone scan can be helpful in identifying and clarifying the sources of pain. There is also a predilection for chondrocalcinosis and marked osteoarthropathy later in life (Whyte et al., 1982a).

## Histopathology

In the infant, bone histomorphometry reveals a marked excess of osteoid volume and an osteomalacic pattern of tetracycline labelling in dynamic

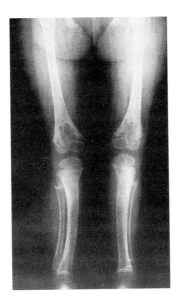

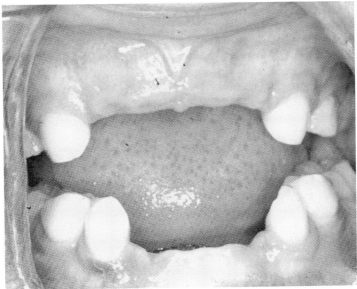

**Fig. 11**  Childhood Hypophosphatasia
A) Radiographs showing osteolytic changes, with marked metaphyseal notching at the ends of the long bones. Bowing and demineralization are also evident (Courtesy of R. J. Gorlin, Minneapolis, MN). B) Early loss of deciduous teeth resulting from lack of cementum (Courtesy of R. J. Gorlin, Minneapolis, MN).

studies (Fallon *et al.*, 1984). Bone alkaline phosphatase is usually undetectable and electron microscopy shows otherwise normal subcellular architecture of osteoblasts and their associated matrix vesicles (Fallon *et al.*, 1984; Ornoy *et al.*, 1985). Iliac crest biopsies in adults show less dramatic and more variable changes (Fig. 13). The severity of the osteomalacia, as measured by relative osteoid volume, is inversely correlated with the amount of detectable alkaline phosphatase and with the concentrations of serum alkaline phosphatase activity. In shed teeth, marked deficiency or absence of cementum is a striking characteristic, accounting for the ready loss of teeth (Beumer *et al.*, 1973; Bruckner *et al.*, 1962; Pimstone *et al.*, 1966; Rasmussen, 1983). This appears to be the result of aplasia, since resorption of cementum has never been observed. Dentin formation is delayed and less appears to be formed. Interglobulin dentin and osteodentin have also been observed (Breumer *et al.*, 1973; Bruckner *et al.*, 1962; Pimstone *et al.*, 1966).

Delayed dentition, premature loss of deciduous teeth, and spontaneous loss of permanent teeth are distinctive characteristics of hypophosphatasia (Fig. 11B). They may be the only clinical signs of disease, giving rise to the term odontohypophosphatasia for this variant condition (Pimstone *et al.*, 1966). The anterior deciduous teeth are more likely to be affected and the most frequent loss involves the incisors (Beumer *et al.*, 1973; Brucker *et al.*, 1962). The process is that of relatively painless extrusion and does not invoke periodontal inflammation (Beumer *et al.*, 1973). Dental X-rays show reduced alveolar bone, enlarged pulp chambers and root canals, but normal enamel (Beumer *et al.*, 1973; Bruckner *et al.*, 1969; Pimstone *et al.*, 1966).

## Biochemical Phenotype

### Diagnostic Indices

In the classical forms of hypophosphatasia, total serum alkaline phosphatase activity is markedly reduced. This does not appear to be the result of increased degradation, since the half-life of infused alkaline phosphatase is normal (Posen and Grunstein, 1982; Whyte *et al.*, 1982a; Whyte *et al.*, 1984). Nor it is due to an endogenous inhibitor, since co-incubation experiments show no inhibition of exogenous alkaline phosphatase by serum from hypophosphatasia patients (Whyte, 1989a). Rather, it reflects a failure of liver and bone to contribute the usual amounts of activity to the serum. Even in the most severe cases, some degree of alkaline phosphatase activity is detectable in serum. This may be due to: 1) presence of circulating placental or intestinal isoenzyme; 2) true residual activity of the TNSALP; or 3) contributions from other phosphomonoesterases (e.g., 5'-nucleotidase) to the phosphatase activity measured *in vitro*. Other tissues that show a

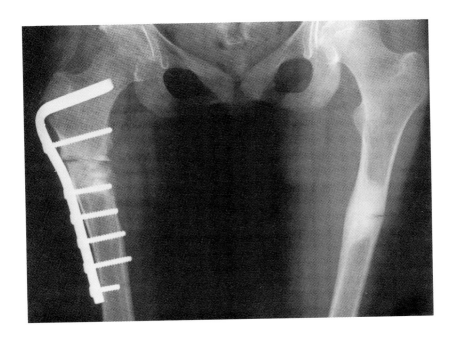

**Fig. 12** Adult Hypophosphatasia
Radiograph of femurs and pelvis with reduced mineralization, bilateral pseudofractures (right femur—treated by internal fixation), and increased trabeculation typical of an osteomalacic process.

deficiency in alkaline phosphatase include granulocytes, bone itself, liver, kidney and cultured skin fibroblasts (Mueller *et al.*, 1983; Brydon *et al.*, 1975; Smith *et al.*, 1985; Gainer and Stinson, 1982; Milivor *et al.*, 1978; Whyte *et al.*, 1982b; Whyte *et al.*, 1983).

In pseudohypophosphatasia, serum alkaline phosphatase activity towards artificial substrates is normal but there is accumulation of natural substrates

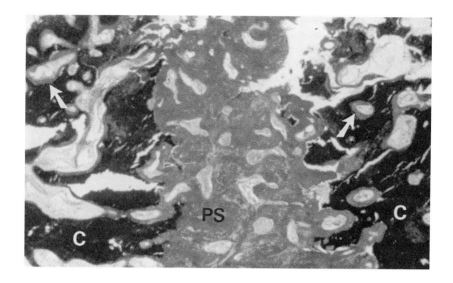

**Fig. 13**   Hypophosphatasia — Bone histopathology
Trichrome stain of an undecalcified section showing abundant osteoid formation (arrows) in mineralized bone (B). The vertical band of unmineralized bone is a zone of pseudofracture (PS) running between zones of completely calcified (C) matrix. (Courtesy of M. Fallon, Philadelphia PA)

and decreased catalytic activity towards them in cultured fibroblasts (Scriver and Cameron, 1969; Mehés et al., 1972; Cole et al., 1986; Fedde et al., 1986).

   Phosphoethanolamine was the first phosphoester found to be increased in hypophosphatasia (McCance et al., 1955; Rasmussen, 1968). Patients show increased concentrations in serum and urine. Quantitation of urinary ex- cretion by amino acid analysis has been a useful confirmatory test for hypophosphatasia (Rasmussen, 1968; Eastman and Bixler, 1982; Eastman and Bixler, 1983), but it should be recognized that phosphoethanolaminuria has been observed in association with other metabolic bone diseases, and that some patients with hypophosphatasia may have normal excretion

(Licata *et al.*, 1978). Similarly, most patients with hypophosphatasia have increased serum and urinary concentrations of pyrophosphate (Russell, 1965; Russell *et al.*, 1971), although the accurate measurement of this metabolite is by no means simple.

More recently, Whyte and colleagues have shown that an increased level of serum pyridoxal 5'-phosphate (PLP) may be a sensitive marker of hypophosphatasia (Whyte *et al.*, 1985; Coburn and Whyte, 1989). Although supplementation with large amounts of pyridoxine (vitamin $B_6$) can be a confounding artifact, $B_6$ loading in hypophosphatasia patients shows a significantly exaggerated response and may be useful in carrier detection (Whyte, 1989b). Although serum PLP is increased, tissue levels are normal and vitamin $B_6$ nutritional status is undisturbed in affected individuals (Whyte *et al.*, 1988). In most other bone diseases, where serum alkaline phosphatase activity may be elevated, serum PLP concentrations tend to be lower than normal, thus providing increased diagnostic discrimination in the case of the affected individual (Fig. 14).

## Prenatal Diagnosis

Most of the alkaline phosphatase activity found in human amniotic fluid originates from the fetal intestine (Moss and Whitaker, 1987; Stinson and McPhee, 1987). This isoenzyme has biochemical characteristics that distinguish it from the adult form and it is readily quantitated by immunoassay, a feature which has been used successfully for prenatal diagnosis. Monoclonal antibodies may be helpful for analysis of chorionic villus samples (Warren *et al.*, 1985), but amniotic fluid TNSALP is normally so low under the usual conditions that routine enzyme assays are of little diagnostic value by themselves (Mulivor *et al.*, 1978; Rudd *et al.*, 1976). Most severe forms of hypophosphatasia can be diagnosed by second-trimester ultrasonography and confirmed by assay of TNSALP in cultured amniocytes. Amniotic fluid alkaline phosphatase, measured with the more sensitive fluorometric assay (Rattenbury *et al.*, 1976; Rudd *et al.*, 1976; Mulivor *et al.*, 1978), may be significantly depressed in those forms of the disease that cannot be detected by fetal ultrasongraphy, suggesting that several methods may be required for optimal diagnostic discrimination.

## Molecular Genetics

Until very recently, it was not certain that the TNSAP locus itself need be the locus of the hypophosphatasia mutation. However, studies by Greenberg and co-workers have shown a linkage between the Rh locus and the infantile hypophosphatasia found in an isolated Mennonite population

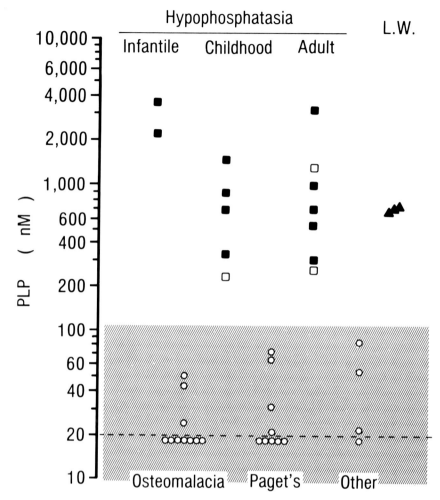

**Fig. 14** Hypophosphatasia — Serum PLP
Plasma pyridoxal-5′-phosphate (PLP) concentrations for infants, children and adults with classic hypophosphatasia (closed squares) or odontohyposphosphatasia (open squares) are above the normal range (shaded area) as are those for the patient (LW) with pseudohypophosphatasia (triangles — far right). Values for patients with other bone diseases and metabolic diseases (open circles) are in the normal range or at the lower limit of sensitivity (20nM, broken line). [Reproduced with permission]

in Manitoba (Chodirker *et al.*, 1987). They obtained a conservative estimate of linkage with a recombinant fraction of 0.09 with LOD scores of greater than 5, which constitutes good evidence for genetic proximity. Subsequently, these investigators have used restriction fragment length polymorphisms (RFLP's) for the TNSALP gene itself and found tight linkage (confidence interval for recombination: 0 to 4%) with the hypophosphatasia genotype in their Mennonite kindreds (Greenberg *et al.*, 1988).

Recent studies by Weiss and colleagues (1988b) provide the first direct evidence of TNSALP gene involvement in hypophosphatasia. They identified a point mutation in the TNSALP gene from a child that died of infantile hypophosphatasia. The G to A transition mutation at base pair 711 results in substitution of a threonine for the alanine-162 residue (Fig. 15). When spliced into a transfection vector and expressed in culture cells, alkaline phosphatase is absent, although inactive protein is still immunologically detectable. The site of the mutation is in a domain that is extensively conserved (Fig. 8) and close to the active site of the folded protein, and

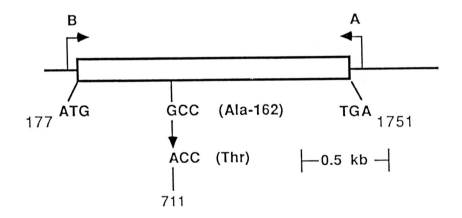

**Fig. 15** Infantile Hypophosphatasia—gene defect
Schematic showing the single base-pair (G to A) mutation at position 711 leading to a substitution of threonine for alanine-162 and resulting in a non-functional enzyme. The numbers indicate the size of the sequence amplified (using oligonucleotide primers at positions A and B), for detection of the point mutation. [Reproduced with permission from Weiss *et al.*, 1988]

provides the final proof that mutation of alkaline phosphatase enzyme is the origin of the hypophosphatasia phenotype. Subsequently, this has been used to provide accurate genetic counselling to other family members at risk (Cole *et al.*, unpublished observations).

## Osteosarcomas and the *c-fos* proto oncogene

## Osteosarcoma

### Introduction

Osteosarcoma is a malignant tumor of bone in which the neoplastic cells *directly* produce osteoid (in contrast to reactive bone surrounding a tumor). The neoplasm has a variable histologic picture and both fibrosarcomatous and chondrosarcomatous elements may be observed; the presence of primary osteoid anywhere in the lesion makes it, by definition, an osteosarcoma (Fig. 16). Diagnosis is by histopathologic evaluation. Polarizing light may aid in identifying osteoid. Uncalcified osteoid may be difficult to differentiate from collagen produced by fibroblastic spindle cells. Histochemical methods can be used to establish alkaline phosphatase activity in tissue sections of osteosarcoma (Brozmanova and Skrovina, 1973; Jeffree, 1972; Jeffree and Price, 1965; Mori *et al.*, 1968); in contrast, alkaline phosphatase activity is entirely absent in fibroblastic lesions that produce collagen.

### Natural History

Osteosarcoma usually arises in bone, but extraskeletal soft-tissue examples are known to arise by osseous metaplasia. Except for plasma cell myeloma, osteosarcoma is the most common primary bone neoplasm. Males are affected slightly more commonly than females. The most frequent occurrences of osteosarcoma correspond to the period of peak skeletal growth during childhood and adolescence. Furthermore, the growth potential of each individual long bone influences the frequency of tumor occurrence for specific bones. Thus the femur, tibia, and humerus—in that order—are the most common sites for osteosarcoma. Fraumeni (1967) showed that osteosarcoma tends to arise in bones that grow very rapidly and produce taller individuals. Tjalma (1966) observed that large breeds of dogs were more susceptible to osteosarcoma than smaller breeds. That large size with increased mitotic activity is related to osteosarcoma is not surprising since rapidly dividing cells are a prerequisite for both processes. With respect to neoplasia, cells are most vulnerable to structural changes in DNA, disrupted

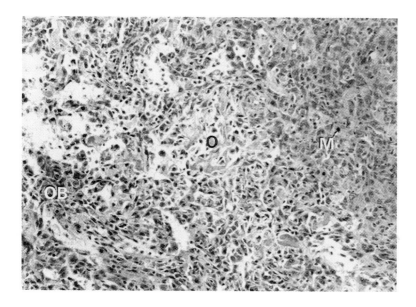

**Fig. 16**  Osteosarcoma — histopathology
Histologic section showing malignant osteoblasts (OB) and osteoid formation (O). Note
frequent mitotic figures (M). [Courtesy of C. Neave]

transcription to RNA, and altered translation into protein-enzyme synthesis
during mitotic activity. Mitosis is also required to produce clones of altered
cells that make up neoplasms (Bolande, 1973).

## Etiology and Pathogenesis

Various DNA and RNA viruses are known to induce osteosarcoma in
experimental animals. For example, SE polyoma, a DNA virus, produces
osteosarcoma in mice (Stewart, 1960). SV40 virus, another DNA virus,
produces osteosarcoma when injected into Syrian golden hamsters
(Diamandopoulos, 1973) and induces dominantly transmitted osteosarcomas

(as well as atrial tumors) in mice when introduced via transgenic transduction (Behringer *et al.*, 1988). Various RNA murine sarcoma viruses, which have a C-type virus particle morphology, can produce osteosarcoma in animal species different from the species that originally supplied it (Fujinago *et al.*, 1970; Soehner and Dmochowski, 1969). The oncogenicity of FBJ and FBR viruses in specific strains of mice (Finkel and Biskis, 1968; Finkel *et al.*, 1975; Finkel *et al.*, 1976) appears to be the result of the *v-fos* oncogene, as discussed below. Other protooncogenes also appear to be expressed above control levels in a variety of murine osteosarcomas (Schön *et al.*, 1986).

The etiology of most cases of human osteosarcoma is unknown. Many clinical reports suggest trauma as a cause, but this is highly unlikely. Because many osteosarcomas arise in the femur or tibia, a region in which minor traumatic injury commonly occurs during childhood and adolescence, it is not surprising that a history of trauma can frequently be elicited. However, it is far more likely that the injury drew the patient's attention to an already existing neoplasm. Thus, trauma probably reveals more malignant growth than it produces (Ewing, 1935).

Although there is no direct evidence for a viral cause of human osteosarcoma, several studies are highly suggestive. Cell-free extracts from human osteosarcomas injected into Syrian hamsters can produce osteosarcomas in them (Finkel *et al.*, 1976). Additional supporting evidence that the hamster lesions result from human cell-free osteosarcoma extracts has been provided by immunofluorescence assays (Pritchard *et al.*, 1971; Reilly *et al.*, 1972) and cytotoxicity tests (Pritchard *et al.*, 1974).

It is therefore likely that human osteosarcomas are both etiologically and pathogenetically heterogeneous (Fraumeni, 1975). Table 5 lists various conditions known to be associated with a number of cases of osteosarcoma and appropriate references are provided. Some appear to cause and others appear to predispose to osteosarcoma. Familial aggregations are divided into three basic types with several subtypes. An autosomal recessive gene in the homozygous state may be responsible for many of the instances of affected sibs (usually two sibs but as many as three and even four sibs have been reported). Affected parent and child suggests the possibility of an autosomal dominant gene. Some familial aggregations of osteosarcoma are associated with various other types of neoplasms which suggests the possibility of an autosomal dominant gene with pleiotropic effects. Finally, the Mulvihill type of familial aggregation appears to be a unique, possibly autosomal recessive condition.

Osteosarcoma may arise as a pleiotropic effect in the autosomal dominant form of retinoblastoma. Several instances of osteogenesis imperfecta have been recorded with osteosarcoma. Paget's disease shows a predilection for osteosarcoma. Ionizing radiation is a known cause of osteosarcoma in some

**Table 5**

Conditions Associated With Osteosarcoma

| Condition | Comments | References |
|---|---|---|
| Familial aggregation, isolated type | Affected sibs | Harmon and Morton, 1966<br>Lee and MacKenzie, 1964<br>Matejovsky, 1977<br>Pohle *et al.*, 1936<br>Roberts and Roberts, 1935<br>Swaney, 1973 |
| | Affected cousins | Robbins, 1967 |
| | Affected parent and child | Swaney, 1973 |
| Familial aggregation of osteosarcoma with other types of tumors in family | Polyposis coli (familial) | Hoffman and Brooke, 1970 |
| | Other cancers | Epstein et al, 1970<br>Lee and MacKenzie, 1964<br>Miller and McLaughlin, 1977 |
| Familial aggregation, Mulvihill type | Three affected sibs with osteosarcoma, skeletal defects, erythrocytic macrocytosis, and immunodeficiency | Mulvihill *et al.*, 1977 |
| Autosomal dominant retinoblastoma | Osteosarcoma as pleiotropic effect | Kitchen and Ellsworth, 1974<br>Friend *et al.*, 1986 |
| Osteogenesis imperfecta | True osteosarcoma (not exuberant callus formation) | Hatteland, 1957<br>Jewell and Lostrom, 1940<br>Klenerman *et al.*, 1967<br>Werner, 1930 |
| Paget's disease | Predeliction for osteosarcoma. Giant cell tumors of bone and multiple myeloma have also been associated. | Huvos, 1979 |
| Ionizing radiation | Thorotrast (radioactive contrast medium) | Altner *et al.*, 1972<br>Tsuya *et al.*, 1963 |
| | External high dose irradiation for cancer therapy | Sim *et al.*, 1972<br>Tucker *et al.*, 1987 |

**Table 5    (Continued)**

| Condition | Comments | References |
|-----------|----------|-----------|
| | Internal bone-seeking radioisotopes from occupational or medical use | Loutit, 1970 |
| Rothmund-Thomson syndrome | Infantile poikiloderma, cataracts, hypogonadism, skeletal anomalies, short stature, autosomal recessive inheritance | Dick *et al.*, 1982<br>Kozlowski *et al.*, 1980<br>Roschlau, 1962<br>Starr *et al.*, 1985<br>Tokunago *et al.*, 1976 |
| Werner syndrome | Short stature, premature graying of hair, baldness, scleropoikiloderma, trophic leg ulcers, juvenile cataracts, hypogonadism, diabetes mellitus, calcification of blood vessels, osteoporosis, autosomal recessive inheritance | Rosen *et al.*, 1970 |
| Parry syndrome | Waardenburg-like features, cataracts, small head size, joint abnormalities, hypogonadism, osteosarcoma, sporatic occurence to date | Parry *et al.*, 1978 |
| Schuman-Burton syndrome | Frontal bossing, low-set ears, prominent nose, micrognathia, genitourinary anomalies, osteosarcoma, family history of breast cancer, sporadic occurrence to date | Schuman and Burton, 1979 |

instances and chemotherapy in children has also been implicated (Tucker *et al.*, 1987). Finally, there are several syndromes — two of them autosomal recessive — with a predisposition for the development of osteosarcoma (Table 5).

Despite this heterogeneity, it seems likely that human osteosarcomas, like other neoplastic conditions, arise from altered function of specific genes, particularly those related to cell differentiation and replication. Recent studies of the *v-fos* oncogene isolated from murine viral tumors offer the first glimpse of the molecular events that give rise to osteosarcoma.

## Murine Viral Osteosarcomas

The discovery of viral induction of osteosarcomas had its origins in the study of tumorogenesis by the radionuclides required for atomic bomb construction during World War II (Finkel and Biskis, 1968). The first successful isolation of a viral agent in 1966 was from a spontaneously appearing well-differentiated osteosarcoma appearing in a 260-day old male animal from a colony of the CF1 inbred strain of mice (Finkel *et al.*, 1975). The virus, referred to as FBJ after the discoverers (Finkel, Biskis and Jinkins), was serially transmitted through multiple generations of mice. This was followed in 1973 by the isolation of a similar virus from a radiation-induced osteosarcoma in the tumor-resistant X/Gf line of inbred mice, now called the FBR (Finkel, Biskis and Reilly) virus. Subsequent experiments with FBJ demonstrated bone tumors that closely resemble the gross and microscopic features of human juxtacortical osteosarcoma (Ward and Young, 1976).

Both the FBJ and FBR viruses are generally replication incompetent and are passaged with a helper or replication-competent virus. In association with a helper virus, they induce osteosarcomas with a latency period as short as 30 days (Finkel *et al.*, 1975; Lee *et al.*, 1979). The tumors arise anywhere along the bones and begin as focal proliferations in the periosteum and grow peripherally to involve the adjacent soft tissues and eventually invade the osseous cortex. Individually, the FBJ and FBR viruses by themselves appear to be responsible for both the transformation and immortalization steps in oncogenesis.

The two viruses were identified as homologs of replication competent RNA retroviruses by Curran and colleagues (Curran *et al.*, 1982; Curran and Verma, 1984). However, tumor viruses of this type containing genes that transform cells (oncogenes) appear to have originated by recombinant mutation with viruses containing genes to ensure viral replication (Bishop, 1983; Friend *et al.*, 1988). This small but profound change has its origins in the unique life cycle of the RNA retroviruses (Varmus and Swanstrom, 1985) (illustrated in Fig. 17). This begins with DNA replication from the viral RNA template (achieved by the reverse transcriptase, coded for by the *pol* gene) to form a provirus with host cell transcription of the proviral DNA sequence, the synthesis of RNA viral elements that are packaged with capsid protein(s) (coded for by the *gag* gene), and envelope protein(s)

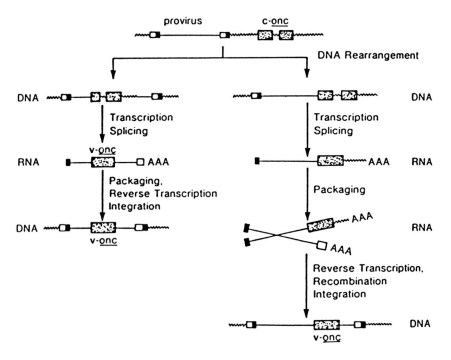

**Fig. 17** Oncogene transduction

Two models for transduction of cellular oncogenes (*c-onc*) by retroviruses. The provirus genes (straight line) are flanked by long terminal repeats (black and white boxes) that promote integration into the host DNA (jagged lines). In the first model, the DNA rearrangement places *c-onc* directly within the provirus (left); in the second, more likely scenario (right), fusion of the two loci results in usurpation of host regulatory elements by the retroviral equivalent. This appears to be the case with the FBJ virus, which expresses a *gag-fos* fusion product (Curran and Verma, 1982). The *c-onc* exons (stippled boxes) are transcribed to RNA and spliced together by the host machinery, but packaging of the virus, recombination with other viral elements at the RNA level and subsequent re-integration into host DNA are controlled by the retroviral genome, ultimately leading to transcription from a condensed viral oncogene (*v-onc*) lacking introns. (Reproduced with permission from Bishop 1983)

(coded for by the *env* gene) are completed and new retroviral virions are released. Special sequences, known as long terminal repeats (LTR's) or recombination functions (RJ's) direct the insertion of the viral DNA into the host genome, an essential step in the transcription process. This genetic recombination is highly efficient but non-specific with respect to integration site in the host. Host genomic sequences may be accidentally incorporated into the virus at a high rate. Moreover, the genes in the host sequence may undergo genetic recombination themselves and subsequently express altered gene products, a process known as transduction (Fig. 17). This process can be deduced from examining the relationship between the oncogenes in tumor viruses (called *v-onc*) and the homologous sequences in host cells, known as protooncogenes (called *c-onc*). These proto-oncogenes appear to have important roles in the regulation of cellular differentiation and replication, and clearly constitute important targets for the genetic mutations underlying carcinogenesis (Bishop, 1983; Müller and Verma, 1984; Müller, 1986a).

## The Genetics of *c-fos*

Sequencing of the FBR and FBJ viral genomes show a specific oncogene, *fos* (*F*BR or *F*BJ *o*steosarcoma), is central to the induction of these tumors in mice (Bishop and Varmus, 1985; Müller, 1986b). The cellular gene, *c-fos*, encodes a single peptide of 380 amino acids that is found in a variety of evolutionarily divergent eukaryotes, including man (MIM#16481). The gene contains upstream and downstream consensus sequences for transcription activation, polyadenylation of the mRNA and a 3' site that regulates transcription (Fig. 18). The expression of *c-fos* shows a complex pattern dependent on tissue, cell type, and stage of differentiation (Fig. 19). In the mouse, it it initially synthesized as a 54 kDa protein which rapidly undergoes posttranslational glycosylation. This glycoprotein remains restricted to

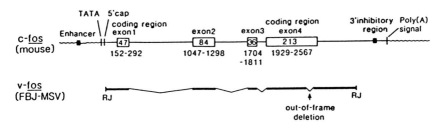

**Fig. 18** Structure of the *c-fos* and *v-fos* genes
Genomic structure of the murine *c-fos* is shown at the top. Starting from the 5' (left) end, are enhancer (bp −332 to −276) and "TATA" box (−31 to −26) sequences of the promotor, and the 5' cap. The exons (boxes with number of encoded amino acids) are separated by 3 introns and followed by a 3' untranslated region which plays an important role in regulation of transcription (see text). The crucial inhibitory region [black box (bp +3138 to +3172)] just 5' to the poly(A) signal (bp +3361 to +3366)] is required for messenger RNA processing. Other numbers below refer to the distance (in base pairs) from the 5' start. The *v-fos* of the FBJ virion (heavy lines) is shown with recombination junctions and introns (light lines) that are deleted. The out-of-frame deletion in exon 4 results in an altered C-terminal peptide that runs into the 3' untranslated region and transcription terminates in another junction before the crucial 3' inhibition region. [Reproduced with permission from Müller 1986]

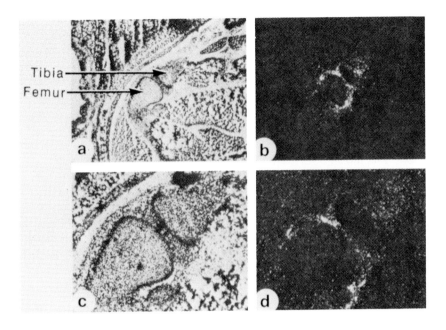

**Fig. 19** Prenatal expression of *c-fos*
*In situ* hybridization [at low (a and b) and high (c and d) power magnification] of a *fos*-specific
RNA probe in 17 day old mice. Bright (a and c) and dark (b and d) field photographs of the
tibia and femur show marked expression only at the ends of the long bones. [Reproduced with
permission from Dony and Gross 1987]

the nucleus but becomes associated with an unidentified protein (p39)
derived from the cytoplasm. Its half-life is only 30 minutes, in keeping with
a rapidly-responsive regulatory role and it undergoes cAMP-stimulated
phosphorylation at serine and threonine residues, indicating that it may be
a target for cell-signal activated protein kinases (Curran *et al.*, 1987).

Structure-activity relationships have been probed by means of genetic constructs and suggest that the N- and C-terminals are relatively dispensible for constitutive function (Jenuwein and Müller, 1987). The middle portion (amino acids 111 to 219), whose structure is completely conserved in man and mouse and intact in the FBR virus, is clearly required for biological activity. However, key recognition sequences for cAMP-dependent binding are found in both these domains and may serve as specific inducible or regulatory elements. The c-fos protein appears to have DNA binding properties and probably functions as part of an early nuclear response to cytoplasmic signals activated by a wide variety of extracellular stimuli. The cellular response to c-fos expression is tissue-specific but the molecular details remain to be determined (Müller, 1986b; Hunt et al., 1987; Rollins et al., 1987; Sassone-Corsi and Verma, 1987).

The relationship between cellular and viral genes is also under active investigation (Miller et al., 1984; Curran et al., 1984; Müller, 1986b). The FBJ v-fos gene (Fig. 19) differs in four ways: i) the 5′ untranslated sequence is viral; ii) the three protooncogene introns are deleted; iii) there is a single base-pair out-of-frame deletion so that the C-terminal 49 amino acids of the virus are completely different; iv) the 3′ untranslated sequence is interrupted and lacks a key inhibitory element. In the FBR viral genome, more complex rearrangements have taken place, but both FBR and FBJ v-fos proteins appear to induce transformation by virtue of the loss of regulatory elements in the 3′ untranslated end of the gene. Only a single amino acid substitution is needed to realize the immortalizing potential of the fos protein once the 3′ untranslated sequence is interrupted (Jenuwein and Müller, 1987) and the malignant progression of otherwise transformed lines can be enhanced by incorporation of v-fos into the host genome (Kawano et al., 1987)

## c-fos and Bone Development

The discovery of the fos gene through the analysis of viruses responsible for mouse osteosarcomas suggests that it may have a special role in the formation of bone. This possibility has been studied by examining the amount of transcribed c-fos messenger RNA in tissues of inbred mouse strains (Müller, 1986b). For the first two weeks of the 21-day gestation period, murine c-fos is expressed primarily in extra-embryonic tissues, including placenta, amnion and visceral yolk sac. Increased c-fos transcription in the embryo itself is not observed until day 16 but it increases rapidly thereafter. Autoradiographic studies with the probe on histologic sections in late-gestational embryos shows very specific localization to the most actively growing regions of bone and connective tissue webs of the fore and hind feet (Dony and Gross, 1987). On day 17, when the murine skeleton is wellchondrified and ossification is already well established, enhanced c-fos transcription activity is most prominent in the ends of the long bones and the interzones of associated joints (Fig. 19).

The spatial and temporal specificity of this response is at odds with the ubiquity and non-specificity of c-fos activation by extracellular stimuli in various cultured cell lines (Hunt et al., 1987; Sassone-Corsi and Verma, 1987; LaTour et al., 1988). Thus, there appears to be an "organ-specific window of susceptibility" for the cellular actions of the c-fos gene. This concept receives support from an elegant series of transgenic experiments by Rüther and colleagues (1987). They generated a DNA sequence that expresses a c-fos gene in response to the human metallothionein promotor. This promotor is a unique DNA sequence that enhances transcription of associated genes when stimulated by the addition of a metal, particularly cadmium. The chimeric sequence of mouse protooncogene and human promotor was cloned and microinjected into isolated fertilized mouse eggs under conditions that maximize integration of foreign DNA into the embryonic genome. The transformed eggs were then implanted into pseudopregnant surrogate mothers and the resulting growth and development of the transgenic animals were studied. Because the normal c-fos promotor has been removed, constitutively high levels of c-fos transcription and expression are found. As a consequence, a disturbed pattern of bony development emerges. The affected animals first present with visible swellings in both hind legs. Radiographs (Fig. 20) show altered conformation and increased mineralization in both tibias and forearms. When these long bones are sectioned, increased trabecular bone formation, bone marrow fibrosis and bony resorption are all visible, but neoplastic changes are not observed (Fig. 21). Once introduced, this trait is faithfully transmitted to subsequent generations, confirming the integration of the mutation into the host genome. Otherwise, the animals do not appear to be adversely affected.

These experiments do not offer an explanation for tissue specificity with respect to the effects of altered c-fos genes. The response appears to be restricted to a small developmental field (proximal ends of the long bones) for a short period of time. Postnatally, c-fos expression becomes highest in the marrow elements, particularly the macrophage, and it seems likely that the gene also has an important role in regulating hematopoiesis (Müller, 1986a). However, sensitivity of the c-fos gene to extracellular stimuli has recently been demonstrated in cultured osteoblast-like cells (LaTour et al., 1988). Moreover, the oncogenic potential of c-fos mutations (including v-fos and a number of artificially created mutants) and the known predilection of human osteosarcomas for sites of rapid growth in the long bones suggests that both may share a common pathogenic mechanism. Although fos mutations have been shown to be directly responsible for human tumor devel-

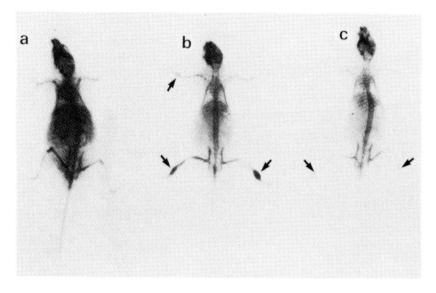

**Fig. 20** Expression of *c-fos* in transgenic mice
Radiographs of controls (a), affected transgenic offspring (b) with visible lesions in the tibia and forearm bones (arrows), and unaffected offspring (c). [Reproduced with permission from Rüther *et al.* 1987]

opment, they constitute a new paradigm for bony malformations as a predictable consequence of a precisely defineable genetic alteration. At the same time, the delineation of protoocogene structure and expression will undoubtedly offer important new insights into the nature of skeletal growth and development.

## Acknowledgments

We thank Karen Moore and Elfreida Schneider for preparing the typescript. We also thank M. Whyte, M. Weiss, and C. Greenberg for permission to quote their unpublished material.

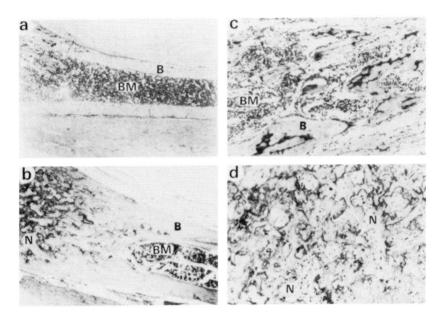

**Fig. 21** Expression of *c-fos* in transgenic mice
Histology of bone lesions in affected transgenic offspring. Different magnifications of normal
mouse tibia are shown at the top (a,c). The low magnification view (b) of affected bone (B)
reveals changes localized to the metaphysis, including proliferation of trabeculae, excessive
new bone (N) formation and fibrosis of the bone marrow (BM). Higher magnification (d)
demonstrates a distinctive mosaic pattern of bone development. Newly woven bone (N;
slightly stained) appears between lamellae undergoing resorption. Original magnifications: 30x
and 120x respectively. [Reproduced with permission from Rüther *et al.* 1987]

## References

Ackerman, L. V. (1958). Extra-osseous localized non-neoplastic bone and cartilage formation
(so-called myositis ossificans). *J. Bone Joint Surg.*, **40A**: 279.
Altner, P. C., Simmons, D. J., Lucas J. F. Jr. (1972). Osteogenic sarcoma in a patient injected
with Thorotrast. *J. Bone Joint Surg.*, **54A**: 670–675.

Allan, C. J., Soule, E. H. (1971). Osteogenic sarcoma of the somatic soft tissues — clinicopathologic study of 26 cases and review of the literature. *Cancer*, **27**: 1121—1133.

Anderson, H. C. (1985). Matrix vesicle calcification: Review and update. In: *Bone and Mineral Research/3*, W. A. Peck (ed). Elsevier, North Holland, 109—150.

Behringer, R. R., Peschon, J. J., Messing, A., Gartside, C. L., Hauschka, R. D., Palmiter, R. L., Brinster, R. L. (1988). Heart and bone tumors in transgenic mice. *Proc. Natl. Acad. Sci. (USA)*, **85**: 2548—2552.

Beratis, N. G., Kaffe, S., Aron, A. M., Hirschhorn, K. (1976). Alkaline phosphatase activity in cultured fibroblasts from fibrodysplasia ossificans progressiva. *J. Med. Genet.*, **13**: 307—309.

Berger, J., Garattini, E., Hua, J., Udenfriend, S. (1987). Cloning and sequencing of human intestinal alkaline phosphatase cDNA. *Proc. Natl. Acad. Sci. USA* **84**: 695—698.

Besman, M., Coleman, J. E. (1985). Isozymes of bovine intestinal alkaline phosphatase. *J. Biol. Chem.*, **260**: 1190—1193.

Beumer, J., Trowbridge, H. O., Silverman S. Jr., Eisenberg, E. (1985). Childhood hypophosphatasia and the premature loss of teeth. *Oral Surg.*, **35**: 631—640.

Bishop, J. M. (1983). Cellular oncogenes and retroviruses. *Ann. Rev. Biochem.*, **52**: 301—354.

Bishop, J. M., and Varmus, H. (1985). Functions and origins of retroviral transforming genes. Supplement 9 *In: Molecular Biology of Tumor Viruses: RNA Tumor Viruses* (2nd ed), R. Weiss, N. Teich, H. Varmus, J. Coffin eds. Cold Spring Harbor Laboratory, p. 291—294.

Bolane, R. P. (1973). Relationships between teratogenesis and oncogenesis. In: *Pathobiology of Development*, E. V. D. Perrin and M. J. Finegold (eds). Williams and Wilkins Co., (1973), pp. 114—134.

Bourne, G. H. (1973). Phosphatase and calcification. In: *The Biochemistry and Physiology of Bone*, (2nd ed), G. H. Bourne (ed), Academic Press, New York, 79—120.

Bradshaw, R. A., Cancedda, F., Ericsson, L. H., Neumann, P. A., Piccoli, S. P., Schlesinger, M. J., Shriefer, K., Walsh, K. A. (1981). Amino acid sequence of *Escherichia coli* alkaline phosphatase. *Proc. Natl. Acad. Sci. (USA)* **78**: 3473—3477.

Brenner, R. L., Smith, J. L., Cleveland, W. W., Behar, R. L., and Lockhart, W. S. Jr., (1969). Eye signs of hypophosphatasia. *Arch. Ophthalmol.*, **81**: 614—617.

Brozmanovà, E. and Skrovina, B. (1973). Serum alkaline phosphatase in malignant bone tumours (osteosarcoma, chondrosarcoma, fibrosarcoma, Ewing's sarcoma). *Neoplasma*, **20**: 419—425.

Bruckner, R. J., Rickles, N. H., and Porter, D. R. (1962). Hypophosphatasia with premature shedding of teeth and aplasia of cementum. *Oral Surg.*. **15**: 1351—1369.

Brydon, W. G., Crofton, P. M., Smith, A. F., Barr, D. G. D., Harkness, R. A. (1975). Hypophosphatasia: Enzyme studies in cultured cells and tissues. *Biochem. Sci. Trans.*, **3**: 927—929.

Burton-Fanning, F. W. and Vaughan, A. L. (1901).A case of myositis ossificans. *Lancet*, **ii**: 849—850.

Caplan, A. I., Pechak, D. G. (1987). The Cellular and Molecular Embryology of Bone Formation In: *Bone and Mineral Research Annual Review*, Vol. 5, W. A. Peck (ed.), Elsevier North Holland, 117—183.

Caswell, A. M., Whyte, M. P., Russell, R. G. G. (1986). Normal activity of nucleoside triphosphate pyrophosphatase in alkaline phosphatase-deficient fibroblasts from patients with infantile hypophosphatasia. *J. Clin. Endocrinol. Metab.*, **63**: 1237—1241.

Chang, C. N., Kuang, W., Chen, E. Y. (1986). Nucleotide sequence of alkaline phosphatase gene of *Escherichia coli. Gene*, **44**: 121—125.

Chiang, T. M., Postlethwaite, A. E., Beachery, E. H., Seyer, J. M., Kang, A. H. (1978). Binding of chemotactic collagen derived peptides to fibroblasts — the relationship to fibroblast chemotaxis. *J. Clin. Invest.*, **62**: 916–922.

Chodirker, B. N., Evans, J. A., Lewis, M., Coghlan, G., Belcher, E., Philips, S., Seargeant, L. E., Sus, C., Greenberg, C. R. (1987). Infantile hypophosphatasia — linkage with the RH locus. *Genomics*, **1**: 280–282.

Chuang, N. (1987). Alkaline phosphatase in human milk: A new heat-stable enzyme. *Clin. Chim. Acta.*, **169**: 165–174.

Coburn, S. P., Whyte, M. P. (1989). Role of phosphatases in the regulation of vitamin $B_6$ in hypophosphatasia and other disorders. In: *Proceedings of the 3rd International Conference on Vitamin $B_6$*, R. Reynolds (ed.). Alan R. Liss, New York.

Cocivera, M., McManaman, J., Wilson, I. B. (1980). Phosphorylated intermediate of alkaline phosphatase. *Biochemistry*, **19**: 2901–2907.

Coe, J. D., Murphy, W. A., and Whyte, M. P. (1986). Management of femoral fractures and pseudofractures in adult hypophosphatasia. *J. Bone Joint. Surg.*, **68A**: 981–990.

Cole, D. E. C., Salisbury, S. R., Stinson, R. A., Coburn, S. P., Ryan, L. M., and Whyte, M. P. (1986). Increased serum pyridoxal-5'-phosphate in pseudohypophosphatasia (Letter). *N. Engl. J. Med.*, **314**: 992–993.

Coleman, J. E., Gettins, P. (1983). Alkaline phosphatase, solution structure, and mechanism. *Adv. Enzymol.*, **55**: 382–452.

Connor, J. M. and Beighton, P. (1982). Fibrodysplasia ossificans progressiva in South Africa: Case reports. *Sa. Mediese. Tydskrif.*, 13 March: 404–406.

Connor, J. M. and Evans, D. A. P. (1981a). Quantitative and qualitative studies on skin fibroblast alkaline phosphatase in fibrodysplasia ossificans progressiva. *Clin. Chim. Acta.*, **117**: 355–360.

Connor, J. M. and Evans, D. A. P. (1982a). Genetic aspects of fibrodysplasia ossificans progressiva. *J. Med. Genet.*, **19**: 35–39.

Connor, J. M. and Evans D. A. P. (1982b) Fibrodysplasia ossificans progressiva: The clinical features and natural history of 34 patients. *J, Bone Joint. Surg.*, **64B**: 76–83.

Connor, J. M., Evans, C. C., Evans D. A. P. (1981) Cardioplumonary function in fibrodysplasia ossificans progressiva. *Thorax*, **36**: 419–423.

Cramer, S. F., Ruehl, A., Mandel, M. A. (1981). Fibrodysplasia ossificans progressiva: A distinctive bone-forming lesion of the soft tissue. *Cancer*, **48**: 1016–1021.

Cremin, B. et al, (1982). The radiological spectrum of fibrodysplasia ossificans progressiva. *Clin. Radiol.*, **33**: 499–508.

Curran, T., Peters, G., VanBeveren, C., Teich, N. M., Verma, I. M. (1982). FBJ murine osteosarcoma virus: Identification and molecular cloning of biologically active proviral DNA. *J. Virol*, **44**: 674–82.

Curran, T., Verma, I. M. (1984). FBR murine osteosarcoma virus: I. Molecular analysis and characterization of a 75,000-Da *gag-fos* fusion product. *Virology*, **135**: 218–28.

Curran, T., Miller, A. D., Zokas, L., Verma, I. M. (1984). Viral and cellular *fos* proteins: A comparative analysis *Cell*, **36**: 259–68.

Curran, T., Gordon, M. B., Rubino, K. L., Sambucetti, L. C. (1987). Isolation and characterization of *c-fos* (rat) cDNA and analysis of post-translational modification *in vitro*. *Oncogene*, **2**: 79–84.

Currarino, G. (1973). Hypophosphatasia. *Progr. Pediatr. Radiol.*, **4**: 469–494.

Davitz, M. A., Hereld, D., Shak, S., Krakow, J., Englund, P. T., Nussenzweig, V. (1987). A glycan-phosphatidylinositol — specific phospholipase D in human serum. *Science*, **238**: 81–84.

de Bernard, B., Bianco, P., Bonucci, E., Costantini, M., Lunazzi, G. C., Martinuzzi, P., Modricky, C., Moro, L., Panfili, E., Pollesello, P., Stagni, N., Vittur, F. (1986). Biochemical and immunohistochemical evidence that in cartilage an alkaline phosphatase is a $Ca^{2+}$-

binding glycoprotein. *J. Cell Biol.*, **103**: 1615−1623.

Diamandopoulos, G. T. (1973). Induction of lymphocytic leukemia, lymphosarcoma, reticulum cell sarcoma, and osteogenic sarcoma in the Syrian golden hamsters by oncogenic DNA Simian virus 40. *J. Natl. Cancer Inst.*, **50**: 1347−1365.

Dick, D. C., et al, (1982). Rothmund-Thomson case and osteogenic sarcoma. *Clin. Exper Dermatol.*, **7**: 119−123.

Dixon, T. F., Mulligan, L., Nassim, R., Stevenson, F. H. (1954). Myositis ossificans progressiva: Report of a case in which ACTH and cortisone failed to prevent reossification after excision of ectopic bone. *J. Bone Joint. Surg. (Br)*, **36B**: 445−449.

Dony, C. and Gross, P. (1987). Proto-oncogene *c-fos* expression in growth regions of fetal bone and mesodermal web tissue. *Nature*, **328**: 711−714.

Eastman, J. R., Bixler, D. (1977). Serum alkaline phosphatase: Normal values by sex and age. *Clin. Chem.*, **23**: 1769−1770.

Eastman, J. R., and Bixler, D. (1980). Urinary phosphoethanolamine: Normal values by age (Letter). *Clin. Chem.*, **26**: 1757−1758.

Eastman, J. R., and Bixler, D., (1982). Lethal and mild hypophosphatasia in half-sibs. *J. Craniofac. Genet. Develop. Biol.*, **2**: 35−44.

Eastman, J. R. and Bixler, D. (1983). Clinical laboratory, and genetic investigations of hypophosphatasia: Support for autosomal dominant inheritance with homozygous lethality. *J. Craniofac. Genet. Develop. Biol.*, **3**: 213−234.

Eaton, W. L., Conkling, W. S., Daeschner, C. W. (1957). Early myositis ossificans progressiva occurring in homozygotic twins. A clinical and pathologic study. *J. Pediatr.*, **50**: 591−598.

Endo, T. Ohbayashi, H., Hayashi, Y., Ikehara, Y., Kochibe, N., Kobata, A. (1988). Structural study on the carbohydrate moiety of human placental alkaline phosphatase. *J. Biochem.*, **103**: 182−187.

Epstein, L. I., Bixler, D., Bennett, J. E.(1970). An incident of familial cancer. Including 3 cases of ostteogenic sarcoma. *Cancer*, **25**: 889−891.

Ewing, J. (1935). Bulkley lecture: Modern attitude toward traumatic cancer. *Arch. Pathol.*, **19**: 690−728,

Fallon, M. D., Teitelbaum, S. L., Weinstein, R. S., Goldfischer, S., Brown, D. M. and Whyte, M. P. (1984). Hypophosphatasia: Clinicopathologic comparison of the infantile, childhood, and adult forms. *Medicine*, **63**: 12−24.

Farley, J. R., Baylink, D. J. (1986). Skeletal alkaline phosphatase activity as a bone formation index in vitro. *Metabolism*, **35**: 563−571.

Farley, J. R., Chesnut, C. H., Baylink, D. J. (1981). Improved method for quantitative determination in serum of alkaline phosphatase of skeletal origin. *Clin. Chem.*, **27**: 2002−2007.

Fedde, K. N., Oakley, L. M., Cole, D. E. C., Whyte, M. P., (1986). Pseudohypophosphatasia: Identification of defective pyridoxal-5′-phosphate phosphatase in cultured fibroblasts. *Am. J. Hum. Genet.*, **39**: A10, (Abstract).

Finkel, M. P., Biskis, B. O. (1968) Experimental induction of osteosarcomas. *Progr. Exp. Tumor. Res.*, **10**: 72−111.

Finkel, M. P., Reilly, C. A., Jr, Biskis, B. O., (1975). Viral etiology of bone cancer. *Front. Radiat. Therap. Oncol.* **10**: 28−39.

Finkel, M. P., Reilly, C. A. Jr., Biskis, B. O. (1976). Pathogenesis of radiation and virus-induced bone tumors. In: *Malignant Bone Tumors*, Grundmann E. (ed), New York, Springer-Verlag, 97−103.

Fraser, D. (1957). Hypophosphatasia. *Am. J. Med.*, **22**: 730−745.

Fraumeni, J. F., Jr. (1867) Stature and malignant tumors of bone in childhood and adolescence. *Cancer*, **20**: 967−973.

Fraumeni, J. F., Jr. (1975). Bone cancer: Epidemiologic and etiologic considerations. *Front. Radiat. Therap. Oncol.*, **10**: 17−27.

Friend, S. H., Bernards, R., Rogelj, S., Weinberg, R. A., Rapaport, J. M., Albert, D. M., Dryja, T. P. (1986) A human DNA segment with properties of the gene that predisposes to retinoblastoma and osteosarcoma. *Nature*, **323**: 643−646.

Friend, S. H., Dryja, T. P., Weinberg, R. A. (1988). Oncogenes and tumor-suppressing genes. *N Engl. J. Med.*, **318**: 618−22.

Fujinaga, S., Poel, W. E., Dmochowski, L. (1970). Light and electron microscope studies of osteosarcomas induced in rats and hamsters by Harvey and Moloney sarcoma viruses. *Cancer Res.*, **30**: 1698−1708.

Gainer, A. L., Stinson, R. A. (1982). Evidence that alkaline phosphatase from human neutrophils is the same gene product as the liver/kidney/bone isoenzyme. *Clin. Chim. Acta*, **123**: 11−17.

Garba, M., Marie, P. J. (1986). Alkaline phosphatase inhibition by levamisole prevents 1, 25-dihydroxyvitamin D$_3$-stimulated bone mineralization. *Calcif. Tissue Int.*, **38**: 296−302.

Gaster, A. (1905). Discussion in meeting in West London Medico-Chirurgical Society, 7 October 1904. *W. London. Med. J.*, **10**: 37.

Gonchoroff, D. G., and O'Brien, J. F. (1988). Liquid-chromatographic separation of liver and bone alkaline phosphatase in human serum. *Clin. Chem.*, **34**: 1518.

Greenberg, C. R., Chodirker, B. N., McKendry-Smith, S., Redekopp, S., Haworth, J. C., Coglan, G., Sus, K., Seargeant, L. E., Weiss, M. J., Harris, H. (1988). Evidence equating the disease locus *HOPS* with the *ALPL* locus. *Pediatr. Res.*, **23**: 329A (Abstract).

Griffin, C. A., Smith, M., Henthorn, P. S., Harris, H., Weiss, M. J., Raducha, M., Emanuel, B. S. (1987). Human placental and intestinal alkaline phosphatase genes map to 2q34−q37. *Am. J. Hum. Genet.*, **41**: 1025−1034.

Griffiths, J., Black J. (1987). Separation and identification of alkaline phosphatase isoenzymes and isoforms in serum of healthy persons by isoelectric focusing. *Clin. Chem.*, **33**: 2171−2177.

Hall, A. D., Williams, A. (1986). Leaving group dependence in the phosphorylation of *Escherichia coli* alkaline phosphatase by monophosphate esters. *Biochemistry*, **25**: 4784−4790.

Harmon, T. P., and Marton, K. S. (1966). Osteogenic sarcoma in four siblings. *J. Bone Joint, Surg.*, **48B**: 493−498.

Harris, H, (1983). Applications of monoclonal antibodies in enzyme genetics. *Ann. Rev. Genet.*, **17**: 279−314.

Hatteland, K. (1957) Osteosarcoma ven osteogenesis imperfecta. *Tidsskr. Nor. Laegeforen.*, **77**: 70−73.

Hawrylak, K., Stinson, R. A. (1987) Tetrameric alkaline phosphatase from human liver is converted to dimers by phosphatidylinositol phospholipase C. *Febs. Lett.*, **212**: 289−291.

Henthorn, P. S., Knoll, B. J., Raducha, M., Rothblum, K. N., Slaughter, C., Weiss, M., Lafferty, M. A., Fischer, T., Harris, H. (1986). Products of two common alleles at the locus for human placental alkaline phosphatase differ by seven amino acids. *Proc. Natl. Acad. Sci. (USA)*, **83**: 5597−5601.

Henthorn, P. S., Raducha, M., Edwards, Y. H., Weiss, M. J., Slaughter, C., Lafferty, M. A., Harris, H. (1987). Nucleotide and amino acid sequences of human intestinal alkaline phosphatase: Close homology to placental alkaline phosphatase. *Proc. Natl. Acad. Sci. (USA)*. **84**: 1234−1238.

Herrmann, J., Schuster, M., Walker, F. A., White, E. F., Opitz, J. M., Zurhein, G. M. (1969). Fibrodysplasia ossificans progressiva and the XXXY syndrome in the same sibship. *Birth Defects*, **19 (5)**: 43−49.

Higashi, Y., Tanae, A., Inoue, H., Fuji-Kuriyama, Y. (1988). Evidence for frequent gene conversion in the steroid 21-hydroxylase P-450 (C21) gene: Implications for steroid 21-hydroxylase deficiency. *Am. J. Hum. Genet.*, **42**: 17−25.

Hoffmann, D. C., and Brooke, B. N. (1970). Familial sarcoma of bone in a polyposis coli family. *Dis. Colon Rectum*, **13**: 119−120.

Hösli, P., Vogt, E. (1979). High alkaline phosphatase activity in isoproterenol stimulated fibroblast cultures from patients with numerically unbalanced chromosomal aberrations. *Clin. Genet.*, **15**: 487−494.

Howard, A. D., Berger, J., Gerber, L., Familletti, P., Udenfriend, S. (1987). Characterization of the phosphatidylinositol-glycan membrane anchor of human placental alkaline phosphatase. *Proc. Natl. Acad. Sci. (USA).* **84**: 6055−6059.

Hua, J., Garattini, E., Pan, Y. E., Hulmes, J. D., Chang, M., Brink, L., Udenfriend, S. (1985). Purification and partial sequencing of bovine liver alkaline phosphatase. *Arch. Biochem. Biophys.*, **241**: 380−385.

Hua, J., Berger, J., Pan, Y. E., Hulmes, J. D., Udenfriend, S. (1986). Partial sequencing of human adult, human fetal, and bovine intestinal alkaline phosphatases: Comparison with the human placental and liver isozymes. *Proc. Natl. Acad. Sci. (USA).* **83**: 2368−2372,

Hunt, S. P., Pini, A., Evan G. (1987). Induction of *c-fos*-like protein in spinal cord neurons following sensory stimulation. *Nature*, **328**: 632−634.

Huvos, A. G. *Bone Tumors: Diagnosis, Treatment and Prognosis*, W. B. Saunders, Philadelphia, (1979), pp. 116−126.

Imai, Y., Rodan, S. B., Rodan, G. A. (1988). Effects of retinoic acid on alkaline phosphatase messenger ribonucleic acid, catecholamine receptors, and G proteins in ROS 17/2.8 cells. *Endocrinology*, **122**: 456−463.

Ishino, Y., Shinagawa, H., Makino, K., Amemura, M., Nakata, A. (1987). Nucleotide sequence of *iap* gene, responsible for alkaline phosphatase isozyme conversion *Escherichia coli*, and identification of the gene product. *J. Bacteriol*; **169**: 5429−5433.

Jeffree, G. M. (1972). Enzymes in fibroblastic lesions. A histochemical and quantitative survey of alkaline and acid phosphatase, β-glucuronidase, non-specific esterase and leucine aminopeptidase in benign and malignant fibroblastic lesions of bone and soft tissue. *J. Bone Joint Surg.*, **54B**: 535−546.

Jeffree, G. M. and Price C. H. G. (1965). Bone tumours and their enzymes. A study of the phosphatases, non-specific esterase and β-glucuronidase of osteogenic and cartilaginous tumors, fibroblastic and giant-cell lesions. *J. Bone Joint Surg.*, **47B**: 120−136.

Jelke, H. (1960). Hypophosphatasia. *Acta Pediatr. Scand.*, **49**: 297−308.

Jemmerson, R., Low, M. G. (1987). Phosphatidylinositol anchor of HeLa cell alkaline phosphatase. *Biochemistry*, **26**: 5703−5709.

Jenuwein, T. and Rolf Müller. (1987). Structure-function analysis of *fos* protein: A single amino acid change activates the immortalizing potential of *v-fos Cell*, **48**: 647−657.

Jewell, F. C., and Lofstrom, J. E. (1940). Osteogenic sarcoma occurring in fragilitas ossium. A case report. *Radiology*, **34**: 741−743.

Kam, W., Clauser, E., Kim, Y. S., Kan, Y. W., Rutter, W. J. (1985). Cloning, sequencing, and chromosomal localization of human term placental alkaline phosphatase cDNA. *Proc. Natl. Acad. Sci. (USA)* **82**: 8715−8717.

Kaneko, Y., Hayashi, N., Toh-e, A., Banno, I., Oshima, Y. (1987). Structural characteristics of the PHO8 gene encoding repressible alkaline phosphatase in *Saccharomyces cerevisiae*. *Gene*, **58**: 137−148.

Kawano, T., Taniguchi, S., Nakamatsu, K., Sadano, H., Baba, T. (1987). Malignant progression of a transformed rat cell line by transfer of the *v-fos* oncogene. *Biochem. Biophys. Res. Commun.*, **149**: 173−179.

Kewalramani, L. S. (1977). Ectopic ossification. *Am. J. Phys. Med.*, **59**: 99−121.

Kitchin, F. D. and Ellsworth, R. M. (1974). Pleiotropic effects of the gene for retinoblastoma. *J. Med. Genet.*, **11**: 244−246.

Klenerman, L., Ockenden, B. G., Townsend, A. C. (1967). Osteosarcoma occurring in osteogenesis imperfecta. Report of two cases. *J. Bone Joint Surg.*, **49B**: 314−323.

Knoll, B. J., Rothblum, K. N., Longley, M. (1987). Two gene duplication events in the evolution of the human heat-stable alkaline phosphatases. *Gene*, **60**: 267−276.

Komoda, T., Koyama, I., Nagata, A., Sakagishi, Y., Deschryver-Kecskemeti, K., Alpers, D. H. (1986). Ontogenic and phylogenic studies of intestinal, hepatic, and placental alkaline phosphatases. *Gastroenterology*, **91**: 277−286.

Kozlowski, K., Sutcliffe, J., Barylak, A., Harrington, G., Kemperdick, H., Nolte, K., Rheinwein, H., Thomas, P. S. and Uniecka, W. (1976) Hypophosphatasia. *Pediatr. Radiol.*, **5**: 103−117.

Kozlowski, K., et al, (1980). Osteosarcoma in a boy with Rothmund-Thomson syndrome. *Pediatr. Radiol.*, **10**: 42−45.

LaTour, D. A., Merriman, H. L., Kasperk, C. H., Linkhart, T. A., Mohan, S., Strong, D. D., Baylink, D. J. (1988). The proto-oncogene *c-fos*−a potential regulator of bone cell proliferation− is induced by bone growth factors [Abstract]. *J. Bone Miner. Res.*, **3(1)**: S207.

Lee, C. K., Chan, E. W., Reilly, C. A. Jr., Pahnke, V. A., Rockus, G., Finkel, M. P. (1979). *In vitro* properties of FBR murine osteosarcoma virus. *Proc. Soc. Exp. Biol. Med.*, **162**: 214−220.

Lee, E. S. and MacKenzie, D. H. (1964). Osteosarcoma: A study of the value of preoperative megavoltage radiotherapy. *Br. J. Surg.*, **51**: 252−274.

Licata, A. A., Radfar, N., Bartter, F. C., Bou E. (1978). The urinary excretion of phosphoethanolamine in diseases other than hypophosphatasia. *Amer. J. Med.*, **64**: 133−138.

Loutit, J. F. (1970). Malignancy from radium. *Br. J. Cancer*, **24**: 195−207.

Low, M. G., Ferguson, M. A. J., Futerman, A. H., Silman, I. (1986). Covalently attached phosphatidylinositol as a hydrophobic anchor for membrane proteins. *TIBS* **11**: 212−215.

Low, M. G., (1987). Biochemistry, of the glycosyl-phosphatidylinositol membrane protein anchors. *Biochem. J.*, **244**: 1−13.

Low, M. G., Saltiel, A. R. (1988). Structural and functional roles of glycosylphosphatidylinositol in membranes. *Science*, **239**: 268−275.

Low, M. G., Prasad, A. R. S. (1988). A phospholipase D specific for the phosphatidylinositol anchor of cell-surface proteins is abundant in plasma. *Proc. Natl. Acad Sci. (USA)*. **85**: 980−984.

Lutwak, L. (1964). Myositis ossificans progressiva−mineral, metabolic and radioactive calcium studies of the effects of hormones. *Am. J. Med.*, **37**: 269−293.

Maesaka, H., Niitsu, N., Suwa, S., Fujiia, T. (1977). Neonatal hypophosphatasia with elevated serum parathyroid hormone. *Europ. J. Pediat.*, **125**: 71−80.

Matejovsky, Z. (1977). Familial occurrence of osteosarcoma. *Acta Chir. Orthop. Traumatol. Cech.*, **44**: 24−27.

Maxwell, W. A., Spicer, S. S., Miller, R. L., Halushka, P. V., Westphal, M. C., Setser, M. E. (1977). Histochemical and ultrastructural studies in fibrodysplasia ossificans progressiva (myositis ossificans progressiva). *Am. J. Pathol.*, **87**: 483−492.

McCance, R. A., Morrison, A. B., Dent, C. E. (1955). The excretion of phosphoethonolamine and hypophosphatasia. *Lancet*, **1**: 131.

McComb, R. B., Bowers, G. N. Jr, Posen, S. (1979). *Alkaline phosphatase*, Plenum Press, New York.

McKusick, V. A. (1972). Fibrodysplasia ossificans progressiva. In: *Heritable Disorders of Connec-*

*tive Tissue.* 4th ed. St. Louis: C. V. Mosby, 400−415.

McKusick, V. A. (1988). *Mendelian Inheritance in Man.* 8th ed., Johns Hopkins Univ Press, Baltimore MD.

McLean, F. M., Keller, P. J., Genge, B. R., Walters, S. A., Wuthier, R. E. (1987). Disposition of preformed mineral in matrix vesicles. *J. Biol. Chem.,* **262**: 10481−10488.

Méhes, K., Klujber, L., Lassu, G. and Kajtár, P. (1972). Hypophosphatasia: Screening and family investigations in an endogamous Hungarian village. *Clin. Genet.,* **3**: 60−66.

Micanovic, R., Bailey, C. A., Brink, L., Gerber, L., Pan, Y. C. E., Hulmes, J. D., Udenfriend, S. (1988). Aspartic acid-484 of nascent placental alkaline phosphatase condenses with a phosphatidylinositol glycan to become the carboxyl terminus of the mature enzyme. *Proc. Natl. Acad. Sci. (USA).* **85**: 1398−1402.

Millán, J. L. (1986). Molecular cloning and sequence analysis of human placental alkaline phosphatase. *J. Biol. Chem.,* **261**: 3112−3115.

Millán, J. L. (1987). Promoter structure of the human intestinal alkaline phosphatase gene. *Nucl. Acid Res.,* **15**: 10599.

Miller, C. W. and McLaughlin, R. E. (1977). Osteosarcoma in siblings. Report of two cases. *J. Bone Joint Surg.,* **59A**: 261−262.

Miller, R. L., Maxwell, W. A., Spicer, S. S., Halushka, P. V., Varner, H. H., Westphal, M. C. (1977). Studies on alkaline phosphatase activity in cultured cells from a patient with fibrodysplasia ossificans progressiva. *Lab. Invest.,* **37**: 254−259.

Miller, A. D., Curran, T., Verma, I. M. (1984). *c-fos* protein can induce cellular transformation: A novel mechanism of activation of a cellular oncogene. *Cell,* **36**: 51−60.

Misumi, Y., Tashiro, K., Hattori, M., Sakaki, Y., Ikehara, Y. (1988). Primary structure of rat liver alkaline phosphatase deduced from its cDNA. *J. Biochem.,* **249**: 661−668.

Miura, M., Matsuzaki, H., Sakagishi, Y., Komoda, T. (1987). Partial characterization of human ileal alkaline phosphatase: Differences between human ileal and duodenal enzymes. *Clin. Chim. Acta,* **163**: 279−287.

Mori, M., Fukuda, M., Tsukamoto, S. (1968). Enzyme histochemistry of osteogenic sarcoma, chondrosarcoma, and giant-cell lesions in jawbones. *Oral Surg.,* **26**: 103−117.

Moss, D. W. (1982). Alkaline phosphatase isoenzymes. *Clin. Chem.,* **28**: 2007−2016.

Moss, D. W. (1986). Multiple forms of acid and alkaline phosphatases: Genetics, expression, and tissue-specific modification. *Clin. Chim. Acta,* **161**: 123−135.

Moss, D. W., Whitaker, K. B. (1987). The physical characteristics and enzymatic modification of fetal intestinal alkaline phosphatase in amniotic fluid. *Clin. Biochem.,* **20**: 9−12.

Mueller, H. D., Leung, H., Stinson, R. A. (1985). Different genes code for alkaline phosphatases from human fetal and adult intestine. *Biochem. Biophys. Res. Commun.,* **126**: 427−433.

Mueller, H. D., Stinson, R. A., Mohyuddin, F. and Milne, J. K. (1983). Isoenzymes of alkaline phosphatase in infantile hypophosphatasia. *J. Lab. Clin. Med.,* **102**: 24−29.

Mulivor, R. A., Mennuti, M., Zackai, E. H. and Harris, H. (1978). Prenatal diagnosis of hypophosphatasia: Genetic, biochemical and clinical studies. *Am. J. Hum. Genet.,* **30**: 271−282.

Mulivor, R. A., Hannig, V. L., Harris, H. (1978). Developmental change in human intestinal alkaline phosphatase. *Proc. Natl. Acad. Sci. (USA).* **75**: 3909−3912.

Müller, R., Verma, I. M. (1984). Expression of cellular oncogenes. *Curr. Top. Microbiol. Immunol.,* **112**: 74−115.

Müller, R. (1986a). Proto-oncogenes and differentiation. *Trends Biochem. Sci.,* **11**: 129−32.

Müller, R. (1986b). Cellular and viral *fos* genes: structure, regulation of expression and biological properties of their encoded products. *Biochim. Biophys. Acta,* **823**: 207−225.

Mulvihill, J. J., Gralnick, H. R., Whang-Peng, J. (1977). Multiple childhood osteosarcomas in an American Indian family with erythroid macrocytosis and skeletal anomalies. *Cancer*, **40**: 3115−3122.

Nair, B. C., Majeska, R. J., Rodan, G. A. (1987a). Rat alkaline phosphatase I. Purification and characterization of the enzyme from osteosarcoma: Generation of monoclonal and polyclonal antibodies. *Arch. Biochem. Biophys.*, **254**: 18−27.

Nair, B. C., Johnson, D. E., Majeska, R. J., Rodkey, J. A., Bennett, C. D., Rodan, G. A. (1987b). Rat alkaline phosphatase II. Structural similarities between the osteosarcoma, bone, kidney, and placenta isoenzymes. *Arch. Biochem. Biophys.*, **254**: 28−34.

Noda, M., Yoon, K., Rodan, G. A., Koppel, D. E. (1987). High lateral mobility of endogenous and transfected alkaline phosphatase: a phosphatidylinositol-anchored membrane protein. *J. Cell Biol.*, **105**: 1671−1677.

Opshaug, O., Maurseth, K., Howlid, H., Aksnes, L., Aarskog, D. (1982). Vitamin D metabolism in hypophosphatasia. *Acta Pediat. Scand.*, **71**: 517−521.

Ornoy, A., Adomian, G. E., Rimoin, D. L. (1985). Histologic and ultrastructural studies on the mineralization process in hypophosphatasia. *Am. J. Med. Genet.*, **22**: 743−758.

Parry, D. M., Safyer, A. W., Mulvihill, J. J. (1978). Waardenberg-like features with cataracts, small head size, joint abnormalities, hypogonadism, and osteosarcoma. *J. Med. Genet.*, **15**: 66−69.

Pimstone, B., Eisenberg, E. and Silverman S. (1966). Hypophosphatasia: Genetic and dental studies. *Ann. Intern. Med.*, **65**: 722−729.

Pitt, P. and Hamilton, E. B. D. (1984). Myositis ossificans progressiva. *J. Royal Soc. Med.*, **77**: 68−70.

Pohle, E. A. Stovall, W. D., Boyer, H. N. (1936). Concurrence of osteogenic sarcoma in two sisters. *Radiology*, **27**: 545−548.

Posen, S., Doherty, E. (1981). The measurement of serum alkaline phosphatase in clinical medicine. *Adv. Clin. Chem.*, **22**: 165−245.

Posen, S., Grunstein, H. S. (1982). Turnover rate of skeletal alkaline phosphatase in humans. *Clin. Chem.*, **28**: 153−154.

Pritchard, D. J., Reilly, C. A. Jr., Finkel, M. P. (1971). Evidence for a human osteosarcoma virus. *Nature*, **234**: 126−127.

Pritchard, D. J., Reilly, C. A. Jr., Finkel M. P. (1974). Cytotoxicity of human osteosarcoma sera to hamster sarcoma cells. *Cancer*, **34**: 1935−1939.

Rasmussen, K. (1968). Phosphorylethanolamine and hypophosphatasia. Studies on urinary excretion, renal handling and elimination of endogenous and exogenous phosphorylethanolamine in healthy persons, carriers, and in patients with hypophosphatasia. *Dan. Med. Bull.*, **15**: (suppl. II): 1−110.

Rasmussen, H. (1983). Hypophosphatasia In: *The Metabolic Basis of Inherited Disease (5th ed)*, Stanbury WB et al., (eds) McGraw Hill, New York, 1497−1506.

Rathbun, J. C. (1948). Hypophosphatasia, a new development anomaly. *Am. J. Dis. Child*, **75**: 822−831.

Rattenbury, J. M., Blau, K., Sandler, M., Pryse-Davies, J., Clark, P. J., Pooley, S. S. (1976). Prenatal diagnosis of hypophosphatasia. *Lancet*, 306.

Ray, K., Weiss, M. J., Dracopoli, N. C., Harris, H. (1988b). Probe 8B/E5' detects a second RFLP at the human liver/bone/kidney alkaline phosphatase locus. *Nucl. Acids Res.*, **16**: 2361.

Reddi, A. H., Gay, R., Gay, S., Miller, E. J. (1977). Transitions in collagen types during matrix induced cartilage, bone and bone marrow formation. *Proc. Nat. Acad. Sci. (USA)* **74**: 5589−5592.

Reddi, A. H. (1985). Regulation of bone differentiation by Local and systemic factors, In: *Bone and Mineral Research/3*, W. A. Peck (ed.) Elsevier North Holland, 27−48.

Register, T. C., McLean, F. M., Low, M. G., Wuthier, R. E. (1986). Roles of alkaline phosphatase and labile internal mineral in matrix vesicle-mediated calcification. *J. Biol. Chem.*, **261**: 9354−9360.

Reilly, C. A. Jr., Pritchard, D. J., Biskis, B. O. (1972). Immunologic evidence suggesting a viral etiology of human osteosarcoma. *Cancer*, **30**: 603−609.

Rettinger, S. D., Whyte, M. P. (1985). Normal circulating acid phosphatase activity in hypophosphatasia. *J. Inher. Metab. Dis.*, **8**: 161−162.

Robbins, R. (1967). Familial osteosarcoma. Fifth reported occurrence. Letter to the editor. *JAMA*, **202**: 1055.

Roberts, C. W. and Roberts, C. P. (1935). Concurrent osteogenic sarcoma in brother and sisters. *JAMA*, **105**: 181−185.

Rodan, G. A., Rodan, S. B. (1984). Expression of the osteoblast phenotype. In: *Bone and Mineral Research Annual/2*. W. A. Peck, ed. Elsevier, North Holland, pp. 244−285.

Rogers, J. G. and Chase, G. A. (1979). Paternal age effect in fibrodysplasia ossificans progressiva. *J. Med. Genet.*, **16**: 147−148.

Rogers, J. G. and Geho, W. B. (1979). Fibrodysplasia ossificans progressiva. *J. Bone Joint Surg.*, **61A**: 909−914.

Rollins, B. J., Morrison, E. D., Stiles, C. D. (1987). A cell-cycle constraint on the regulation of gene expression by platelet-derived growth factor. *Science*, **238**: 1269−71.

Romero, G., Luttrell, L., Rogol, A., Zeller, K., Hewlett, E., Larner, J. (1988). Phosphatidylinositol-glycan anchors of membrane proteins: Potential precursors of insulin mediators. *Science*, **240**: 509−511.

Roschlau, G. (1962). Rothmund-Syndrome. kombiniert mit Osteogenesis imperfecta tarda und Sarcom des Oberschenkels. *Z. Kinderheilkd.*, **86**: 289−298.

Rosen, R. S. (1970). Werner's syndrome. *Br. J. Radiol.*, **43**: 193−198.

Roth, S. I., Stowell, R. E., Helwig E. B. (1963). Cutaneous ossification. *Arch. Pathol.*, **76**: 44−54.

Rubecz, I., Méhes, K., Klujber, L., Bozzay, L. Weisenbach, J., Fenyvesi, J. (1974). Hypophosphatasia: Screening and family investigation. *Clin. Genet.*, **6**: 155−159.

Rudd, N. L., Miskin, M., Hoar, D. I., Benzie, R., Doran, T. A. (1976). Prenatal diagnosis of hypophosphatasia. *New Engl. J. Med.*, **288**: 146−148.

Ruderman, R. J., Leonard, F., Elliott, D. E., Hungerford, D. S., Siggers, D. C. (1979). A possible etiologic mechanism for fibrodysplasia ossificans progressiva. *Birth Defects*, **10**: 299.

Russell, R. G. G. (1965). Excretion of inorganic pyrophosphate in hypophosphatasia. *Lancet*, **2**: 461−464.

Russell, R. G. G., Bisaz, S., Donath, A. & Morgan, D. B., Fleisch H. (1971). Inorganic pyrophosphate in plasma in normal persons and in patients with hypophosphatasia, osteogenesis imperfecta, and other disorders of bone. *J. Clin. Invest.*, **50**: 961−969.

Russell, R. G. G. (1976). Metabolism of inorganic pyrophosphate (PP$_i$). *Arthr. Rheum.*, **19**: 465−478.

Rüther, U., Garber, C. Komitowski, D., Müller, R., Wagner, E. F. (1987). Deregulated *c-fos* expression interferes with normal bone development in transgenic mice. *Nature*, **325**: 412−416.

Sargeant, L. Z., Stinson, R. A. (1979). Evidence that three structural genes code for human alkaline phosphatases. *Nature*, **281**: 152−154.

Sassone-Corsi, P. and Verma, I. M. (1987). Modulation of *c-fos* gene transcription by negative and positive cellular factors. *Science*, **326**: 507−510.

Schiele, F., Henny, J., Hiltz, J., Petitclerc, C., Gueguen, R., Siest, G. (1983). Total bone and liver alkaline phosphatases in plasma: Biological variations and reference limits. *Clin.*

*Chem.*, **29**: 634−641.

Schneider. E. L., Mitsui, Y., Au, K. S., Shorr, S. (1977). Tissue specific differences in cultured human diploid fibroblasts. *Exp. Cell Res.*, **108**: 1−6.

Schön, A., Michiels, L., Janowski, M., Merregaert, J., Erfle. V. (1986). Expression of proto-oncogenes in murine osteosarcomas. *Int. J. Cancer*, **38**: 67−74.

Schuman, S. H., Burton, W. E. (1979). A new osteosarcoma−malformation syndrome. *Clin. Genet.*, **15**: 462−463.

Scriver, C. R. and Cameron, D. (1969). Pseudohypophosphatasia. *New Engl. J. Med.*, **281**: 604−606.

Shephard, M. D. S., Peake, M. J. (1986). Quantitative method for determining serum alkaline phosphatase isoenzyme activity I. Quanidine hydrochloride: New reagent for selectively inhibiting major serum isoenzymes of alkaline phosphatase. *J. Clin. Pathol.*, **39**: 1025−1030.

Schwartz, R. I., Bissell, M. J. (1977). Dependence of the differentiated state on the cellular environment: Modulation of collagen synthesis in tendon cells. *Proc. Nat. Acad. Sci. (USA).* **74**: 4453−4457.

Sehgal, H. L., Sehgal, L. R., Rosen, A. L., Gould, S. A., Dalton, L., Moss, G. S. (1980). Urinary phosphoethanolamine: Normal values by age. *Clin. Chem.*, **26**: 1757−1758.

Shipton, E. A. Retief, L. W., Theron, H. Du T., de Bruin, F. A. (1985). Anaesthesia in myositis ossificans progressiva: A case report and clinical review. *S. Afr. Med. J.*, **67**: 26−28.

Sim, F. H., Cupps, R. E., Dahlin, D. C., Ivins, J. C. (1972). Postradiation sarcoma of bone. *J. Bone Joint Surg.*, **54A**: 1479−1489.

Skogg, T. (1967). The use of periosteum and surgical for bone restoration in congenital clefts of the maxilla. A clinical report and experimental investigation. *Scand. J. Plast. Reconstr. Surg.*, **1**: 113−130.

Smith, D., Zeman, W., Johnston, C. C., Deiss, W. P. (1966) Myositis ossificans progressiva−Case report metabolic and histochemical studies. *Metabolism*, **15**: 521−528.

Smith, R. (1975). Myositis ossificans progressiva. *Sem. Arth. Rheum.*, **4**: 369.

Smith, M., Weiss, M. J., Griffin, C. A., Murray, J. C., Buetow, K. H., Emanuel, B. S., Henthorn, P. S., Harris, H. (1988). Regional assignment of the gene for human liver/bone/kidney alkaline phosphatase to chromosome 1p36.1−p34. *Genomics*, **2**: 139−143

Smith, G. P., Sharp, G., Peters, T. J. (1985). Isolation and characterization of alkaline phosphatase-containing granules (phosphasomes) from human polymorphonuclear leucocytes. *J. Cell Sci.*, **76**: 167−178.

Soehner, R. L. and Dmochowski, L. (1969). Induction of bone tumours in rats and hamsters with murine sarcoma virus and their cell-free transmission. *Nature*, **224**: 191−192.

Sorensen, E., Flodgaard, H. (1975). Adult hypophosphatasia. *Acta Med. Scand.*, **197**: 357−360.

Sorimachi, K., Yasumura, Y. (1988). The autorelease of alkaline phosphatase from the plasma membrane during the incubation of cultured liver cell homogenates. *J. Biochem.*, **103**: 195−200.

Sowadski, J. M., Handschumacher, M. D., Murthy, H. M. K., Foster, B. A., Wyckoff, H. W. (1985). Refined structure of alkaline phosphatase from *Escherichia coli* at 2.8 A Resolution. *J. Mol. Biol.*, **186**: 417−433.

Spiess, Y. H., Price, P. A., Deftos, J. L., Manolagas, S. C. (1986). Phenotype-associated changes in the effects of 1,25-dihydroxyvitamin $D_3$ on alkaline phosphatase and bone GLA-Protein of rat osteoblastic cells. *Endocrinology*, **118**: 1184−1340.

Starr, D. G. (1985). Non-dermatological complications and genetic aspects of the Rothmund-Thomson syndrome. *Clin Genet*, **27**: 102−104.

Stepán, J. J., Tesarová, A., Havránek, T., Jokl, J., Formánková, J., Pacovsky V. (1985). Age and sex dependency of the biochemical indices of bone remodelling. *Clin. Chim. Acta*, **151**: 273–283.

Stewart, S. E. (1960). The polyoma virus. In *Advances in Virus Research, Vol. 7*, K. M. Smith and M. A. Lauffer (eds), Academic Press, New York, pp. 61–90.

Stigbrand, T. (1984). Present status and future trends of human alkaline phosphatases. In: *Human Alkaline Phosphatases*, T. Stigbrand, W. H. Fishman (eds), Alan R. Liss, New York, 3–14.

Stinson, R. A., McPhee, J., Lewanczk, R., Dinwoodie, A. (1985). Neutrophil alkaline phosphatase in hypophosphatasia. *New Engl. J. Med.*, **321**: 1642–1643.

Stinson, R. A., Gainer, A. L., Chai, J., Chan, J. A. (1986). Substrate specificity of alkaline phosphatase from human polymorphonuclear leukocytes. *Clin. Chim. Acta*, **161**: 283–291.

Stinson, R. A., McPhee, J. L., Collier, H. B. (1987). Phosphotransferase activity of human alkaline phosphatases and the role of enzyme $Zn^{2+}$. *Biochim. Biophys. Acta*, **913**: 272–278.

Stinson, R. A., McPhee, J. L. (1987). Isoenzymes of alkaline phosphatase in amniotic fluid: Implications in prenatal screening for cystic fibrosis. *Clin. Biochem.*, **20**: 241–244.

Stout, A. P., Lattes, R. (1967). Tumors of the soft tissues. In: *Atlas of Tumor Pathology*. Second Series, Fascicle I. Armed Forces Institute of Pathology, Bethesda, p. 162.

Sty, J. R., Boedecker, R. A. and Babbitt, D. P. (1979). Skull scintigraphy in infantile hypophosphatasia. *J. Nucl. Med.*, **20**: 305–306.

Sumikawa, K., Saeki, K., Okochi, T., Adachi, K., Nishimura, H. (1987). Hydrolysis of phosphatidate by human placental alkaline phosphatase. *Clinica Chimica Acta*, **167**: 321–328.

Sussman, H. H. (1984). Structural analysis of human alkaline phosphatase. In: *Human Alkaline Phosphatases*, T. Stigbrand, W. H. Fishman (eds), Alan R. Liss, Inc., New York, pp. 87–103.

Swaney, J. J. (1973). Familial osteogenic sarcoma. *Clin. Orthop.*, **97**: 64–68.

Sympson, T. (1886). Case of myositis ossificans. *Br. Med. J.* **ii**: 1026–1027.

Takahashi, K., Shimidzu, M., Shindo, H., Kawamoto, T., Nishi, M. Matsumoto, U., Taniguchi, S. (1987). Tyrosine-specific dephosphorylation-phosphorylation with alkaline phosphatases and epidermal growth factor receptor kinase as evidenced by $^{31}$P NMR spectroscopy. *J. Biochem.*, **101**: 1107–1114.

Takami, N., Ogata, S., Oda, K., Misumi, Y., Ikehara, Y. (1988). Biosynthesis of placental alkaline phosphatase and its post-translation modification by glycophospholipid for membrane-anchoring. *J. Biol. Chem.*, **263**: 3016–3021.

Terao, M., Mintz, B. (1987). Cloning and characterization of a cDNA coding for mouse placental alkaline phosphatase. *Proc. Natl. Acad. Sci. (USA)*. **84**: 7051–7055.

Teree, T. M. and Klein, L. (1968). Hypophosphatasia: Clinical and metabolic studies. *J. Pediatr.*, **72**: 41–50.

Terheggen, H. G., Schürer, S. W., vanSande, M., Bützler O. (1972). Congenital hypophosphatasia. *Monogr. Hum. Genet.*, **6**: 188.

Thickman, D. (1982). Fibrodysplasia ossificans progressiva. *AJR*, **139**: 935–941.

Thiede, M. A., Yoon, K., Golub, E. E., Noda, M., Rodan, G. A. (1988). Structure and expression of rat osteosarcoma (ROS 17/2.8) alkaline phosphatase: Product of a single copy gene. *Proc. Natl. Acad. Sci. USA*, **85**: 319–323.

Tjalma, R. A. (1966). Canine bone sarcoma: Estimation of relative risk as a function of body size. *J. Natl. Cancer Fnd.*, **36**: 1137–1150.

Tsavaler, L., Penhallow, R. C., Kam, W., Sussman, H. H. (1987). Pst I restriction fragment length polymorphism of the human placental alkaline phosphatase gene in normal placentae and tumors. *Proc. Natl. Acad. Sci. (USA)*. **84**: 4529–5432.

Tokunaga, M. (1976). Rothmund-Thomson syndrome associated with osteosarcoma. *J. Jap.*

*Orthop. Assoc.*, **50**: 287−293.

Tsuya, A., Tanaka, T., Mori, T. (1963). Four cases of Thorotrast injury and estimation of absorbed tissue dose in critical organs. *J. Radiat. Res.*, **4**: 126−145.

Tucker, M. A., D'Angio, G. J., Boice, J. D. Jr., Strong, L. C., Li, F. P., Stoval, M., Stone, B. J., Green, D. M., Lombardi, F., Newton, W., Hoover, R. N., Fraumeni, J. F. Jr. (1987). for the Late Effects Study Group, Bone sarcomas linked to radiotherapy and chemotherapy in children. *N. Engl. J. Med.*, **317**: 588−593.

Tünte, W., Becker, P. E., von Knorre, G. V. (1967). Zur Genetik der Myositis ossificans progressiva. *Humangenetik*, **4**: 320−351.

Uddstromer, L., Ritsila, V. (1978). Osteogenic capacity of periosteal grafts. A qualitative and quantitative study of membranous and tubular bone periosteum in young rabbits. *Scan. J. Plast. Reconstr. Surg.*, **12**: 207−214.

Varmus, H. and Swanstrom R. (1985). Replication of retroviruses. In: *Molecular Biology of Tumor Viruses: RNA Tumor Viruses* (2nd ed), R. Weiss, N. Teich, H. Varmus, J. Coffin, eds. Cold Spring Harbor Laboratory, p. 75−134.

Vastine, J. A., Vastine, M. F., Arango, O. (1948). Myositis ossificans progressiva in homozygotic twins. *AJR*, **59**: 204−212.

Ward, J. M. and Young, D. M. (1976). Histogenesis and morphology of periosteal sarcomas induced by FBJ virus in NIH Swiss mice. *Cancer Res.*, **36**: 3985−3992.

Warren, R. C., Rodeck, C. H., Brock, D. J. H., McKenzie, C. F., Moscoso, G., Barron, L. (1985). First trimester diagnosis of hypophosphatasia with a monoclonal antibody to the liver/bone/kidney isoenzyme of alkaline phosphatase. *Lancet*, 856−858.

Weinstein, R. S., Whyte, M. P. (1981). Heterogeneity of adult hypophosphatasia: Report of severe and mild cases. *Arch. Int. Med.*, **141**: 727−731.

Weiss, M. J., Henthorn, P. S., Lafferty, M. A., Slaughter, C., Raducha, M., Harris, H. (1986). Isolation and characterization of a cDNA encoding a human liver/bone/kidney-type alkaline phosphatase. *Proc. Natl. Acad. Sci. (USA).* **83**: 7182−7186.

Weiss, M. J., Spielman, R. S., Harris, H. (1987). A high-frequency RFLP at the human liver/bone/kidney-type alkaline phosphatase locus. *Nucl. Acid. Res.*, **15**: 860.

Weiss, M. J., Henthorn, P. S., Ray, K., Lamb, B., Kadesch, T. (1988a) Structure of the human/liver/bone/kidney alkaline phosphatase gene. *J. Biol. Chem.*, **263**: 12002−12010

Weiss, M. J., Cole, D. E. C., Ray, K., Whyte, M. P., Lafferty, M. A., Mullivor, R. A., Harris, H. (1988b). A missense mutation in the human liver/bone/kidney alkaline phosphatase gene in a lethal form of hypophosphatasia, *Proc. Nat. Acad. Sci. (USA).* **85**: 7666−7669.

Werner, R. (1930). Mehrfaches Vorkommen einer Neigung zu Knochenbrüchen und Sarkomentwicklung in einer Familie. *Z. Krebsforsch.*, **32**: 40−42.

Whyte, M. P., Teitelbaum, S. L., Murphy, W. A. and Avioli, L. V. (1978). Adult hypophosphatasia dominant inheritance in a large kindred. *Trans. Assoc. Am Phys.*, **91**: 144−155.

Whyte, M. P., Murphy, W. A., Fallon, M. D. (1982). Adult hypophosphatasia with chondrocalcinosis and arthropathy. *Am. J. Med.*, **72**: 631−641.

Whyte, M. P., Seino, Y. (1982). Circulating vitamin D metabolite levels in hypophosphatasia. *J. Clin. Endocrinol. Metab.*, **55**: 178−180.

Whyte, M. P., Valdes, R. Jr, Ryan, L. M., McAlister, W. H. (1982a). Infantile hypophosphatasia: Enzyme replacement therapy by intravenous infusion of alkaline phosphatase−rich plasma from patients with Paget bone disease. *J. Pediatr.*, **101**: 379−386.

Whyte, M. P., Vrabel, L. A., Schwartz T. D. (1982b). Adult hypophosphatasia: Generalized deficiency of alkaline phosphatase activity demonstrated with cultured skin fibroblasts. *Trans. Assoc. Am. Phys.*, **45**: 253−263.

Whyte, M. P., Vrabel, L. A., Schwartz T. D. (1983). Alkaline phosphatase deficiency in cultured skin fibroblasts from patients with hypophosphatasia: Comparison of the infantile, childhood, and adult forms. *J. Clin. Endocrinol. Metab.*, **57**: 831—837.

Whyte, M. P., McAlister, W. H., Patton, L. S., Magill, H. L., Fallon, M. D., Lorentz, W. B. Jr., Herrod, H. G. (1984). Enzyme replacement therapy for infantile hypophosphatasia attempted by intravenous infusions of alkaline phosphatase—rich Paget plasma: Results in three additional patients. *J. Pediatr.* **105**: 926—933.

Whyte, M. P. Mahuren, J. D., Vrabel, L. A., Coburn, S. P. (1985). Markedly increased circulating pyridoxal-5'-phosphate levels in hypophosphatasia. *J. Clin. Invest.*, **76**: 752—756.

Whyte, M. P., Magill, H. L., Fallon, M. D. and Herrod, H. G. (1986). Infantile hypophosphatasia: Normalization of circulating bone alkaline phosphatase activity followed by skeletal remineralization. *J. Pediatr.*, **108**: 82—99.

Whyte, M. P., Vrabel, L. A. (1987). Infantile hypophosphatasia fibroblasts proliferate normally in culture: Evidence against a role for alkaline phosphatase (tissue nonspecific isoenzyme) in the regulation of cell growth and differentiation. *Calcif. Tissue Int.*, **40**: 1—7.

Whyte, M. P., Mahuren, J. D., Fedde, K. N., Cole, F. S. McCabe, E. R. B., Coburn, S. P. (1988). Perinatal hypophosphatasia: Tissue levels of vitamin B6 are unremarkable despite markedly increased circulating concentrations of pyridoxal-5'-phosphate. *J. Clin. Invest.*, **81**: 1234—1239.

Whyte, M. P. (1989a). Hypophosphatasia, In: *The Metabolic Basis of Inherited Disease*, 6th ed., C. R. Scriver et al (eds), McGraw Hill, New York, 2843—2856

Whyte, M. P. (1989b). Alkaline phosphatase: Physiological role explored in hypophosphatasia. In: *Bone and Mineral Research/6*, W. A. Peck (ed), Elsevier North Holland. [IN PRESS]

Wolff, C. and Zabransky, S. (1982). Hypophosphatasia congenita letalis. *Eur. J. Pediatr.*, **138**: 197—199.

Wyckoff, H. W., Handschumacher, M., Murthy, H. M. K., Sowadski, J. M. (1983). The three dimensional structure of alkaline phosphatase from *E. coli. Adv. Enzymol. Mol. Biol.*, **55**: 453—480.

Yora, T., Sakagishi, Y. (1986). Comparative biochemical study of alkaline phosphatase isozymes in fish, amphibians, reptiles, birds and mammals. *Comp. Biochem. Physiol.*, **85B**: 649—658.

Zernik, J., Stover, M. L., Thiede, M. A., Rodan, G. A., Rowe, D. W. (1988). Isolation and characterization of a genomic clone corresponding to the promotor of the gene for rat bone alkaline phosphatase. *J. Bone Min. Res.*, **3**: S207. (Abstract).

# Index

## A

acid glycerophosphate 90, 92, 96, 97
acid phosphatase 98-100, 180, 183, 356
acidic fibroblast growth factor, *see*
fibroblast growth factor
acromegaly 222
adenosine triphosphate 82, 85, 87
adenylate cyclase 87
ageing 220, 224-229, 232-235, 382, 390-391, 395
alkaline phosphatase
androgen stimulation of, 257
calcitriol stimulates, 409
circadian rhythms and, 258
gene for, 445-446
Il-1 stimulates, 338
in marrow cells, 46, 47
in osteoblasts, 73-75, 77-86, 172, 181, 182, 201-204
in periosteal cells, 49, 50
isoenzymes, 443-444, 451-452
isoforms, 451-452
and mineralization, 208
as osteogenic cell marker, 54,133,177, 179, 181,185,186, 261, 308,
parathyroid hormone reduces, 332
TGF- stimulation of, 115
zinc inhibits, 264
alpha 2HS-glycoprotein, 211, 216
aluminium, 262
amorphous calcium phosphate, 218, 219
angiogenesis, 126, 238
aryl sulfatase, 99
ascorbic acid, *see* Vitamin C
ATP, *see* adenosine triphosphate
autocrine factors, 63, 179; *see also*
growth factors

## B

basic fibroblast growth factor (bFGF), *see*
fibroblast growth factor
BDGF, *see* bone-derived growth factors
biomineralisation, *see* mineralisation
biorhythms, *see* circadian rhythms
B$_2$-microglobulin, 128, 131, 245, 249, 335-336
bone,
alveolar, 225, 329, 384
cancellous, 355, 388, 391
compact, 195

cortical, 232-235, 237, 356, 363, 372, 375, 380
ectopic, 211, 433, 435-437
formation rate, 222-237, 363-369
lamellar, 353, 385
metaplastic, 436
trabecular, 195, 237
woven, 353, 385, 400
bone-derived growth factors, 129-133, 165-166, 245-247, 335
bone formation, 10, 41-63, 193-266, 303-320, 369-382; *see also* osteoinduction
bone growth, 112, 146, 245
bone lining cells, 9, 23, 389
bone morphogenetic protein, 57, 61-63,144, 213-215, 221, 245; *see also*
demineralized bone matrix
bone phophoproteins, 210-211
bone remodelling, *see* remodelling
bone resorption, *see* resorption
bone sialoprotein, 54, 211, 214, 237; *see
also* osteopontin
boron, 262-263
brushite, 217, 218, 389

## C

calcidiol, 400
calcification, *see* mineralisation
calcitonin, 202-205, 254, 389, 416
calcitriol, 401, 409: *see also* vitamin D
calcium phosphate, 217
calvarium, 173
cell lines derived from, 126,177,179,180, 184, 311, 316-319, 335, 338, 342
clonal MC3T3-E1 cell line from, 175, 186, 202, 251, 312, 330, 337
calvarial cells *in vitro*, 49, 132, 200, 202, 203, 216, 240-242, 305, 306, 309, 339
fibronectin and, 215
hypophosphatasia and, 453
type III collagen from, 206
cartilage induction factor, 62, 116, 131
cell cycle, 108-109, 137
cement line, 366
centrioles, 21
*c-fos* proto oncogene, 107, 109, 462-473
chlortetracycline, 222
cholesterol, 261
chondrocalcinosis, 454
chondrocytes, 195, 196, 215, 216, 240
*in vitro*, 311